Setting Up Healthcare Services Information Systems

A Guide for Requirement Analysis, Application Specification, and Procurement

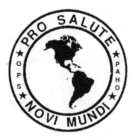
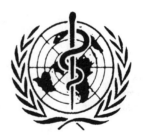

July 1999

Essential Drugs and Technology Program
Division of Health Systems and Services Development
Pan American Health Organization
World Health Organization

PAHO Library Cataloguing in Publication Data

Pan American Health Organization.
  Setting up Healthcare Services Information Systems: A Guide
for Requirement Analysis, Application Specification, and Procurement.
Washington, D.C. : PAHO, © 1999.
624 p.

        ISBN 92 75 12266 0

I.   Title.
1. INFORMATION SYSTEMS.   2. TECHNOLOGY, MEDICAL.
3. INFORMATION MANAGEMENT.   4. QUALITY OF HEALTHCARE.
5. MANUALS

NLM W26.5

ISBN 92 75 12266 0

Editorial Team

Pan American Health Organization

Roberto J. Rodrigues, *Editorial Team Coordinator, HSP/HSE*
César Gattini, *HSP/HSO*
Gisele Almeida, *HSP/HSO*

Collaborators

Pan American Health Organization

Carlos Gamboa, *HSP/HSE*
Antonio Carlos Azevedo, *HSP/PWR Chile*
David Taylor, *HSP/CPC Office*
Ana Rita Gonzalez, *HSP/PWR Peru*
Eduardo Guerrero, *PWR/Brazil*
Dale Ifill, *CPC Office, Barbados*
Gerald Lucas, *PWR/Jamaica*
Antonio Hernandez, *HSP/HSE*
Carlos Albuquerque, *HSP/HSO*
Hugo Chacón, *PWR/Costa Rica*
Oscar Salinas, *PWR/El Salvador*
Rosanne Marchesich, *HSP/HSR*

Collaborators

Acknowledgements

This publication is the result of an extensive review of many sources and a compilation of collective and individual contributions made by an international group of distinguished professionals. It represents the conclusion of more than two years of work, consultations, and expert meetings. We were very fortunate to be able to access professionals from public and private health organizations, academic institutions, and industry, with extensive experience in the area of health services information systems design, implementation, and operation. To them we would like to declare our recognition and thankfulness.

This undertaking was conceived and conducted in the framework of a partnership between the Pan American Health Organization and the IBM Corporation aimed at the investigation of health services information systems and technology, with emphasis directed to the requirements of Latin America and the Caribbean countries. We express our special gratitude to IBM Brasil Ltda. and IBM Healthcare Industry, for providing invaluable technical input and partial financial support to this endeavor.

We thank Dr. Daniel Lopez-Acuña, Director of the Health Systems and Services Development Division, for his suggestions and encouragement throughout the execution of this challenging project. We could not end without expressing our sincere appreciation for the skilled assistance provided by the staff of the former PAHO Health Services Information Systems Program in handling consultants' schedules, contracts, and travel, and in the organization of two international consultative meetings held respectively in São Paulo, Brazil, and in Washington, D.C.

The Editors
July 30, 1999
Washington, D.C.

Foreword

It is a pleasure to write a brief foreword to this book *Setting Up Healthcare Services Information Systems*. It is billed as a guide for requirement analysis, application specification and procurement, but it goes beyond that and gives much of the background necessary for understanding the nature of the tasks involved in setting up the systems that are required. I have stressed repeatedly, here in the Pan American Health Organization (PAHO), that information is a critical resource for our work. Our technical cooperation must be based on good information about those areas in which we will cooperate with our Member States. It is essential that we have information about the health status of the people of the Americas and that part of our technical cooperation be also directed towards strengthening the national capacity to collect the needed data on health status and transform them into useful information.

But we are well aware that it is not enough to have information on health status or morbidity conditions; it is also crucial that there be information on those factors that have been deemed to be determinants of health. Many of these factors are outside the range of activities that fall within the purview of those institutions, which have traditionally been included in the health sector. But there is no doubt that the health services, which represent one of those determinants, have to be the constant concern of the health sector.

The importance of the health services does not only depend on their intrinsic value for health, but also because they represent a major cost — particularly those services that are responsible for the restoration of health. The growth of technology has made healthcare services increasingly complex and with this growth in complexity has come more difficulty in managing the multiple resources that must contribute to the function of the services. Competent management of the services requires that there be efficient and effective information systems. The information systems have themselves grown in sophistication and the net effect of the changes and developments has been to create the need for understanding the systems within the services as interlocking and for appreciating the extent to which information technology can assist.

Thus a publication which guides the manager in understanding the needs for the information technology is most useful. But, in addition, this publication performs the essential task of helping those who have managerial responsibility in the healthcare services to understand the steps necessary to definite needs and then to acquire the information technology to satisfy those needs. The responsibility of disseminating information that is important for various aspects of management of the health systems and services, is also an important facet of our technical cooperation.

Another attractive aspect of this publication is that it represents the product of a partnership with a private sector organization. This is a trend that must continue, as it becomes ever clearer that all sectors and a wide range of actors are to be involved in finding solutions to the pressing problems of health.

I hope that this publication will have the widest possible circulation and be a useful reference for all those who are involved in providing healthcare.

Dr. George A. O. Alleyne
Director
Pan American Health Organization

Executive Summary

Setting Up Healthcare Services Information Systems: A Guide for Requirement Analysis, Application Specification, and Procurement contains practical guidelines and suggestions to be used by healthcare and systems professionals when embarking in the initial stages of planning and developing healthcare services information systems and information technology (IS&T) applications.

Setting up information systems in healthcare involves some key preparative technical tasks: requirements analysis; technical specification of computer-based applications; preparation of Request for Proposals (RFP) for information systems, technology, and services; evaluation and selection of providers; and contracting aspects when acquiring IS&T for healthcare services.

It is expected that the judicious use of the concepts and recommendations detailed in this publication will contribute to improved decisions regarding IS&T design, acquisition, and deployment at all levels of management. The material was prepared considering the specific planning and execution requirements of tasks related to systems design, such as reaching consensus regarding desired functions in computerized applications, and to the complex process of procurement and acquisition of equipment and services. In addition, these guidelines may prove to be of great usefulness to those involved in making policies or to anyone who desires to develop a critical vision of healthcare services information systems and related technology.

Although general principles for requirement analysis and procurement can be applied to any healthcare information project, special consideration was given in this work to the technical knowledge components needed by healthcare professionals involved in IS&T institutional projects. The document describes current developments occurring in the field of information systems and technology, with appropriate emphasis on its implications for healthcare and projection of trends. Highlights of successful ingredients of an IS&T implementation plan are covered, including development of a strategic plan, processes and roles, implementation phases, and application modules.

This publication seeks to balance the readiness for long-term decisions with the practical needs of today's diverse healthcare institutions in the area of IS&T. To that end, it should be viewed as a general source of information, with references to applicable World Wide Web sources for further details. It is not the purpose of this document to provide highly specific guidelines for individual application systems or users, or the promotion of a specific set of standards.

After a short introductory presentation of the objectives, audience, and description of how this publication was envisioned and written, a Quick Reference chapter facilitates the identification of topics and the navigation throughout the work.

Basic principles of IS&T implementation are discussed from the broad perspective of healthcare services requirements, followed by a comprehensive review of information systems and information technology solutions where project management, market, and commercial aspects are examined. The general and technology solutions where project management, market, and commercial aspects are examined. The general and institutional IS&T development framework presented considers healthcare services as productive organizations operating in particular settings with specific functionalities and content requirements that must be defined in each case. In particular, healthcare networks, involving several stakeholders and different levels of clinical and managerial decision-making, must be supported by integrated IS&T solutions. Healthcare-related indicators have been included, representing a range from basic (PAHO Core Data Indicators) to more detailed indicators, involving higher level of information systems development (OECD Healthcare Indicators).

The review of information systems and information technology solutions covers the state of the art and trends. It includes the area of health services automation, features of health services information networks, issues regarding the structuring of the information chain, computer-based patient records, and information project management and implementation aspects of interest to health and systems professionals involved in information systems project development. Components involved in developing, deploying, and operating IS&T are detailed. These components are inter-related in a dynamic process, through project management, project operation, and project development teams. For the purposes of this document, discussions are focused in three basic components: *planning, preparation,* and *procurement.* Legal, confidentiality, and security aspects of health information systems and databases are addressed, and references on those important areas are reproduced, including a set of recommendations of functional requirements for healthcare documentation.

Procurement and contracting of IS&T services and products are described. Those topics encompass pertinent details related to the technological and market aspects of systems acquisition, including essential aspects of technology and services outsourcing, preparation of Request for Proposals (RFP), evaluation of proposals and providers, and the negotiation and contracting of services, products, and technological resources.

The core contribution of the document is the description of healthcare services applications functional specifications (Part D). This highly technical chapter lists the basic functionalities that each application area should consider. It includes a systematic categorization of functions in different formats, with the objective of assisting decision makers in the preparation of RFP, in evaluating existing products, and as a departure point for the discussion with users of desired functions when planning systems acquisition or development. The proposed desired functionalities also assist developers and users, in each implementation environment, to reach a consensus regarding which basic data elements would be needed for each application. Suggested basic data elements follow recommendations of the National Committee on Vital and Health Statistics, U.S. Department of Health and Human Services.

An electronic database of application functionalities in MS-Acess format (APFUNC.MDB) is included as a file in the CD-ROM version — with it developers and other interested parties will be able to generate a variety of reports and printouts. The database also can be used as a departure point for the construction of databases of functional descriptions tailored to particular projects.

The heterogeneous development level of societies and health services throughout Latin America and the Caribbean Region is associated with different degrees of infrastructure, organization, and quality

Standards are a central element of open systems — without reliable, approved ways to connect the necessary components, open systems cannot work. Within the healthcare industry there are a very large number of categories of information that require standardization. There is an extensive examination of the complex issue of standards on data, communication, software, and hardware, at a highly specialized and technical level, and four annexes are added as references. The knowledgeable healthcare executive will do well to stay current on healthcare standards development. In addition, vendors demonstrating present and future commitment to standards are those most likely to survive in the very competitive healthcare IS&T marketplace, and should be given top consideration by healthcare enterprises in the process of systems selection.

Finally, references related to the issue of setting up information systems are also included: a listing of World Wide Web sites for Health and Medical Informatics and Standards Organizations, and a listing of Pan American Health Organization and World Health Organization publications in the area of Health Informatics.

This work is the successful result of a collaborative study conducted in the context of a partnership between the Pan American Health Organization and the IBM Corporation directed to the study of health information issues in Latin America and the Caribbean. The study was enriched by the collected experience reflected in several reference sources and by the contributions of a large panel of international experts from public and private organizations. Funding for the organization and conduction of consultation meetings, preparation and editing of manuscripts, translation, and publication was shared by the partners.

The final product is organized in a modular electronic format intended to provide a logical and step-wise framework for study and practical utilization. The electronic format allows the reader to have dynamic access to the different chapters and sections, according to the individual interest of each reader.

Introductory Remarks

The concern over information systems is solely that they should support health and health services, and the purpose of technology is that it should support the necessary information system.

George A.O. Alleyne
Director of the Pan American Health Organization

The implementation of healthcare information systems and technology has become critical to the delivery of cost-efficient and quality healthcare. Information systems applications have contributed to better health service management and delivery of care by creating an environment conducive to increased access and quality of patient care and by supporting the knowledge base required for clinical and administrative decision making.

Indeed, the dominant objectives for the deployment of information systems are: facilitation of the logistical aspects of healthcare; enabling health institutions to function efficiently; assisting care providers to act effectively; improving access to individual and collective administrative, clinical, and epidemiological data; and simplifying the access to biomedical reference. These benefits are achieved through automated patient and clinical data management, support to diagnostic and therapeutic services, image-based systems, resource management, integration of administrative and clinical data, remote access to medical information, access to knowledge databases, and appropriate physical resource and financial management.

1. The Relevance of a Cautious IS&T Implementation

In the area of information systems and technology (IS&T), health services seek appropriate responses to issues related to the possibilities offered by IS&T and want to be advised on feasible expectations, benefits, and constraints associated with the introduction of information systems and technologies.

In what is becoming increasingly known as the Information Society, the public, politicians, and professionals all expect information to be readily available to improve services, and thus to improve health and healthcare. However, information and the organization, resources, and technology to make it happen are not cheap — they are expensive commodities that rapidly become obsolete. Information *per se* is a perishable asset and one that can be hazardous, if misused. Data collection and information generation, storage, and retrieval cost money and time to establish and process in a consistent manner. Information is also perishable, and must therefore be regularly maintained and updated. It has no intrinsic value, but becomes invaluable in the appropriate utilization setting. Its utility is in the illumination it provides to problems under consideration, or which should be considered. Investment in successful information systems has a high cost-benefit ratio. Furthermore, investment in information collecting, processing, and archiving activities has to compete for financing against other healthcare activities with more immediately obvious and immediate benefits.

Moreover, the past investment experience in information systems has been sometimes disappointing. In the United States, it has been said that the healthcare industry's significant investments in patient information systems over the last thirty years failed to meet many expectations, and a large-scale study showed that only one-quarter of the built-in functionality of hospital information systems was actually used. Many projects resulted in disillusionment with information systems that were built with little regard to user's day-to-day needs. Lack of relevance to actual practice or clear-cut benefit to operational staff results in systems that are not properly used, and thus are prone to deliver inaccurate information. Therefore, though there are compelling reasons for investment in information systems, there are also significant risks to avoid.

The broad spectrum of country and institutional development level requires implementation strategies that range from very basic to very sophisticated. The variety of requirements and possible solutions demands that each project must be approached in a unique and individualized manner. Any strategy, however, must consider the long-term outlook of healthcare IS&T and focus on practical and tactical implementation issues directed to the solution of immediate informational problems faced by countries, organizations, and healthcare services. The reform processes of the last years, occurring in the healthcare sector and the society in general, and the fast-paced advances of information systems industry, mean an increased level of complexity, detail, and interdependency of decisions and actions.

In order to assist Latin American and Caribbean countries and their local decision-makers in developing appropriate and effective information systems, the Pan American Health Organization has described very clearly in an earlier document[a] the challenges and potential solutions for the introduction of information systems and technology. The subsequent and practical companion document is the present publication.

2. Emphasizing the Role of Information in Healthcare

Information systems should be related to need, in exactly the same way that health services should be needs-led rather than provider-driven. The essential first task of setting up any information system is, therefore, the identification of the healthcare issues under consideration, and the factors that may influence them, so as then to define the appropriate information requirements. When investing in information systems, the core purpose ("the business") of the organization must be clearly identified. In the case of health services, the core purpose is to improve the state of health of individual citizens and the health of communities, by improving the systems of health and healthcare. This core purpose should always be kept in mind when designing information systems — as it is not at all rare for

---

[a] Information Systems and Information Technology in Health: Challenges and Solutions for Latin America and the Caribbean. July 1998. 113 pp. ISBN 92 75 12246 6

health managers to permit systems technical staff to come to crucial decisions in the design of systems that are technically driven and may result in inappropriate applications.

Decisions made without good information may be appropriate decisions or may be very inappropriate ones, and the need and value of information relates directly to their contribution to decision making. The availability of relevant and appropriate information is the essential ingredient that transforms a decision into an *informed decision* — and one that is thus much more likely to be the correct one. It is of significance to understand how the resource of *Information* relates to *Data* and to *Knowledge*.

- *Data* are the raw items, such as a blood pressure reading, a temperature, the name of a pharmaceutical product, the date of a patient's hospital discharge. By themselves, data have no meaning; they are totally isolated facts.

- *Information* is produced when data are grouped by a specified set of common factors. Thus an assembly of biometric facts becomes information about a patient's vital signs or the serial grouping of discharge dates related to one individual patient becomes the pattern of hospitalization, whereas dates of discharge for different persons within a specified calendar period indicate a hospital's rate of activity. Information, in many circumstances is also the "middle part" of an information continuum, being both a product and an input.

- *Knowledge* is created when information is put into an overall setting. For instance, it relates to the expected pattern of vital signs for a particular illness, the available pharmaceutical products and their known side effects, or the level of activity of a hospital as it relates to budget and catchment population.

The key issue is, therefore, *context* — information can be described as data put into a specific context, whilst knowledge is information put into a general context. Thus definition of the context for which information is required is essential to developing appropriate information systems, and relates directly to wider decision-making processes.

From the perspective of health services, three broad levels of information are required for decision support: *Clinical, Operational,* and *Strategic.* These can be further refined to five core functions: *Case Management, Caseload Management, Operational Management, Strategic Management,* and *Political Accountability.* The actual utilization of information by clinical and administrative managers can be further refined considering the specific areas of application.

Having defined the nature and role of information, one should consider the development of a systematic approach to both the production and use of information. This is important for two reasons:

- In the health sector, the responsibility and burden for nearly all data capture fall squarely to the clinical and operational levels. Staff responsible for primary data capture may not understand the objectives or problems to be addressed, nor see it as important and the original data supplied may be inaccurate and thus the information compiled will be either incorrect or of limited usefulness. One-off-a-kind data collection to provide information for a specific decision is difficult, expensive, and a burden to line staff and should rarely be employed.

- In many decision-making situations, not least with regard to health status itself, a key technique is the analysis and interpretation of trends. This means that information must be compiled and compared on a regular basis to standardized definitions.

To meet both these challenges, a methodical approach to information is required to ensure that data flows regularly and smoothly to meet the desired objectives and purposes of implemented systems.

3. The Institutional Context of Information Systems

If information systems must be developed considering context, what are the settings that determine requirements? In this direction, five important contextual aspects of healthcare must be examined when designing information systems:

- Healthcare model
- Patterns of healthcare provision
- Primary care and community orientation
- Information infrastructure
- Appropriateness

There are a number of models of healthcare, with regard both to funding and delivery. Healthcare may be funded publicly, it may be insurance-based, or consumers may pay directly (with or without co-payments from a third party). Those alternatives are not mutually exclusive — for instance, insurance companies may offer supplementary services in situations where there is a basic publicly funded service. Similarly, the supply of healthcare may be rendered by public sector services, by private or not-for-profit providers, or by a combination of them.

It is the prevailing model of care of a defined country that will ultimately determine the types of decisions being made, and thus the requirements for information. Most Latin American and Caribbean (LAC) countries have models which are more closely aligned to European, Canadian, or Australian models, and indeed many countries in the LAC region have already established fruitful links with agencies and information service suppliers in these countries. The examination of the installed healthcare infrastructure shows the relatively small size of most LAC hospitals. In the 1996/1997 period, 76% of the region's 16,500 hospitals were 100 beds or fewer (with 61% having 50 beds or fewer) and only 215 hospitals (1%) had more than 500 beds. Most ambulatory care is provided in offices or clinics with rather limited diagnostic resources. This suggests that advanced hospital information systems modeled on those of highly industrialized countries will not be appropriate for those institutions.

The challenge is to identify the health provision infrastructure and their information requirements, as it enables to focus where priority information systems are mostly needed — in secondary or tertiary sites, or at primary care at the community or local level. Focus at the patient level and the development of patient-based and community-oriented health information systems is in accordance to the World Health Organization recommendations, which have global endorsement. This perspective should underpin our thinking in all strategic healthcare information solution development. It is within primary care that the greatest volume of healthcare activity takes place, including almost all preventive healthcare, and thus where health status is determined. Also, it is at the community level that basic information about the health of citizens and communities should reside, and it should constitute the core information for policy and service development at all levels.

There is a tendency to consider information systems in terms of high-technology computerized systems, but this is likely to be inappropriate in many settings in developing areas or small organizations. Latin America and the Caribbean has the lowest per capita expenditure on information technology, and with the growth of communications-based information applications, essential infrastructures such as telephone lines are still a major problem — telephone lines range from 1.7 telephones per 100 persons in Nicaragua to 31.8 in Barbados, whereas in developed countries telephone connectivity reaches 70 to 80 per 100 persons. Power supply is also variable in many places and power outages may be a daily occurrence. Unsuitable technical investment will simply be a waste, and even when the capital cost is donated, as in many international cooperation projects, the time and effort of trying to operate inappropriate systems will merely divert resources from more productive tasks, as well as creating a bad image for information systems generally.

Another important concept is that of appropriateness, particularly regarding the selection and deployment of technology. Many places in the region are already too familiar with other inappropriately deployed technologies, such as clinical equipment that cannot function without reliable physical infrastructure or for which replacement components cannot be obtained, or cannot be maintained. One should avoid replication of this situation with regard to information technology, and appropriateness of technological components and potential use must be a principal guiding element.

4. Purposes and Nature of the Guidelines

This publication contains practical guidelines to be used by health and systems professionals when embarking in the technical activities related to requirement analysis and the initial technical specification of computer-based applications. These include a number of tasks which health professionals are expected to have a minimum level of competence and be prepared to manage: preparation of Request for Proposals (RFP) for information systems, technology, and services; evaluation and selection of providers; and contracting information systems and technology (IS&T).

4.1. Objective and Scope

It is expected that the judicious use of the concepts and recommendations detailed in this publication will contribute to improve decisions regarding IS&T design and acquisition, and the deployment of information systems and technology at all levels of management and clinical settings. The material was prepared considering the needs of health executives and practitioners and systems professionals involved in the definition of user requirements, in reaching consensus regarding desired functions in computerized applications, and immersed in the complex process of procurement and acquisition of information equipment and services. Although the principles for requirement analysis and procurement hereby described can be applied to any health information project, they were specifically written considering the needs of healthcare services professionals. In addition, this text may prove to be of great usefulness to those involved in policy making or to anyone who desires to develop a critical vision of healthcare services information systems and related technology.

The experts that participated in the writing of the document and in the development of recommendations and guidelines were concerned with the following realities:

- *Lack of a comprehensive source for guidelines* — There are many written publications that can be used by healthcare and systems professionals to assist their work in user requirement analysis, technical specification, and the procurement of information systems and technology. Unfortunately, few are related to the health sector area of application.

- *The need for a comprehensive source for desired functionalities of health services operation and management computerized applications* — To be used as a departure point for user requirement analysis and as a template for the preparation of Requests for Proposals and evaluation of provider bids, proposals, and products.

- *The demanding changes occurring in the health sector in Latin America and the Caribbean* — These changes include the merger of the traditional vertically constructed and frequently overlapping stakeholders of the healthcare process (regulators, providers, payers, employers, and consumers) into new and integrated organizations, whether virtual or real. These are known as integrated delivery systems (IDS), health maintenance organizations (HMO), preferred provider organizations (PPO), managed care organizations (MCO), and others. The consequent impact on information needs is enormous and changing at a fast rate.

- *The rapid developments in the information technology industry* — Improvements in all aspects of computers and communications are enabling health and healthcare organizations to link together disparate sources of data, share information electronically across previously impassable distances and borders, and bring clinical practice and administration alike to the healthcare professional's environment as never before.

Against this changing backdrop, the current state of readiness for the deployment of modern information systems in Latin America and Caribbean countries lies across a wide range. In some areas or sub-sectors, users already enjoy a high degree of sophistication, many with pioneering clinical information systems and networks. In others, well-established, stand-alone, and relatively straightforward departmental systems such as laboratory, radiology, pharmacy, basic medical records, and others are still awaiting initial automation.

The scope of this publication is to balance preparation for long-term decisions with the practical needs of today's diverse healthcare institutions. The publication is intended to serve as a guideline to the planning and initiation of healthcare service IS&T implementation. To that end, it should be viewed as a general source of information, with references to applicable sources for further details. It is not the province of this document to provide highly specific guidelines for individual systems or users, or even the endorsement of specific standards.

4.2. *Intended Audience and Utilization*

- The document was written for the technically initiated and conceived as a manual with a utilitarian objective.

- This publication does not delve into general conceptual aspects of IS&T, with healthcare services managerial models, or the operational aspects of healthcare organizations or services.

- It is specifically targeted to healthcare executives, health services administrators, information technology professionals and managers, and other interested professionals working in healthcare institutions with an immediate and pragmatic interest in information systems and related technology.

- The reader is expected to have a fair knowledge about information systems and information technology, about health services organization and management, and to be comfortable with technical terms related to the above areas.

- The Editors and Collaborators earnestly expect that this documentation will be profitably used as an instrument to assist health organizations currently involved with or anticipating the planning of IS&T in their services.

- Guidelines and recommendations, regarding infrastructure and dealing with technology and service suppliers, were drafted considering the particular needs of health managers, care providers, and policy makers in the Latin America and the Caribbean Region.

4.3. *How this Document Was Developed*

The recommendations and concepts hereby presented grew out of a review of the voluminous published material in the subject and from extensive consultations with prominent healthcare professionals, IS&T experts, and interested vendors and consultants, from Latin America, the Caribbean, the United States, and Europe.

The consultations and writing of the document followed a structured approach. A number of prominent health sector IS&T experts from Latin America and the Caribbean were identified and commissioned to prepare extensive individual position papers for preliminary input. These consultants were later interviewed for additional details and clarification. A team of health IS&T professionals from Latin America, the Caribbean, United States and Europe was then commissioned to edit the material, combine it with other publicly available information on healthcare IS&T trends, and then to assemble the voluminous material into a cohesive set of technical reviews, guidelines, and references. The resulting draft was brought before a panel of managers, health professionals of different levels and fields of expertise, clinicians, consultants, and vendors for a thorough review and subsequent revision.

The document is, therefore, the collaborative product of a large number of professionals. A great amount of time was spent by the Editorial Team in bringing a unified format to the variety of viewpoints and experiences related to information systems in the Region.

Quick Reference

Knowledge is of two kinds. We know a subject ourselves,
or we know where we can find information upon it.
Samuel Johnson (1709-1784)

Setting Up Healthcare Services Information Systems: A Guide for Requirement Analysis, Application Specification, and Procurement provides a systematic introduction to the most important knowledge components required by decision makers when embarking in the initial stages of healthcare services information systems and information technology planning and development.

The changes in both the healthcare industry in the Region and the information systems industry itself mean an increased level of complexity and detail. In addition, the broad range of development in the Region, from very basic to very sophisticated implementations, calls for a unique approach. Accordingly, this manual has been designed to guide the audience — healthcare administrators and clinical practitioners, and IS&T executives and professionals — along two paths:

- One is the long-term *outlook of healthcare IS&T*, as forecasted by the consensus perspective of the document's contributors. Particular attention is devoted to the development of the Computer-based Patient Record and Healthcare Information Networks.

- The second is the focus on *practical, tactical implementations* found in many current systems throughout the Region and the world. Considerable detailed information is included that speaks to the potential functional specifications for those systems.

With these two concepts in place, the document guides the audience through the current developments occurring in the field of information systems and technology, with appropriate emphasis on its implications for healthcare, and projection of trends. Planning for the IS&T implementation is emphasized. Highlights of successful ingredients of a plan are covered, including development of an IS&T strategic plan, processes and roles, implementation phases, and application modules.

Document Structure

The publication consists of *seven parts* in a modular format that is intended to provide a framework for study and practical utilization.

- Part A was written with the general reader in mind, one that is interested only in the basic principles and a broad perspective of the area of healthcare services information systems. If a deeper understanding of the technology and market aspects is desired, one may progress to Part B.

- Part B is dedicated to the presentation of the state of the art and trends in the area of health services automation, the features of health services information networks, issues regarding the structuring of the information chain, computer-based patient records, and information project management and implementation aspects of interest to health and systems professionals involved in information systems project development.

- Part C describes in detail the technological and market aspects of systems acquisition, including essential aspects of outsourcing information technology and services, preparation of Request for Proposals (RFP), evaluation of proposals and providers, and negotiating and contracting services and technology.

- Part D describes in detail the basic functionalities that each application should have — it presents a systematic categorization of functions in different formats, with the objective of assisting decision makers in the preparation of request for proposals, in evaluating products, and as a departure point for the discussion with users of desired functions. The focus on the definition of desired functionalities will assist the users in each implementation environment to reach a consensus regarding which basic data elements will then be needed in each application. Part C is the technical core of this document.

- Part E examines particular issues related to the implementation of information systems in the health sector of Latin America and the Caribbean.

- Part F, a highly specialized and technical chapter, addresses the complex issue of data, communication, software and hardware standards, the central element of open systems. Without reliable, approved ways to connect the necessary components, open systems cannot work, and within the healthcare industry there are a number of categories of information that each have separate standards. Four annexes enrich the information presented. This is a technical part, intended to be used as a reference. The knowledgeable healthcare executive will do well to stay current of healthcare standards development. In addition, vendors demonstrating present and future commitment to standards are those most likely to survive in the very competitive healthcare IS&T marketplace, and should be given top consideration by healthcare enterprises in the process of systems selection.

- Part G contains a listing of World Wide Web sites for Health and Medical Informatics and Standards Organizations. Also there is a listing of Pan American Health Organization and World Health Organization publications in the area of Health Informatics.

Intended Audience

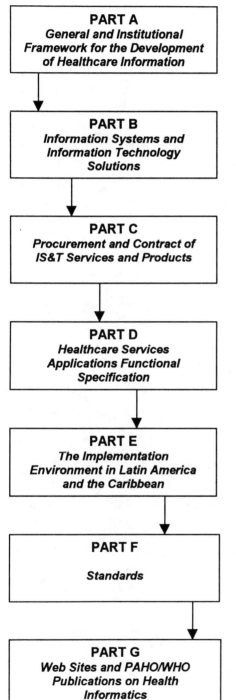

PART A
General and Institutional Framework for the Development of Healthcare Information

Oriented towards the general reader, interested in the basic principles and in acquiring a broad perspective of the area of healthcare services information systems.

PART B
Information Systems and Information Technology Solutions

This chapter was written for readers that wish to have a deeper understanding of the hardware, software, organizational, and implementation issues in health services information systems design and deployment.

PART C
Procurement and Contract of IS&T Services and Products

Reader interested in understanding the technological and market aspects of systems acquisition, including essential features of a Request for Proposals (RFP), evaluation of proposals and providers, and the contracting of services.

PART D
Healthcare Services Applications Functional Specification

Systematic categorization and description of functions for each healthcare service application area with the objective of assisting the preparation of RFP, evaluating products, and for the discussion of desired functionalities.

PART E
The Implementation Environment in Latin America and the Caribbean

This chapter discusses issues of interest to readers involved in the implementation of healthcare information systems in Latin America and the Caribbean.

PART F

Standards

This is a specialized technical chapter to be used as initial source of reference for the complex issues related to data, communications, software, and hardware standards.

PART G
Web Sites and PAHO/WHO Publications on Health Informatics

List of World Wide Web sites of Medical/Health Informatics and Standards organizations sites. List of PAHO and WHO publications in the area of Health Informatics.

PART A
General and Institutional Framework for the Development of Healthcare Information

---

Section A1
Conceptual Framework for Information Systems Development

Section A2
Infrastructure for Health Services Information Systems and Technology (IS&T)

Section A3
Organizational Environment and Content Requirements for Health Promotion and Care Information

---

Section A4
Evolution and Current Challenges for Healthcare Information Systems

---

References

1. PAHO Core Data Indicators
2. OECD Healthcare Indicators
3. Health Databases Protection and Confidentiality
4. Functional Requirements for Healthcare Documentation
5. Health Insurance Portability and Accountability Act Security Standards

Part A. General and Institutional Framework for the Development Of Healthcare Information Systems

Part A. General and Institutional Framework for the Development of Healthcare Information Systems

> *The first glance at History convinces us that the actions of men proceed from their needs, their passions, their characters and talents; and impresses us with the belief that such needs, passions and interests are the sole spring of actions.*
>
> **Georg Wilhelm Friedrich Hegel** (1770—1831)

A.1. Conceptual Framework for Information Systems Development

Information Systems and related Technology (IS&T) are necessary in order to create, "democratize", and apply knowledge. Information systems function at many levels of sophistication and complexity — from very specific to very general. The goal is to improve the health of individuals and populations through the appropriate application of knowledge created through organized information systems.

Before embarking in the process of setting up information systems, one must clearly and explicitly identify the objectives of the system, i.e., determine the expected results. The following questions must be answered regarding what is desired from the information system: is the objective to facilitate care?; are the implemented systems going to be used to manage resources, in this case from a single organization or for the whole healthcare system?; is the system going to be utilized to allocate and control resources?; are the systems expected to contribute to preventive care and in the promotion of health of a defined population?

In order to ensure that Information Systems add value (i.e., *do something good* and "*keep one out of trouble*") by implementing systems that are the best possible answer — technically, cost-wise, and deployed effectively — *it is necessary to follow a defined and logical process.* Also, one must be aware of the technical, human, and financial resources required to carry out each stage of the process.

A.1.1. Concepts and Goals of Information Systems in Healthcare Delivery Organizations

When dealing with the issue of Healthcare Information and Technology, it is useful to start by defining certain terms. The most common term in use to refer to information systems for the support of the operation and management of healthcare services is *Healthcare Information System* (HIS). Although some experts have advocated abandonment of this common term, it is ubiquitous and simple enough to prove useful for the present discussion. A Healthcare Information System may be defined as a computerized system designed to facilitate the management and operation of all technical (biomedical) and administrative data for the entire healthcare system, for a number of its functional units, for a single healthcare institution, or even for an institutional department or unit.

The establishment and operation of an information function component in the context of organizations involve the development and management of three interrelated areas: Information Systems (IS), Information Technology (IT), and Information Management (IM).

- *Information Systems (IS)* — Represented by the collection of administrative and technical tasks realized with the objective of ascertaining the demand for the application portfolio of the organization. Information Systems are, therefore, concerned with "what" is required (demand issues).

- *Information Technology (IT)* — Represented by the collection of technical knowledge and tasks with the objective of satisfying the demand for applications. It involves creating, managing, and supplying the resources necessary for the development and operation of the applications portfolio of an organization; it is concerned with "how" what is required can be delivered (supply issues).

- *Information Management (IM)* — The strategic organization-wide involvement of four components: data, information systems, information technology, and information personnel.

Information Technology (IT), in a more strict sense, is a machine-based technology that actively processes information. IT is just one of a set of information-related technologies that share some characteristics. The definition, however, does not separate active information processing from other technologies, such as the telephone and the television, and from non-technological information-handling activities.

The special characteristics of IT — hardware and software, — as "physical" and "abstract" machines distinguish it from other similar technologies. Hardware and software are alternative yet complementary aspects of IT; both aspects are required for any IT system and they share a flexible symbiotic relationship. Further, the development of new instances of IT depends directly on existing hardware and software, among other factors, meaning that IT is essential to its own development.

Health information systems, to be useful, must allow for a wide scope of health data. Information is an essential element in decision making, and the provision and guidance of healthcare are a complex enterprise, highly dependent on information for a great variety of clinical and managerial decisions. To be useful, information systems must capture and process health and health-related data of broad diversity, scope, and level of detail. All organizations have always had some form of information system to help them record, process, store, retrieve, and present information about their operations.

At all sector levels, the greatest need remains the establishment of continuous information systems that enable the recovery of patient-oriented, problem-oriented, and procedure-oriented data. It has been only in the last twenty-five years that organizations have come to realize that information is a most valuable asset — the quality of managerial decision making, which depends on their success in a very competitive world market, is directly related to the quality of the information available to their managers.

This realization has been gradually forcing organizations to perceive information systems in a different light, more as decision-support tools than as mere registry of past activities. Information systems are, accordingly, gradually moving out of the "back room" to which they have for so long been relegated and into the "front office" of executive suites.

Information, and the technology used to support its acquisition, processing, storage, retrieval, and dissemination, have, as a consequence, acquired strategic importance within organizations, ceasing to be elements that had to do only with operational and administrative support. The ultimate goal of computerized information systems is to improve the way we work, by increasing efficiency, quality of data, and access to stored information.

The technological basis of automated information systems is the computer program — the application software — that enables us to achieve that goal. Application, in broader terms, is defined as the use of systems resources (equipment, computer programs, procedures, and routines) for a particular purpose or in a special way to provide the information required by an organization. All hardware and operating systems, however, are worthless without properly designed and written programs that address and answer, as completely as possible, the requirements of users.

Figure 1. Data, Information, and Knowledge Relationships

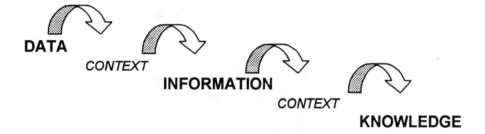

The role of information systems is to capture, transform, and maintain three levels of facts: raw data, processed data, and knowledge. Processed data, traditionally referred to as *information*, conveys intelligence about a particular topic. Knowledge represents an intellectual construct of a higher order, where evidence and information from various fields and sources are linked, validated, and correlated to established scientific truths and thus becoming a generally accepted body of wisdom. We could say that information is data in context and knowledge is information in context (Figure 1).

A.1.2. The Process of Setting Up Information Systems

Development and implementation of information systems is seen by many decision makers as a paradoxical mixture of opportunities to harness modern solutions and gain new technology and, at the same time, an intimidating situation, as they become aware of the limitations of their own understanding and knowledge of the variety and complexity of issues brought forth by IS&T. From the identification of the simple essential steps through to reference material on many technical details there is a wealth of available published materials to assist in those processes.

Fundamental to the understanding of the process of setting up IS&T is the concept of added value — all participants must get out of an information system at least as much as they put in, as well as the system — it must generate benefits greater than its own cost, otherwise the system by definition becomes a burden. Information systems are almost totally dependent upon the staff who provide and record the information, yet these are usually the lowest valued and least involved. If this fact is not recognized and benefits realized for these contributors, there is a high probability of building inaccuracy, instability, and future failure into any information system. Good practice and positive guidelines do exist and some are reproduced in this Guide, along with lists of positive learning points as well as warnings of hazards to avoid.

A.1.2.1. The Process

Figure 2. Dynamics of the Process of Developing and Operating IS&T

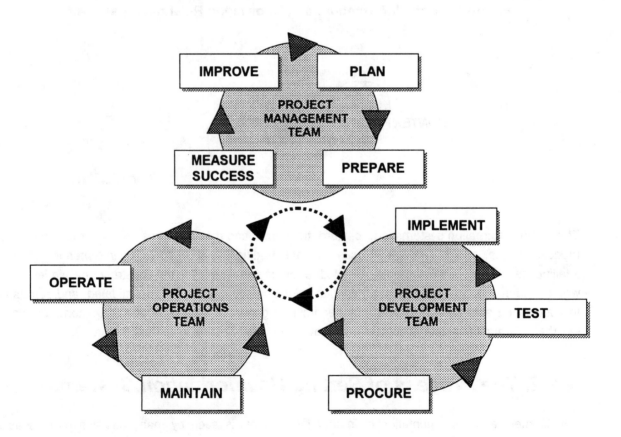

The nine components (Figure 2) involved in developing, deploying, and operating IS&T are:

- Plan
- Prepare
- Procure
- Test
- Implement
- Operate
- Maintain
- Measure Success
- Improve

There follows a brief description of each of the first three components (Plan, Prepare, and Procure), which are pertinent to the initial phase of systems development. They will be discussed in detail throughout this document.

Component 1. PLAN

[a] Define knowledge needs
   - define information outputs
   - define data needs and sources

[b] Define scope of the project
   - is it too large?
   - is it feasible?

[c] Understand legacy information systems — electronic or not

[d] Do cost/benefit analysis (business case)

[e] Identify Resources

[f] Do process analysis

[g] Identify appropriate technical experts

[h] Define users

[i] Define indicators of success

[j] Ensure top level commitment

[k] Define project management methodology
   - all viewpoints
     • business
     • technical
   - user

[l] Identify Change Agent
   - is there someone with the SKILLS internally or externally?
     • respected
     • knowledgeable
     • energetic

Component 2. PREPARE

[a] Design new/refined processes (if required)
[b] Designate project director
[c] Define functionalities required
[d] Identify training needs (immediate and continuing)
- IT staff
- operations staff

Component 3. PROCURE

[a] Write RFP specifications
- technology
- capabilities
- training
- accountabilities (both parties)
- maintenance needs
- project management responsibilities
    • vendor
    • purchaser
    • guarantees, etc.
[b] Prepare negotiation strategy - "buy", don't be "sold"
[c] Prepare proposal evaluation and selection process
[d] Identify possible vendors
- advertise
[e] Distribute RFP
[f] Short list responses
[g] Demonstrations on site - define expectations
[h] Select according to predefined process
- ensure decision is defensible
[i] Manage unsuccessful vendors
[j] Write contract

A.1.2.2. Standards — the Principal Strategic Issue

The most important strategic issue in information systems is standards. Data processing, technical, and electronic standards are essential if equipment is to be able to interconnect. Data definitions and terminologies will be essential if health professionals are to communicate. Specific technical components such as the recording and transmission of images have their own international standards. And in the country-specific setting, the requirements for statistical and other analyses to be passed upwards to support informed decision making must be compatible and follow specific standard definitions.

This Guide gives a wide range of references to international standards, enabling local decision makers to draw directly upon best international practice. Failure to adhere to open technical standards will result in isolated "islands of automation"; failure to adopt data and terminological standards will result in "islands of information". Only compliance with recognized standards, which are too complex for local development, will ensure an integrated information system.

A.1.2.3. Cost-Benefit Analysis

The only justification for any information system, or particular component, is that the benefits justify the costs. Those benefits must be identified, being justified not only in monetary terms but also considering improvement of access, quality of care, better return of resource utilization, better clinical end results, user satisfaction, and improvement of the overall community health status.

There may be more than one way of meeting an information need; there will almost certainly be competing calls for application of information system development funds; and there will certainly be other competing demands such as for diagnostic equipment or increased pharmaceutical supplies. Given limited and finite resources, the right decisions can be reached only by appraising the alternative options to see which gives most added value, as well as being affordable within budget.

A.1.2.4. Incremental Development

Rarely can one develop a complete Information System in less than two years. Even in the most industrialized countries, where fully integrated electronic patient record systems are appropriate in very large hospitals, attempts to specify and implement major systems in one exercise have been fraught with difficulties and have often gone seriously over budget. A stepped approach, adding compatible components in a phased basis, has major attractions.

A.1.2.5. Stakeholder Support

Obtaining the support of key stakeholders and their interests is essential. Good and bad experiences abound; Canada has considered it worthwhile to invest heavily in identifying local views and obtaining stakeholder support — by contrast, the Department of Health in England minimized this step, which led to mistrust of some of the perceived objectives and technical standards of the strategy and consequent definition of requirements and project implementation delays. Key amongst stakeholders are staff, whose understanding and commitment are essential to information system success, commencing with the data recording process. In the U.S. a high failure rate of technically sound medical information systems has been identified due to user or staff resistance. Systems must therefore be defined, then procured or developed, using organizational methods that are openly focussed on all user needs.

A.1.2.6. Security and Confidentiality

Given the very sensitive nature of health care information, and the high degree of reliance by health professionals in particular on reliable records, security and confidentiality must be seen to be clearly and effectively addressed. Security relates to the physical safety of information, including protection against accidental loss as well as against unauthorized alteration. Confidentiality relates to ensuring that only persons with a clinical responsibility see patient-specific information. At the same time, the regulations and technical standards developed must be realistic in terms of recognizing the realities of health care delivery.

A.1.2.7. Education and Training

The importance of education and training cannot be overemphasized. Education relates to change in professional practice, as information systems often give opportunity to work in a new and more appropriate manner. This can apply as much to finance staff, maintenance staff, and pharmacists as it can to clinical health professionals, and the education in new ways of healthcare practice must be undertaken through professional channels. Training, on the other hand, is specifically related to the information system itself, for which all staff must be trained on how to use the equipment, how to enter data, and how to get out appropriate analyses. Training in particular must be ongoing, both to give update training as staff become more familiar with the system and wish to make better use of the functionality, and also to ensure that new staff are trained in information system use as part of their induction training.

A.1.2.8. Project Management

Information systems projects are notorious for running over-time, and over-budget, yet often still failing to deliver all the specified functions satisfactorily. This could be largely avoided by effective project management, including planning, quality assurance, and resource management components. Obtaining an effective system is not simply a process of competitive tendering, local development, or acceptance of an externally funded donated system. The procurement process should be planned and structured, in order to match the solution to the need and circumstances. This in turn needs a systematic approach to defining the requirements and the available resources, including running costs and staff availability.

A.1.2.9. Ongoing Evaluation and Development

Information systems must never become static, or they lose their value. The context in which they operate, the clinical patterns they support, and the policy environment will all change, and therefore so must the information systems. Additionally, the development and progressive roll-out of new technical infrastructures means that new opportunities will also arise, which should be exploited when cost-benefit analysis shows this to be justified. Scientific evidence from formal evaluations should be sought for any health information technology application. Equally important, and more within the control and responsibility of the operational implementing organization, is ensuring that information systems are evaluated and adjusted in the light of how they are perceived, and how they change practice within the organization, and ultimately change the organization itself. Evaluation of the use and effects within the organization should therefore start from the time of implementation, using structured approaches.

Beginning Automation: A Case Study

Background

A hospital of 120 beds, located in a major city, decided to automate information. At the time, the hospital had two desktop computers and three laptops, and only a few of their personnel knew how to use a computer to perform basic tasks. The administration was willing to make another effort to create a network to automate all the information. It is important to mention that the same administration had tried to develop systems in the past few years, but the vendors had provided solutions that led to poor results, creating a very skeptical environment for any new companies trying to offer products or services.

The Plan

Needs assessment is performed and creation of a three-year project is suggested to the administration, following priorities and budget limitations:

1. First-year objectives were to buy some workstations, start training personnel, and to develop a Human Resources/Personnel and a Financial-Billing module.

2. Second year, start installing a network and initiate the development of an Admission module and Medical Inventory.

3. During the third year, integration of all the modules and completion of training all the necessary personnel.

Results

The first year of the plan started on schedule, equipment was bought, training was provided and requirements were gathered for the HR/Personnel and Financial-Billing modules. Development of the modules started slowly due to the lack of experience of some engineers, and precious time was lost setting standards and getting everyone at the same level. Modules were implemented on schedule.

continues next page...

---

continuation from previous page...

In the second year there were problems with the budget, several months were lost, and installation of the network was left behind. The Admission and Medical Inventory modules were developed and implemented. By the end of this year, people were getting tired and the interest from management and employees was very low.

Training was provided for the new modules but problems persisted because employees were expecting that the modules would make work easier and not so much detail oriented and complex. Also, duplication of data and concomitant added effort to record data was being questioned by some employees.

At the beginning of the third year, problems with the quality of data started to appear. Employees were careless about data entry and management was getting reports with very questionable results. Management started to question the quality of work of the modules and the integration was postponed. A few months later the administration of the hospital changed, and due to the questionable results of the data in the modules, no priority and budget were assigned for the next year.

Commentary

Expectations in data automation are too high in many of our institutions. It is incredible the amount of money and effort involved not only in development but also in maintenance and training in corporations and governments. This amount of effort never ends, technology is taking us into a very complex environment where only the people with a realistic, systematic, and objective-oriented vision will accomplish the goals and expected results proposed for IS&T implementation.

Lessons Learned

- Vendors will provide anything to anyone. Selection of vendors should be done using a very objective evaluation, and by getting professional help to make your selection a successful one. Poor design in computer systems creates future complex automation problems.

- Full commitment from management is indispensable, and integration of employees into the automation process will make for better acceptance of new working procedures, due to a better understanding of the institution goals, while automation will be accepted as a normal process of institutional development.

- Consistency in every automation process is necessary to guarantee good data and analysis information.

A.2. Infrastructure for Health Services Information Systems and Technology (IS&T)

The future of Information Technology (IT) as a whole could not be brighter, particularly as it concerns health services and its users, patients, and other constituents. Virtually every category of IT is experiencing progress that promises to bring powerful processing and problem solving to the industry. New technologies are emerging and rapidly maturing, in some cases even faster than users can absorb and integrate them. Developments in technology are divided into the categories of hardware, software, and systems architecture.

A.2.1. Hardware and Software

The ongoing improvements in hardware technology — the oldest element of computing — show no signs of letting up. Computer hardware consists of these main components:

- *Processors* - The logic and arithmetic units of computers will continue to see strong advances. In fact, the physics of silicon and circuitry promise to yield an additional 100-fold increase in processor speed and power before reaching the natural barrier of the individual atom as a unit of data storage. Recent breakthroughs in the semiconductor industry involve the use of higher performance copper chips in integrated circuits. This could increase processor speed and power by an order of magnitude over the aluminum wiring traditionally used in chip manufacturing. In health services IS&T this means faster processing for less cost for all applications, but particularly for such data-intensive functions such as patient chart access and update, image retrieval and manipulation, and chronological retrieval of clinical laboratory data. It also means improved workstations for both healthcare providers and administrators, available at lower cost for dispersal over the enterprise.

- *Storage* - Research and development in files has been no less dramatic, producing unprecedented advances in capacity, performance, and price. Already on the market are hard disk drives that can store a billion characters on a square inch, with additional three-fold increases in the laboratories. Also, new 3½ inch devices are now available which allow storage of over 13 gigabytes of data on 10,000 RPM drives with average seek times of 6.3 milliseconds. In addition, optical storage has been rapidly developing in all key aspects. Traditional tape storage systems have also continued to see improvements. All of these devices have enjoyed better engineering, with fewer moving parts, higher reliability, and less energy consumption. For health services IS&T this means faster, better, more reliable storage media for the very large files required by the large, integrated health services organizations seeking to provide the continuum of care. It also means improved capacity for the enormous amounts of data generated, for example, by radiographic images, and for the massive data mining requirements generated by outcomes research and clinical studies.

- *Displays* - The trend in video display technology is toward larger, thinner screens, higher resolution, better use of color, and improved price/performance. There are now available a number of models thin enough to fit onto a wall, and which display thousands of color combinations. On the other end of the spectrum, very small hand-held devices are available inexpensively. While limited in their ability to deliver large amounts of data, they provide easy, quick, portable access to many kinds of information. All these improvements are required for health services IS&T, since high-quality, low-cost displays are needed to present the data-rich information commonly found in the clinical setting. These include charts and graphs such as ICU flow sheets and ECG waveforms, and radiographic images requiring very high resolution. Display screens must be thin and compact enough for mounting in limited-space environments such as inpatient rooms. They must be inexpensive enough to station at all relevant points of care, not only inpatient rooms, but also outpatient clinic treatment rooms and care givers' offices and homes.

- *Multimedia* - This is a catchall category for the efforts to integrate data, text, voice, and full-motion video. It is also perhaps the most visible and popular point of interest in the industry at present. While still emerging and relatively expensive, multimedia has promise for providing integrated information. This is good news for health services IS&T, since the industry has excellent application potential for this technology. A typical use of multimedia might be to present a full-motion video of a patient's beating heart, alongside an ECG wave form moving in conjunction with the video, together with data from laboratory results, problem lists, and demographics, all accompanied by a voice playback of the cardiologist's assessment and diagnosis.

- *Personal Identification Devices* - Technology of all types continues to improve. Magnetic-stripe badge readers have been in use for some time, and will continue to play a large part of many systems. They currently enable employee identification and controlled access. The development of denser data storage in badges heralds the advent of the so-called "chip card or smart card", in which a patient will be able to carry a credit card that contains coded clinical data (allergies, problems, medications, physicians, etc.), demographics, and coverage data. Other technologies include fingerprint recognition devices, which are already replacing magnetic-stripe readers for employee identification and controlled access, and newly emerging retina scanners, which promise even more speed, accuracy, and ease of use.

- *Bandwidth Technology* - Communications technology will grow the size and speed of data transmission, especially over fiberoptic cable, microwave links, and satellites. This is especially important to healthcare since much clinical data, such as radiographic images, consists of very large packages. A typical mammogram, for instance, requires 64 megabytes for storage. Compression technologies may reduce the file size and improve transmission rates.

- *Connectivity Equipment* - An entire business segment has sprung up around the requirement to link together different portions of a network. Hubs, routers, and their kin are now integral parts of a powerful communications system that supports the health services enterprise of today and tomorrow.

- *Other Input/Output Devices* - Traditional hardware systems for data entry and output will also see improvement, albeit not as dramatically as those in the other categories. Printers and fax machines will continue to become more compact, quieter, and less expensive while printing faster, in a broader range of colors. This has direct application in sending rich patient data to healthcare providers and administrative offices located remotely. Relatively new devices like scanners will experience the same improvements, enabling the capture and transmission of clinical and administrative data across and between enterprises.

Just as important as hardware to the utilization of information technology is the progress in software. In this respect health services IS&T is very much like other industries, which depend on a variety of programs to perform the industry-specific tasks that give computers their value. While there are many types of software for many functions, we have chosen to list the ones pertinent to the health services industry, as follows:

- *Software Languages* - Although the progress in software language development has not equaled that of hardware, advances have nonetheless been steady and sure. Recent times have seen new languages and techniques designed to exploit new hardware and networking technology. Other types of software enable programmers to "paint" screens with data from other applications and databases. Health services IS&T benefits from progress in software language development by acquiring applications sooner, that run faster, over a variety of computing environments. These applications are just in time to support the explosion in application development brought about by the changes in healthcare described in Chapter 5.

- *Systems Software* - While the development of mainframe operating systems has proceeded quietly but steadily over the years, there have been quantum leaps in systems software for workstations, client/server systems, and devices. In particular, personal computer multitasking, multi-programming operating systems have enjoyed tremendous growth, as have graphical user interfaces (GUI). The significance of software to health services IS&T is paramount, since these capabilities are necessary to permit healthcare providers an easy and powerful use of workstations for patient-centric work.

- *Software Enablers* - Recent years have seen significant growth in software that logically operates between the systems software and the application layer. They include database management systems, security systems, interface engines, messaging systems, and a variety of software generally known as "middleware", to name the most prominent. Health services IS&T requires the latest in this technology to enable complex processing to take place without the IS&T staff having to concern itself with development and maintenance of complex, system-wide functions.

- *Communications Software* - This category includes network programming like Ethernet, Token Ring, ATM (Asynchronous Transfer Mode), and other software designed to manage the flow of data along communication lines. In addition, we have elected to include in this category most of the software developed for the Internet, such as hypertext markup language (HTML), web browsers, and other programs for connectivity. These are vital to health services IS&T as the industry joins others in the leap to electronic commerce.

- *Application Software* - Nowhere, however, is there more focus and excitement than in application software development. This is understandable, since this is the primary emphasis of the user; and the user — the health services administrator or healthcare provider — is now involved in IS&T as never before. The new emphasis on the Computer-based Patient Record has seen application development expand to include not only the traditional billing and accounting functions but also clinical applications for clinical users. The new emphasis on Healthcare Networks has seen new applications for linking the traditional payer and provider functions into a single network. Whole new types of applications have arisen, such as speech recognition, with programs written to handle domain-specific vocabularies such as radiology and pathology.

Table 1 summarizes the hardware and software developments, some key examples, and their chief applicability to the health services industry:

Table 1. Software and Hardware Developments

Computer Hardware	Applicability to Health
Processors	Data-rich clinical functions
Storage	Longitudinal medical records
Displays	Ubiquitous placement, intuitive presentation of many clinical data types
Multimedia	Single-point presentation of multiple patient data types; distance learning
Personal Identification Devices	Employee identification, patient "smart card"
Bandwidth	Longitudinal medical record transmission
Connectivity Equipment	Transmission of high-volume patient data
Other Input/Output Devices	Transmission of patient data to clinical points of care
Computer Software	**Applicability to Health**
Software Languages	Faster development of software for a rapidly changing industry
Systems Software	Easier presentation of data to healthcare providers
Software Enablers	Health services IS&T developers focus on applications
Application Software	New applications improve the value of health services IS&T to the healthcare process
Communications Software	Construction of Healthcare Networks

A.2.2. Systems Architecture

Systems architecture goes beyond hardware and software, including additional components and factors that blend into the IS&T design process. The best analogy is that of a *blueprint* for an IS&T system. The blueprint takes into account key elements such as networking infrastructure, connectivity and communications. Standards loom large in importance when considering architecture. There are many features that could fall into the category of systems architecture. This document focuses on two with particular application to the health services industry: open systems and network computing.

> *Designing the right systems architecture for a health services institution is likely to be the most important technical step. From an information technology perspective, systems architecture serves the same purpose as a blueprint when applied to the construction of a physical building. The blueprint defines the end point, what the building will look like when completed, and what standards are to be applied during construction. Once you have an agreed-to blueprint, you can begin building with the confidence that the completed solution will all fit together. The same is true for the design of a health services IS&T solution. One could broaden the building metaphor even further in the context of health services IS&T:*

>> *Think of an IT architecture in terms of planning a city rather than just building a house. Architecture provides building codes that limit near-term design options for the sake of the community, but these codes do not tell individuals what kind of buildings they need. Like building codes, an IT architecture should consist of a set of standards, guidelines, and statements of direction that permit step-by-step business-driven implementation without sacrificing integration.*

When an organization picks a proprietary system the vendor automatically chooses the architecture. Indeed, many institutions, particularly smaller ones, choose proprietary systems because they do not want to focus resources on questions of systems architecture definitions. Nevertheless, since the *overwhelming emphasis in today's IS&T environment is on open systems*, and since an open system usually requires more up-front planning, institutions that aspire to open architectures will want to outfit themselves with detailed technical information on the subject. Here again, there is a considerable amount of easily accessible publications, but an overview of open systems selection criteria is in order.

Detailed pros and cons of open versus proprietary systems will be highlighted later, but here it suffices to say that a well-defined open systems architecture, in combination with a good health services business strategy, offers the following advantages:

- It enables *sharing of resources*, a critical role in evolving health services institutions today.

- *The* linkage *between the institution and technical strategies enables better decision making, by clearly identifying key business issues and demonstrating linkages between the business strategy and the IS&T strategy.*

- Having a defined set of *standards* allows users to assemble the necessary modules more quickly and take advantage of market opportunities as they appear.

- It offers support for *transparent end user access* to system resources (single log-on and security, for example).

- Common services (reusable building blocks) can help *reduce future maintenance costs.*

- It can *simplify systems administration and reduce costs* through use of common distribution and communication services.

- The transparent access to resources helps application developers in *deployment of new solutions*.

- Using a technical architecture *helps eliminate potential technology integration issues* in the future.

- A technical architecture *clearly defines the technologies for the organization*, which allow development of competencies in selected areas.

A.2.2.1. Open Versus Proprietary Systems

Information systems were initially introduced with software components — including operating systems, enablers, and even some languages — that were proprietary to the vendor. Indeed, there are many health services information systems still on the market that are proprietary. Generally, the terms "proprietary" and "closed" are used interchangeably in this discussion, to mean system characteristics kept from the public domain by the vendor.

An analogy lies in the area of stereo components. In the 1960's, manufacturers of stereo equipment agreed to make most of their component parts interchangeable by making the connections standard, so one vendor's speakers would connect to another vendor's tuner, etc. Nowadays the trend is actually reversed, with manufacturers building whole systems, including tuners, speakers, amplifiers, tape and CD decks all connected together — a closed or proprietary system.

That proprietary systems in the health services IS&T arena still enjoy continued success due to some very tangible assets of proprietary systems that are discussed in the next section. However, the worldwide trend is inexorably toward open systems that utilize recognized standards.

The current and most accepted definition of open systems is an environment that implements sufficient open specifications for interfaces, services, and supporting data formats to enable all properly written applications to do the following:

- Allow porting with no changes or minimal changes across a variety of hardware architectures

- Inter-operate with applications on both local and remote systems having various architectures

- Interact with users in a common manner that allows user skills to transfer easily among different hardware architectures

Open specifications are public specifications maintained by an open, public consensus process. They usually contain international standards as they are adopted. They can also contain specifications developed by private companies or consortia when maintenance of the specification is transferred to some public consensus or control process.

There are many influences to help drive the open systems environment. These influences fall into four major categories:

- *De Facto Standards* - A *de facto* standard is a specification that is widely implemented and used. *De facto* standards can be either open or proprietary. The public can generally obtain the specification for an open-system *de facto* standard. There is a process for the public to control the future content of the specification. Microsoft Windows and Systems Network Architecture (SNA) from IBM are examples of proprietary *de facto* standards. An example of an open *de facto* standard would be the Hypertext Markup Language (HTML), used for presenting information on the Internet.

- *De Jure Standards* - *De jure* standards are produced by a group with legal status, such as sanctions by a government body or by a recognized international organization. To create the standard, the *de jure* group must follow an open process that allows anyone to participate in forming a consensus. This consensus building process is the longest of all the open systems processes. The World Health Organization International Classification of Diseases (ICD) is an example of de *Jure Standards*.

- *Consortia* - Since 1988, many open systems consortia have formed. Consortia are usually not-for-profit organizations funded by members with a common interest in defining some aspect of the open systems environment. Consortia often incorporate existing *de facto* and *de jure* standards; they then address other user needs with an open process. In this process, members define profiles and standards for areas that have no *de facto* or *de jure* standards. Health Level 7 (HL7), for instance, is a prime example for healthcare provider data message format standards.

- *Technology Providers* - Technology providers actually produce a usable technology (source code) for an open systems environment, incorporating existing *de facto*, *de jure*, and other consortia specifications.

The pros and cons of open and proprietary systems are captured in Table 2, where the checkmark denotes the type of system generally acknowledged to have the advantage. In considering the acquisition of a health services information system, the decision of whether to purchase an open system, a vendor proprietary system, or something in-between is often difficult. The fast-moving world of health services IS&T demands the versatility of the "plug and play" environment of open systems. It is, however, impossible to say unequivocally that all health services IS&T systems should be open.

The advantages enjoyed by users of proprietary systems are substantial enough to require at least a comparison of relative strengths and weaknesses. Technology — in the form of faster and less expensive hardware and software, combined with widening standards development and acceptance — will with great probability result in predominately open systems in the future.

Table 2. Open Versus Proprietary Systems

CHARACTERISTIC	PROPRIETARY SYSTEMS	OPEN SYSTEMS
Best performance	√	
Fewest interfaces	√	
Lowest maintenance	√	
Fewest number of vendors	√	
Easier to answer user requirements		√
Least reliance on a single vendor		√
Widest choice of applications, technologies		√
Fastest time to application development		√
Ease and speed of growth		√

Open systems have the benefit of being attractive for institutional top management. As in the stereo analogy, managers can make strategic decisions without worrying about whether a particular health services IS&T vendor can supply the needed computer-related solution. Moreover, reliance on a single vendor carries increased risk in today's fast-moving environment. Recent industry events have seen some vendors pass out of existence overnight, as a result of faulty planning, poor product performance, or acquisition. Open systems provide the opportunity to spread the risk among several strong players. These issues are further detailed in the section below regarding selection of systems architecture.

There is no question that the trend in IS&T is to open systems. The majority of IS&T suppliers have demonstrated tangible commitment to openness by bringing new technology to market with a wide spectrum of open features and adherence, in one degree or another, to open standards. The standards are what make open systems possible. The subject of standards in the health services industry is involved and important enough to warrant its own section, later in this document.

The software industry is also approaching a new paradigm: the industry of software components. This new approach depends on the ability of transportable and reusable components to communicate with each other according to standardized interfaces. The Object Management Group (OMG) is a large consortium of individuals, companies, and developers with the mission of developing such standards. The specification is described by CORBA (Common Object Request Broker Architecture), which is expected to allow the development of pieces of software that can be easily expanded and replaced without jeopardizing the whole application.

A.2.2.2. Network Computing

The second major architectural trend is toward network computing. In fact, there is arguably no more prominent topic in IS&T architecture today. The term is distinct from "Healthcare Networks" described previously. Healthcare Networks is an organization and application concept, while network computing is an IS&T implementation. Network computing in the IS&T sense *enables* Healthcare Networks. A subtle feature of the term "network computing" is that it is frequently used interchangeably with "the Internet." This is because the Internet has grown so large and so visible as an example of network computing. While networks have been in common use in health services for over ten years, the Internet has seen its explosive growth over just the last few years. This document uses the terms network computing and the Internet interchangeably.

The move to network computing represents an evolution to a form of computing that has the power to significantly alter the business process itself. It is a combination and extension of other forms of computing — centralized, distributed, and personal computer oriented. In network computing, applications and data reside in the network, allowing, as we have already seen, health services enterprises to merge into large, vertical and horizontal organizations that share comprehensive information to provide the continuum of care. The continuous movement toward network computing raises the demands placed on applications. The *World Wide Web* is a network computing application that works with almost any workstation. This aspect alone has huge significance for health services IS&T, since it means that many networked health services institutions can enjoy the benefits of integrated systems and applications using inexpensive terminals and workstations.

Thousands of graphics are transmitted daily over the Web to millions of users worldwide, many of them in health services and many of them in Latin America and the Caribbean. Some have a smaller number of users but require extensive network resources, such as the Intranet, which is an Internet that limits access to a selected group of people or resources and uses the same communication protocols as the Internet. Wider use of applications and their increasing use of graphic and multimedia content are driving the need for more bandwidth. And, because bandwidth can be costly, efficiency is critical. The most striking example of network computing is the estimate that by 2000, more than *150 million people in more than 100 countries will have connected to the Internet*. The number of users increases by 1 million each month, and 60 percent of the users are business people (Figure 3). In 1997, about 15% of the U.S. population used electronic mail and 12.8 million households had E-mail connectivity. Over 100,000 companies were conducting business worldwide using the World Wide Web and over 15,000 business concerns were listed in the Commercial Sites Index — and, on average, 73 new entries were being added daily. By the end of the next decade it is expected to be upwards of 800 million users on the Internet, over 1 million networks, and over $1 trillion per year in Internet-based transactions.

Much has been said about the impact of computers and the Internet on society. The question remains if we really will transform society through the use of computers and the Internet. Certainly the potential is there, but it will be realized only if we can get access in the hands of everyone. Otherwise, we are not likely to see the much-heralded revolutionary changes expected from the generalized use of the Internet resources. We still will have the schisms and chasms in society where there will be sectors of society in which people are able to partake of the wonderful riches online while, at the same time, other groups are effectively excluded. Effective change will require getting entire countries — especially developing countries and societies — online.

Figure 3. The Growth of the Internet

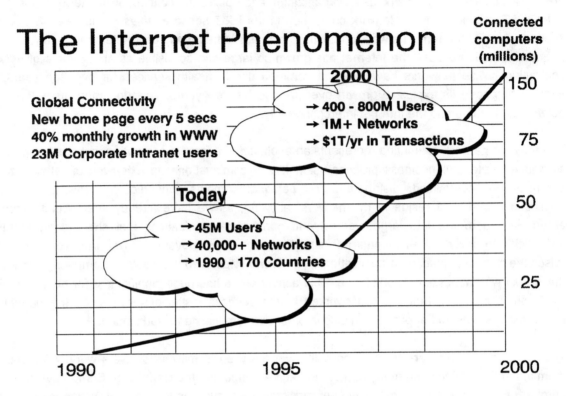

Without network computing, Healthcare Networks would not be possible and network computing promises exciting functionality and a whole new world of features and capabilities.

A quick summary of network computing requirements includes:

- *Network Provider* - These are organizations that provide integration, management, and delivery of networked applications. They typically offer a range of multi-protocol requirements, EDI (Electronic Data Interchange) transmission, and network speed.

- *Network Application Services* - These include the functional applications such as patient registration, master patient indexes, professional communication, and many others.

- *Professional Services* - Networks usually require significant up-front consulting for systems design and planning, customization of education and training for users, and services for network management.

- *Network Enabling Products* - Networks require special languages and tools, web servers and clients, various gateways, and network systems management programs.

- *Servers* - Servers are the computers, both the hardware and the operating system environment that will act as the central hub of the network.

- *Security* - The network is the logical place to install the health services enterprise's security system and all its components. Since this topic is so important to the health services industry, it is included in a separate section.

As with systems architectural considerations, health institutions must understand and plan for their respective regional idiosyncrasies. From the community level to the institutional level, networks depend on individual members for success. Proper interregional planning by all affected members is necessary for networks to achieve their promise.

A.2.3. Human Resource Infrastructure

The key to success in the implementation of information systems of any kind is the existence of a skilled and motivated workforce with competence in the use of information. Considering the requirements for technical (systems and programming) expertise and, above all, of specialized professional management, an assessment must be made of the number, level of experience, and balance of skills required. Especially in less developed countries, the identification and recruitment of competent professionals and difficulties with staff retention may be a major hindrance to systems development and operation.

The existence of an appropriate behavioral and institutional infrastructure implies that a framework must exist to allow information to be used in a way that encourages individuals to work towards the overall objectives of the organization. Unless such an appropriate framework is in place, information cannot be translated into action. It should include:

- Clearly defined responsibility and accountability structure,

- Setting of objectives and targets for individuals and departments,

- Mechanisms for motivating individuals and for providing feedback about their achievements,

- An environment in which managers are able to take action to influence events in their areas of responsibility.

Work patterns will have to be modified and considerable training both of line staff and management will be required. They will have to learn to work with the new system's technology and to use the better information available to improve decision making and the provision of health services. In addition to these demands, there also will be a change in the role of information services. In the past, information services have been organized entirely on a national or regional basis, but now districts require a defined information management function. Initially the information management function of the organization may be invested in an existing manager but eventually an appropriate team of skilled people will be required — the Information Systems Committee. The role of this group will be to plan, steer, and undertake the implementation of systems. It will also play a leading role in defining information needs and interface with the systems professionals.

A.2.3.1. Data Management Activities

There are two key human organizational components to the successful production of data: the health service line manager and the system manager. The line manager has a well defined responsibility for the timeliness and accuracy of data captured by the health staff, and the system manager is responsible for developing policies, procedures, and standards, and for monitoring activities to ensure that these are adhered to. Both should respond directly to a formal organizational body (Information Systems Committee or equivalent).

Line Manager Responsibilities - Line Managers must assume explicit responsibility for ensuring that data captured in their sphere of activity are within the agreed standards of accuracy, completeness, and timeliness. They are also responsible for appropriate staff training to carry out their data production tasks.

Information Systems Manager Responsibilities - Information Systems Managers are to be responsible, from the user's viewpoint, for the operation of implemented applications, whether manual or computerized, and to serve as an intermediary for questions related to existing or desired applications. They play key roles in:

- Formulation of operational policies for systems,

- Development of procedures and routines in cooperation with the systems staff (analysts and programmers),

- Responsibility for organizing and providing training,

- Coordination of systems introduction or reorientation,

- Setting performance targets and monitoring standards,

- Supervision of the execution of procedures and routines, and

- Establishing liaison with systems technical personnel and with the higher levels of the health organization structure.

A.2.3.2. User Education and Training

The involvement in and acceptance of computerized system by staff is the most important and challenging part of its implementation. In general, the direct care staff does not have a real understanding of either the role or the value of information technology in medical care and health services administration and the effort, in terms of time, commitment, and resources needed for the deployment of effective information systems. Even administrators may be surprisingly ill equipped to discern such issues. Paradoxically, they all state that they are aware of the importance of information for decision making and that there is "not enough" information.

After appropriate hands-on training, users should be able to visualize the benefits of better information with better patient care and the many issues attendant to IS&T. A structured human resource development program must be defined to increase awareness, to assess training needs, and to involve the staff in all aspects of systems design and implementation with the objective of developing an understanding of the methodologies and the technology of information systems, without which it would be very difficult to make appropriate use of data and deployed processing capabilities. Individuals in the organization who generate, collect, and use data and information must be educated and trained, so they can effectively participate in the management of information.

The training support staff should be involved throughout all the nine steps of systems design and implementation (see A.2.1.). Practical actions regarding the establishment of a human resource development and training program include:

- Ensure, as soon as possible, that those staff involved in all levels of systems implementation and operation are identified and selected to receive appropriate training, both theoretical and practical, in health information systems and systems technology,

- Consider the issues associated with the organizational environment in which systems will be deployed and utilized,

- Develop training strategies for health information systems, which take account of the issues associated with their development, the organizational environment in which they are expected to operate, and the specific circumstances of the organization.

The following guidelines on training strategies for health are recommended:

- Identify target groups on the basis of user functions.

- Analyze expected user performance requirements associated with the new system using a participatory model that calls upon all professional categories.

- Assess training needs, including current level of comfort and skill with technologies to be used.

- Develop training programs to meet identified target groups' needs.

- Establish a network of training focal points, which take account of the organization health units' requirements and undertakings.

- A training strategy for modern forms of information processing and analysis must cover all those involved in healthcare and be interdisciplinary, while taking account of the specific needs of the different functional and professional groups.

The following target groups must be considered: those who originate, collect, and supply data; operational decision makers (direct healthcare professionals and administrators); managers, planners, and policy makers; and information systems managers. Each organization must develop its own strategy for initial and continuing training in health information systems, which takes into account, on the one hand, the overall development of health information systems and, on the other hand, its particular healthcare and market environment. Attention must be given to:

- Training should take place in a multidisciplinary setting;

- Advanced technological teaching tools should be used wherever practicable;

- In-service training should be provided at all levels to meet day-to-day requirements;

- Education and training should be closely linked to practical experience of health services to motivate users.

- Depending on the target group, great attention must be given to avoid excessive use of jargon and complexity of concepts.

- Define minimum levels of competency.

- Provision of resources to support the preparation of teaching aids and to allow for the adaptation of training material to meet the needs of target groups at various levels. The training should include hands-on basic computer skills, application-specific training, and individual role and functions in systems operation.

- Test training programs prior to full-scale use.

- The methodology used for presentation should allow for interaction of participants. Training should be done away from distractions from the daily work environment and as close as possible to the actual implementation. Group activities will help to reduce the tedious development of some technical issues. Simulated situations, group or individual presentations should be devised to determine to what extent participants achieved the level of knowledge or mastery of skills indicated by the objectives.

- Evaluate effectiveness of training programs by considering user satisfaction and feedback, manager feedback, pre- and post-testing, audit trails, and the frequency and type of calls for assistance during systems use.

The knowledge basis necessary to provide to trainees, in each category, must necessarily be related to the expected competencies required for optimal performance of the non-automated and automated systems to be developed and implemented. Besides a core knowledge requirement needed for all professionals of the same category, each in turn will demand training specifically oriented to their operational needs. The concept of training modules arranged in "tracks", specifically developed and appropriate to each professional category, is considered as the most suitable approach to the question of diversity of training required.

Case Study
User Training

Background

The facility involved is a 250 bed regional hospital that has emergency services, an intensive care unit, obstetrics, pediatrics, and adult medical and surgical care. The existing information system application was a 15-year-old financial system. The system was networked with all nursing units, supply office, and the billing office. The administration decided to implement a new application, an Admissions, Discharge, and Transfer (ADT) system that integrated with the financial system. The new system utilized a graphical user interface (GUI) and introduced the mouse as an input device. The system tracked patients' location from admission through to discharge, providing real time status of every bed in the hospital.

Prior to implementation, the location of the patient was difficult to track because the manual system for tracking was maintained in the Admitting office, but was not kept current as patients moved throughout the hospital. The nursing units were supposed to call Admitting with every patient transfer and discharge, but the calls were often late or forgotten. There was never an accurate count of the available beds at any given time

The Plan

An ADT system had been purchased from a national vendor that has installed this system in seven other regional hospitals.

- *Duration* -The time frame for installation was 3 months and utilized the vendor's training packet to establish the institutional training program.
- *Parameters* - Each nursing unit, the admitting office and the administration office, and the Emergency Room needed to have new hardware.
- *Expected Outputs* - Every patient that was admitted to the hospital would have a retrievable trail location and duration of stay. Additional information was also obtained including diagnosis and care providers, providing staff with a basic history of the patients' admissions and diagnoses.

continues next page...

continuation from previous page...

Clinical View

Current users of the billing system are clerical staff who track hospital charges and generate patient billing. They have basic keyboarding skills and are comfortable with the current billing application. They have not used any Windows-like applications or data input using a mouse.

The clerical staffs on the nursing units and the Emergency Room have no experience with a computer but are efficient at typing dictated reports. The professional nursing staff, a total of 10 Registered Nurses, are also users of the new ADT system. They hold supervisory and administrative jobs.

IS&T View

Prior to the installation of the new ADT system, the hospital had a computer network that linked the nursing units and the billing and supply office. A contract was initiated with a local IT business to upgrade the network to all patient care units, the admitting office, administration, and the emergency room. The training responsibilities for implementing this new system were assigned to an IT staff member whose other responsibilities included scheduled maintenance of the current network.

Training Needs Analysis

Identified users were surveyed, through a written questionnaire to assess their level of experience, comfort, and skill in using computers and/or keyboards — a sample survey form is reproduced at the end of this discussion. Survey results indicated that the billing office clerical staff had basic keyboarding skills and were comfortable with the mainframe application that had been in place for 15 years. None of them, however, had used the GUI applications or mouse devices.

The clerical and professional nursing staff on the patient units were, in general, less proficient with computers than the billing office staff. The majority had no more than basic keyboarding skills. The survey feedback also revealed that most nursing staff were anxious about using a computer. The following training needs were identified based on the survey results and the vendor recommendations for skills and knowledge required for use of the new system:

continues next page...

continuation from previous page...

[a] Basic Computer Skills
Input devices:
- Keyboarding skills
- Use of mouse

Operating system and GUI
- Screen set-up
- Navigation

Output
- Reports for tracking, auditing
- Printing capabilities

[b] System-Specific Skills
- Purpose of ADT system
- Implications for patient care
- Responsibilities of users: clerical staff and professional staff

The training plan included provision of basic computer skill education by the IT staff member and system-specific education based on the vendor-provided materials. Staff members were assigned to attend one or both of the above sessions during the four-week period prior to the system implementation date. Training sessions were offered in a centrally located classroom away from the patient units.

During the four-week training period, approximately 75% of the identified users actually completed the training. The remainder, although scheduled for classes appropriate to their needs, were unable to complete the training for a variety of reasons.

Commentary

The system implementation was only partially successful. Twenty-five percent of the staff had been unable to complete training prior to the target date, delaying implementation by two additional weeks. This delay further complicated the process in that the staff who had been trained early, four to six weeks prior to actual implementation, found that they forgot some of what they had been taught before the system was in place on their unit. Early weeks were more stressful than they needed to be because the anxiety of the users had not been addressed.

continues next page...

continuation from previous page...

Lessons Learned

- Schedule training as close as possible to implementation. Offering training on a new system four weeks or more before the system is available will not be sufficient. Users will forget what they learned if they do not use the information and skills immediately after receiving the training.

- Consider super user/ train the trainer approach in order to support the staff using the system. This can provide staff who have an interest and/or skills with computers with a specific role in supporting the implementation of new systems. These staff members can be given more in-depth training and can then provide one-on-one training and/or support to the rest of the staff during the initial implementation process. The super users can also provide ongoing support to staff and can participate in orienting new staff as they are hired. These staff members may also be resources to the IS&T department for other system selections and installations.

- Address computer anxiety prior to training by creating introductory activities such as e-mailing, searching the Internet, and solitaire.

- Begin planning for the training as soon as the system selection has taken place. Whenever possible, the system selection process should even consider training issues as a part of the decision-making process. The importance of this, alone, cannot be over-emphasized.

continues next page...

continuation from previous page...

Model for a basic computer literacy assessment form:

Basic Computer Literacy Assessment

Please complete the following:

Date: _____/_____/_____   Unit:

Job Title: _____

1.   Do you own a Personal Computer (PC)?   _____Yes   _____No

2.   Have you ever used a Personal Computer (PC)? _____Yes   _____No

3.   If yes, for how many years, approximately?   _____Years

     If yes, have you used any of the following applications?

Word Processing	_____Yes	_____No
Spreadsheet	_____Yes	_____No
Internet	_____Yes	_____No

4.   Do you "surf " the Internet?   _____Yes   _____No

5.   <u>On a scale of 1-5, please rate the following based on your level of comfort or familiarity:</u>

	Least		Moderate		Most
Computers in the workplace..............	1	2	3	4	5
The external parts of a computer........	1	2	3	4	5
The mouse.....................................	1	2	3	4	5
Windows based applications............	1	2	3	4	5
Handling diskettes..........................	1	2	3	4	5
The computer keyboard....................	1	2	3	4	5
Laser printers.................................	1	2	3	4	5
Label printers.................................	1	2	3	4	5

6.   Would you be interested in taking a basic computer literacy class developed to help you be comfortable with PCs?   _____Yes   _____No

     If yes, what days and times would be convenient for you?
     _____Days of the week

     _____Times

A.2.4. Security and Confidentiality

Healthcare organizations face a great variety of security and confidentiality risks and are fully responsible for maintaining all aspects of security and confidentiality of data and information, and the eventual conflicts between data sharing and data security and confidentiality must be addressed early in the process of systems procurement and development. The prudent healthcare enterprise automating application modules will want to consider a number of system-wide security and confidentiality implementation factors that cross application boundaries. Two factors make the subject a preeminent concern in the healthcare industry today: the intrinsically sensitive nature of patient data, and the growing use of network computing, particularly the Internet, for healthcare information processing. These two items in combination have frequently made headlines in the healthcare industry in the last few years.

Selling the importance of security to managers and developing security awareness in physicians and administrative staff, and writing, implementing, and monitoring security policies are functions of the systems manager working in close collaboration with the Information Systems Committee, the high administration and the legal counsel of the organization. The terminology used in the areas of "security", "safety", and "data protection" is far from uniform and frequently confusing. All issues can be, however, grouped under four areas:

- Integrity - the prevention of unauthorized modification of information,

- Access - the prevention of the unauthorized entry into information resources, and

- Physical protection - the protection of data and data processing equipment against intentional or accidental damage.

- Confidentiality - the prevention of unauthorized disclosure of information.

None of the issues related to systems security and confidentiality is unique to the health sector; it is, however, the combination of some of these aspects that justifies special consideration in the case of health information systems. Among the many characteristics of health data some are very particular:

- Health information systems store identified data on the health of people, and some of the information is highly sensitive,

- Because of the team nature and frequent interdisciplinary activities in health, confidential individual data are needed by many professionals and access control and authorization become special problems,

- Recorded individual data play an essential role in healthcare delivery and may even be critical to the patient. Availability, even on-line, and quality of such data deserve special attention and the balance of access and integrity control is a serious problem in these circumstances.

- Remote access to medical records and other healthcare data is being granted to increasing numbers of service providers, payers, controllers and clerical workers — the challenge is to simultaneously provide required levels of access, while ensuring protection for internal systems, confidentiality, meaningful authentication of users, and the ability to audit systems utilization.

- Patient data are important for research and the statistical analysis of groups of patients is important for planning and improvement of medical practice and of social interest. Confidentiality, one of the aspects of data security, includes balancing the demand for healthcare information with patient privacy rights and the establishment of fair principles of privacy of individual data — limits of use of health records by public health authorities, police, and researchers.

- In keeping with the growing focus on the patient as the centerpiece of medical care is the notion of ownership of the medical record. More and more, the trend is to promote the patient as the owner of his/her medical record data. However, the actual legal instruments to enforce this perspective are lagging. In most countries of the Americas the healthcare institution is the legal owner of the medical record created at that entity, just as the institution owns other "business records" it creates. And while the majority of independent healthcare organizations, user groups, consultants, and affiliations encourage providers, payers, and employers to invest ownership with their constituents, the reality is mixed at the present time.

Each organization must determine the level of security and confidentiality for different categories of information, and which access to each category of information is appropriate to the user's title and job function. An effective way to deal with the questions of security and confidentiality includes the following definitions:

- Who has access to data or information?

- Definition of data or information sets to which a particular professional has access,

- Establishment of mechanisms to educate and compel (via disciplinary action) the individual who has access to information to keep it confidential,

- Rules for the release of health-related information,

- Establishment of physical barriers and systems deterrents to secure data and data processing equipment against unauthorized intrusion, corruption, disaster, theft, and intentional or unintentional damage.

There are many features under the umbrella topic of security that bear review by the healthcare enterprise. Security can be implemented at the hardware or software levels, and a secure remote access architecture may combine a variety of technologies: firewalls, authentication, virtual private networks, filters, backdoor software security flaw prevention, encryption, passwords, etc., but the features of security that bear directly on the confidentially and protection of electronic patient data use fall into five basic categories:

- Physical Security. Lightning, power fluctuations, flooding, fire, static electricity, and improper environmental conditions constitute the most common problems. Theft of equipment and data media is less common but can be disastrous. A contingency plan for disaster recovery and backup of data and redundant equipment are the ways to deal with problems of this nature.

- Authentication. This is the most basic method. It entails a user sending user identification code, along with a password, to the network the user is interrogating. The network security system matches the identity to the password, and "authenticates" the user in the case of a match, or denies the user access if there is no match. Different levels of access can be defined for the same record.

- Encryption. Encryption is the method of encoding a message, a field, forms, data, or an entire network, using alphanumeric keys to scramble the data so that only the individuals possessing the appropriate key can decrypt and read the information. The end result is secured data. The encryption key can be a string of digits that have a mathematical relationship to a decryption corresponding key, so that one is used to encrypt, the other to decrypt, or the same key can be used to encrypt and decrypt.

- Digital Signature. This is an identification mark provided by the sender/composer in each communication transaction to prove that he/she really sent the message. Digital signatures meet the following conditions: they are impossible to fraudulently imitate, authentic, not alterable, and not reusable. They have the potential to have greater legal authority than handwritten signatures. This feature has clear-cut potential in the healthcare industry for enabling electronic physician signatures.

- Access Control. This is a sophisticated form of security that has wide applicability in the healthcare industry. Access control systems work by allowing the enterprise to define a number of roles. Examples of roles are patients, attending physicians, consulting physicians, nurses, therapists, administrators, etc. Different roles are allowed access by to different levels of data, beyond the simple requirement for authentication. Access control methods have excellent potential for protection of sensitive patient data.

Within each of these categories there are many features, some subtle, some obvious (Table 3). The healthcare enterprise automating security on a network should thoroughly investigate the specifics of vendors supplying electronic security. However, the human factor is the weakest link in the prevention of security and confidentiality faults in any setting. Most episodes of breach of systems security and unauthorized access to confidential records are related to absent or poorly implemented or monitored procedures and malicious use or damage to systems by insiders, disgruntled employees, fraudulent or criminal activity, and espionage. Recently, security experts have been cautioning organizations to the increasing risk of external attacks and the risks represented by downloading executables (Java Applets, Active X) and recommend that non-trusted code should never be allowed to be executed on the corporate network.

Table 3. Administrative Procedures to Guard Data Integrity, Confidentiality, and Availability

Requirement	Implementation
Certification. Chain of trust partner agreement. Contingency plan (all listed implementation features must be implemented).	Applications and data criticality analysis. Data backup plan. Disaster recovery plan. Emergency mode operation plan. Testing and revision.
Formal mechanism for processing records. Information access control (all listed implementation features must be implemented).	Access authorization. Access establishment. Access modification.
Internal audit. Personnel security (all listed implementation features must be implemented).	Ensure supervision of maintenance personnel by authorized, knowledgeable person. Maintenance of record of access authorizations. Operating, and in some cases, maintenance personnel have proper access authorization. Personnel clearance procedure. Personnel security policy/procedure. System users, including maintenance personnel, trained in security.
Security configuration mgmt. (all listed implementation features must be implemented).	Documentation. Hardware/software installation & maintenance review and testing for security features. Inventory. Security Testing. Virus checking.
Security incident procedures (all listed implementation features must be implemented).	Report procedures. Response procedures. Security management process (all listed implementation features must be implemented). Risk analysis. Risk management. Sanction policy. Security policy.
Termination procedures (all listed implementation features must be implemented).	Combination locks changed. Removal from access lists. Removal of user account(s). Turn in keys, token, or cards that allow access.
Training (all listed implementation features must be implemented)	Awareness training for all personnel. Periodic security reminders. User education concerning virus protection. User education in importance of monitoring log in success/failure, and how to report discrepancies. User education in password management.

A recovery plan should be defined for offsetting the effects of an unpredictable disaster or data loss. Such a contingency operation can take the form of a document that delineates the steps necessary for recovery, including a listing of critical operations, financial or otherwise, that must be resumed immediately and a listing of all software items (applications and data files) needed for carrying out the organization's critical operations. Equipment listings, vendor delivery considerations, communications linkage specifications, and the people to contact must be also incorporated in the document.

Government intervention and legal constraints have been introduced in many countries, especially in Europe. A set of security recommendations was developed by the U.S. Government and directed to the improvement of security measures in healthcare organizations.

A.2.5. *Legal Issues Related to Software*

A well-defined policy and guidelines regarding the acquisition, development, distribution, and support of computer software must be conceived concerning technological, legal, social, and marketing considerations.

Many problems exist, with potentially significant and costly legal implications, regarding the acquisition, distribution, and utilization of software products. Among the most common issues, mention is made of: the use of illegal copies of commercial packages; disregard of copyright issues and ownership rights in contracting external software development; inappropriate agreement provisions with contracted external systems developers; lack of guidelines regarding the selection, testing, and evaluation of software products, and the lack of guidelines regarding the transference of software products.

A.2.5.1. Some Relevant Definitions

- "Source code" means the set of instructions as written by the programmer in one or more computer languages.

- "Object code" means any instruction or set of instructions in machine-executable form, also referred to as "compiled code". Object code is generated by processing the source code with specialized programs called compilers.

- "Technical documentation" means any printed, magnetic, or optical media material containing a detailed description of the internal organization, procedures, and sequencing of machine operations related to one specific computer software product and should include a copy of the source code.

- "User documentation" means any standard manuals or other related materials used for user instruction or reference in use of the licensed program.

- "Licensed program" means the object code version of the program and related program user documentation.

- "Use" means copying of any portion of the licensed program from a storage unit or media into the designated equipment and execution of the licensed program on that equipment.

- "Copy-protected software" does not, as it may appear, relate to copyright regulations, but to the existence of software or hardware solutions that make it difficult or impossible for users to make copies of the object code or prevent installation of the programs except for a pre-determined number of times. There are many copy protection schemes as well as many ways to by-pass such limitations. Much used in the past, presently very few commercial programs still use such resources.

A.2.5.2. Trends in Software Design and Developer's Rights

In the first-generation electric tabulators and electronic computers, the instructions ("software" or "programs") were hard-wired by the physical connection of rows of contacts. Because of the desire to be able to run multiple unrelated applications without the bother of rewiring the contacts every time, removable panels with wiring were later introduced. This approach was later improved by the introduction of the "loaded-program concept", using removable boards with appropriately connected cables and plugs similar to the ones utilized by early hand-operated telephone exchanges. Subsequently, decks of punched cards, initially only used for data entry, storage, and loading, were also employed for loading the instructions to be used by the electronic circuitry to execute a defined set of sequential operations.

Eventually, magnetic media of varied formats (disks and tapes) and optical media (laser disks) became the support elected for general use in the distribution of software and data storage. Up to about a decade ago, commercial programmers relied on secrecy and on the strict enforcement of copyright laws to ensure competitiveness of their programs. The arcane command structure of early programming languages also provided a significant barrier for outsiders to copy or emulate such early products.

Based on the origins of programming, patent lawyers argued that the software was just another way of wiring up a machine. This concept deemed the duality computer-software not much different from any other piece of equipment and thus free to be patented. By 1995 some 12,000 software patents were been issued, and about 3,000 more awaited review. Software developers found trespassing on other firms' intellectual property have been sued and large sums have been paid as settlement for such litigation cases.

More recently, the trend has been to get away from patenting and move towards the implementation of strong copyright protection and its enforcement. The concept, however, is fully valid only for what is usually labeled as "generic" or "development" software. Such products, usually programming languages, are employed in the development of "applications", i.e. software written in one or more of the generic products with the object of performing a predetermined sequence of data manipulations with a well-defined purpose. The burden of proving the occurrence of copyright infringement is much more complex in the case of an application software product.

From the point of view of patent rights, in contrast with the generic products or development programming languages, an application software is built out of thousands of lines of source code that rely on standard expressions that are part and characteristic of the programming language syntax, rules, and conventions (e.g., sort values, select the larger of two values, compare a set of variables, write to the video monitor, or transfer to a printing device, etc.). Similarly to what happens in literature, it is the way known ideas are expressed — not the ideas themselves — that makes a computer application program useful. Here, the issue becomes the protection of the intellectual production of software developers, in a manner not dissimilar to the one afforded to writers, musicians, and movie or video directors. Although the issue of software property rights is still very cloudy, the prevailing view is that such a computer program is entitled to copyright "as a literary work".

Radical innovations in the way applications were developed occurred in the 80's. That decade witnessed a confrontation between the traditional role of the Data Processing Department, as the omnipotent master of information technology, and end-users who could, for the first time, afford to buy their own systems, including development software, and design and write their own applications. The growing power of desktop computers and user-oriented languages empowered the users to turn data into information, information into decisions, and, through communication, decisions into knowledge. However, the tools of the 80's were crude and cumbersome to use, and the deployment of systems was limited by cost considerations, the slow learning curve, and the quality of the applications. More recently, with the introduction of a large variety of productivity tools designed to work in conjunction with many of the available programming languages, the property rights situation of applications software became a great deal more complicated. Those highly efficient tools assist programmers in the technical definition and documentation of systems and in the generation of programs ("application generators"). They can produce code that will control everything in a program, from the code used to drive the data-related procedures and reporting to the construction of the user interface with all the "bells and whistles" that may be desired.

In the development of applications, the "programming without programmers" became a reality. Over the next decade it is expected that open standards will become generalized and user interface and programming tools will evolve to become more and more user-oriented. They will incorporate cognitive elements such as object-oriented programming, authoring tools, extensive use of neural networks and knowledge navigators, integration of multimedia and systems built on small, portable code, with many layers of high-level interfaces. Object-oriented technology will allow greater freedom to assemble skeleton routines or components into a solution that could be tailored to very specific implementation environments.

While traditional development focused on the optimization of the application for the most efficient use of the hardware, next-generation development software will continue to emphasize optimization based on users' needs, even when this may require larger programs and more lines of code. The source code of routines of different applications, generated by software development and productivity tools utilized by different developers, will certainly have large portions that may be identical. In these circumstances, the question of the confines of the developer's intellectual property becomes more difficult to ascertain or justify for a specific product.

The appearance of multimedia created new, and broader, legal enforcement problems. The combined use of a scanner, sound board, and a multimedia authoring software allow a user to incorporate a large quantity and variety of data from the surrounding environment. It is rather improbable that someone will end up being prosecuted for digitizing and using a "stolen" segment of music or a scanned picture from, for instance, the National Geographic Magazine in his or her microcomputer production, although the fact remains that the contents of virtually every book or magazine are copyrighted, as are films, TV programs, tapes, CDs, etc.

A.2.5.3. Ownership Rights

Software ownership and attending rights fall into two categories: *proprietary* and *public domain.*

Proprietary Software

"Proprietary software" corresponds to products, usually developed for commercial purposes, where copyright or, more rarely, patent protection applies. Proprietary software can be distributed through a variety of outlets: computer manufacturers, software houses, retail software businesses, and special distribution schemes as is, for instance, the case of "shareware".

Shareware distribution gives users a chance to try software before buying it. If you try a shareware program and continue using it, you are expected to register and pay for it. Individual programs differ on many details — some do not need mandatory registration, while others require it, some specify a maximum trial period. With registration, anything from the simple right to continuing use of the software to an updated program with printed manual could be had. Copyright laws apply to both shareware and commercial software, and the copyright holder retains all rights, with maybe a few specific exceptions. Shareware authors are accomplished programmers, just like commercial authors, and the programs are of comparable quality. The main difference is in the method of distribution. The author specifically grants the right to copy and distribute the software, either to all or to a specific group of users.

Commonly the user of a proprietary system is licensed for one or more installations of each product. A "site license" is a relatively inexpensive way for more than one person to legally use one copy of a program on more than one computer at a time. Site licenses are designed for companies, offices, or workgroups where more than one person in the organization needs to use a product. A site license does not require the acquisition of additional original installation disks.

All programs are distributed as a licensed product for use and very rarely sold to users. A licensee understands and agrees that the source code for the licensed program and all related documentation constitute property and trade secrets of the developer, owner of the copyright to the licensed program, embodying substantial creative efforts which are secret, confidential, and not generally known by the public. A licensee usually is supposed to agree that, during the term of the corresponding license, he will hold the licensed program, including any copies and any documentation related to it, in strict confidence and not permit any person or entity to obtain access to it except as required for the licensee's own internal use. It is required, under the law of most countries, that the licensee shall inform the developer promptly and in writing of any actual or suspected unauthorized use or disclosure of the licensed programs or related documentation.

Public Domain Software

This type of product is distributed free of charge although the developer may charge the cost of the distribution media, printing of documents, and mailing. There are a very large number of products in this category and many specialized catalogs of public domain software are regularly published. Many international, governmental, and non-governmental organizations have been instrumental in developing and distributing public domain software and the tendency has been to have products developed with public or international resources to be considered in this category.

A.2.5.4. Understanding Software Copyright Protection

The licensee of a copyrighted product is granted a nontransferable, nonexclusive right to use an agreed number of copies of the licensed program. In general, the licenser will deliver one copy of the licensed program to the licensee. The licensee may make additional copies of the licensed program, up to the number of copies licensed, provided that each copy of the program contains the developer's copyright notice and any other proprietary legends deemed appropriate and necessary.

In general, each copy of the licensed program provided under a license may be used on only one computer at any one time. If used on a network system, each terminal user is frequently considered to be using a distinct copy of the licensed program whether or not he is actually using it.

It is understood, under copyright protection agreements, that the licensee shall not use, copy, rent, lease, sell, modify, decompile, disassemble, reverse engineer, or transfer the licensed program, except as provided in the pertinent agreement. Any such unauthorized use may result in immediate and automatic termination of the license and eventual legal prosecution. A license is effective until terminated unilaterally or by failure to abide by the conditions of the license agreement. The licensee may terminate his binding agreement at any time, by destroying the licensed program and all copies of it. In some cases, he or she may be required to notify the developers in writing and, on termination, the licensee is supposed to erase or destroy the magnetic media containing the program and may be bound to return part of or all materials not destroyed to the developers, together with a written declaration that the eventual remaining materials have been indeed destroyed.

In the past, the extent of software copyrights was interpreted as protection to the source code, any translation of the source code into another language as well as the structure, sequence, and organization of the source code, including routines and subroutines and the order in which they are called by the sets of instructions written by the developer. The protection of the structure and organization of a software product is equivalent to the protection against plagiarism awarded to the plot or ideas in a written work, even if the actual text may not be identical.

Cases have been brought to court in the U.S. and the U.K. where these matters were taken well beyond copying the structure, sequence, and organization of the program code itself — and copyright infringements have been found when programs do no more than exhibit close similarities at the user level interface, even when the structure of the underlying code is completely different. The commercial computer software industry has long been advocating that the user interface should be entitled to copyright protection.

With the appearance and widespread utilization of application generators and other software development aids, the question of protection of the structure, internal organization, and user interface of programs becomes, however, very difficult to justify. Much controversy around this matter is expected to occur in the future.

A.2.5.5. Copyright Issues in Contracted Software Development

It has been a general understanding that in the absence of any specific assignment of ownership and copyright to the customer, the product development work done for a customer by someone who is not directly employed by the customer carries limitations on the contractor's ownership rights. In this situation, the ownership and copyright rests with the developer, independent of the fact that the developer may have given the contractor an unrestricted right of use of the developed product. Even if the commissioned work represents just the rewriting of portions of an existing program or making improvements, the contractor may be faced with a property claim by the developer.

Too many instances occur of contracted software development carried out without proper attention to the above principle and organizations have found themselves, with products that they paid for, without technical documentation or access to the source code. The caveat here is that a written agreement, dealing specifically with copyright ownership, must always be secured before development work is initiated.

Similarly to the situation observed with the introduction of photocopiers, which created a generalized and mostly uncontrollable infringement of copyright regarding printed works, the ease of copying magnetic media has facilitated the illegal reproduction of copyrighted software. It has been claimed that in some countries 90% of generic commercial software in use consists of illegal copies. Enforcement is a major problem and there are many who believe that copyright protection of software products should be revised considering the realities brought forth by modern software development tools and the prevailing attitudes and practices.

A major problem in many organizations, and potentially costly from the legal point of view, is the rampant infringement of copyright requirements for proprietary software. This situation emulates the also generalized illegal copying of software in private computers. Users and managers have become too complacent with the practice and this may put their organizations in an exposed situation if the software developers or legal owners decide to prosecute. Many episodes of legal action taken against organizations in the U.S. and other countries should be considered as a serious warning.

A clear definition of the responsibilities of the organization and the introduction of controlling mechanisms to deal with the problem of illegal software utilization must be addressed. It must be clearly established that proprietary software acquired, installed, or distributed by an organization should conform to existing legislation, and efforts should be made to enforce such regulations. The responsibility to establish and enforce such actions should be left to the information systems manager or, when one does not exist, to the chief executive or manager.

As a distributor of proprietary, commercial products or in the case of transference of products developed by other organizations or individuals, the organization assumes the legal liabilities related to improper utilization as well as the responsibilities regarding product registration and dealing directly with the developer or supplier, if eventual problems do occur.

A.2.5.6. Developer's Responsibilities

There are technical and ethical obligations of the developer or legal owner to support the user and provide maintenance of the software for a reasonable period of time. A few pertinent points must be stressed:

- A developer, even in proprietary or commercial products, never warrants that the program is free from coding errors. Usually programs are distributed or licensed "as is". However, program problems reported to the developer and determined to be actual coding errors should be corrected within a reasonable time.

- The limited warranty that usually accompanies a program also does not apply to the extent that any failure of the licensed program to perform as warranted, if the program is not used in accordance with the user documentation or modified by any person other than authorized personnel.

- If existing, the liability of developers or suppliers for any claim or damage arising out of the use of their products is commonly limited to direct damages which do not exceed the license fee(s), which have been paid by the licensee for the specific product that is the subject of such claim or damage.

- It is a standard clause in agreements that no developer is liable for damages, including lost profits, lost savings, or other incidental or consequential damages arising out of the use or inability to use the software product in question.

- In transfer or license agreements, the agreement or any rights or obligations cannot be assigned or otherwise transferred by the licensee to other parties without prior written consent of the developers, providers, or distributors.

Proprietary software developers maintain great secrecy of their trade products. There are, however, many possibilities of obtaining source code from independent developers and other sources. Most developers, even of non-commercial products, usually do not share freely the code of their applications. In general it is not advisable that the source code and complete technical documentation, even in the case of public domain products, should be made indiscriminately available. The responsibilities of the developer regarding software maintenance and upgrading and the interests of maintaining standards of data definition, programming routines, reporting, and quality may be impaired by the proliferation of many "copy-cat" versions of the original product.

In very specific circumstances and after assurances regarding the technical qualification of the recipient and clear definition of intended use, source code and technical documentation may be provided to other parties with the clear understanding that the alterations will be the total responsibility of the new owner. Although credits may be given, the changed products should be clearly differentiated from the original ones to avoid confusion to the end-user.

A.3. Organizational Environment and Content Requirements for Health Promotion and Care Information

Health promotion and care information systems and technology adopt different roles and characteristics, depending on multiple determinants, such as: the goals pursued by the healthcare delivery systems, particular day-to-day clinical, educational, and managerial needs, and the level of development and integration reached by single healthcare organizations. This chapter focuses on the variety of implementation environments at different levels of decision and action, and the content of required information for each level of management and data aggregation.

A.3.1. Information and Healthcare Services

The importance of information in health services relates to its support to the aspects of management and operation:

- Sustaining the day-to-day operation and management of health services and healthcare network, and support of diagnostic and therapeutic functions.

- Facilitate the clinical and administrative decision making at various levels of action and decision.

- Support the monitoring and evaluation of healthcare interventions; the health status of populations and the conditions of the environment; the production and utilization of the health care services; and the impact attributable to the action of the health services and other health-related interventions.

Figure 4. Functions and Information Systems in Health Services

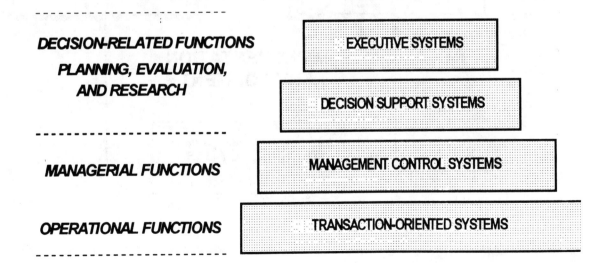

In health services, information systems and their associated technological infrastructure are oriented to the support of two functional levels (Figure 4):

[a] *Systems for the support to the operational and management functions*:

- Management of Transactions - logistics of healthcare; flow, registry, processing, and recovery of clinical and administrative data; operation of diagnostic and therapeutic support services.

- Managerial Control - administrative operation, accounting, financing, and human and physical resources management.

[b] *Systems that utilize operational data arising from the operation of health systems and services in support of decision functions — planning and evaluation — and for research*:

- Support for decision making - support for the administrative and clinical decision making based on evidence.

- Executive Systems - support to the tasks of planning, evaluation, and research.

The operational and managerial control data, isolated or in combination with other organizational data or originating from external sources, constitute the basis of the systems for the managerial support and for high-level decisions.

Figure 5. Integrated Components of Health Information Systems

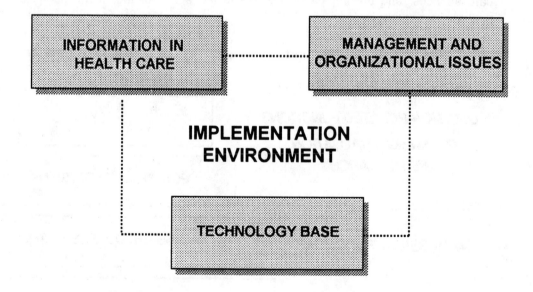

Three IS&T components (Figure 5) are required:

[a] *Information* - needs assessment, definitions of data, production of information (flow; processing; analysis, products or outputs), and adequate contents;

[b] *Management and organizational* - including pertinent resources that are necessary for the implementation and operation of applications (organizational infrastructure); and

[c] *Technological infrastructure* - processing and communication.

The operationalization of the three components is achieved in a different manner in each implementation environment, in accordance with the characteristics, needs, and local resources. When we colloquially speak about "information systems", actually we refer to the integration of the three aspects described above: systems as such, the management of the information function in the organization, and the technological infrastructure for data capture, processing, and communication. This concept orients the functional and strategic perspective of the present document.

A.3.1.1. Health Services as Object of Investigation and Evaluation

Information systems are strategic components of the health services and contribute to informed action on:

- planning, supervision, and control of care
- evaluation and monitoring of the state of health of populations
- evidence-based clinical and administrative decision making
- assessment of outcomes
- education and health promotion
- research

A.3.1.2. Healthcare and Health Promotion Productive Processes and Indicators

Healthcare organizations determine the particular environment for the possible purposes and implementation strategies of information systems. This is summarized in Figure 6.

As in other commercial and industrial areas of application, information on the productive process of a particular health service is related to *input* such as resources, organization, knowledge, and technology and to *outputs*, such as products and effects. Monitoring and evaluation of the *outputs* of the productive processes of healthcare is a useful tool, but it depends on opportune and dynamic information generated from the capture and processing of quantitative and qualitative data. Health services information data capture and processing are, however, extremely more challenging. The content of information of healthcare activities being mainly obtained by ongoing measurement of performance, fulfillment of tasks, and quality of the process, deals with the delivery of heterogeneous and complex health products and services. The goals of healthcare being well beyond simple *outputs* (products and services) involve outcomes and effects, on individual and group health, which are of difficult measurement.

Figure 6. The Organizational Health Promotion and Care Environment of Information Systems and Technology

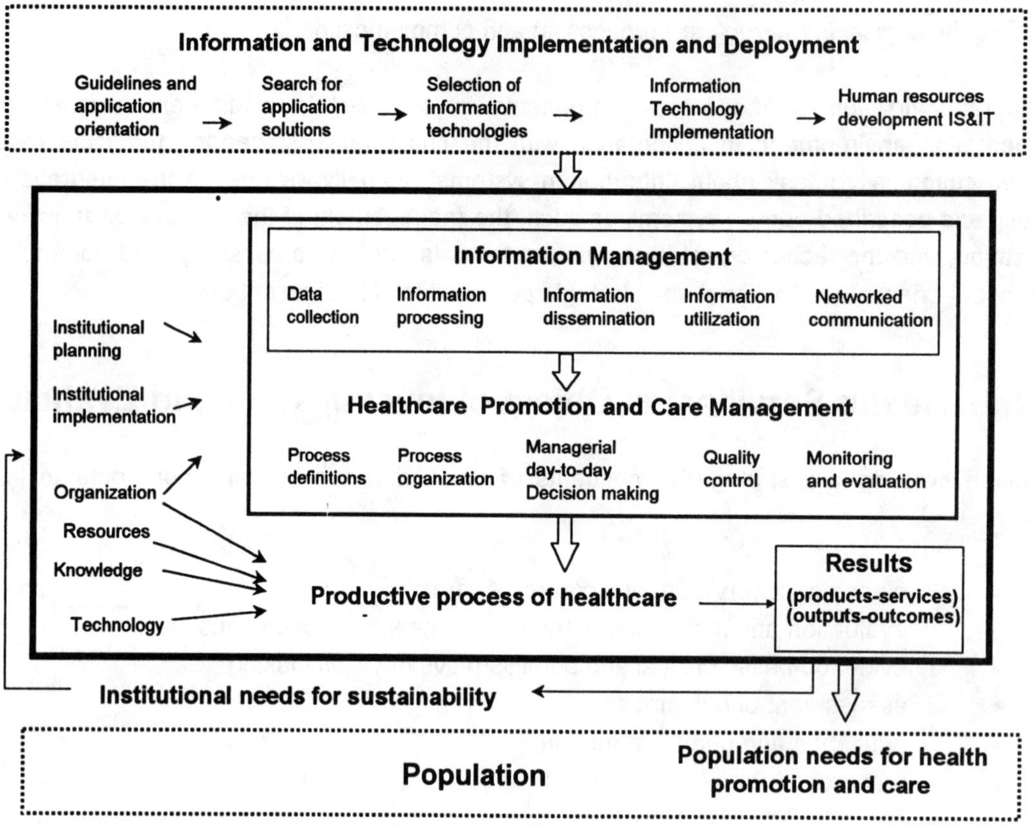

Information and Technology Implementation and Deployment

| Guidelines and application orientation | → | Search for application solutions | → | Selection of information technologies | → | Information Technology Implementation | → | Human resources development IS&IT |

Information Management

| Data collection | Information processing | Information dissemination | Information utilization | Networked communication |

Healthcare Promotion and Care Management

| Process definitions | Process organization | Managerial day-to-day Decision making | Quality control | Monitoring and evaluation |

Institutional planning
Institutional implementation
Organization
Resources
Knowledge
Technology

Productive process of healthcare

Results
(products-services)
(outputs-outcomes)

Institutional needs for sustainability

Population Population needs for health promotion and care

As an illustration of the issues involved, the quantity of vaccine applications is the routine measurable output of an immunization drive, but the number of vaccinated individuals who were effectively immunized, i.e., acquired an appropriate level of antibodies and the concomitant reduction of infections, should be the real measurable effect (outcome) of the initiative. Further difficulties in establishing measurable outputs are related to the fact that there are outcome measurements of quality of care and health promotion that involve judgmental criteria. Satisfaction of users, understanding of drug utilization, how to prevent infirmities, perception of health improvement, prevention of avoidable events (avoidable deaths and hospital infections), and fulfillment of quality norms and guidelines constitute variables difficult to categorize and quantify.

The variety of implementation environments of the sector also poses many problems to information systems developers. Information for management must be applicable to different definitions of "local" level: primary health care centers, hospital internal productive (intermediate or final) services, and health care delivery networks (health services organized in a multi-centered pattern), and information must support the different specific functions related to decision making in each level.

Different levels of care and management require distinct aggregation and display of processed data. Health information at the "local" level uses an amalgam of detailed mixed data from patients, local resources, and procedures, with the objective of providing more exact parameters of administrative or clinical details, whereas aggregated data from groups of patients or institutions are many times adequate only to the macro levels (district, region, province, state, national). Macro-level aggregated data, with few exceptions, consist of both simple and compound collective indicators.

The overall information resulting from compound indicators, although of common use, is in general not sufficient to provide a true vision of the reality of the health status and appropriateness of healthcare of a population group. An example of this problem is the case of child health status, which usually is approached through a set of indicators such as infant mortality, incidence of transmissible diseases, and anthropometric parameters. Such a set of indicators provides just a simplistic and incomplete knowledge of the real world.

Despite the limitations of information in representing the realities of health and healthcare, the information needs for research, planning, and decision making justifies the use of diagnostic approaches based on sets of simple and compound indicators.

A.3.1.3. Healthcare Networks

Healthcare delivery systems, mainly in the public sector, tend to be organized in a multilevel basis according to technical complexity and degree of specialization. As long as referral from one level to another is based on needs, this can provide appropriate access to primary healthcare and to more complex technological levels of care.

Within the healthcare network model (Figure 7), primary healthcare (PHC) is the normal gate to the system. Primary healthcare has great importance and a priority role in promotion and prevention, with emphasis in prevention-oriented services, although it also provides simple cure-oriented services and refers those patients that are beyond local solving capability to higher complexity levels of care, including curative, rehabilitative, and palliative care.

Organized PHC is found more frequently in the public sector, because private healthcare tends to be concentrated in specialties that deal with complex medical conditions, using modern and high-cost care technologies. They are located in large cities and are mostly hospital centered. The higher organizational care levels (secondary, tertiary) have reduced population coverage and are usually concentrated in larger urban areas.

Complex hospitals and clinical specialties, as well as more sophisticated equipment used to support medical specialties, are at the top level of the referral hierarchy. In this situation, the patient referral system and coordination between levels are key issues.

Figure 7. The Healthcare "Complexity/Coverage" Organized Delivery Network

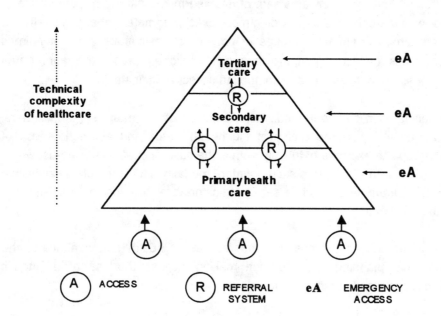

A.3.2. *Information Requirements and Levels of Management*

At the health promotion and patient care level, information supports mostly clinical and educational actions and clinical management, based on detailed data, and local administrative management. In a wider geographic or administrative area, such as in networked health services, information is commonly used in an aggregated format, and addresses administrative management. At national level, an information system uses different sources of aggregate data, including sources outside the health sector, addressed mainly to macro administrative and normative roles, such as planning, national monitoring, and control of financial flows. A national system of information involves four areas supporting planning, management, and evaluation for national and regional, province, state, or district levels:

- *epidemiology and demography*

- *regulatory actions in health promotion and care*

- *public health services; collective interventions that are not based on vital statistics*

- *health promotion*

- *individual healthcare, in support of clinical and management areas.*

This document focuses mainly in the last area, and is concentrated on the functionalities needed for individual health promotion and care and detailed management of physical resources. It must be stressed that in most comprehensive multilevel information systems, data collected at the care site and community are the necessary primary input for further construction of aggregated indicators and variables, used by the higher organizational levels.

From the user's perspective, the key issues related to the need for information are the determination of the specific data requirements and the search for adequate technical answers. Some of the main phases in the implementation of information systems and technology, addressed by clinical, educational, and managerial needs are:

- *determining the need for information according to clinical, educational, and managerial requirements*

- *specifying of variables and indicators (aggregated measures)*

- *defining which are the primary sources of data needed to develop the required indicators*

- *defining how the information system is organized and how processing and delivering of information will be accomplished*

- *defining what information technology supporting the system is appropriate and how it will be implemented*

- *developing human resources for implementing and managing the system.*

A.3.3. Operational and Management Support

The objective of the information system application in the operation and management of health services considers that systems and computer technology, when designed, implemented, and handled appropriately, contribute to reach the goals and expected results of the health system:

- equitable access to services
- better technical and administrative management
- improvement of service and quality of individual care
- support for preventive actions
- facilitation of health promotion and self-care
- access to knowledge bases
- clinical decision making based on evidence
- expansion of the opportunities for professional education

Systems in this area are oriented towards administrative and financing efficiency, emphasis on cost control, and facilitation of reimbursement schemes; the maintenance of data inventories for shared use by organizations and individuals; support of services with the objective of knowledge and resource management; individual clinical care; and the support of public health interventions at both individual and population levels. In this area IS&T represent the principal organizational asset for operation, planning, control, and competitiveness.

A.3.4. The Decision-Making Requirements

An ongoing feature of all Latin American and Caribbean countries, and indeed of most countries in the world, is that of health sector reform. The realization is that centrally driven and standardized health systems are not flexible enough to provide needs-led and appropriate healthcare to meet the differing priorities and volumes in individual localities within any country. For purposes of information system development two key features become challenges and opportunities in identifying the need for information, and in deciding on the creation of information systems. These are:

- Decisions will be devolved to the lowest possible level, within such policy criteria.

- Many services will be outsourced on a contractual basis, including clinical as well as support services.

A.3.4.1. Autonomy without Fragmentation

Not least in information systems, autonomy of decision making has the potential risk of fragmentation. This cuts across the key principles of information gathering, where information from one level should be summarized to provide the raw input for information at the next level upwards using standard definitions. Indeed, a strategic United Kingdom policy group indicated that it was impossible to think of any information relevant at one level that was not required in more detail at the lower level. In information system development, this means that whilst systems must be acquired and implemented at the local level to meet local need, this must be within an overall strategic framework devised at the national level.

A.3.4.2. Levels of Decision-Making and Information Systems

In increasingly devolved health services, levels of organization and geographical aggregation involve different types of decision making. They can be summarized as shown in Table 4.

Understanding these levels and types of decisions is key to identifying information needs and thus meeting those needs. It also indicates the levels at which implementation of information systems occurs. There is an important national role in defining a strategic framework, but implementation within this must be at the lower levels. On occasion, there may be an important role at the regional level either for coordination, where the smaller units see advantage in a collaborative approach, or for pilot studies, but it is important that these are requested and supported at the devolved level. Imposed solutions will not work effectively, but requested support can be beneficial.

Table 4. Type of Decision and Health Services Organizational Levels

AGGREGATION LEVEL	PREVAILING STRATEGIC POLICY
NATION/REGION/PROVINCE	Resource Allocation; Secondary and Tertiary Services
OPERATIONAL UNIT (Primary Care Unit; Hospital)	Operational Management; Local Strategic Development
HEALTHCARE PROFESSIONAL	Treatment Delivery
POPULATION	Lifestyle and Health Behavior

A.3.4.3. Decision-Making Processes

In order to make effective health decisions a systematic approach is necessary, and this in turn will be instrumental in identifying the information requirements. Helpfully, the discipline of public health provides a valuable model, with the three key tasks of Assessment, Policy Development, and Assurance of delivery and of effect. Application of this conceptual framework should help to define the necessary information needs.

The core purpose of the process is to enable decision-makers at all levels to make appropriate decisions about development of information systems in their settings. This process starts with identifying the levels of decision making and needs for information, specific to the issues, which are relevant in that setting in that country.

A.3.5. Content Requirements for Healthcare Information

The primary input data for the information system should consider the components of the health promotion and care delivery (structure, process, and results). Several factors determine the characteristics of the information required, planned, collected, or produced:

- Specific issues to be covered related to the healthcare organization, the institutional aspects, the process of health education and care, the population, and the environment.

- Operational utilization of the information. The users, mainly those responsible for clinical, educational, and managerial decisions, must define each specific application and utility of information.

- Options regarding the use of new data, to be generated, or use of already existing data, either from internal or external sources.

- Level of aggregation (individual, local center, health care network, national level)

- Expectations for the quality and adequacy of the resulting information. Expectations are linked to the feasibility of collecting and producing adequate information.

A.3.5.1. Patient-Based Data

Individual data are focused in identification, administrative, and clinical data captured for each patient:

- Identification: unique coded identification, name, age, gender, address

- Administrative data: insurance type, insurance healthcare number

- Clinically useful data: pre-existing diseases and risk status, disabilities, anthropometric measures, diagnoses, and clinical performance tests

- Healthcare process data: consultations, hospital admissions, examination procedures, clinical procedures for treatment, clinical findings, and the patient's perception about the health problem

- Resources used in clinical procedures and the production of intermediate activities

- Procedures and norms: clinical guidelines applicable to patients

- Social health-related useful data: income, type of work, family structure, ethnicity, language

- Degree of patient knowledge about the health problem, how to avoid it, the treatment and satisfaction with healthcare: past and current individual opinions and survey results on perceptions and experiences with healthcare delivery

A.3.5.2. Aggregated Variables and Indicators

Health and healthcare indicators are currently relevant for supporting the role of the state and the new models of health promotion and care. Issues such as health unit autonomy, management, and contracting for services require dynamic and opportune information in order to allow the whole health promotion and care delivery system to operate appropriately.

Health and healthcare indicators can be categorized according to the thematic area of information to which they are related; the healthcare dimension to be evaluated; or the health situation they intend to represent. Some of the types of indicators currently used are:

- *Indicators related to health situation* - such as dwelling, socioeconomic and educational level, clean water and waste disposal, contacts with animals, etc.

- *Indicators related to health needs* - such as those of socioeconomic deprivation, differential ill-health status and risk situations,

- *Indicators of health promotion and care delivery* - from structure (resources and organization), the process of care, and results (outputs and outcomes),

- *Indicators of population access, coverage, and use of healthcare* - access, coverage of resource, coverage of activities, and use of services. Some of these indicators are used for equity analysis,

- *Indicators for efficiency assessments* - indicators used to assess how efficiently the resource is allocated between areas or groups of the population; indicators for cost-benefit analysis; performance or productivity of the resource used (compared to standards for comparison),

- *Indicators for effectiveness assessment* - related to outcomes of health interventions and impacts in the global health status of population groups,

- *Indicators of quality of health education and care* - related to structure and process of health promotion and care, from the technical and scientific perspectives,

- *Indicators of user's and health workers' satisfaction* - involving physical and human conditions of the environment and process of care,

- *Indicators of social participation* - degree of involvement of community groups and other stakeholders,

- *Indicators of adherence to specific health programs* - related to specific curative and preventive services.

The main components involving different groups of indicators according to the different dimensions of health promotion and care (institutional, population, socioeconomic, and geographical) that are commonly used in the description and analysis of health systems and services are:

- *Systems macro context* – political, economic, and social context,

- *Geographic environment* - climate; natural determinants to lifestyle and health,

- *Health systems* - system organization, normative and financial framework; role of the State; role of the market; insurance and financing,

- *Change process in health systems* - sector development; sector reform; specific adjustment,

- *Health services structure, organization, and functions* - type of health promotion and care provider; public/private sector; administrative organization; health promotion and clinical care organization; health promotion and care financing; human resources, physical structure and equipment; inpatient and outpatient services; preventive-oriented services; collective actions of prevention and promotion, and

- *Population and health conditions* - demography (including structure and geographic distribution); health, ill-health and risk; socioeconomic circumstances; other determinants; population factors influencing differential access and use of services.

A listing of indicators used in health care is given in References 1 and 2. They include variables currently utilized by the Pan American Health Organization Core Data Set (PAHO Core Data), based on data produced by the countries of the Region of the Americas, and variables used by the Organization for Economic and Cooperation Development (OECD) database.

A.4. Evolution and Current Challenges for Healthcare Information Systems

As discussed in the previous Chapter, healthcare delivery systems share similar characteristics with most service and productive organizations but also exhibit specific characteristics, which are related to the complexity and diversity of healthcare production, including the dissimilar ways healthcare professionals discharge their clinical tasks.

New requirements and technological advances occurring in healthcare, information systems, and information technology have influenced the evolving role of healthcare information systems and related technology. Relevant aspects that took place in the evolution of systems and technology in order to appropriately support healthcare organizations are:

- The diverse organizational healthcare environment of information systems, which need to be adapted to multiple types of healthcare organizations.

- Dynamic changes in the required role of information systems, following changes in the role and dynamics of all levels of healthcare delivery and management.

- The need for integration of information systems within healthcare organizations, which are also organized as networks.

- Technological advances in systems structure and communications, facilitating the implementation of integrated healthcare networks.

The healthcare information network, when centered on the patient, allows the comprehensive and coordinated management of detailed individual data. Patient originated information also may be used as input for the development of collective databases. Aggregate clinical and administrative data may be applied to the process of planning, management, and evaluation. As these components use data arising from detailed patient care clinical and administrative data, resources utilized, and procedures performed, the development of common criteria and standards on data is fundamental to ensure quality and completeness of resulting collective indicators. The important subject of data standards is dealt with in Chapter 4. Data standards recommendations also make up the bulk of the appended material of this publication.

A.4.1. Evolution and Dissemination of Healthcare Information Systems and Technology

Healthcare Information Systems (HIS) have evolved according to the new role implied by changing demands to healthcare and healthcare information, and supported by the possibility to apply new technological advances to healthcare organizations. The vast majority of issues addressed until the early 80's were those associated with how to "supply" information for business operations. As the supply issues became better understood and the price-performance of computers dropped dramatically, attention turned to more imaginative applications of the technology.

This shift of attention has highlighted new issues, now associated with the "demand" for information systems in organizations. With this change of paradigm, from supply to demand, no longer are organizations content to focus upon the obvious. The mid-80's saw the development of several techniques to help analyze an organization's objectives and methods of operation in order to reveal more innovative opportunities based on information systems. From being concerned primarily with the logic used in computerized processes, the focus shifted to information and its use.

For the past 30 years organizations have been developing computer-based information systems and before this, people paper, pencils, calculators, and mechanical punch card tabulators were the main tools available for data manipulation. The tasks undertaken by the early, cumbersome, and expensive computers were those which were the most obvious to identify and the easiest for the computer to improve, such as accounting, inventory control, billing, and other labor-intensive office activities.

Healthcare Information Systems have followed the general evolutionary trends of all information systems: an extensive central computer station, the appearance of microcomputers allowing the replacement of passive terminals, the connection of these components into a network, and the development of multimedia and workstations. Such systems have developed for many decades; most currently in use are still based on concepts originated almost 30 years ago. The history of the development and implementation of HIS in Latin America and the Caribbean is not very different from that in other parts of the globe. After using data processing service bureaus in the late 1960s and early 70's, healthcare institutions started to purchase and install commercially available information systems based on heavily centralized architectural designs. With the advent of microcomputers, networks, and client/server architectures, HIS evolved to a more flexible and decentralized framework.

Activities covered by traditional HIS systems also evolved from mundane tasks such as admission, discharge and transfer, to patient billing, then to more sophisticated tasks such as clinical information management, advanced laboratory systems, simulation, and image processing. Lack of integration and difficulties in obtaining key information have led to a number of major HIS revisions. As information becomes increasingly more important for cost containment and improving efficiency and efficacy, more pressure is put on HIS to deliver solutions that assist organizations to achieve the strategic goals of the healthcare enterprise of providing services with better quality effectively and efficiently in a financially sustainable environment.

There has been a major paradigm shift in healthcare information processing, corresponding to changes in the goals of the organization. The traditional emphasis on data has now given way to emphasis on information. Central control has now evolved to empowerment. Healthcare organizations are now much more concerned with each other and how they can exchange services, and necessarily patient information. This has forced information systems to leave the traditional healthcare institutions' physical boundaries. Now, more than ever, healthcare enterprises wield HIS to provide strategic, connected information to reduce costs, improve patient care, and increase service levels to their customers.

Despite the many dozens of Healthcare Information Systems (HIS) hat can be found on the market, only a very small number of products cover all requirements of a particular institution or unit, and provide adequate integration with the potentially vast healthcare networking needs. The varieties of tasks, the players involved, the existing organizations, and the technical possibilities substantiate this situation. In any case, the installation of a HIS is universally viewed as a necessity that must be adequately and widely supported by all participants in the health system.

Until recently, they have done so almost exclusively for accounting and fiscal purposes. Among the factors that have been associated with the dissemination of Information Systems and Information Technology (IS&T) in the organizations, the following were most contributory:

- *Technological convergence* - Characterized by the integration of a variety of related developments in electronics, industrial production of integrated circuits, the introduction of new computer languages that fostered the increasing availability of easily operated low-cost systems with greater processing capacity, and the use of powerful user-oriented database management systems.

- *Diffusion of computer-related skills* - Increasing the number of non-technical individuals with basic computer knowledge and training in its operation.

- *Increased productivity and quality in application development* - Large number of generic software products that allow the development of complex applications.

- *Appreciation of the benefits of information* - Recognition of the effectiveness and efficiency of information systems as planning, operation, and control tools for managers.

- *Acceptance of technology* - Recognition that modern IS&T resources are appropriate technology for less developed countries and small organizations.

Information resources and commodities display four general economic characteristics:

- Information cannot be appropriated; the "seller" of information is not deprived of its possession.

- Information is non-divisible in use; some, if not all, sets of information must be complete if they are to be usable. For example, half of an algorithm or half of an application program would not be usable commodities.

- Information is heterogeneous; unlike quantities of homogeneous physical resources, "more information" means different items of information, not further copies of the same items.

- Information is context-dependent; the value of an information set as a resource depends on the context of its interpretation, use, or exchange.

This host of new requirements calls for fundamental change in the way information systems and information technology are deployed, used, and managed today — changes that capitalize on how technology can support the continuum of care are necessary.

The sharing of patient clinical and administrative data is a prime example of those new requirements. Healthcare providers traditionally approach their work on an episodic basis, treating patients for specific medical problems as they occur according to the realms of medical specialties. One goes to a family practitioner for a minor upper respiratory infection, to an orthopedist for lower back pain, and to a surgeon for an operation. Unfortunately, those involved in providing medical care frequently do not have the means to easily access and share patient information. The emerging development of the Computer-based Patient Record (CPR), while significant enough in itself, still does not solve the entire problem. From the patients' perspective, problems associated with the lack of information sharing are basic — they still must recite their present and past medical histories again and again as they move from one physician's office to another, one facility to the next. On top of it, a lot of important clinical data is lost or remains buried in individual patient files in different sites.

The focus on information that relates to administrative and financial issues, such as payer transactions, on an episodic basis, has been in general better addressed when there is an economic interest involved, as is the case of private health insurance. Characteristically, this aspect has been present in the public sector. Even less attention has been paid to developing an overall electronic health planning capability that focuses on all aspects of a member's wellness and includes plans to manage member care from birth through adulthood.

With the changes occurring in the context of the health sector reform processes information systems must have the ability to:

- Capture and deliver data at the point of service

- Support concurrent and multicentric clinical and administrative information utilization and exchange

- Support intensive data manipulation

- Provide facilities to support synchronous, as opposed to retrospective, decision making

A.4.2. Challenges in the Deployment of Healthcare Information Systems and Technology

In order to support its constituent enterprise in Latin America and the Caribbean and deliver appropriate solutions, IS/IT/IM face two broad challenges: the complex, dynamic nature of today's healthcare enterprise, and the generally unsophisticated, unprepared state of healthcare information systems development across the Region.

A.4.2.1. Dynamics of Technological Changes

A great deal of debating about current and future economic development and the reorganization of the health sector is centered on the implications of rapid technological change. In this context, information technology is seen as the means for catalyzing the radical transformations required.

Different from past forms of technology, which processed physical resources and economic commodities, information technology processes an abstract resource and one cannot assume that innovation in this area has necessarily the same characteristics as previous forms of technological progress. Indeed, the inputs, the scale of investment, the relationship between the scale of input and output, and even the time scale of information technology development place it outside the scope of mainstream thought on technology, which is still fixed to the physical resource processing paradigm.

Three reasons account for the significance of information technology innovation as a radically new or "revolutionary" as opposed to "evolutionary" phenomenon:

- Rate and extent of technological change that is unique in terms of the pace of development.

- Vast extent of applicability of this new technology, certainly the most general technology ever developed.

- The peculiar nature of the technology itself. Not only does it process abstract resources but also the technology is, in itself, partly information. Innovation in this technology occurs typically through the production of new information resources that include abstract machines, as software, rather than the development of new physical components.

A.4.2.2. Complexity and Changes in Healthcare Organizations

The nature of the healthcare enterprise, particularly as regards information, is markedly different from most other industries. For example, in the banking industry information is very well structured; the number of possible transactions is limited to a dozen or so; their vocabularies are also very limited; and there are well-established standards for data exchange among banks and their partners. Customer records contain a few, simple data types. Procedures in banks are easy enough that nowadays most transactions can be performed by the customers themselves, with many benefits accruing to the banks.

Specialization and hierarchical considerations in a distributed healthcare system, departmentalization according to the technical qualifications of providers, and the stated goal of delivering integrated cost-efficient healthcare services to the whole population highlight the multiple challenges to be confronted by health managers and professionals when developing information systems.

In addition to the evolutionary nature of HIS in the Region as noted earlier, it should be plain that the various characteristics deemed to be important to healthcare activities require an extensive review for the majority of the HIS now in use. Most of these systems were conceived according to the prevailing philosophy of 15 to 20 years ago, which meant a different healthcare system focus. The vision then was generally healthcare institution-centered and focused on administrative and financial aspects, and the healthcare institution was considered as a collection of service-rendering units. These, from the point of view of the system as a whole, were required to access requirements for information for the purposes of following up on service orders, from the requisition of the needed inputs to the delivery of services and corresponding billing. In some instances, this collection of procedural functions was even more abbreviated, to the degree that it required not more than the recording of a given service (for example, the basic act of examination by a specialist), for the subsequent bill processing and collection. Most of the reports produced also pertained to a *posteriori* type of follow-up on the healthcare institution's earnings.

The purpose here is not to regard activities of this sort as invalid. On the contrary, institutions that control these processes can indeed improve their operational efficiency. Knowing what was performed, what was spent, and where such amounts were spent and, above all, the ability to collect timely reimbursement for services provided, are essential for the survival of most institutions.

A.4.2.3. The Healthcare Delivery Process

The organizational and operational processes of even a relatively uncomplicated healthcare institution, such as a long-term care facility or a home health agency, are many and complicated. Much thought and research have gone into the study and analysis of healthcare processes, resulting in a great deal of useful literature available to the industry professional. One view of the organizational structure of an enterprise seeks to align processes according to the needs of either the institution or the patient (Table 5).

Integration of the inherent variety of functions expected from information applications requires two operation environments: first, an environment characterized by a shared database of collective access and utilization; and second, an environment made up by subsystems of predominantly local or departmental use. At the technological level, two data processing environments are required in the development and implementation of the desired functional integration at systems level:

- An integrated common data environment not necessarily physically centralized, as data can be logically centralized in a distributed physical system, and

- A distributed environment in which each functional unit manages and processes data of local interest as well as systems of common use.

Vertical integration is achieved by defining data flows, reporting responsibilities, and integration of data generated and processed at each functional unit around an informational framework with three interacting areas for the generation and reporting of decision support oriented information: client-oriented managerial information, economic and administrative (utilization and production), and clinical and epidemiological.

Table 5. Organizational Structure and Processes of a Typical Healthcare Organization

Services Management	Patient Management
Resources Administration	*Logistics of Care Delivery*
Finances	Patient Identification
Personnel	Admissions/Discharges/Transfers
Materials and Support Services	Orders
Bed Management	Appointment Scheduling
Staffing and Benefits	Service Scheduling
Assets Management	
Facility Management	
Technical Equipment Maintenance	
Drugs and Medical Materials	
Evaluation and Planning	*Primary Clinical Data*
Activities	Automated Digital Instrumentation
Medical Care	Digital Images
Clinical Epidemiology	
Clinical Research	
Quality Assurance	
Information Management	*Medical Records Administration*
Data Files	Medical Records
Access to Data Bases	Insurance and Legal Documentation
HIS Architecture	Clinical Audit

A.4.2.4. The Variety and Detail of Healthcare Information

Healthcare institutions could not be more different from banks. For example, healthcare institutions automating their "customer records" first face the task of computerizing a daunting array of data types, as shown in Table 6.

The variety and requirements specification problems found in many healthcare data types is exacerbated by the size and complexity of the medical vocabulary, the codification of biomedical findings, and the classification of health conditions and interventions. Nomenclature issues include concepts such as procedures, diagnoses, anatomical topography, diseases, etiology, biological agents such as classification of microorganisms, drugs, causes for healthcare contact, symptoms and signs, and many others. Possible combinations and detailing represent a staggering number of possible identifying coding requirements.

Table 6. Typical Patient Health Record Data Types

Data Types	Typical Examples
Coded Data	Diagnosis, Procedures, Laboratory Results
Text	Radiology, Pathology Reports, Notes
Document Images	Optically Scanned Medical Records
Biological Signal Records	ECGs, EEGs, Spirograms
Voice Objects	Dictated Reports
Still Images	X-rays, MRIs, CATs, Mammograms, Photos
Full-motion Video	Cardiac Catheterization, Sonograms

Apart from difficulties with vocabularies, the very nature and structure of clinical documents such as prescriptions and medical records are not standardized for automated data processing. Attempts have been made to define a structured format for such documents. The Problem-Oriented Medical record is an example of an early attempt to deal with the standardization required for data processing. Many models have been defined since then but as yet there is no universally accepted paradigm.

Current approaches for recording medical data fall into two broad categories: free text and controlled vocabularies. In free text doctors and other professionals simply write what they want, using their own words. Usually these documents are later coded manually by other professionals, who use standard vocabularies to describe the most important parts of the document, such as primary diagnosis and procedures. Several approaches to automatically extracting information from free-text records, using the relatively new method called Natural Language Processing, have only partially solved the many problems associated with codification. The second basic method for recording medical data involves the use of controlled vocabularies. In this approach health professionals must use words and concepts that have been previously determined to be the standard, or "canonical" terms for the health enterprise. Certainly, this method achieves uniformity at the expense of professional freedom and is extremely difficult to implement. Even purely administrative applications — patient billing, accounts receivable, general accounting, personnel, materials management, fixed assets, etc. — all have their own databases with their particular data elements and rules for processing and for information generation.

A.4.2.5. Different Perspectives in Provider- and Procedure-Oriented Sources

Specific provider and procedure-oriented information systems have a different scope as they are, as a rule, concerned with the utilization and the financial aspects of health delivery. They are generally imposed from the top administrative level and, in most cases, are directed to the reimbursement for services provided and financial control. They utilize standardized data sets that typically record patient identification, reimbursement category, length of hospital stay, diagnostic data and the utilization of special services. One criticism regarding most provider- and procedure-oriented systems is related to the fact that they have given little attention to the lower echelons of the healthcare structure in terms of supporting service operation and improvement.

Most databases are highly aggregated and have minimal value to clinical decision-makers, at individual or community level, or as a source of support information for individual patient care, surveillance, and monitoring. The aggregation or averaging of data over large groups may hide variations and can conceal important information, such as those related to the poor quality of primary data and failures or inadequacies of specific health program components. Many health information systems of this type produce only highly aggregated data directed to centralized bureaucratic control and supervision.

There is a growing trend in developing event-based patient-oriented systems, as the basis for unit, organizational, or regional information systems. Such systems demand the extensive training and continuous collaboration of physicians, nurses, and other direct care providers. A large amount of information is produced and needed where people live and make contact with the health services. Focusing on local information and local decision making and action involves finding answers that cannot be provided by information systems directed to central planning and supervision, typically based on highly aggregated data.

Patient-oriented systems consider clients as the central observational unit and reference of the information system. They can provide production, utilization, diagnostic, and epidemiological information of great importance to managers and direct care professionals. The major problems in designing such systems are related to:

- Definition of the data set to be processed

- Integration of unobtrusive data capture instruments into routine health practice

- Data procedures that are acceptable to direct healthcare professionals

- Common specifications, data dictionaries, and the agreement upon a minimum data set to be utilized by all healthcare professionals in any care unit

A.4.2.6. The Need for National Policies and Strategies

Technology developers and suppliers, users, and decision-makers must be aware of national policies and strategies that may affect their judgment regarding the acquisition, development, deployment, and operation of health information systems. Policy establishes the rules that an organization must follow in carrying out its work. Establishing an information management and technology (IM&T) for the health sector ensures that the development and use of systems will proceed in a coordinated manner. The policy must, necessarily, be in consonance with any overall informatics policies in force in a country as well as with its overall health sector policies. The national health IM&T policy, in turn, sets limits to any policies that may be established lower in the hierarchy, at regional or local levels. Once formulated, a policy must be implemented in a coordinated manner. It is highly recommended that a formal organizational entity be established to organize the strategy for the implementation of the national policies. A health IM&T policy may require legislation, operational regulations, and guidelines. As part of a national informatics policy, it should support established priorities and should also define linkages, common standards, and procedures for sharing information with other sectors.

The goal of establishing national strategies for IM&T is to provide a coherent national arrangement directed to facilitating projects, infrastructure development, maximizing the benefits for invested financial resources, and enabling people to function more effectively. The success of the strategy depends largely on people in all functions and levels. They must be computer-literate and have good awareness of the principles of information systems management. Success depends critically on the existence of an information systems staff with the right mix of skills.

Elements incorporated in a national set of policies consider the definitions regarding the following information system components:

- Identification of benefits,

- Technological standards (hardware and software),

- Common data sets and dictionaries based on a fixed structure of registries and forms — in particular a thesaurus of coded clinical terms,

- Procedures, data flow, and communication standards between sites and equipment,

- Measures and standards for ensuring reliability, privacy, and security of data,

- Policies for human resources development, allocation, and utilization,

- Financial requirements, and

- Plans for training and developing staff.

Since it is natural that strategies will differ from one country to another, and possibly between different health authorities or institutions within the same country, each implementation must be carefully evaluated under the following strategy-related aspects:

- Systems specifications and architecture,

- Shared and local applications,

- Distribution of responsibilities and resources,

- Skills required, and

- Standards of compatibility.

The strategy must outline the architecture of the systems in terms of hardware, software, and method to be used for application development and communication protocols. Applications must be defined in terms of priorities and the time frame in which they are to be developed. Lines of responsibility and the allocation of human, financial, and material resources must be clearly defined and understood.

Health services, unlike most other social and human endeavors, have an additional complicating factor because of the potential clashes between those with responsibility for individuals (e.g., direct patient care) and those with responsibility to the organization and the community at large (managers). Human resources development through awareness programs, education of health staff, continuous training, and career opportunities must be institutionalized from the inception of the developmental effort. The obvious rationale for standards is to facilitate the exchange of programs and data. Technical standards relate to data definition and format, security, media utilized, systems and applications software, and equipment and training.

National, regional, and institutional health information systems committees have an essential role in the definition and enforcement of policies and strategies. Ideally they should have a rotating membership and be formed by users and producers of health information at all levels. Membership should be as broad as possible and, when possible, include: health statisticians from operating agencies and universities, epidemiologists, demographers, economists, sociologists, administrators, planners, community representatives, information specialists, representatives of industry, physicians, and nurses.

The committee should recommend policies and guidelines for overall development of the system. In many settings the committee will be, at the highest level, advisory to the Ministry of Health, and in some settings there will be an analogous internal standing committee to deal with practical problems of implementation at the institutional level. Practical activities of the national committee and analogous committees can include the use of working parties and external technical consultant panels, such as international organizations and agencies, to deal with a wide variety of special problems. The committee should publish a periodical, possibly annual, report commenting on health information systems issues and proposing changes, additions, and, especially, deletion of useless data and procedures.

REFERENCE 1

PAHO CORE DATA INDICATORS

Component	PAHO Code	Indicator
Demographic	A1	Population
	A2	Life expectancy at birth
	A3	Total fertility rate
	A4	Annual population growth rate (%)
	A5	Percent urban population
	A6	Number of births registered
	A7	Estimated crude birth rate
	A8	Number of deaths registered
	A9	Estimated crude death rate
	A10	Population under 15 year as % of total population
	A11	Proportion 65 years and over, as proportion of total population
Socio-Economic	B1	Availability of calories (kcal/day per capita)
	B2	Literacy rate, in population 15 years and older
	B3	Average years of schooling of the population
	B4	Gross domestic product per capita, in constant 1990 US$
	B5	Gross domestic product per capita, US$ adjusted by purchasing power parity (PPP)
	B6	Ratio of 20% highest / 20% lowest income
	B7	Percent of population living in poverty
	B8	Percent of population living in extreme poverty
	B9	Rate of unemployment
	B10	Inflation: annual change in the consumer price index
Mortality	C1	Infant mortality rate
	C2	Neonatal mortality rate
	C3	Postneonatal mortality rate
	C4	Perinatal mortality rate
	C5	Estimated death rates
	C6	Mortality rate under 5 years of age (UNICEF)
	C7	Percent deaths < 1 year of age, certain conditions originating in the perinatal period
	C8	Number of registered deaths under 5 years of age due to measles
	C9	Number of registered deaths < 5 years of age due to other diseases preventable by immunization
	C10	Estimated deaths rate among children < years, intestinal infectious diseases

	C11	Estimated deaths rate among children < years, acute respiratory infections
	C12	Number of registered deaths due to tetanus neonatorum
	C13	Maternal mortality rate
	C14	Estimated deaths rates due to communicable diseases
	C15	Number of registered deaths from tuberculosis for the year
	C16	Number of registered deaths from AIDS for the year
	C17	Estimated deaths rates due to diseases of the circulatory system
	C18	Estimated deaths rates due to ischemic heart disease
	C19	Estimated deaths rates due to cerebrovascular disease
	C20	Estimated deaths rates due to neoplasm (all types)
	C21	Estimated deaths rates due to malignant neoplasm of lung, trachea and bronchus
	C22	Estimated deaths rates (female) due to malignant neoplasm of uterus
	C23	Estimated deaths rates (female) due to malignant neoplasm of the breast
	C24	Estimated deaths rates due to malignant neoplasm of the stomach
	C25	Estimated deaths rates from external causes
	C26	Estimated deaths rates due to accidents, excluding transport
	C27	Estimated deaths rates due to transport accidents
	C28	Estimated deaths rates due to suicide and self-inflicted injury, age >15 years
	C29	Estimated deaths rates due to homicide, age 15 years and over
	C30	Estimated deaths rates due to cirrhosis and chronic liver disease
	C31	Estimated deaths rates due to diabetes mellitus
Morbidity	D1	Percent of live births weighting less than 2.500 grams
	D2	Proportion of children < 5 years weight/age less than 2SD from WHO reference median
	D3	Percent of infants exclusively breasted through 120 days of age
	D4	Average of diseased, missing or filled teeth at age 12
	D5	Number of confirmed cases of poliomyelitis registered during the year
	D6	Number of measles cases registered during the year among children <5 years of age
	D7	Number of cases of diphtheria registered during the year among children <5 years of age
	D8	Number of cases of whooping cough registered during the year in children <5 years of age
	D9	Number of cases of tetanus neonatorum registered during the year
	D10	Number of cases of yellow fever registered during the year
	D11	Number of cases of plague registered during the year
	D12	Number of cases of dengue registered during the year
	D13	Number of cases of human rabies registered during the year
	D14	Number of cases of congenital syphilis registered during the year
	D15	Number of yellow fever registered during the year
	D16	Malaria annual parasite index
	D17	Number of cases of syphilis registered during the year
	D18	Number of cases of tuberculosis registered during the year

	D19	Number of cases of AIDS cases registered during the year
	D20	Prevalence of leprosy cases
	D21	Proportion of women of childbearing age currently using any type of contraceptive method
	D22	Adolescent fertility rate (%)
	D23	Incidence of malignant neoplasm of lung
	D24	Incidence of malignant neoplasm of stomach
	D25	Incidence of malignant neoplasm of female breast
	D26	Incidence of malignant neoplasm of cervix uteri
	D27	Prevalence of hypertension
	D28	Prevalence of diabetes mellitus type 2
	D29	Prevalence of overweight among adults (20-74 years)
	D30	Proportion of 15-19 years of age who smoke
Health Services	E1	Percent of population with access to health services
	E2	Percent of urban population with potable water through house connections
	E3	Percent of urban population with reasonable access to public sources of potable water
	E4	Percent of rural population with reasonable access to potable water
	E5	Percent of urban population with house connection to public sewer systems
	E6	Percent of urban population served by individual systems of excreta disposal
	E7	Percent of rural population having adequate sanitary means of excreta disposal
	E8	Percent of population with access to disinfected water supplies
	E9	Percent of urban population with regular collection of solid waste
	E10	Percent of children under 1 year attended by trained personnel
	E11	Percent of children under 1 year vaccinated against diphteria, whooping cough, tetanus
	E12	Percent of children under 1 year vaccinated against measles
	E13	Percent of children under 1 year vaccinated against poliomyelitis (OPV3)
	E14	Percent of children under 1 year vaccinated against tuberculosis (BCG)
	E15	Percent of pregnant women attended by trained personnel during pregnancy
	E16	Percent of pregnant women attended by trained personnel during first trimester pregnancy
	E17	Percent of deliveries attended by trained personnel
	E18	Cumulative % of women of childbearing age living at risk
	E19	Ambulatory care consultations (any type) per inhabitant per year
	E20	Number of hospital discharges per 100 population
	E21	Population per physician
	E22	Number of graduates in medicine
	E23	Population per university-professional nurse
	E24	Number of university graduates in professional nursing
	E25	Population per non-university-professional nursing personnel

A

	E26	Population per dentist
	E27	Population per hospital bed
	E28	Number of ambulatory care establishments
	E29	National health expenditure as percent of GNP
	E30	Public hospital expenditures as percent of government health expenditure
	E31	Government health expenditure as percent of national health expenditure
	E32	Under-registrations of births (%)
	E33	Percent of birth registrations which are for children under 1 year old at time of registration
	E34	Under-registrations of mortality (%)
	E35	Deaths with medical care as % of registered deaths
	E36	Deaths due to signs, symptoms and ill-defined conditions as % of registered deaths

REFERENCE 2

OECD HEALTHCARE INDICATORS

Component	Indicator
Life expectancy	Life expectancy (both genders, at birth and 40, 60, 65 and 80 years of age)
Potential years of life lost	Potential years of life lost (by selected causes)
Premature mortality	Perinatal mortality
	Infant mortality
	Mortality by accidental fall
	Mortality by liver cirrhosis
	Mortality by lung-trachea-bronchial cancer
	Mortality by medical complications
	Mortality by adverse effects from medicine
Morbidity	Low weight at birth
	Spina bifida
	Transposition of the great vessels
	Limb reduction
	Down Syndrome
	Decayed missing filled teeth (DMFT)
	Edentulous population
	Absenteeism due to illness
	Road traffic injuries in accidents
	Incidence of AIDS
Perceptual indicators	Self-evaluation as "less than good"
	Health system perceived as excellent
	Health system perceived as good
	Health system perceived as bad
Inputs and throughputs	Beds in in-patient care
	Beds in acute care
	Beds in physiatric care
	Beds in nursing home
	Beds in privately-owned hospitals
	Beds in private for-profit beds
	Bed-days in in-patient care
	Bed-days in acute care
	Occupancy rate in in-patient care

	Occupancy rate in acute care
	Hospital turnover rate in acute care
	Hospital staff ratio in acute care
	Nurse staff ratio in acute care
	Patient contacts per physician
	Doctor consultations per capita
	Dental services per capita
	Laboratory and biological tests
	Births in hospitals
	Deaths in hospitals
Health employment	Total health employment
	Active (practicing) physicians
	Female physicians
	General family practitioners
	Specialists (consultants)
	Active (practicing) dentists
	Active (practicing) pharmacists
	Certified (registered) nurses
	Total hospital employment
Medical education and training	Enrolment in Paramedical and Medical Schools
	Enrolment in Paramedical Schools
	Undergraduate enrolment (Medical/Paramedical)
	Postgraduate enrolment (medical/biomedical)
	New entrants in Paramedical and Medical Schools
	New entrants in Paramedical Schools
	New entrants in undergraduate level
	Paramedical and medical degrees
	Paramedical degrees
	College degrees (medical/paramedical)
	Postgraduate degrees (medical/biomedical)
High technology medical facilities	Scanners
	Radiation treatment equipment
	Lithotriptors
	Magnetic resonance imaging equipment
Medical research and development	Total expenditure on health for medical research and development
	Public expenditure on health for medical research and development
	Pharmaceutical industry R&D expenditure
	Government budget outlays for health R&D

Trade in medical goods and services	Pharmaceutical goods exports
	Pharmaceutical goods imports
	Medical equipment exports
	Medical equipment imports
	Therapeutical equipment exports
	Therapeutical equipment imports
	Medical services exports
	Medical services imports
Health expenditure	Total expenditure on health
	Public expenditure on health
	Total investment on medical facilities
	Public investment on medical facilities
	Total current expenditure on health
	Public current expenditure on health
	Total expenditure on health administration
	Public expenditure on health administration
	Expenditure on occupational health care
	Expenditure on military health services
	Expenditure on school health services
	Expenditure on prison health services
	Expenditure on maternal and child health care
	Expenditure on screening and monitoring health services
	Expenditure on food, hygiene and standards monitoring
	Expenditure on health education and training
	Expenditure on environmental health
	Expenditure on health promotion and prevention
	Total expenditure on personal health care
	Public expenditure on personal health care
Health expenditures (Economic Classification)	General government final consumption
	Transfer to household (health)
	Subsidies to medical producers
	Private consumption on health
Expenditure on in-patient care	Total expenditure on in-patient care
	Total expenditure on acute care
	Total expenditure on psychiatric care
	Total expenditure on nursing homes
	Total expenditure on home care
	Public expenditure on in-patient care

	Public expenditure on acute care
	Public expenditure on psychiatric care
	Public expenditure on nursing homes
	Public expenditure on home care
Expenditure on ambulatory care	Total expenditure on ambulatory care
	Total expenditure on physician services
	Total expenditure on dental services
	Total expenditure on laboratory tests
	Total expenditure on X-rays and imaging diagnosis
	Total expenditure on dental prostheses
	Total expenditure on patient transport
	Public expenditure on ambulatory care
	Public expenditure on physician services
	Public expenditure on dental services
	Public expenditure on laboratory tests
	Public expenditure on X-rays and imaging diagnosis
	Public expenditure on dental prostheses
	Public expenditure on patient transport
	Total expenditure in pharmaceutical goods
	Total expenditure in therapeutical appliances
	Public expenditure in pharmaceutical goods
	Public expenditure in therapeutical appliances
	Expenditure on prescribed medicines
	Expenditure on OTC products
Expenditure by age group	Expenditure on population 65+ / population 0-64
	Expenditure on population 75+ / population 0-64
	Expenditure on population 65-74 / population 0-64
Health care financing	General revenue
	Social security contributions and payroll taxes
	Employer payroll taxes
	Health-related tax expenditures
	Private health insurance
	Out-of-pocket outlays (household)
Cost of illness	Cost of illness in all hospitals
	Cost of illness in ambulatory care
	Cost of illness in pharmaceuticals
	Cost of illness in each ICD group of diseases
Social protection	Social protection in total medical care
	Social protection in in-patient care
	Social protection in ambulatory medical care
	Social protection in pharmaceutical goods
	Social protection in therapeutical appliances

	Social protection in sickness cash-benefits
Lifestyle and environment	Alcoholic beverage intake
	Tobacco consumption
	Total sulphur oxide emissions (SO)
	Total nitrogen oxide emissions (NO)
	Total carbon oxide emissions (CO)
	Access to waste water treatment
	Road transport noise exposure
	Energy consumption
	Total land surface
	Number of dwellings
	Dwelling size 1 Room
	Dwelling size 2 Rooms
	Dwelling size 3 Rooms
	Dwelling size 4 Rooms
	Dwelling size 5 Rooms and more
	Dwelling equipment central heating
	Dwelling equipment bath or shower
	Dwelling equipment refrigerator
Nutrition and biometrics	Total calories intake
	Crop calories intake
	Animal calories intake
	Total protein intake
	Crop protein intake
	Animal protein intake
	Fats and oil from land animals
	Butter consumption
	Sugar consumption
	Overweight persons over 20 years old
	Average height of the population
Pharmaceutical activity	Pharmaceutical production
	Pharmaceutical value added
	VAT rates on prescribed drugs
	Pharmaceutical industry gross capital performance
	Pharmaceutical industry gross rates of return
	Pharmaceutical industry net rates of returns
	Pharmaceutical industry exports
	Pharmaceutical industry imports
	Pharmaceutical industry employees
	Pharmaceutical labor compensation
	Pharmaceutical wholesale labor costs
	Pharmaceutical retail sales labor costs

Pharmaceutical consumption per person	DDD: Anti-acids
	DDD: Anti-peptics
	DDD: Anti-diabetics
	DDD: Mineral supplements
	DDD: Anticoagulants
	DDD: Cholesterol reducers
	DDD: Cardiac glycosides
	DDD: Systemic anti-arrythmics
	DDD: Cardiac sympathomimetics
	DDD: Myocardial Therapy
	DDD: Hypotensives
	DDD: Diuretics
	DDD: Beta-blocking agents
	DDD: Corticoids
	DDD: Systemic antibiotics
	DDD: Analgesics
	DDD: Benzodiazepines
	DDD: Psychoanaleptics
	DDD: Antiasmathics
	DDD: Antihistaminics
Pharmaceutical deliveries	Pharmaceutical sales on the domestic market
	Digestive tract and metabolic procedures sales on the domestic market
	Cardiovascular pharmaceutical sales on the domestic market
	Genito-urinary system and sex hormones sales on the domestic market
	Anti-infective for systemic use sales on the domestic market
	Musculo-skeletal system pharmaceutical sales on the domestic market
	Antiparasitic products sales on the domestic market
	Sensory organs preparation pharmaceutical sales on the domestic market
	Blood and blood forming organs products sales on the domestic market
	Dermatological products sales on the domestic market
	Systemic hormonal preparations sales on the domestic market
	Anti-neoplastic & immuno-modulating sales on the domestic market
	Central nervous system pharmaceutical sales on the domestic market
	Respiratory system pharmaceutical sales on the domestic market
	Other products of pharmaceutical sales on the domestic market
ALOS and discharge rate	Average length of stay (for each ICD disease group)
	Discharge rate (for each ICD disease group)
	Average length of stay case-mix (for each ICD disease group)
	Discharge rate case-mix (for each ICD disease group)

Surgical and medical procedures	All surgical and medical procedures
	Operations on the nervous system
	Operations on the endocrine system
	Operations on the eye
	Lens procedures
	Cornea transplants
	Operations on the ear
	Tympanotomy
	Surgery on nose, mouse, pharynx
	Tonsillectomy
	Thyroidectomy
	Adenoidectomy
	Operations on the respiratory system
	Pulmonary lobectomy
	Operation on cardiovascular system
	Hemorroidectomy
	Coronary bypass
	Heart (heart-lung) transplant
	Stripping and ligation varicose veins
	Angioplasty (dilatation coronary artery)
	Operations on hernia and lymphatic system
	Bone marrow transplant
	Operations of the digestive system
	Appendectomy
	Inguinal herniorraphy
	Cholecystectomy
	Gastrectomy
	Exploratory laparotomy
	Liver transplants
	Pancreas transplants
	Operations of the urinary system
	Prostatectomy
	Surgery on the male genital organs
	Surgery on the female genital organs
	Hysterectomy
	Mastectomy
	Obstetrical procedures
	Episiotomy
	Artificial rupture of membranes
	Manually assisted delivery
	Cesarean section
	Repair of current obstetric laceration
	Fetal EKG & fetal monitoring
	Other obstetric procedures

	Operations of the musculo-skeletal system
	Hip replacements
	Operations on the integumentary system
Ambulatory surgery	All ambulatory surgical and medical procedures
	Inguinal hernia repair
	Excision of breast lung
	Anal procedure
	Dilatation and curetage
	Circumcision
	Excision in Dupuytren's contraction
	Carpal tunnel decompression
	Knee arthroscopy
	Cholecystectomy, laparoscopic
	Cataract extraction
	Squint surgery
	Myringotomy
	Sub-mucous resection
	Inguinal and femoral hernia repair
	Laparoscopic sterilization
	Lachrymal duct procedures
	Tonsilectomy, adenoidectomy
	Procedures on lymphatic structures
	Ventral hernia repair
	Vasectomy
	Vaginal hysterectomy
	Implanted devices removal
	Vein ligation and stripping
	Orchiopexy-varicocele
	Hemorroidectomy
	Gynecological procedures
	Other hand or foot procedures
	Skin/subcutaneous procedures
	Laparoscopy w/o sterilization
	End-stage renal failure
	Dialysis
	Kydney transplants
	Functioning transplants
	Dyphteria, tetanus, polio immunization
Medical services fees	Microscopic urine examination fees
	Extraction grinder fees
	X-ray unit fees
	Electrophoresis fees
	Electroencephalogram (EEG) fees

	Bilateral; tonsillectomy on children < 10 y. fees
	Hospitalization for delivery fees
	Scintigraphy of the thyroid fees
	Total tooth prosthesis (1 Jaw) fees
	Brains abscess by a neurosurgeon fees
	Anesthesia by special stereotaxic technique fees
	Intracardiac surgery under hypothermia fees
	Numeration of cholesterol fees
	Hemoglobin numeration fees
	Electrocardiogram fees
	Echography fees
	Colonoscopy fees
	Computerized scan of the skull fees
	Operation of the cataract fees
	Cholecystectomy fees
	Herniorraphy fees
	Menisectomy fees
	General practitioner home visit fees
	Office visit by a General Practitioner fees
Demographic references	Population (per age structure)
	Mean age of the population
	Median age of the population
	Fertility
	Birth
	Deaths
	Dependency
Household status	Household single, unmarried
	Household married
	Household single, divorced
	Household single, widowed
Labor force	Labor force
	Unemployment
	Total employment
	Employment females
	Employment males
	Wage and salaried employment
	Female labor force participation
	Part-time employment
	Fixed-term employment contracts
	Employment, agriculture
	Employment, industry
	Employment, market services
	Employment, general government
	Man-hours worked by and per employee

Occupational status	Professionals and technical-related workers
	Administrative, managerial workers
	Clerical and related workers
	Sales workers
	Service workers
	Agriculture, forestry, fisher workers
	Production and related workers
	Enrolment Secondary and Higher education
	Enrolment Secondary level
	Enrolment undergraduate level
	Enrolment post-graduate level
	New entrants Secondary and Higher education
	New entrants Secondary level
	New entrants undergraduate level
	Degrees awarded Secondary and Higher education
	Degrees awarded Secondary level
	Degrees awarded undergraduate level
	Degrees awarded post-graduate level
	Total education attainment
	Attainment in lower secondary education
	Attainment in upper secondary education
	Attainment in non-university enrolment
	Attainment in university education
Macro-economic references	Total domestic expenditure
	Gross domestic product
	Trends in gross domestic product
	Potential gross domestic product
	Public revenue
	National disposable income
	Compensation of employees
	General government deficit
	Gross public debt
	Public debt servicing
	Net rates of return
	Government budget outlays for total R&D
	Total factor productivity
	Labor productivity
	Capital productivity
Private consumption	Private final consumption
	Expenditure on food and beverages
	Expenditure on clothing and footwear
	Expenditure on gross rent, fuel, power

	Expenditure on furniture, equipment
	Expenditure on personal care
	Expenditure on transport and communication
	Expenditure on entertainment and education
	Expenditure on miscellaneous services
Monetary conversion rates	Exchange rate per US$
	Exchange rate per ECU
	GDP purchasing power parities US$
	GDP purchasing power parities ECU
	Health purchasing power parities US$
	Health purchasing power parities ECU
	Medical services purchasing power parities US$
	Medical services purchasing power parities ECU
	Pharmaceutical purchasing power parities US$
	Pharmaceutical purchasing power parities ECU

REFERENCE 3

HEALTH DATABASES PROTECTION AND CONFIDENTIALITY

ABBREVIATED AND EDITED RECOMMENDATIONS FROM THE

Council of Europe
DIRECTORATE OF LEGAL AFFAIRS
Public and International Law
Division "Data Protection" Section

Introduction to the Legal Aspects of Health Databases

1. The use of computers in medicine serves the interests of the individual and of the community. In the first place, computers contribute towards better medical care by automating techniques, reducing the burden on the doctor's memory and facilitating the establishment of medical records. Medical computer systems are an answer to the increasing demand, caused by specialization and teamwork, for quick and selective access to information on the patient and his treatment, thus ensuring the continuity of medical care.

2. Medical data processing also brings a major improvement to hospital management and in this way it can help to reduce the cost of health care. Computers are used for recording the admission, transfer and release of patients, keeping track of diagnostic and therapeutic activities, medication, laboratory analyses, accounting, invoicing, etc. Lastly, medical data processing represents an indispensable instrument for medical research and for a policy of early and systematic diagnosis and prevention of certain diseases.

3. Accordingly, the data concerning an individual's health appear in many files, which can be recorded on a computer. The holders of these files vary: the attending physician, the hospital doctor, the school doctor, the works doctor, the medical consultant of an insurance company, hospital administrator, social security offices, etc. Usually the recording of medical data occurs in the context of the doctor-patient relationship. It takes the form of a medical record, which will help to establish the diagnosis and facilitate the supervision and care of the patient. The information is obtained with the patient's consent by the doctor or a member of the medical team who is required to observe confidentiality under the ethical rules of his profession. Health records may also be established outside the context of the doctor-patient relationship and may include data concerning perfectly healthy persons. The recording of information is sometimes imposed by a third party, perhaps even without the explicit consent of the person concerned.

4. The quality and integrity of information is extremely important in matters of health. At a time of increasing personal mobility, the exchange of accurate and relevant information is necessary for the individual's safety. Furthermore, the development of medical science takes place thanks to a transfrontier flow of medical data and the setting up of specialized information systems across considerable geographical distances (such as the Eurotransplant organization for the transplantation of human organs).

5. The needs which medical data processing systems have to satisfy are often contradictory. Indeed, information must be made rapidly available to duly authorized users whilst remaining inaccessible to others. The obligation to respect the patient's privacy places certain restrictions on the recording and dissemination of medical data, whereas the right of each individual to health implies that everyone should benefit from the progress made by medical science thanks to extensive use of medical data.

6. Certain of the contents of medical files may harm the patient if used outside the doctor-patient relationship. Medical data comes within the individual's most intimate sphere. Unauthorized disclosure of personal medical particulars may therefore lead to various forms of discrimination and even to the violation of fundamental rights.

7. Apprehension about abuse of medical information is not due to computer technology as such, for it is generally acknowledged that the use of computers makes it possible to improve considerably the reliability and security of medical data. It is rather a consequence of the awareness that the high technical quality of automated medical records makes it possible to use them for a great variety of purposes.

8. Furthermore, access to medical files is not restricted to doctors alone or to members of the health care staff who are bound to observe medical secrecy. Medical data processing requires the co-operation of numerous persons in other professions outside the medical field, not all of who are bound by rules of professional secrecy. The use of computers may imply a shift of responsibility between the medical profession and other professions, so that the possibility of an indiscretion is a real danger.

9. Moreover, the emergence of automated data banks has given rise in most countries to a reform of the law according to which individuals will be entitled to know what information is stored about them in computers. The application of this rule in the medical field may cause certain difficulties on account of medical ethics. It should therefore be subject to special safeguards and, as the case may be, restrictions in the interest of the data subject.

10. In view of these problems, it is highly desirable to make the operation of every automated medical bank subject to a specific set of regulations. The general purpose of these regulations should be to guarantee that medical data are used not only so as to ensure optimum medical care and services but also in such a way that the data subject's dignity and physical and mental integrity is fully respected.

11. Although such regulations will be adopted by the person or body in charge of each data bank (hospital management, faculty of medicine, etc), it is desirable that they should follow a common pattern and conform to general principles of data protection. This follows, *inter alia*, from the fact that in most countries data protection is, or will be, the subject of legislation. Some laws recently adopted in this field provide that every automated data bank, or at least those data banks which store sensitive information, should have its own regulations. Consequently, it is up to public authorities to give general guidelines for the drawing up of medical data bank regulations.

12. There are a number of data processing problems which are peculiar to medicine, such as, for example:

- the structuring of computerized medical records so that they can be put to various uses;

- the need to keep medical data for periods which are generally very long;

- the problem of the applicability in the medical field of the general rule that it must be possible for the individual to be notified of computerized data concerning him.

13. Several of these problems arise outside the field of data processing. Data processing had, however, intensified the need for a solution.

Recommendation No.R (81) 1

OF THE COMMITTEE OF MINISTERS TO MEMBER STATES ON REGULATIONS FOR AUTOMATED MEDICAL DATA BANKS

1. Scope and purpose of the regulations

1.1. The following principles apply to automated data banks set up for purposes of medical care, public health, management of medical or public health services or medical research, in which are stored medical data and, as the case may be, related social or administrative data pertaining to identified or identifiable individuals (automated medical data banks).

1.2. Every automated medical data bank should be subject to its own specific regulations, in conformity with the laws of the state in whose territory it is established. The regulations of medical data banks used for purposes of public health, management of medical and health services, or for the advancement of medical science should have due regard to the pre-eminence of individual rights and freedoms.

1.3. The regulations should be sufficiently specific to provide ready answers to those questions likely to arise in the operation of the particular medical data bank.

1.4. Where a medical data bank combines several sets of medical records or sub-systems of medical data, each of these elements may require separate supplementary regulations relating to its special features.

1.5. The requirements and obligations following from this recommendation are to be taken duly into account not only with regard to medical data banks, which are operational, but also those, which are in the development phase.

2. Public notice of automated medical data banks

2.1. Plans for the establishment of automated medical data banks as well as plans for the fundamental modification of existing banks should be brought to the notice of the public in advance.

2.2. When an automated medical data bank becomes operational, a public notice thereof should be given, relating at the very least to the following features:

 a. the name of the medical data bank;

 b. reference to the instrument pursuant to which the medical data bank has been established;

 c. a summary of the data bank's regulations and an indication of how the complete regulations can be obtained or consulted.

3. Minimum contents of the data bank's regulations

3.1. The data bank's regulations should at least contain provisions on:

 a. it's specific purpose(s);

 b. the categories of information recorded;

 c. the body or person for whom the data bank is operated and who is competent to decide which categories of data should be processed;

 d. the person(s) in charge of its day-to-day running;

 e. the categories of persons who are entitled to cause data to be placed in storage, modified and erased ("originators of the data");

 f. the person or body:

      - to whom certain decisions must be submitted for approval;

      - who supervises the use of the data bank;

- to whom appeal may be made in the event of dispute;

g. the categories of persons who have access to the data bank in the course of their work and the categories of data to which they are entitled to have access;

h. the disclosure of information to third parties;

i. the disclosure of information to the individuals concerned ("data subjects");

j. the long-term conservation of data;

k. the procedure concerning requests for use of data for purpose other than those for which they have been collected;

l. the security of data and installations;

m. whether and on which conditions linking with other data banks is permitted.

4. Recording of data

4.1. The person or body responsible for establishing and/or managing a medical data bank should ensure that:

a. data are collected by lawful and fair means;

b. no data are collected other than those which are relevant and appropriate to the declared purpose(s);

c. so far as is practicable the accuracy of the data is verified; and

d. the contents of the record are kept up to data as appropriate.

4.2. In order to ensure on the one hand selective access to the information in conformity with paragraph 5.1 and on the other hand the security of the data, the records must as a general rule be so designed as to enable the separation of:

a. identifiers and data relating to the identity of persons;

b. administrative data;

c. medical data;

d. social data.

A distinction between objective and subjective data is to be made with regard to the data mentioned under c and d above.

Where, however, it is unnecessary or impossible to achieve such separation, other measures must be taken in order to protect the privacy of individuals and confidentiality of the information.

4.3. A person from whom medical information is collected should be informed of its intended use(s).

5. Access to and use of information

5.1. As a general rule, access to the information may be given only to medical staff and, as far as national law or practice permits, to other health care staff, each person having access to those data which he needs for his specific duties.

5.2. When a person mentioned in the previous paragraph ceases to exercise his functions, he may no longer store, modify, erase or gain access to the data, save by special agreement with the person or body mentioned in paragraph 3.1.f.

5.3. A person referred to in paragraph 5.1 who has access to data in the course of his work may not use such data for a purpose different from that for which he originally had access to those data, unless:

a. he/she puts the information in such a form that the data subject cannot be identified, or

b. such different use has been authorized by the person or body referred to in paragraph 3.1.f., or

c. such different use is imposed by a provision of law, it being understood that national law or practice may impose an additional obligation to obtain the consent of the data subject (or, should he be deceased, of his family) or his physician.

5.4. Without the data subject's express and informed consent, the existence and content of his medical record may not be communicated to persons or bodies outside the fields of medical care, public health or medical research, unless such a communication is permitted by the rules on medical professional secrecy.

5.5. Linking or bringing together information on the same individual contained in different medical data banks is permitted for purposes of medical care, public health or medical research, provided it is in accordance with the specific regulations.

6. The data subject and his medical record

6.1. Measures should be taken to enable every person to know of the existence and content of the information about him held in a medical data bank.

This information shall, if the national law so provides, be communicated to the data subject through the intermediary of his physician.

No exception to this principle shall be allowed unless it is prescribed by law or regulation and concerns:

a. data banks which are used only for statistics or scientific research purposes and when there is obviously no risk of an infringement of the privacy of the data subject;

b. information the knowledge of which might cause serious harm to the data subject.

6.2. The data subject may ask for amendment of erroneous data concerning him and, in case of refusal, he may appeal to the person or body referred to in paragraph 3.1.f.

When the information is amended, it may nevertheless be provided that a record will be kept of the erroneous data so far as knowledge of the error may be relevant to further medical treatment or useful for research purposes.

7. Long-term conservation of data

7.1. As a general rule, data related to an individual should be kept on record only during a period reasonably useful for reaching their main purpose(s).

7.2. Where, in the interest of public health, medical science, or for historical or statistical purposes, it proves desirable to conserve medical data that have no longer any immediate use, technical provision is to be made for their correct conservation and safekeeping.

8. Professional obligations

In addition to the members of the health care staff, the data processing personnel and any other persons participating in the design, operation, use or maintenance of a medical data bank, must respect the confidential nature of the information and ensure the correct use of the medical data bank.

9. Extended protection

None of the principles in this appendix shall be interpreted as limiting the possibility for a member state to introduce legal provisions
granting a wider measure of protection to the persons to whom medical data refer.

10. Detailed comments

10.1. Scope and purpose of the regulations

10.1.1. The recommendation concerns medical data contained in medical records established in the context of the doctor-patient relationship or in health records established for other purposes. The term "medical data" includes information concerning the past, present and future, physical or mental health of an individual, as well as related social or administrative information. The latter type of information may relate to a person's address, profession, family circumstances, psychological factors, etc. The information may refer to a data subject who is sick, healthy or deceased. The recommendation is concerned only with such data as can be attributed to identified or identifiable individuals, not with anonymous or aggregate information.

10.1.2. In so far as the removal of substances of human origin, or the grafting and the transplantation of tissues or organs have led to the constitution of a medical record, the problem of the protection of the anonymity between the donor and the donor will be covered by this recommendation, since it extends to an individual's past health. Such protection of anonymity between donor and recipient is provided for in general terms in Resolution (78) 29 of the Committee of Ministers of the Council of Europe on harmonization of legislation of member states relating to removal, grafting and transplantation of human substances.

10.1.3. Medical data may appear together with other information in non-medical records, for example insurance or employment records. Such data banks are not covered by the recommendation. However, it is clear that such records may raise important problems in regard to individual freedoms. It should be noted that Article 6 of the Convention for the Protection of Individuals with regard to Automatic Processing of Personal Data stipulates that personal data concerning health may not be processed automatically unless domestic law provides appropriate safeguards. Under that convention, therefore, it is for contracting states to provide appropriate safeguards for the protection of individuals in cases where data relating to health are processed in data banks not covered by this recommendation. It is of course highly desirable, in so far as possible, for medical information to be recorded in special data banks and not integrated with
general data banks.

10.1.4. Automated data banks generally offer better safeguards for the protection, confidentiality and integrity of data than manual systems. However, computerized systems raise specific problems because of the co-operation necessary between members of the medical profession and data processing experts, and because they permit a wider range of uses. One should not, however, exclude the possibility that the effort expended on this recommendation, which is restricted to computerized systems, may also bear fruit in the sphere of non-computerized medical records.

10.1.5. Unlike Resolutions (73) 22 and (74) 29, which provided for two separate series of principles applying to the public and the private sectors, this recommendation applies to medical data banks in both sectors, since they must meet the same requirements and since there is a frequent transfer of data between the two sectors.

10.1.6. Further, it is to be observed that the recommendation is designed to allow for the use of medical data for research purposes. In this respect it should be noted that, at the time of publication of this explanatory memorandum, more detailed recommendations for the protection of personal information used for research purposes were being examined by the Council of Europe's committee of experts on data protection. Of course, the recommendation does not apply to collections of medical statistics, which cannot in any way be related to identified or identifiable persons.

10.2. Public notice of automated medical data banks

10.2.1. In some member states, no automated medical data bank may be established unless the authorities and the public at large have been notified of the fact. It is desirable that, in countries where there is as yet no legal obligation to make a declaration or give public notice of the existence of a medical data bank, those responsible for medical data banks should give such notice in an appropriate form (e.g., by a notice in the press).

10.2.2. Publicity of this kind is first and foremost aimed at guaranteeing protection of the individual's rights and freedoms in matters of health. It would also help to make the public aware of the usefulness of computerized medical data systems and, furthermore, may encourage the public to support the introduction of such systems.

10.2.3. It is important to note in this connection that the recommendation applies not only to existing operational data banks, but also to those, which are in the process of development (project, transition from manual to computerized system, trial installation, etc). Timely notice of a project for the establishment of a new medical data system will allow interested circles to make their views known before substantial funds have been spent and thereby prevent their being faced with a fait accompli.

10.3. Minimum contents of the data bank's regulations

10.3.1. Access to the information in a medical data bank must be carefully controlled. This must not result in the medical data bank becoming shrouded in mystery; on the contrary, its regulations must contain such elements as to enable outsiders to obtain an accurate idea of its purpose, the categories of information recorded, its way of operation, etc.

10.3.2. For this reason, it must be quite clear from the regulations of the data bank who is the person or body on whose behalf the data bank is operated, who is its manager, who can store information in it, which body exercises supervision over it, to whom requests for information and possibly complaints can be addressed, what is the exact nature and purpose of the data recorded, who are the users, etc.

10.3.3. While mention may be made of the fact that security measures exist, no precise details must of course be given, in the interests of security itself. Mention will also be made of the method of erasing obsolete data, the storing of data, which no longer serve any immediate purpose and the procedure governing the use of data for purposes other than those for which they were collected. The preservation of medical records may be required for much longer periods even going beyond the lifetime of the data subject - than is the case with other kinds of personal records. This is an additional reason why there must be sound data security methods.

10.4. Recording of data

10.4.1. The data recorded must be accurate and the content of records kept up to date. As regards accuracy, it is obvious that in medicine, errors or inaccuracies may well cause serious damage. However, the consequences of error (e.g., regarding a blood group) can be neutralized if the information provided by the computer is verified with other clinical data submitted for the doctor's assessment. Cross-checking procedures should be used in order to eliminate errors made within the computer system. It is pointed out that detection of an error does not always necessitate a correction (see in this connection paragraph 6.2 of the recommendation). The requirement that medical data should be up to date derives from the fact that the medical record is intended to guarantee continuity of treatment.

10.4.2. Information must be obtained by lawful and fair methods. The present methods of obtaining information from patients are regarded as being generally satisfactory because the patient normally knows what he is being asked for and why. However, there always remains a risk of abuse, having regard to the fact that a patient may be in a state of dependence vis-à-vis the doctor or medical establishment.

10.4.3. One of the distinct advantages of computerized records over manual records is that they permit the separation of different types of information (name of the person concerned, administrative, medical or social data, etc) and that by various technical methods access by the various categories of personnel (medical and paramedical staff, researchers, hospital administrators, etc) can be restricted, each having access only to such parts of the file as he needs for his specific duties. Furthermore, objective medical and social data (temperature, blood group, treatment prescribed, social background, profession, etc) must be kept separate from subjective data (probable diagnosis, likely development of the disease, behavior, aptitudes, etc). The words "As a general rule" indicate that the separation of identifying information and other data is not mandatory in all cases. It would be meaningless in the case of a medical data bank, which is accessible only to a small number of physicians who all know the identity and illness of the patients.

10.5. Access to and use of information

10.5.1. As the patient is the source of the information, his consent is the basis for the use of information and the conservation of his file by the doctor or the hospital administration.

10.5.2. In the interests of the care of patients, the recommendation allows states to grant access to a patient's medical record to members of the medical profession who, because of their functions, are required to observe professional secrecy. A reference to national law and practice is made with regard to access to information by other health care staff (nurses, physiotherapists, etc), since the definition of that category of personnel and their legal status differs from one country to another, and sometimes even within one country (e.g., in the case federal states).

10.5.3. Since the originator of the data is not the owner of the record, a change in his status or that of any other person having right of access will terminate the possibility for such persons to have access to the data or to record, alter or erase data, without special authorization.

10.5.4. With regard to the use of medical data for purposes other than those originally envisaged, the recommendation draws a clear distinction between persons who have access to the data in the exercise of their functions, and others. The former, consisting mainly of the medical and health care staff (see paragraph 5.1), may use the information for other purposes (research, teaching, scientific publications, statistics, etc) provided it is either in anonymous form or by special consent of the person or body named to that effect in the data bank regulations. If it is a person that decides on the follow-up to be given to requests for secondary uses of medical information (see paragraph 3.1.1), he should preferably be a physician. Where this function is entrusted to a collegiate body, it is desirable that not only the medical profession but also the representatives of other interests (patients, social security, etc) are included in the body's membership. Requests for secondary uses should be duly justified.

10.5.5. Under the law or ethical practice of some countries the sole person who can authorize secondary uses of medical information which was obtained in a doctor-patient relationship is the treating physician.

10.5.6. Paragraph 5.3.c covers the case where other uses of medical information are imposed by provisions of law (compulsory reporting of a contagious disease, injury caused by an animal suspected of rabies, etc). Some of these measures are taken as a result of directions from international organizations, such as the World Health Organization.

10.5.7. Paragraph 5.4 deals with the communication of data to other persons or bodies. Since professional secrecy guarantees that the information disclosed to a doctor will remain confidential, no medical record may be circulated outside the doctor-patient relationship, hospital management, public health services or medical research without the consent of the person concerned, unless such a communication is permitted under the medical profession's rules on secrecy. The doctor-patient relationship naturally includes the patient's relationship with the whole medical team. The circulation of information within this team is in fact essential in the interests of the patient himself.

10.5.8. The records sometimes include administrative data, which are not automatically covered by professional secrecy. But certain data of an administrative nature, such as the presence of a person in the hospital or the prices charged for a medical act, reveal that an individual is or has been under treatment and may make it possible to establish the nature of the disease. In some cases, the disclosure of information of this kind may be harmful to the individual. It therefore seems reasonable to allow an individual to request that the examinations, medical treatment or operation which he has undergone should not be divulged.

10.5.9. It is provided in paragraph 5.3 in fine and 5.4 that the communication of medical data outside the medical or health context will be possible under certain conditions and especially with the proviso that the data subject should give his consent. However, this does not prevent the law from explicitly prohibiting the communication of certain data, even if the data subject does not object. Such is, for example, the tendency with regard to matters concerning artificial insemination.

10.5.10. Respect for the purposes of information should not be an obstacle to a possible link between records storing information on the same patients at different times or in different places, in so far as the information exchanged is medically useful and in particular guarantees the continuity of care. However, this linking must take place in accordance with the data bank's specific regulations.

10.6. The data subject and his medical record

10.6.1. One of the most important principles in the field of data protection is the right of every person to know the information that is stored about him by other persons. In the medical field, there are two obstacles to the application of this principle. On the one hand, it may be extremely detrimental to the treatment of a patient if he is given the full facts about his case. Moreover, medical information as such may make little sense to the layman.

10.6.2 Paragraph 6 of the recommendation provides as a general rule that every person should be enabled to know of the existence of information about him in a record. Exceptions to this rule should be reduced to a minimum; as an example of such an exception, it might be detrimental for a patient to know that he is on record in a cancer registry. The data subject should also be enabled to obtain the information itself, but it may be provided that such information should be communicated to him through the intermediary of his physician.

10.6.3. A general principle in the field of data protection is that erroneous data must be corrected. The recommendation provides, however, that when knowledge of the error could be relevant to further medical treatment, a record of the erroneous data may be kept. Accordingly, in this specific case, it was decided against "over-writing" that is erasure of an item of information in a record and its replacement with new information.

10.6.4. It should be pointed out that if the data subject is incapable (a child, or a legally or mentally incapacitated person), his legal representative will exercise his rights set out in this paragraph, as well as the right of consent mentioned in paragraph 5.

10.7. Long-term conservation of data

10.7.1. Finally, the recommendation gives attention to a point on which medical data banks must be treated differently from most other types of data banks. As a general rule computerized information should not be stored longer than is strictly necessary, for it is a threat to privacy if information relating to any individual is allowed to accumulate as the years go by. However, the interests of public health and scientific research may justify the long-term conservation of medical data, even after the death of the persons concerned. Specific regulations exist in a number of countries for the conservation of medical archives. The present recommendation, in paragraph 7, permits the long-term conservation of data, provided that adequate safety and privacy safeguards are given.

10.8. Professional obligations

10.8.1. The use of medical data processing requires the co-operation of many professional people who take part in the design and operation of medical data banks. But, although professional liability and the doctors' code of ethics are clearly defined, the position of computer experts and other persons involved in the running of data banks should be established more precisely. At the time of publication of this explanatory memorandum, the Council of Europe's committee of experts on data protection was drawing up more detailed recommendations on the question of rules of conduct for data processing experts.

10.8.2. The essential co-operation between the medical profession, data processing experts and other persons sometimes involves the transfer of responsibility. In the case of an error in the transmission of information or the breakdown of the data processing installations assisting the patient, a problem arises concerning the apportionment of liability. Therefore, the duties and responsibilities of the various persons involved should be set out clearly in the regulations.

10.8.3. Recorded medical data must be accurate and the contents of records kept up to date. This involves the responsibility of the doctor at the time the data are stored and of the data processing expert when the program is designed and implemented. Staff responsible for the
processing of data are also in charge of installations, programs and premises, and must, just as members of the medical staff, be required to respect the confidential nature of medical and personal information of which they acquire knowledge in the exercise of their profession.

10.9. Extended protection

10.9.1. It should be noted that the recommendation does not prevent states from introducing a wider measure of protection to the persons to whom medical data refer.

REFERENCE 4

Swedish Institute for Health Services Development (Spri)

Set of Recommendations on Functional Requirements for Healthcare Documentation (1996)

The Swedish Institute for Health Services Development (SPRI) in Stockholm, has been responsible for a variety of developments in the area of health informatics. Although computerized systems of patient records have existed in Sweden since the beginning of the seventies, it was not until the end of the eighties that their use became generalized and, up to the end of 1992, around 500 systems were installed. The next years showed a marked increase in the number of installations and, by the end of 1995, over 2,200 systems were in use. The majority of systems have been installed in the primary care setting, which at present has approximately 85 per cent coverage. Conversely, the corresponding figure for institutional care is less than 15 per cent. However, at the beginning of 1996 many hospitals and county councils were at the procurement stage, and the number of systems installed (and, as a result, investments) are expected to further increase in the next few years.

The Swedish Commission of Enquiry into Information Structure for Health and Medical Care pointed out the need for a common and well-defined information structure for health and medical services as a whole, based on local databases. A prerequisite for the viability of a common structure is that the concepts, definitions, classifications and technical standards employed should be uniformly defined and described and related to target structures. Among the areas prioritized by the Board of SPRI in 1993 were computerized patient record systems. The project "Computerized Care Documentation" (DVD in Swedish), started in the spring of 1994 with a feasibility study. The outcome of the study included an inventory of existing computerized systems of patient records and a plan for carrying out the main study. The latter commenced in October 1994 and was completed at the beginning of 1996.

The goal laid down for the project was to produce a list of essential as well as desirable functional requirements for computer-supported health documentation. The approach chosen was to collect all the requirements considering four categories of users: primary care, institutional care, psychiatric care, and those related to common (shared) needs. In order to gain support for the specification of requirements, a total of nine seminars were held, each attended by 60-80 delegates, representing all categories of care providers, information specialists, and healthcare managers. At those seminars the requirements were reviewed and suggestions regarding their formulation and new ones were identified. In order to gain further support for the requirements, the initial listing was sent out for consideration to a total of 550 professional groups.

The original idea was that the list should only contain requirements originating from users. This proved impossible since in certain areas essential requirements relating to computerized documentation systems were lacking. This was the case, in areas such as security, confidentiality, technical platforms, methods of identifying patients and documentation and needs relating to the retrieval of information. The final list of functional requirements identified by SPRI is intended to ensure that future computerized healthcare documentation systems serve as an aid to the process of care, and have a modular structure. The list contains basic requirements and additions will be needed during procurement in order to arrive at a system that is suited to a particular application environment.

The listing of functional requirements for computerized health documents hereby presented was adapted from the publication "User Requirements on Electronic Health Care Records", Swedish Institute for Health Services Development, Stockholm 1996, ISSN 0281-6881. Please note that many functionalities are specific to the legal framework of Sweden or apply only to the clinical and administrative documentation used in the Swedish healthcare system where concerns related to privacy, confidentiality, accountability, and data security are paramount.

A. General Requirements

1. Common Patient Record

1a. The record system shall facilitate a multiprofessional and multimedia record where all people who are required to record/document register data can do so.

1b. The data can be stored in different locally distributed databases, but it shall be possible to compile and present it in the form of a common record.

1c. It shall not be necessary to re-register data that are already in the system or that can be retrieved from other systems.

2. System Structure

2a. It shall be possible for the record system to act as a module of a larger system comprising areas like Patient Administration, Funds, Bookings, Referrals and Answers to Requests.

2b. The patient record module shall be able to exchange information with other modules.

2c. The modules shall be able to use common data, not just exchange information w1th each other.

3. Simultaneous Access

3a. Several persons shall be able to access the record at the same time.

3b. A person who reads a record shall be made aware of the fact that someone else is currently writing in the record when this happens.

3c. Simultaneous writing/updating of the same record shall not be possible.

4. Patient Treatment Plan

4a. Treatment plans shall be displayed and accessible at any time.

4b. The system shall support the adding of care protocols and patient instructions.

4c. The system shall support local treatment plans with related instructions, for example databases of exercises and other care programs or protocols.

4d. The system shall allow the usage of different types of care assessment/result scales.

4e. As a decision support function it shall be possible to include specific treatment and rehabilitation programs for prevailing diagnoses.

5. User Training

5a. The system shall contain a training database for standard and common care situations.

5b. The system shall be built in such a way that it is as self-explanatory as possible. Clear guidance shall be present by the use of selection buttons and logical actions.

5c. The system shall contain interactive support that can be used during training.

B. User Interface

1. Graphic User Interface

1a. The interface shall be based on graphic windowing technique.

1b. The system shall have a common user interface that can adapted to future standards for the basic functions of the system.

1c. All functions shall be based upon existing standards, or according to established procedures.

1d. Activation of commands shall be by the use of either a pointing device or from the keyboard.

1e. Irrespective of what procedure/routine or module of the system the user is in, there shall be standard commands that always apply to the same functions.

2. Window Management

2a. The system shall be able to have a number of windows open for the same patient at one time. Patient's identity shall be clearly stated in each window.

3. Shortcuts

3a. A function which enables direct movement to a patient's record, e.g., the ability to "jump" to a specific function or field.

3b. A shortcut for reaching another module for the current patient, patient account, service scheduling, etc.

3c. A quick choice for reaching another patient's record, but with a "read only" restriction. It shall be possible in the system to quickly "set aside" the current record in order to be able to view another patient's record. It shall also be easy to return quickly to the previous record.

3d. It shall be possible to move around easily between specific functions in the record without being tied to navigate up and down in a tree structure.

4. Information Display

4a. It shall be possible to present information in chronological order or reversed chronological order in one sequence and covering all patient's treatments.

4b. It shall be possible to present the information either as source or problem orientated.

4c. It shall be possible to retrieve detailed information from images/clinical investigation.

4d. It shall be possible to present different types of clinical investigations for different staff and patient categories in a flexible way.

4e. It shall be possible to compile and present information via index (key) words.

4f. It shall be possible to use different timeframes in order to increase the overall perspective, for example in the lab list, progress notes, clinical measurements (e.g. weight, fluid and caloric intake, etc.)

5. Selective Display

5a. There should be the possibility to choose the scope of information display broken down into care category and/or per given time period. It should be clearly evident that there is more information available.

6. System Messages

6a. The system shall automatically inform the user the status of message processing, such as printing.

6b. Error messages shall be presented directly on the screen.

6c. All error messages shall be in Swedish.

7. Warning Functions

7a. Warning functions are to be displayed according to directives from the National Board of Health and Welfare SOSF (M) 1982:8 on how non-tolerance and hypersensitivity to medication shall be indicted. For further details see under heading safety/security.

8. Recording Clinical Data

8a. It shall be possible to indicate differing values or medical interactions in the system. The indication shall show at printout or when storing on a different medium. For further details see under heading safety/security.

8b. It shall be possible to record as text important medical, epidemiological, and social facts.

8c. The system shall allow a caregiver to indicate that specific data or text shall only be available to another authorized caregiver and hidden for unauthorized users. A log of each transaction shall be stored. The receiving caregiver shall, when the record is opened be made aware of the fact that information has been received.

9. Word Processing

9a. Simple word processing functions shall be integrated into the system.

9b. Change of font should be avoided. It should only to be done by the system administrator and it is to be common to the unit.

9c. Copying and pasting function may only be used within the same record.

9d. Functions for spelling checking, including medical terminology, shall be available in the system.

10. Contents and Scope

10a. It should be possible to organize the contents and scope of the different parts of the patient record graphically.

C. Data Capture

1. Data Entry Tools

1a. Input shall be possible either by pointing device or from the keyboard.

1b. A scanning function for images and text as image shall be included.

1c. Input shall be possible via bar codes

1d. Input shall be possible via cards with magnetic stripe.

1e. Input shall be possible via smart (chip) cards.

1f. Input shall be possible via optical cards.

1g. Input shall be possible via voice input.

1h. It shall be possible to import files in different file formats, for example EDIFACT, ODA/ODIF, RTF, SGML, SQL2.

1i. It shall be possible to register information via a hand terminal, which then transfers information on-line to the patient record.

2. Mandatory Information

2a. In some forms/images it shall be possible to indicate certain fields as compulsory. In these fields you are required to enter data.

3. Template and Form Design

3a. It shall be possible for users to be able to design their own input templates on delivery of the system and later after the system has become fully operational.

4. Default and Pre-defined Values

4a. There shall be a function in the system that facilities certain fields to be set automatically by the system (default values), date for example. It shall be possible to change these values.

5. Out-of-Range Warning

5a. There shall be a function, which tells the user that he/she tried to register an unreasonable value. A reference value limit value should be presented. Overriding shall be possible.

D. Support Functions

1. Shared Databases

1a. The system shall be able to retrieve information from specialized databases, such as drug reference, population registries, diagnosis registries, etc.

2. Text Recognition

2a. It shall be possible to create text strings linked to a user-defined dictionary/codes that can be retrieved automatically when entering text. These strings can be both personal and/or of a general nature.

3. Automatic Recording of Standard Actions

3a. Health administrative actions such as referrals, prescriptions, medical certificates, and other standard routine actions, shall generate an automatic note under the appropriate index word in the current record referrals. It shall possible to make simple additions or to clarify this note when necessary.

4. Anonymous Patients

4a. The system shall be able to handle patients who do not have a personal identification number.

5. Handling of Alternative Identification Numbers

5a. It shall be possible to use a reserve number if the patient's identity is not known. The system shall have functions to link an alternative number with individual identification numbers, if such a link is requested.

6. Updating of Personal Identity

6a. The record module should facilitate linking of information between an "old" and new identity.

E. Security and Confidentiality

1. Common Requirements

1a. The following laws and regulations shall be followed:

> The Data Act SFS 1973:289, 1992:446.
> The Confidentiality Act SFS 1980. 1989:713, 1991:246, 1992:890.
> The Patient Record Act SFS 1985:562.
> The Archive Regulation.
> The Social Services Act.
> The Support and service Act (LSS). -
> The Data Inspection Board's regulations, general advice.
> National Board of Health and Welfare's regulations (SOSF 1982:8).
> Healthcare Act SFS 1982:763.
> Freedom of the Press Act 1991.1500, SFS 1994:1476.
> Code of Practice for Physicians (Allmänna läkarinstruktionen).
> The Royal Archive Regulations Records.

1b. When there are local rules for handling security issues, these shall be taken into consideration when designing the system.

1c. Deletion of a complete record or a part there of (including backup copy and copies) shall be possible according to the legal requirements that are applicable. It shall be possible to verify that destruction has been has been carried out by log of a transactions.

2. Notes

2a. The system shall be able to handle missed appointments, discontinued medication, hypersensitivity, medication etc.

2b. "Observation Note" shall ensure that a message is to be shown on the screen. The message display shall be so evident that the user is fully aware of the event.   X

3. Access Control and Identification

3a. The system shall have an access control function that includes:

- Identification and authentication of given identification
- Access control to system resources including stored data
- Logging of systems activities.

3b. The access control system function shall be flexible in order to meet law changes and/or changes in the organization. It shall be possible to process an entire health unit as an activity unit for a record or, alternatively, split up into smaller units.

3c. The system shall work with identifiers (user names, codes) that guarantee a unique identification of users, even after a long period of time.

3d. The identifier shall include the full name and preferably the personal identification number.

3e. A shorter form of user id can be used in many functions, but it should to be possible to obtain a reference to the full identification.

3f. The given identity shall be authenticated by a method that corresponds to specific security requirements specified by the user.

3g. It shall be possible to perform strong authentication with smart cards and cryptographic methods (RSA). A European standard for this area is being developed. Temporarily, the ASL specifications made by the Agency for Administrative Development's Allterminal Project should be used. These specifications will be complemented to form a specification for a Swedish electronic identification card.

3h. If strong authentication is used the system should allow single sign-on. The local system/work station shall support secure identification in all functions, both at the level of the operative system and applications, and also with different computers in the network.

3i. If authentication using a password is used, the European standard shall be used. Medical Informatics - Secure User Identification for Health Care: Management and Security of Passwords Health Care Orientated IT Security Functionality Class (CENITC 25 11WG6 N 95-02).

4. Access Control

4a. Access control shall encompass both the operating control system and the database manager and in many cases the applications.

4b. The system shall have such a protective shell that access control is concrete.

4c. The access control shall cover all resources, not only data access. (It is especially important to give attention to the possibilities of copying to a diskette, or the use of communication networks and printers.)

4d. The system shall facilitate access for different users to different functions and data stored in the system.

4e. It shall be possible to combine a shared and a divided record, so that certain parts can be common, a warning list, for example.

4f. Each user shall get access to the functions and information he/she needs to perform his/her task.

4g. Users that need access to the information system in a similar way shall be gathered into one category/role with the same rights in order to facilitate access administration. (Category can involve a general group of staff, such as physicians, nurses within a unit, but can also be a more advanced concept. See below.)

4h. The system should be able to handle the definition of access rights both on the level of single user and on the level of category/role-privilege.

4i. The system shall be able to handle a dynamic role concept for providers that, for example, links a certain number of patients to a group of users (role category). The system shall also contain functions for defining the rights of the group in a simple and safe way and compel individual users to maintain the current role concept for a period of time.

4j. Complex systems should be able to handle a distributed access authorization administration with a central control via special security servers.

4k. The system shall automatically switch off the screen and demand a new authentication with a card or a password after a pre-defined period of inactivity.

4l. The system shall automatically log out after a predefined period of inactivity.

4m. The system should allow a user who logs-in after a forced log-out to return to the previous transaction location without the integrity of the database being threatened.

4n. The system should allow overriding of the normal access rules within certain pre-defined limits. Only users that are securely identified and registered with special authorization will have the right to override the system in the event of a state of emergency. The use of the function shall generate a message direct to the access administrator in charge and be specially recorded in the systems log and in the patient record. The system shall make sure that messages are acknowledged by the access administrator in charge.

5. Classification According to Sensitivity

5a. It shall be possible to classify all pieces of information in the database according to its sensitivity.

5b. It shall be possible to make a basic classification of sensitivity in a catalogue of object classes/keywords or in a catalogue of terms containing attributes that can be applied to a single patient.

5c. It shall be possible to change the classification according to sensitivity when stored in the database.

5d. It shall be possible to control the classification according to sensitivity for an individual patient.

5e. It shall be possible to control access to information so that only the chosen care giver(s) get access to it.

5f. Classification according to sensitivity means that for certain groups of users the information will be filtered during search and presentation. The user shall be made aware of the fact that this is being done, without sensitive information being revealed.

5g. It shall be possible to classify data in other ways, as local/global information, for example. The local information is available within the local unit, the global is available for several units.

6. Logging

6a. The system should log all usage with start and finishing times.

6b. It shall be possible to control logging of activities with respect to: unit, category, role, time period or function including the amount of data involved.

6c. It shall be possible to control logging concerning a single patient.

6d. The system shall be able to log whatever part of a database that has been affected by reading and writing.

6e. There shall be tools for follow-up of the audit trail.

7. Security Protection for External Communication

7a. Data shall always be encrypted when it is communicated outside a safe physical domain.

7b. Fiberoptic cabling for all main networks should be used when control over cabling is not satisfactory.

7c. Separation of different security domains with routers that allow control of access lists. For Internet connection "firewalls" should be used in each server.

8. Data Integrity

8a. The system shall include a signing function.

8b. The system shall facilitate counter signing for certain types of data, for example discharge notes. There shall also be the possibility for making a "vidi mark" (vidi = I have seen).

8c. The system shall make sure that medical information is signed with a reminder to the person responsible for the registration. It should also be possible to get an overview of the different types of notes that are waiting to be signed/counter signed/vidi-marked.

8d. If signing is not done within a certain time there shall be the possibility of locking the text automatically.

8e. It must be evident if record information is signed, locked or open (unsigned).

8f. Erasure or changing locked or signed text shall be marked on the screen and printouts and all earlier versions shall be retraceable.

8g. The signing function must clearly make the person aware of the fact that he/she is responsible for the contents.

8h. It shall be possible to perform signing by digital signature and a user's smart (chip) card.

9. Accountability and Reliability

9a. The system shall make sure that the system makes backup copies regularly.

9b. The system shall have protective functions against voltage irregularity.

9c. It should be possible to run the system without main power supply for a short period of time.

F. Output

1. Report Generator

1a. The system shall have a report generator, which makes it possible the concomitant search by several criteria/keywords.

1b. It shall be possible to generate several reports while without significantly influencing the system's performance.

1c. The search template shall be reported as an appendix to the requested/produced report.

1d. It shall be possible to store for later use the defined search criteria. It shall be possible to give the reports understandable names.

2. Standard Reports

2a. Pre-defined standard reports shall be delivered together with the record module.

3. Export Function

3a. It shall be possible to export data (file transfer) to other modules, systems and programs according to current rules, taking into account current laws and regulations. This shall only be possible at the system administration level.

3b. It shall be possible to remove patient identifiers from all information that is exported.

4. Record Printouts

4a. The length of the printouts shall not be predefined in the record module, but shall be flexible, for example, the whole report, chosen parts, lab list, medications list etc.

4b. It shall be possible to discontinue the printout with a simple command.

4c. Date, time, who is responsible for the decision to release the information, who requested the printout, what has been transferred and who is the receiver of the printout should automatically be registered in the record and presented on the printout.

4d. When record information is printed on paper, it should be evident on the printout if it is signed or not.

4e. The system shall contain form, letter, work and support templates, death certificates, and other standard document formats. The system should accept pre-printed forms or plain paper.

4f. The system shall be able to produce documents that are based on SPRI's basic record concept.

5. Follow-up, Quality Assurance, Evaluation, and Target Results Achievement

5a. Follow-up of treatment and results of treatment shall be possible via access to the patient database aided by a report generator. The same access control used for the patient record module will be utilized.

5b. It shall be possible to plan individual care schemes and then follow up the result by individual patient.

5c. It shall be possible to define and register treatments/actions and time spent per treatment/action. It shall be possible to sum up the time spent by patient, intervention, provider, and diagnosis.

6. Labels and Barcodes

6a. The patient record module shall support functions and barcodes for printing labels.

6b. It shall be possible to add barcodes to labels and other documents with bar codes containing the patient's identity.

7. Archive Function

7a. The system shall have functions for the transfer of information to a different storage medium. When the information is extracted from the system there shall be references in the record system module, which gives information about where the information can be found.

7b. There shall be a surveillance function that automatically transfers information to a different storage medium if the record has not been activated during a preset timeframe.

G. Communication

1. Communication with Other Systems

1a. The system shall be able electronically to exchange information with other modules/systems, such as primary care, in and outpatient care, and dental care. The transfer shall be done according to set standards.

1b. There shall be the possibility of having a master index for x-ray images, photographs, audiograms etc.

2. Decision Support Systems

2a. Should be an independent module where the record system can retrieve pertinent information.

2b. Integrated with the record system and thereby acting as an interactive support for decision making.

3. Individual Patient Medical Images

3a. It shall be possible to store individual images in the record module of the patient.

4. Templates

4a. To be able to visualize where a clinical change is located, there shall be functions to show templates over the different parts of the human body. It shall be possible to add marks and save those.

5. Multimedia

5a. It shall be possible to show video clips via the patient record system.

5b. It shall be possible to record and reproduce different clinical sounds in the system.

5c. Hypertext facilities, i.e. to able to click on separate words in free text and get further information, for example a dictionary, protocol, image, video.

H. Record Structure

1. Term-based/Keyword Structuring

1a. Record notes shall be structured in the form of predefined terms and keywords. Each term/keyword shall have a unique code, which is made up of a searchable key in a patient database. It shall be possible to define terms and keywords hierarchically so that a complex term may be built up of several simple terms. Keyword notes shall be related to time and the person responsible for the note and be connected to a logical unit, for example a signing-in note or reception. It shall be possible to have terms and keywords oriented to problems (problem-oriented).

2. Database of National Terms

2a. Concepts, terms and keywords shall originate from a national database, which is to be fully, or partly housed in the system. Updating to later versions of the national database shall be possible.

3. Patient Record Module

3a. The patient record module shall be able to exchange record information with a process-oriented health administrative module. This shall facilitate planning, target implementation, surveillance, results, evaluation, and started and finished treatment plans.

4. Nursing Documentation

4a. It shall be possible to document nursing history, status diagnosis, targets, and nursing plan. It shall also be   possible to register nursing results and record discharge notes for each patient.

4b. It shall be possible to enter nurses notes, including procedures, intravenous therapy, medication, and checklists for patients.

5. Classification/Coding Systems

5a. It shall be possible to implement different established coding schemes, such as ICD, ICIHD, SNOMED etc.

5b. It shall be possible to include local user-defined classification and coding schemes.

5c. The system shall allow recording of time per activity.

5d. The system shall allow validation against entered records.

5e. There shall not be any limitations in the number of codes that can be registered in the system.

5f. There shall not be any limitations in the number of items that the system is able to reserve. This will enable own detailing of codes to be made.

5g. It shall be possible to give a diagnosis in plain text and code with information about main diagnosis, and secondary diagnoses, procedures, etc.

5h. It shall be possible mark the diagnosis with certain qualifiers: preliminary, single sided, right sided, left-sided etc.

5i. The system shall enable plain text attached to the diagnosis code to be edited when entering patient data. It shall be possible to store both code and plain text. The basic register shall not be changed.

6. Notes Without Visit

6a. It shall be possible to make notes without there being a visit registered on the patient, for example by letter, telephone prescriptions and telephone contact.

I. Documentation

1.Training

1a. When delivered the system shall contain a training database in normal environment together with easy-to use instructions in Swedish.

1b. The system shall be built in such a way that it is as self-instructional as possible.

2. Installation Instructions

2a. There shall be detailed installation instructions in Swedish.

3. User Documentation

3a. There shall be an instruction manual in Swedish.

4. Troubleshooting

4a. There shall be a chapter on troubleshooting in the user documentation.

4b. There shall be a troubleshooting quick table including clear solutions, including detailed explanation on how to deal with encountered problems.

5. System Reference Manual

5a. There should be a detailed technical reference manual in manual for the system.

6. Help Function

6a. There shall be help functions in Swedish on forms, functions, as well as at the entry field level.

7. Operating Procedures

7a. In the operating documentation it shall be described how to enter basic data.

8. Technical Documentation

8a. In the technical description it shall be described how auxiliary equipment is connected to the system.

9. Data Model

9a. The data model shall describe objects and terms that occur in the system.

10. Protocols

10a. It shall be the possible of including treatment and procedure protocols and patient instructions in the system.

J. Special Requirement for Psychiatric Care

1. Surveillance and Alarm Functions

1a. Alarm functions for handling legal aspects of psychiatric care shall be included.

1b. The system shall be able to handle routines in connection with reporting to the National Board of Health and Welfare.

1c. It shall be possible in the system to record the risk of violent behavior, enforcement actions, risk of suicide, etc.

K. Special Requirements for Paramedical Activity

1. Follow-up, Quality Assurance, Evaluation, and Target Results Achievement

1a. The possibility to follow up treatment and results of treatment, individual care plans, flow of referrals, queuing times by cause for contact or diagnosis, number of patients, time spent by action, etc., linked to a report generator.

2. Care and Rehabilitation

2a. When entering patient data there shall be access to pre-defined general care programs and rehabilitation plans related to specific diagnoses.

3. Classification Standards

3a. It shall be possible to detail present coding within the officially adopted classification of interventions and procedures.

3b. The system shall allow time spent per action to be recorded.

4. Rehabilitation Equipment

4a. The system shall include a registration function for equipment including surveillance, tracking, and reminder handling.

5. Home Care

5a. The system shall include support for local programs with instructions, data banks with exercises and examples or rehabilitation programs.

REFERENCE 5

White Paper
Health Insurance Portability and Accountability Act: Security Standards; Implications for the Healthcare Industry

Shannah Koss, Program Manager, IBM Government and Healthcare

This white paper is for general informational purposes only and does not constitute advice by IBM as to any particular actual set of facts, nor does this white paper represent any undertaking by IBM to provide customers with legal advice. Instead, this white paper is designed only to get customers started in understanding the *Health Insurance Portability and Accountability Act (HIPAA) Security Standards*. Therefore, IBM encourages customers to seek competent legal counsel for advice. Note that there is no established schedule for updating this white paper, and IBM is not responsible for the content or frequency of updates.

HIPAA Security Standards

Introduction

Federal security standards and the increased use of the Internet and web technologies in healthcare will require changes in the healthcare industry's information security practices. Whether we like it or not, these changes are inevitable. This paper provides some background information about the emerging Federal requirements, industry implications, and the actions that will be required.

Background

Why focus on Healthcare Security now? The regulatory climate and the increasing use of the Internet

The Health Insurance Portability and Accountability Act (HIPAA), perhaps better known as the Kennedy Kassebaum bill, was passed on August 21, 1996. HIPAA contained a section called Administrative Simplification, which was:

> "intended to reduce the costs and administrative burdens of health care by making possible the standardized, electronic transmission of many administrative and financial transactions that are currently carried out manually on paper."

The Administrative Simplification provisions of HIPAA call for: EDI transaction standards; unique health identifiers for each individual, employer, health plan and healthcare provider; security standards; and, privacy legislation. The logic behind the set of requirements was that standards and unique identifiers would facilitate the exchange of information needed throughout the care delivery system. Making these transactions easier, however, may increase the risk of inappropriate access to sensitive information. Consequently HIPAA also calls for security standards and privacy legislation.

The security standards apply to claims clearinghouses, health plans, employers and healthcare providers; i.e., "any other person furnishing health care services or supplies" (other than those under the statutory definition of "provider") that maintain or transmit automated health information. The purpose section, the security subsection, and the wrongful disclosure penalty section of HIPAA are contained in Appendix A.

The Health Care Financing Administration (HCFA), in the Department of Health and Human Services, is responsible for implementing the Administrative Simplification requirements through notice and comment rulemaking. HCFA developed a draft security matrix and proposed rules that capture the requirements and implementation features the healthcare industry will be expected to meet. HCFA has categorized these requirements as — administrative procedures; physical safeguards; technical security services and technical mechanisms — to guard data integrity, confidentiality and availability. Although the requirements in these categories overlap, they are intended to help organizations understand the different types of requirements needed for a comprehensive security approach.

The core requirements are as follows:

Certification	Media controls
Chain of trust partner agreement	Physical access controls
Contingency plan	Policy/guideline on work station use
Formal mechanism for processing records	Secure work station location
Information access control	Security awareness training
Internal audit	Access control (context based)
Personnel security	Audit controls
Security incident procedures	Authorization control
Security configuration management	Data authentication
Termination procedures	Entity authentication
Training	Communication network controls
Assigned security responsibilities	Digital signature

In the current documents, all requirements, except digital signature, must be addressed for **"All entities, regardless of size, involved with electronic health information pertaining to an individual"**. Recognizing that an industry consensus on security standards does **not** exist, HCFA is trying to establish a flexible framework for security practices that meet the goals of security without prescribing the means. Proposed rules codifying the matrix were published on August 12, 1998. The public comment period ended October 13, 1998. Final rules had a statutory deadline of February 21, 1998, 18 months after the law was passed, the agency has let the time frame slip, but it appears we could have final rules by mid to late 1999. Depending upon their size, plans and providers will have 2 or 3 years from the date the final rules are published to comply. Small plans as defined in the rules will have 36 months to comply. HCFA also has discretion to take into account the needs and capabilities of small and rural healthcare providers (to be defined in the rules) in adopting the security standards; however, the proposed rules did not include any distinct treatment with respect to the compliance time frame.

The HIPAA statute establishes two sets of penalties: one set is for "Failure to comply with requirements and standards" and the second set is for "wrongful disclosure of individually identifiable health information." Penalties for noncompliance are a maximum of $100 for each violation not to exceed $25,000 per year. For "a person who knowingly" discloses individually identifiable health information, however, the penalties range from $50,000-$250,000 in fines and one to ten years in prison. It remains to be seen whether "knowingly" ignoring the rules and failing to establish a security program might be interpreted as "knowingly" causing such a disclosure if it were to occur.

Coincidental to the changing regulatory environment, the healthcare Industry is moving toward consumer and provider online exchange of information. The Internet and intranets are increasingly part of the healthcare IT environment. The use of the Internet in healthcare has heightened anxieties about inappropriate access to healthcare records. The preamble of the proposed rule states: "When using open networks some form of encryption should be employed." Consequently use of the Internet warrants closer scrutiny of the security between internal and external networks.

Privacy, Confidentiality and Security

There is often confusion about the difference between privacy, confidentiality and security. In the context of HIPAA, privacy determines who should have access, what constitutes the patients rights to confidentiality, and what constitutes inappropriate access to health records. Security establishes how the records should be protected from inappropriate access, in other words the means by which you ensure privacy and confidentiality.

HIPAA called for the Secretary of Health and Human Services to submit recommendations to Congress "on standards with respect to the privacy of individually identifiable health information." Congress has until August 21, 1999 to pass privacy legislation pursuant to HIPAA, otherwise the Secretary shall issue final privacy rules by February 21, 2000. The Secretary's recommendations were submitted to Congress on September 11, 1997. They can be downloaded from the HHS website at http://aspe.os.hhs.gov/admnsimp/pvcrec0.htm. Several bills have been introduced in Congress; passage of a law may occur during the current Congress. In any case, it is likely there will be Federal privacy requirements by the year 2000.

Regardless of the timing for Federal privacy requirements, healthcare organizations will need to develop their own confidentiality and privacy policies to have a meaningful security program. In other words, healthcare organizations have to decide who is authorized to have access to identifiable healthcare information, for what purposes, and under what conditions if security plans, policies and procedures are going to have any meaning. Even with a Federal law the level of specificity will not be determined at the institutional level. Developing these policies will facilitate the development of a healthcare organization's security program.

Implications of the Security Standards for the Healthcare Industry

The healthcare industry, like most industries with the possible exception of banking, has not addressed information security in a comprehensive manner. Most healthcare organizations have security features in their information systems. Yet many organizations do not have written policies or procedures for their employees that are authorized to access the information, such as policies on disclosure of sensitive information or personnel policies dictating the types of personnel actions that will be taken if staff members violate the policies. This is not a criticism of the industry, but rather an observation. It describes the extension of information systems into areas that were once paper-based where there was less concern for security because people believed only authorized personnel had access. Automating paper records didn't naturally call for security that wasn't there in the first place. The fear that automated records will make inappropriate access easier for someone intent on gaining access is what has driven the industry to start developing comprehensive security programs.

Automated medical information also highlights concerns about information availability, particularly as more clinical information is stored electronically. Ensuring information availability through appropriate access and data integrity (i.e., knowing that the information in an organization's systems has not been inappropriately or inadvertently changed and that it is not at risk of being lost if the system fails) may be as important as confidentiality. Part of the Administrative Simplification provisions' stated purpose is "encouraging the development of a health information system." Such a system is intended to support access to critical health information when and where it is needed. Automated information systems can support the real-time availability of information on drug allergies, current complicating illnesses and urgent lab results in a way that paper records never could. Information systems can only ensure availability if the systems are working and the information is not easily changed. The goal of information availability supports the proposed HCFA requirement for a contingency plan that includes disaster recovery, an emergency mode operation plan, and a data backup plan.

HCFA's proposed standards imply that healthcare organizations will develop security programs that include technological solutions, but recognize that the persistent risk, regardless of the level of technical security, is through the people who have authorized access rather than "hackers". Consequently a number of the standards address personnel and physical site access, e.g., personnel security, training, termination procedures for both physical and system access and physical access controls.

The planning, policies and procedures driven by the standards will perhaps have the most dramatic effect on healthcare organizations because they will have to develop enterprise-wide security programs and gain organizational support for the programs. It will not be sufficient to have a variety of policies and procedures in each department that may or may not be explicit, documented or known by the rest of the organization. With or without privacy requirements, organizations should review more closely who has access to which information and establish policies and accountability for these decisions. With potential penalties as high as $250,000 and 10 years in prison, not to mention the negative publicity, it behooves everyone to take a proactive approach to security.

The new security standards, once finalized, will probably not have as great an impact on information systems. Most of the technologies needed for compliance are readily available. HCFA has made a conscious decision to not specify technology. HCFA expects healthcare organizations to determine the appropriate technical solutions on the basis of their risk analysis and the level of vulnerability the organization is willing to tolerate. More complex information technology environments may require more attention and internally developed systems may require custom solutions.

The security standards and HCFA's Internet policy may have a significant impact on one information system decision: whether to use the Internet or a private secure network. Effective on November 24, 1998, the HCFA Internet Security Policy removes the prior ban on use of the Internet for transmitting Medicare beneficiary information. However, policy guidelines require that encryption and authentication or identification procedures be used for Internet transmission of HCFA Privacy Act-protected and/or other sensitive HCFA information. These added requirements may tip the balance of the decision in favor of a private network.

As noted previously, HCFA indicated encryption should be employed for open networks. In addition, although digital signature is optional, it is viewed as one of the best means of authentication. Given the pressure on the healthcare industry to enable Internet access, particularly for consumers and practitioners, encryption and digital signature will be a significant technical requirement. Establishing sufficient public key infrastructure and certificate management services that can readily operate across all information technology platforms will be an industry challenge. Interoperability pilots are being developed pursuant to the HCFA Internet policy to help address this challenge.

Another significant technical requirement may be the audit controls and the "accountability (tracking) mechanism." Industry representatives are already expressing concerns that a 100% audit trail of all actions affecting any identifiable records wlll add significant costs to automated health records. This issue is likely to be a topic of debate in the proposed rule public comment process with privacy advocates on the side of complete audit information and industry advocates calling for exception auditing, i.e., mechanisms that track actions that are not consistent with the expected uses of an application or system. At present HCFA is not planning to stipulate the extent of the audit requirement, again relying on the organization's determination regarding the level of appropriate auditing. Certain types of information may warrant 100% audit trail, for instance, organizations may want to closely monitor access to AIDS or substance abuse information.

Some technological developments may significantly change the way people access systems, such as, biometric authentication. It will not be required by the standards, but may emerge as a healthcare industry preference for controlling access by unauthorized users. The advantage of a biometric access control is that it can't be lost, does not require memorizing one of many access codes, and can be linked to site security as well as system security. It is clear that technical breakthroughs such as this will continue to offer methods for addressing inappropriate access once an organization has determined who is or isn't authorized.

For now, time is on the side of those in the industry that see these requirements as just an additional burden that the government has placed upon the industry. Some, however, see this as an inevitable evolution of the information age if we want and expect people to carry out routine and critical business in a network environment. Given that we have two years from the time final rules are issued and the public comment period for the proposed rules recently ended, we can estimate an additional six months to start planning. If healthcare organizations start building security into their strategic planning, they should be able to comply with the requirements without the added expense of a last minute rush.

Next Steps

Depending upon the scope and complexity of the healthcare organization and its information technology environment, compliance with the HIPAA security standards could be quite time consuming. Although the final technical solution may be relatively simple, the security program design and facilitating organizational buy-in to security plans, policies and procedures suggests starting now.

Getting Started

First, assign at least one individual with primary responsibility for security. The person should probably be 100% dedicated, unless it is a very small organization. Although many organizations will tend to choose someone in their IT organization, think about someone with broader responsibilities that can speak to the personnel and administrative requirements as well as the IT solutions. In other words, select someone with authority and visibility in the organization or give them direct reporting responsibilities to a senior executive in the organization.

Next, create a security team that has representation from throughout the organization charging all relevant departments with responsibility for individual health information. This team should help develop the security program and support buy-in within the organization. The team's first task should be to review current policies, procedures and solutions against the most current documentation regarding the emerging security standards to assess how significant an undertaking compliance will be for the organization. Based on this assessment, determine whether the organization has the skills and resources to drive this effort internally or should seek external expertise. Compliance with the security standards has one noted similarity to Year 2000. Security skills and resources are scarce and demand will only increase as the compliance deadline approaches.

Whether the organization chooses to do it in-house or with the help of outside expertise, once a high level assessment of the gaps between the present security initiatives and the standards is completed, a recommended step would be the risk analysis — a required implementation feature of the proposed security management process standard which HCFA currently defines as:

> "a process whereby cost-effective security/control measures may be selected by balancing the cost of various security/control measures against the losses that would be expected if these measures were not in place".

This step should help set parameters for an organization's security program and define its priorities.

With these initial steps and all subsequent steps, be sure actions and decisions are documented. It will only be through documentation that an organization can demonstrate it has addressed many of the requirements.

To be notified regarding the HIPAA implementing rules including the security standards send e-mail to: listserv@list.nih.gov with "HIPAA-REGS *your name*" in the body of the text and no other text or trailers.

For more information on the Administrative Simplification standards go to http://aspe.os.dhhs.gov/adminsimp.

Appendix A

"SEC. 261. PURPOSE.

It is the purpose of this subtitle to improve the Medicare program under title XVIII of the Social Security Act, the Medicaid program under title XIX of such Act, and the efficiency and effectiveness of the healthcare system, by encouraging the development of a health information system through the establishment of standards and requirements for electronic transmission of certain health information."

SEC. 1173. *****

"(D) SECURITY STANDARDS FOR HEALTH INFORMATION.—

(1) SECURITY STANDARDS.—The Secretary shall adopt security standards that—

(A) take into account—

(i) the technical capabilities of record systems used to maintain health information;

(ii) the costs of security measures;

(iii) the need for training persons who have access to health information;

(iv) the value of audit trails in computerized record systems; and

(v) the needs and capabilities of small health care providers and rural health care providers (as such providers are defined by the Secretary); and

(B) ensure that a health care clearinghouse, if it is part of a larger organization, has policies and security procedures which isolate the activities of the health care clearinghouse with respect to processing information in a manner that prevents unauthorized access to such information by such larger organization.

(2) SAFEGUARDS.—Each person described in section 1172(a) who maintains or transmits health information shall maintain reasonable and appropriate administrative, technical, and physical safeguards—

(A) to ensure the integrity and confidentiality of the information;

(B) to protect against any reasonably anticipated—

(i) threats or hazards to the security or integrity of the information; and

(ii) unauthorized uses or disclosures of the information; and

(C) otherwise to ensure compliance with this part by the officers and employees of such person."

"Wrongful Disclosure of Individually Identifiable Health Information

SEC. 1177. (A) Offense. - a person who knowingly and in violation of this part-
(1) Uses or causes to be used a unique health identifier;
(2) Obtains individually identifiable health information relating to an individual; or ,
(3) Discloses individually identifiable health information to another person, shall be punished as provided in subsection (B).
(B) Penalties.- A person described in subsection (A) shall-
(1) Be fined not more than $50,000, imprisoned not more than 1 year, or both;
(2) If the offense is committed under false pretenses, be fined not more than $100,000, imprisoned not more than 5 years, or both; and
(3) If the offense is committed with the intent to sell, transfer, or use individually identifiable health information for advantage, personal gain, or malicious harm, be fined not more than $250,000, imprisoned not more than 10 years, or both."

PART B
*Information Systems and
Information Technology Solutions*

B

Section B1
*Healthcare Information Systems
Outlook*

Section B2
*Information Systems and Technology
Implementation Issues*

Section B3
*Information Systems and Information
Technology Planning Phases*

Section B4
*Defining a Successful
Implementation*

Section B5
*Health Informatics –
Who Leads, Who Represents?*

Part B. Information Systems and Information Technology Solutions

B

Part B. Information Systems and Information Technology Solutions

There are three roads to ruin; women, gambling and technicians.
the most pleasant is with women, the quickest is with gambling,
but the surest is with technicians.

Georges Pompidou (1911–1974)

This section aims to forecast the direction of automation for health services information systems. An inclusive view of the likely technological trends can provide the health services manager and IS&T professional with a useful roadmap for planning the implementation. One central assumption of any information systems design and implementation is that all viable systems must align themselves with the growing trend toward placing the patient at the center of the health services delivery process.

B.1. Healthcare Information Systems Outlook

To provide a sound basis for a high-quality health service, first and foremost healthcare organizations need sufficient and capable staff working in adequate facilities. It also needs proper work processes, including processes for monitoring and improving clinical and service quality essentials. Given those essentials there is now worldwide evidence that modern information and communication technologies can increasingly make a dramatic improvement to healthcare quality. Why is this changing?

The focus of research, applications, and investment in systems has shifted during the 1990's from replacing clerical work to direct clinical support. Similarly, in communication technologies the focus has shifted from sending simple point-to-point messages about laboratory results, for example, to the creation of virtual electronic health records. The use of mobile computing means these can be created and accessible from almost any point. Finally, using large databases to pull together data from health, social, and economic sources at a fraction of their former costs means that the combined health histories of millions of people can be used to predict the future health needs of any given population and to allocate and prioritize resources accordingly. Informatics contribution to the quality of care is therefore about both individuals and populations (Figure 1).

B.1.1. Healthcare Information Networks

From the information perspective, the term "Healthcare Information Network" (HIN) describes many combined systems functions that utilize communication technologies, singly or in concert, to meet the needs of a specific client. HIN applications can provide health services information and integrated functionalities within an institution or throughout multiple institutions and can provide the technical foundation for managing and concurrently accessing clinical and administrative information throughout the continuum of care. It can provide the framework and applications whereby all stakeholders share patient and population information.

Figure 1. Advanced Informatics Improves Quality and Gains

Degree of Sophistication

Cumulative Levels of Healthcare Services Information Systems	Illustrative Improvements in Quality of Care
6. Advanced multimedia and telematics Continuous and remote clinical monitoring Diagnostic images shared remotely for diagnosis and Review Single complete patient record instantly available Improved access to remote expert diagnosis	Immediate alerts to problems Easier access to expert opinion Previous history always available Reduced travelling time and journeys for patients Remote but more frequent, home-care monitoring Images recorded for progress reviews
5. Specialty specific support (shared care system for diabetes, asthma and children, pathways with automated rules-based alerts and prompts, electronic images)	Extensive and detailed pathways set out best practice Faster and more accurate diagnosis Formalized, rapid, and comprehensive communications Greater patient participation in care
4. Clinical knowledge and decision support (simple alerts and prompts, on-line access to knowledge bases, multi-disciplinary care planning)	Immediate access to expert knowledge Alerts to possible drug interactions Faster and more accurate diagnosis Care planning more consistent and complete
3. Clinical activities support (ICU, renal, cardiology services, order-communications systems, electronic prescribing)	Shorter hospital stay Fewer prescribing errors More consistent care Warnings of variations from agreed care plans
2. Integrated clinical diagnostic and treatment support (Pathology & Radiology Systems)	Rapid access to previous diagnostic results and reports Fewer lost case notes Less waiting for new test results
1. Clinical administrative support (Patient Administration System)	Less repetition of personal details Less patient waiting

B.1.1.1. Healthcare Information Network Design

Healthcare information networked applications enable healthcare providers to have up-to-date information on care and services provided to patients — whether they are treated or seen in the family practitioner's office, a specialist's clinic, an inpatient health service, or an emergency facility.

The Healthcare Information Network (HIN) provides an architecture and infrastructure to meet the information needs of numerous constituents. Equally important, it should be designed to be scalable to support the needs of a growing managed care organization, payer, provider, or integrated delivery network.

In a multi-institution environment, HIN can provide the electronic framework to share information and business processes among providers, payers, employers, government agencies, and others touched by the health delivery system, even patients themselves. HIN applications allow integrated delivery networks formed of partners in contracting relationships to manage this "virtual institution" without compromise of data and information availability. In a single institution environment, such network can provide the framework to share information and business processes among departments with disparate information systems and provides the ability to extend information access to physician partners.

Another advantage of a properly designed information network is that it should not require the overhaul of participants' current information systems. Network architects should make every attempt to protect the investment in pre-existing information infrastructure and applications, and end-users need to interact with different legacy environments in a common "look-and-feel" interface. In some cases, this can actually increase the useful life of their current information systems applications.

Research in leading-edge health services institutions around the world has identified these major categories of potential benefits that accrue to the institution establishing a Healthcare Information Network (HIN), ideally including a Computer-based Patient Record (CPR):

- *Improved Clinical Quality* - Physicians, nurses, therapists, and other caregivers, armed with up-to-date information at the points of care, can provide better-quality care in the clinical setting. In addition, it is generally recognized that over the long term, better and more complete clinical data available electronically will produce improved outcomes.

- *Reduced Costs* - Health services institutions can increase administrative efficiency, lower medical costs, and achieve real labor savings by using the network to perform time-consuming manual chores. This is particularly true of traditionally cross-institution transactions such as referrals, claims, eligibility, and even clinical data.

- *Improved Customer Service* - Health services institutions can use the network to provide better, faster information over telephone help lines, reduce waiting time in doctors' offices, and avoid repeated filling out of forms by pre-populating them with information from the HIN.

B.1.1.2. Features of a Healthcare Information Network

Some of the key features of a capable HIN are:

- *Global Registration* - This application overlays or "front-ends" other registration and admission applications. It addresses numerous user requirements including: common access to disparate admission and registration applications; the ability to register a patient for services from remote locations such as physicians' offices or clinics; and simplified registration across multiple systems technologies.

- *Professional Communication* - This provides the ability to communicate with any user on the network through e-mail, bulletin board services for common areas of interest, announcements, and general broadcast information, fax server capabilities to communicate or transmit information from the network to users who are not electronically connected (such as faxing a referral request to a physician who is not connected to the network), and gateway capabilities to other non-HIN electronic mail facilities.

- *Claims Management* - This supports the ability to access, upload, transmit, and support response processing of standard claims forms from physicians, health services institutions, and other provider settings to payers, managed care plans, government plans, and other entities providing payer functions.

- *Clinical Documentation* - This provides authorized users the ability to access clinical information from the source repository/data store of that information, including laboratory results, dictated reports from transcription systems, radiology results, etc. (This can be used in lieu of a fully fledged CPR.)

- *Master Patient Index* - These applications provide an indexing mechanism to identify people and other items of interest throughout the network. The index creates a unique identification number which is "mapped" to all other known identifiers about the item of interest. It provides the ability for the end user to identify a patient in the network by the identifier that the user knows. This makes all the other identifiers, by which that patient may be known in other applications, transparent to the end user. It provides the institution the ability to maintain multiple identifiers to support operations in different user environments, while minimizing invasiveness of legacy applications. It also has the ability to map information of interest throughout the extended health services institution, including physician offices, clinics, health services institutions, payers, employers, and governmental agencies, and the ability to map to different legacy application identifiers both within institution and inter-institution.

- *Health Administration* - These applications provide many aspects of administrative processing of patients and their associated information as they progress through their encounters with the health delivery system. Business issues addressed with these applications include: capturing information only once, at the point of service, and making it available throughout the patient encounter; making information available to the next logical user of the data (workflow support); and smoothing the entire patient encounter with the health system by making information available for verification, rather than requiring redundant capture.

- *Clinical Management* -These are the applications summarily described in the previous section as the components of the Computer-based Patient Record, the key component of a HIN.

B.1.2. First Steps to Integration of Information

Strategies to integrate information around a patient-centered HIN must focus on the establishment of an alliance of stakeholders, restructuring the value chain of healthcare information, and advancing the sometimes challenging process of defining, standardizing, and automating clinical and administrative data elements.

B.1.2.1. Integrating Stakeholders

In order to migrate to a more efficient, patient-centered focus, a linkage must be established among different stakeholders:

- *Employers* - Who wish to provide quality care programs at reasonable costs while minimizing their administrative workload;

- *Payers* - Who want to know the outcome of their members' interactions with the healthcare system — including cost, quality, and patient satisfaction;

- *Managed Care Organizations and Other Health Insuring Institutions* - That are structuring their offerings using new risk assumptions — that is, determining the most cost-effective quality of care in a capitated reimbursement environment;

- *Public Awareness Groups and Local Health Departments and Their Affiliates* - That are promoting wellness, selfcare, primary healthcare, childhood immunizations, preventive interventions, and other programs;

- *Governmental Organizations* - Determined to ensure universal access to quality healthcare while reducing escalating;

- *Direct Healthcare Professionals* - The focal point of patient treatment information, who need easy access to all types of clinical information that can be shared with their colleagues for consults and retrieval across a patient's continuum of access to the health delivery system.

Increasingly, healthcare providers, payers, employers, and governmental officials are realizing that only by working together and sharing patient information can they create the efficiencies in the healthcare system that will contribute to lower costs and to improved services, access, and quality. With the emphasis on providing services across the continuum of care, providers now consider not only how to serve their patients, but what underlies their health conditions. They want to know how well medical interventions worked, if their patients require additional treatments, and the relative effectiveness of different treatments in dealing with disease processes. In short, they require information on every aspect of a person's medical history, from wellness to critical care.

B.1.2.2. Restructuring the Health Services Information Value Chain

Even more anticipated than the traditional assembly of benefits listed above is the ability of healthcare managers to use the vast quantity of comprehensive data coupled to the new software applications, in a way that can dramatically add value to the healthcare process.

Figure 2 illustrates how different categories of health services information supply different levels of value to the process. At the lower value end, the institution simply deals with administrative and financial data, and is satisfied with fragmented, single-department data. Frequently the analysis is strictly retrospective, and its main concern is related to reimbursement for the transactions associated with the services provided for each episode of care.

Moving up one level, the institution launching the Computer-based Patient Record can amass clinical data in real time that centers on the patient. At the next level, the institution integrates financial and clinical data to focus on health improvements and the evaluation and design of best clinical practices and outcomes. At the highest level, the comprehensive patient-centered database is used to focus the health services institution on wellness.

Figure 2. Health Services Information Technology Value Chain

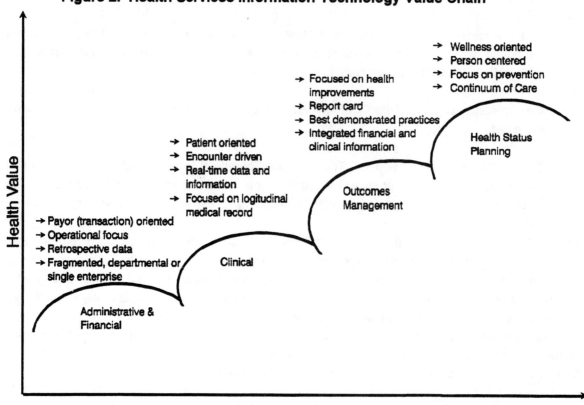

At each level, the value of information increases, since at each higher level the information can simultaneously work to improve patient care while lowering overall healthcare costs, and provide improved services levels to customers. As the sophistication of health services IS&T progresses, so will its ability to provide information to the health services institution that enables it to refocus its efforts on prevention of disease, rather than treatment, wellness instead of illness, and integration of the continuum of care, rather than isolated episodes.

Health services institutions must strike a balance between long-term strategies and near-term tactics. Many health services institutions, whether traditional health services institutions, outpatient treatment centers, or health maintenance organizations, find themselves focused on automation of the traditional applications such as departmental systems, medical records, and other well-defined functions. For such reason this document gives strong emphasis to this traditional portfolio of applications, but doing so in the light of the forecasted direction of the healthcare industry and its IS&T support systems.

B.1.2.3. Automation of Data Elements

The study of health services data has shown a spectrum of automation ranging, on the one hand, from data not yet collected, to data fully automated and standardized. As illustration, Figure 3 provides a depiction of the current availability, automation, and standardization of common data elements in a typical U.S. health institution. In the diagram, the concentric circles represent degrees of automation, standardization, and accessibility of health data.

- The most highly automated data are in the center circle, representing data that are machine-readable and consistently coded across every subsystem. Unfortunately, only a limited number of data types currently meet this threshold.

- The next circle represents data that are manipulated by the typical health information system, but for which there is still no consistent coding scheme.

- Data in the third circle also lack consistent coding, but usually reside in stand-alone information systems.

- The fourth circle includes data that today is recorded only on paper, with no standard format or coding.

- Finally, the outermost circle includes data that would be useful for performance measurement, may reside in non-health information systems, and are generally not recorded in health services information systems.

For each level there is a list of data types that are generally appropriate for that level of automation. For example, progress notes are rarely computerized. They are included in the list associated with the circle for data in paper records. Pharmacy data are commonly automated in the pharmacy provider's system, but are not always incorporated into health databases.

**Figure 3. A Model of Common Data Elements in Health Organizations
Categorized According to Degree of Automation**

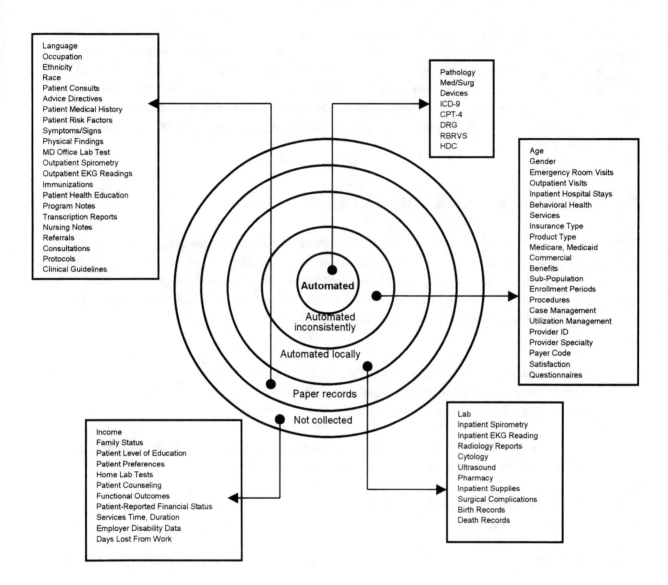

It is likely that in the health services institutions of many Latin American and Caribbean countries, the automation of data has yet to approach even this level of organization. A study of data automation in the Region would likely produce a spectrum comparable to the level of organization of the health services, wherein the wealthiest countries would be those with the highest level of data automation. The challenge for growing health services IS&T systems is to provide more and more automated data for information-intensive clinical and administrative systems.

B.1.3. Patient-centered Vision of Computer Records

The characteristics outlined thus far allow us to claim with certainty that solutions for information systems, such as support for improvements in the quality of healthcare, are closely related to the maintenance of a focus upon the patient through the support given to clinical practice. Maintaining a focus on the patient implies the broadest possible approach in terms of both space and time. Information should never be restricted to a single set of users and should not be seen as property of any institution, each in a real sense contributing to but a portion of the patient's total healthcare.

The particular focus of clinical activity is the critical ingredient for achieving improvements in the quality of healthcare and the economic viability of health services institutions. Access to information, serving as the basic resource in the implementation of medical procedures, grants considerable power to information as a support mechanism for the achievement of these objectives. The clinical record is the tool employed to capture this relationship, thereby rendering indispensable the consideration of the information contained therein.

Beyond this, it is important to remember that health service IS&T systems possess, besides the intrinsic value of the function they exercise, the enormous advantage of serving as a strategic communications link. Some experts even regard the chief function of a health services information system as precisely that of communication among various units and users. Likewise, one of the principal functions of the clinical and administrative individual records is to serve as a medium of communication among professionals. The computerization of health services information implicitly allows for the achievement of this important common purpose.

Application development is at a dramatic new point in health services IS&T. Around the world three significant issues are simultaneously at work to transform the informatics industry. The first is the Computer-based Patient Records, variously called the "electronic medical record", "electronic health record", or "clinical patient record system", among other titles. The second is the integration of the perspectives of the provider, payer, employer, and consumer into Healthcare Information Networks (HIN), already discussed in detail previously. A third is the effort to provide healthcare top management with usable day-to-day information at the desktop — the Executive Information Systems (EIS).

B.1.4. Features of the Computer-based Patient Record

It has already been noted that the complexity, size, and scope of patient data and patient records are daunting, particularly when compared to other highly automated record-management systems such as banking and retail commerce. Only recently has there been affordable, usable technology for computerizing, managing, and storing a variety of medical data items such as voice objects, document images, and radiographic images. In addition, the high-speed networks and communications software needed to speed these data around the health services institution to the points of care have also only recently become available.

A compelling reason for automating patient records involves directly the users of the systems. Experience in other industries — banking, retail, manufacturing — has shown that the most significant advantages of automation accrue when the person responsible for the generation of data is also the one that enters it into the automated system at the point of origin. And while in those other industries the introduction of data-entry-at-the-point-of-service was relatively easy, in health services the data originators are often physicians and other caregivers. It is unarguable that most physicians in particular have been afforded the luxury of clerical staff for data entry, forestalling the development of truly "user friendly" data entry interfaces.

The Computer-based Patient Record (CPR) is indeed an application area whose time has come. The implications of the CPR — the fully automated "customer record" for the health services industry — are enormous. Specifically, the massive shift to managed care with the installation of the primary care physician as the "gatekeeper" to medical resources means that more clinical data are needed from a variety of disparate sources to make informed decisions regarding treatments. In a related trend, the emergence of large, integrated healthcare networks, mentioned above, translates into the requirement to rapidly move around large quantities of clinical data.

The Computer-Based Patient Record Institute describes a CPR as "electronically stored information about an individual's lifetime health status and healthcare". It replaces the paper medical record as the primary record of care, meeting all clinical, legal, and administrative requirements. A CPR system provides reminders and alerts, linkages with knowledge sources for decision support, and data for health outcomes research and improved management of healthcare delivery.

A CPR system is an evolving concept that responds to the dynamic nature of the healthcare environment and takes advantage of technological advances. Despite the compelling reasons for automation of the patient record, substantial challenges still exist, and they are worth mentioning here. Although work on a common definition of CPR contents and CPR management system is still underway by various groups, a universal understanding of the concepts embodied in a CPR does not exist.

Without this clearly understood conceptual framework, users have difficulties in selecting systems that will meet their needs, and vendors have trouble supplying such systems. Of the US$12.8 billion health IS&T market in 1996, the CPR share was only US$180 million. Many developers and vendors became disinterested in CPR development or missed the target, aiming mostly to the inpatient segment rather than the growing outpatient area. They ignored the fact that health managers are more likely to invest in CPR at the points of care where patient volume is increasing and where concomitant access to clinical and administrative data is needed by multiple providers. Also the needs of healthcare institutions related to CPR, but not the focus of most CPR vendors, has changed over the last five years. While the vendor focus remains, in many cases, in the replacement of the paper medical chart by an electronic equivalent, from the user's perspective, the needs have shifted to comprehensive patient management, cost control, decision support, and outcomes analysis.

Most commercial systems are still not intuitive to operate by the healthcare professional. Recent developments in graphical user interfaces (GUIs) have been successful in luring many care givers not only into data entry, but also into many of the other phases of health services application processes, where they can take ownership of data and systems and participate as equal partners in IS&T development. This is not to say that GUI development for healthcare providers has been entirely trouble-free. Poorly designed GUIs are frequently more cumbersome, slower, and provide less information than traditional character-based screens, particularly for experienced users. The slow development of health services informatics departments in health institutions has also been a factor in retarding healthcare provider user acceptance.

The scope of CPR is broad, and it would be beyond the design of this document to describe all of the potential features of the different implementations of the CPR. As a general characteristic, CPRs have two key software components: enabling and application software.

B.1.4.1. Enabling Software for the Computer-based Patient Record

Enabling software involves the following components:

- *Clinical Data Repositories (CDR)* - The data update and access demands on a CPR system require that clinical data be captured, organized, and stored specifically for high-performance clinical use. A CDR may be real (data stored in one place), or virtual (data stored in a number of "legacy" systems, and managed and presented to the user by software as if it were in a single location). A robust CDR will usually have the following features:

  [a] The CDR must be able to contain most or all of the *multiple data types* associated with the patient record. As noted earlier, there could be seven or more types of data elements requiring automation. Some CDR designs allow for storage of certain high-volume data elements, such as radiographic images, in a file separate from the main CDR, but include "foreign keys" or pointers to such data.

  [b] Since clinical practice is patient-centered, the CDR must be *patient-centric*. The CDR should be designed to support the continuum of care by accumulating data longitudinally, or over the patient's lifetime. Physicians are thus able to view data for the current encounter or across all encounters, regardless of the facility within the institution where the encounters occurred.

  [c] In order to support the continuum of care, the CDR architecture should support *multiple episodes of care*. This means that the CDR should permit inclusion of data from multiple caregivers, multiple facilities, and even multiple institutions. It also means that the CDR should be designed with a comprehensive archival and data storage tiering scheme, to permit high-performance access to relevant records, while maintaining historical data at the appropriate level of readiness.

  [d] To allow operation with as many existing HIS systems as possible, a CDR should be designed with *open architecture interfaces*. This means that a good CDR should be easily attachable to databases that it feeds, as well as to applications that exploit it.

- *Vocabulary Management Systems* - It was noted earlier that a significant problem associated with clinical information systems is the lack of a standardized medical vocabulary. A well-designed CPR will include an enabler that attempts to reconcile the need for a homogeneous medical nomenclature with the tendency for individual facilities, providers, and departmental systems to use their own medical terms. The vocabulary manager generally reads medical terms arriving from other systems and matches them against a predetermined, "canonical" term stored in the institution database. A powerful vocabulary manager should have the following features:

  [a] In order to support the large and diverse sets of medical terms, it should have the ability to force *domain completeness*, or the ability to add entire new classes of terms without encountering artificial constraints (e.g., size limitations).

  [b] To counter the problem of multiple terms with the same definition, the vocabulary manager should be able to force *non-redundancy*, a mechanism to provide only one definition of a term.

  [c] It should force *non-ambiguity*, the ability to enable concepts to have a clear, concise meaning.

  [d] It should provide *synonym resolution*, or the ability to handle the different descriptions employed by different health services systems.

  [e] It should force *non-vagueness*, or completeness in meaning, providing the institution with a single, canonical definition for each term.

  [f] In order to address the requirements of many domains of medical terms, and their resulting internal relationships, it should provide support of *multiple classifications* of data, rather than forcing all patient data types into a single hierarchy.

  [g] An advanced vocabulary manager should have the ability to allow definition of explicit, *semantic relationships* between medical concepts, so as to support powerful, user-friendly queries and decision support.

  [h] The vocabulary management system should include an automated *authoring tool* to facilitate mapping the facility terms to institution standard, canonical terms.

B.1.4.2. Computer-based Patient Record Application Software

Application software for CPR involves a number of issues. A large number of software programs have been written and will be written to exploit the CPR. They can be quickly divided into those that support the clinical, patient-centric processes, such as inpatient treatment, and those that search for trends in the clinical database for cross-population analysis, such as outcome research or epidemiological studies. Since the consensus is that the CPR is primarily designed for the former objective, two prominent patient-centric applications, Chart Review and Clinical Decision Support, are mentioned here:

- *Chart Review* - The most natural and most easily justified function of the clinical database is to support the patient care process. This is done with a chart review application that presents the CPR data to physicians and other relevant caregivers. Far from being an easy query function, the chart review subsystem must be able to present a huge variety of data in a format meaningful to healthcare providers. It must perform at "think speed" or risk not being used. It must allow for data entry and update of appropriate information by the caregiver. In addition, a highly functional chart review application has these features:

  [a] To best mimic the manner in which care givers, particularly physicians, work, the chart review application should be able to present information on the screen in a well-developed *chart metaphor*, one that arranges data in the format most likely to follow the healthcare providers workflow, and one that takes advantage of all of the available space on the workstation screen.

  [b] To make the system most usable for healthcare providers, the system should use a sophisticated *graphical user interface* (GUI) that enhances healthcare provider productivity and user friendliness with the proper "look and feel".

  [c] The system should include all the *major healthcare provider functions* and chart information, such as notes, lab results, radiology reports, wave forms, etc. The system should be capable of displaying radiographic images in review quality for attending physicians and diagnostic quality for radiologists.

  [d] The system should allow for *entry of update information* by the caregiver, including progress notes, history and physical data, temperature, pulse and respiration, etc.

  [e] It should allow for *electronic signature* where allowed by law.

- *Clinical Decision Support (CDS)* - CDS is usually implemented as an advanced application, after the health services institution has experienced a relatively mature CPR for a significant time and, more importantly, has enjoyed a good satisfaction rate among the healthcare provider user community. CDS in this context is distinguished from Executive Decision Support, which usually involves data mining over large database samples. CDS, on the other hand, follows the patient-centric theme and processes information based on a single patient. CDS generally produces alerts, reminders, suggestions, and other messages to caregivers. Messages can either be synchronous (real-time, as in an orders application), or asynchronous (after the fact, as in a results application). A high-quality CDS system should have these features:

  [a] It should operate via an *event monitor*, a software program external to the basic application set which reads transactions flowing into the CDR and processes messages based on positive conditions.

[b] It should function based on a portfolio of pre-written *rules*, or *medical logic modules*, small software programs that run in the event monitor and handle specific tasks. For example, a rule might be written to check a patient's history file for ulcers whenever aspirin is ordered, and alert the ordering physician that enteric-coated aspirin would be clinically indicated.

[c] The CDS should include an *authoring facility* that enables rules to be designed and created by healthcare providers to the fullest extent possible.

[d] Rules should be written in *easy-to-use standardized shorthand*, to facilitate exchange of proven rules among health services institutions.

[e] The CDS should exploit the power of the vocabulary management facility, where available, to enable the *construction of rules by class*. For example, if the vocabulary manager maintains the semantic links for acetylsalicylic acid as a class, and all of the 250 or so drugs which contain acetylsalicylic acid, the rule mentioned above could be written using simply the class term "acetylsalicylic acid", leaving the maintenance of the drugs containing such chemical to the pharmacist. These features represents enormous gains in ease-of-use for the healthcare provider, and can result in many more, highly effective rules.

Enabler and application software are only part of a complete CPR system. Numerous system components are still on the drawing board. And the challenges of data automation network architecture and management, and the roll-out of new hardware will mean that many years remain before even the most leading-edge institution can fully implement the CPR. Many vendors have already stepped up to development and delivery of CPR software and the other tools and techniques required for successful implementation. Health services institutions with access to mainstream suppliers should implement today's systems with an eye toward the Computer-based Patient Record as a goal.

B.1.5. Executive Information Systems

In a typical information system environment, the system consolidates and administers many of the day-to-day information functions relating to clerical, administrative, financial, and clinical areas. While many such systems perform their limited functions well, they were never intended to provide the variety of types of management information that senior executives require. The typical information system may produce hundreds of reports daily, but less than a handful may be relevant to the concerns of the health services management team at any specific time. Even with a robust information system, few health services executives are able to fully exploit their organization's existing information to identify trends and support strategic decision-making. As competition continues to intensify, the successful health services organizations will be those that use information as a competitive tool of quality, service, and cost.

One new way to cope with the management of information problems is the development of an *Executive Information System (EIS), designed to integrate data across the entire organization and to deliver information in relevant, intuitive graphs and charts.* EISs are usually built by assembling sets of software designed to run in conjunction with the institution's existing information infrastructure and applications. EISs are designed to make relevant information readily available to executives at all levels of management, so that they can understand past performance and anticipate future trends.

The system should offer real-time reporting and analysis of information throughout the health services organization. It should have easy-to-read, intuitive charts, graphics, and reports that enable managers to track such critical indicators as patient census and current and planned staffing by unit. It should have a simple graphical interface that presents information in easy-to-interpret formats. The EIS should be able to link to, query, and extract data directly from existing systems, eliminating expensive investment in systems integration technology. It should easily accommodate new information, as it becomes available.

The EIS should provide management access to key categories of relevant health services data such as internal data created by the organization, overall institution data, external data (including information about the competition), and worldwide data (using such sources as the Internet). It should allow the institution to view all four kinds of data, at the same time, at one easy-to-use workstation. Using the EIS in this way has enabled some institutions to compare their key data with those of their competitors. It should come with an array of built-in standard reports, and the system's tools should allow management users to create customized reports that can be sent to another workstation or directly to a printer.

B.1.6. The Example of the U.S. Implementation Environment

In contrast with the experience observed in Latin American and the Caribbean Countries, the implementation of Health Information Networks in the United States has been closely linked with the high level of overall development of healthcare. The health sector is undergoing a fundamental change in the alignment of economic incentives with health provision. Under the old model, based on indemnity insurance, the built-in incentive created by the fee-for-service scheme encouraged provider-induced demand, selection of high-cost interventions, and potential over-treatment. Patients with terminal conditions or irreversible organ failure frequently received costly treatment benefiting financially providers, suppliers of equipment and drugs, and inpatient care facilities. This situation resulted in escalating costs not necessarily resulting in proportional better overall improvement of the status of health of the society.

With different forms of managed care emerging as the predominant model for healthcare delivery, the incentives are in the direction of keeping people healthy and lowering costs. The new healthcare models are centered on people and focused on quality, sound financing, and accountability. In this new environment, information system are essential and should be designed and implemented considering the diversity of perspectives of regulators, managers, payers, providers, and clients. The traditional contents of health information systems are not appropriate to the new requirements. The role of clients, for instance, was rarely considered in the past – with the desired increased participation of educated, informed, and empowered consumers, they are a key part of the new models of healthcare. Consumers require information in special formats — when they need it and where they need it, in order that they can take an active role in their own treatment.

There are many Healthcare Networks in implementation in the United States. They are expected to grow rapidly in the near future. Some examples:

- *The Arkansas Health Network* - This organization is a partnership of Arkansas Blue Cross/Blue Shield and two major providers and many physicians in the State of Arkansas. The objective of the network is to share both administrative and clinical information across organizational boundaries. When fully completed, the system will enable physicians to process referrals automatically, administrators to check patient eligibility and handle claims, all without the paperwork previously associated with these "inter-organizational" tasks.

- *BJC Health System* - This 12-hospital corporation centered in St. Louis, Missouri, is developing its own Computer-based Patient Record to support the continuum of care. BJC has begun to automate its patient data types, including laboratory, radiology, and other ancillary data, as well as radiographic images. It uses clinical repositories, vocabulary managers, and clinical decision support tools to provide comprehensive information for caregivers in its system, regardless of where the patient is or has been, or where the caregiver is.

- *Greater Dayton Area Health Association (GDAHA)* - This is a Community Health Information Network (CHIN) located in southwestern Ohio. Although not a corporation, the 15 members of GDAHA plan to automate key functions such as eligibility/certification, referrals, and clinical documents.

- *Kaiser-Permanente* in California - It has more than 4,000 high-end servers and mainframes distributed throughout this organization. The overall information is contained both in mainframes and in thousands of personal computers.

- *United Healthcare* in Minneapolis - This organization has an extensive information-processing network outsourced to IBM, Unisys, and AT&T.

B.2. Information Systems and Technology Implementation Issues

There is a great deal of literature available on the topic of IS&T planning and implementing, and it is not in the scope of this manual to go into the details of the systematic process required by those activities. On the other hand, it is useful to cover the most important elements of planning that are special to the implementation of the health services systems proposed herein, especially to implementations in the Latin American and Caribbean Region, and other elements deemed to be particularly significant and insightful.

B.2.1. Project Management Methodologies

The purchase or development and subsequent implementation of information systems requires the effective use of project management methods or techniques in order to increase the possibility of a successful outcome. In this brief overview of project managing information technology and systems in health care, a range of general project management principles are outlined and advice is provided on their use.

Reference is also made to a specific project management method know as *Projects in Controlled Environments* (PRINCE®). This is the standard project management method for United Kingdom government IT departments and the U.K. National Health Service (NHS) and is approved by the U.K. Central Computer and Telecommunications Agency (CCTA). The latest version of PRINCE is suitable for all types of projects large and small and because the PRINCE method is in the public domain its use is free. It is also scaleable so more or less of the method can be used based on the cost or importance of each project to the organization. Details on how to find more information about PRINCE can be obtained from CCTA, Steel House, 11 Tothill Street, London SW1H 9NF, or via the Internet at the address http://www.ccta.gov.uk/prince/prince.htm

For an in-depth study of project management issues and methodology it is recommended that managers read "A Guide to the Project Management Body of Knowledge", 1996 Edition. Project Management Institute (PMI), which can be downloaded from http://pmi.org/

B.2.1.1. What Is a Project?

Organizations perform work. Work generally involves either operations or projects, although the two may overlap. Operations and projects share many characteristics and they are:

- Performed by people
- Constrained by limited resources
- Planned, executed, and controlled

Operations and projects differ primarily in that operations are ongoing and repetitive, while projects are temporary and unique. A project can thus be defined in terms of its distinctive characteristics — *a project is a temporary endeavor undertaken to create a unique product or service*. Temporary means that every project has a definite beginning and a definite end. Unique means that the product or service is different in some distinguishing way from all similar products or services.

Projects are undertaken at all levels of the organization. They may involve a single person or many thousands. Projects may involve a single unit of one organization or may crossorganizational boundaries, as in joint ventures and partnering. Projects are often critical components of the performing organization's business strategy. They share a certain set of characteristics:

- Are focused on a specific or set of outcomes or deliverables.
- Have an organizational structure, e.g., a Project Committee, Project Team, etc.
- Impact on a range of departments within an organization.
- Bring about a change in the organization.
- Have a number of constraints such as an imposed start or end date, money available, and resources (people and equipment) available.

Projects involve doing something that has not been done before, therefore unique. A product or service may be unique even if the category it belongs to is large. For example, many thousands of office buildings have been developed, but each individual facility is unique — different owner, different design, different location, different contractors, and so on. The presence of repetitive elements does not change the fundamental uniqueness of the overall effort.

B.2.1.2.   Why Do Some Projects Fail?

Many reasons can be cited for why projects do not succeed. Some of the more common reasons include:

- A proper business case is not established at the outset.
- Inadequate identification of the desired end product(s) of the project.
- Scoping of the project is not carried out properly.
- Identification and control of all activities is not adequately addressed.
- The estimate of the effort required for project work is inaccurate.
- No allowance is made for interruptions and non-project activities.
- Change control is not handled effectively.
- Little or no effort is made to identify and manage risk.

B.2.1.3.   What Is a Successful Project?

A project is deemed to be successful if it is completed on time, on or below budget, and provides all the required products or deliverables to agreed quality standards.

B.2.2. Project Management Principles

Project management is the application of knowledge, skills, tools, and techniques to project activities in order to meet or exceed stakeholder needs and expectations from a project. Meeting or exceeding stakeholder needs and expectations invariably involves balancing competing demands among the following elements: scope, time, cost, and quality; stakeholders with differing needs and expectations; identified requirements (needs); and unidentified requirements (expectations).

The term *project management* is sometimes used to describe an organizational approach to the management of ongoing operations. This approach, more properly called *management by projects*, treats many aspects of ongoing operations as projects in order to apply project management to them. Although an understanding of project management is obviously critical to an organization that is managing by projects, a detailed discussion of the approach itself is outside the scope of this document.

B.2.2.1. Project Phases and Project Life Cycle

Because projects are unique undertakings, they involve a degree of uncertainty. Organizations performing projects will usually divide each project into several project phases to provide better management control and appropriate links to the ongoing operations of the performing organization. Collectively, the project phases are known as the project life cycle.

B.2.2.2. Characteristics of Project Phases

Each project phase is marked by completion of one or more deliverables. A deliverable is a tangible, verifiable work product such as a feasibility study, a detail design, or a working prototype. The deliverables, and hence the phases, are part of a sequential logic designed to ensure proper definition of the product of the project. The conclusion of a project phase is generally marked by a review of both key deliverables and project performance in order to determine if the project should continue into its next phase and detect and correct errors cost effectively.

These phase-end reviews are often called *phase exits, stage gates*, or *kill points*. Each project phase normally includes a set of defined work products designed to establish the desired level of management control. The majority of these items are related to the primary phase deliverable, and the phases typically take their names from these items: requirements, design, build, text, start-up, turnover, and others as appropriate.

The project life cycle serves to define the beginning and the end of a project. For example, when an organization identifies an opportunity that it would like to respond to, it will often authorize a feasibility study to decide if it should undertake a project. The project life cycle definition will determine whether the feasibility study is treated as the first project phase or as a separate, stand-alone project. The project life cycle definition will also determine which transitional actions at the end of the project are included and which are not. In this manner, the project life cycle definition can be used to link the project to the ongoing operations of the performing organization.

The phase sequence defined by most project life cycles generally involves some form of technology transfer or hand-off such as requirements to design, construction to operations, or design to implementation. Deliverables from the preceding phase are usually approved before work starts on the next phase. However, a subsequent phase is sometimes begun prior to approval of the previous phase deliverables when the risks involved are deemed acceptable. This practice of overlapping phases is often called fast tracking. Project life cycles generally define:

- What technical work should be done in each phase (e.g., is the work of the systems analyst part of the definition phase or part of the execution phase?)

- Who should be involved in each phase (e.g., concurrent engineering requires that the implementers be involved with requirements and design).

Project life cycle descriptions may be very general or very detailed. Highly detailed descriptions may have numerous forms, charts, and checklists to provide structure and consistency. Such detailed approaches are often called *project management methodologies*. Most project life cycle descriptions share a number of common characteristics:

- Cost and staffing levels are low at the start, higher towards the end, and drop rapidly as the project draws to a conclusion.

- The probability of successfully completing the project is lowest, and hence risk and uncertainty are highest, at the start of the project. The probability of successful completion generally gets progressively higher as the project continues.

- The ability of the stakeholders to influence the final characteristics of the project product and the final cost of the project is highest at the start and gets progressively lower as the project continues. A major contributor to this phenomenon is that the cost of changes and error correction generally increases as the project continues.

B.2.2.3. Project Management Methodologies – The PRINCE Method

The very nature of the definition and characteristics of projects gives some indication as to why projects are sometimes difficult and complicated to manage. In order to help people who are required, as part of their work, to manage projects, a number of project management methods, including formal methods such as PRINCE, have been developed and are becoming more widely used. These methods are based on a common set of project management principles which, when adhered to, will increase the probability of a successful outcome to the project.

Successful projects are those where the following basic areas or activities are implemented and managed effectively.

- Formally starting or initiating the project
- Establishing an organizational structure around the project
- Utilizing a structured planning method
- Applying project control techniques including:
    - Change control
    - Quality control
- Managing the stages of the project
- Executing the project tasks and activities
- Assessing and managing risks which could impact on the project
- Formally closing the project.

Successful project management is aided by a stepped, logical approach, which addresses each of the above areas. All project management methodologies identify a standard set of processes common to all types of project and offer guidance and support on the execution of these processes.

Completing some of the processes below (Figure 4) may seem somewhat heavy going and bureaucratic, but they have been devised as a means of ensuring that the correct amount of detail is applied to the key elements of the project. Lack of attention to detail in projects can lead to expensive time and cost overruns or serious failure in terms of the quality of project deliverables. The damaging effect on the organization and its patients/clients of overruns and low-quality outcomes can far outweigh time saved by cutting corners within projects.

Figure 4.   PRINCE Project Management Processes

- Start-Up the Project (SU)
- Initiate the Project (IP)
- Direct the Project (DP)
- Control the Stage (CS)
- Manage Product Delivery (MP)
- Manage Stage Boundaries (SB)
- Close the Project (CP)

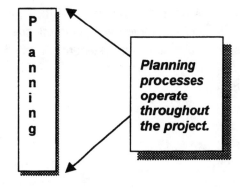

Planning

Planning processes operate throughout the project.

Start-Up the Project (SU)

SU processes remind those who wish to set up a project that time must be given for the activities required to establish a project board and to appoint a project manager. As part of SU, preparation of the project brief and of the detailed plans for the first stage of the project takes place. Starting projects without a clear business case can lead to early failure. These start-up processes help to ensure that the project has a firm foundation in the sense that it is agreed to be worthwhile and viable from the outset.

Initiate the Project (IP)

Project initiation is done at a formal Project Initiation Meeting (PIM). The project brief and plans produced at Start-Up are discussed and agreed upon the PIM. This meeting formally signals start of the project.

Direct the Project (DP)

DP is about ensuring that all of the elements are in place to properly manage the project. Projects sometimes fail because steps are not taken to ensure that staff is released from other duties when required to carry out work on the project. DP creates the lines of communication necessary to authorize the funds and other resources (people and equipment) needed by the project. Sometimes projects are allowed to commence a new project stage before the previous stage has been fully completed. A key element of directing the project processes is to make sure this does not happen.

Control the Stage (CS)

In order to make projects more manageable they should be divided into stages and appropriate mechanisms employed to manage each stage effectively. An example of stages in the development and implementation of a health care system might include the following:

- Specification
- Design
- Development
- Testing
- User training
- Implementation
- Post-implementation review.

Although the PRINCE method involves producing high-level plans for the whole project, the actual work undertaken is approved only one stage at a time. In this way projects in progress which are no longer meeting their original aims or are significantly overspent can, if necessary, be cancelled before any more money or effort is wasted. Staging a project also allows greater focus to be applied to the tasks in the current stage and avoids attention being distracted too much by later stages. Stage plans are produced before the first and each subsequent stage commences. These plans contain details of the tasks to be undertaken, the resources required, and the quality standards to be adhered to during the stage. Controlling a stage involves ensuring that all of the work (or "Work Packages") within a stage is properly authorized and is successfully completed.

Manage Product Delivery (MP)

Products are the "things" or deliverables that the project is to produce. There are two general types of product:

- Final Products - e.g., a fully implemented and operational Patient Administration System within this healthcare institution.

- Interim Products - these are the things that have to be produced throughout the project in order to reach the final product. In the example above, a fully developed and implemented Master Patient Index would be considered as an interim product because it is just one component of the final product.

It is important to ensure that sufficient care and effort are put into the production of each project product. Managing Product Delivery gives guidance on how this can be achieved. This guidance is particularly helpful when products are to be created by suppliers or subcontractors. The customer Project Manager specifies:

- Work packages for the contractor to complete, for instance, developing some reporting software that will be used to monitor patient throughput, and

- The specification of the work package must include the quality standards that must be met by the supplier or contractor.

The contractor must meet this specification before the Project Manager can accept the work package as complete. In this way the customer organization is able to keep control of the development and delivery of project products.

Manage Stage Boundaries (SB)

As already mentioned, projects are more likely to be successful if they are broken into stages. Certain criteria, which assess how well the project is progressing, must be met before a project can proceed from one stage to the next. These criteria should be examined closely at the end of each stage, at the boundary between stages. Senior people in the organization examine the progress of each stage in terms of schedule, costs incurred against budget, and the quality of the products produced so far. In this way, stage by stage, assessment is made of the continuing viability of the project. If it is still viable, then approval to proceed to the next stage can be given.

Close the Project (CP)

When a project is complete it is advisable to conduct a controlled closedown. This allows the formal handing over of the final product of the project to the staff responsible for its continued operation. Closing the project includes steps to ensure that all of the aims have been met.

Formal acceptance and sign off procedures are carried out to check that all the project products meet the required quality standards. The closure processes also include the production of a Lessons Learned Report and a list of recommendations for future actions.

Planning (PL)

This is a common process used by all of the other processes that involve producing plans. Planning is essential — it helps to:

- Communicate what has to be done, when and by whom
- Encourage forward thinking
- Provide the measures of success for the project
- Make clear the commitment of time, resources (people and equipment), and money required for the project
- Determine if targets are achievable
- Identify the activities the resources need to undertake.

Three main types of planning are required within PRINCE projects:

- Project Planning - This is required in order to provide an overview of the whole project.

- Stage Planning - Plans for each stage need to be prepared. These are produced towards the end of the previous stage. Plans are considered at End Stage Assessment meetings. This enables the assessment of the previous stage of the project and consideration of plans for the new stage.

- Exception Planning - This type of planning is used when there are signs that the project is slipping behind schedule or is deviating from budget or quality targets.

B.2.2.4. PRINCE Project Components

The above processes ranging from starting up to closing down a project are backed up by a set of "Components" which take care of other important facets of projects. These are:

- Organization
- Planning
- Controls
- Stages
- Management of Risk
- Quality in a project environment
- Configuration Management
- Change Control

Outlines of some of the processes underpinning the Planning and Controls components have already been provided. A brief overview of the remaining components is provided below.

Figure 5. PRINCE Project Management Organizational Structure
(*arrows indicate accountability*)

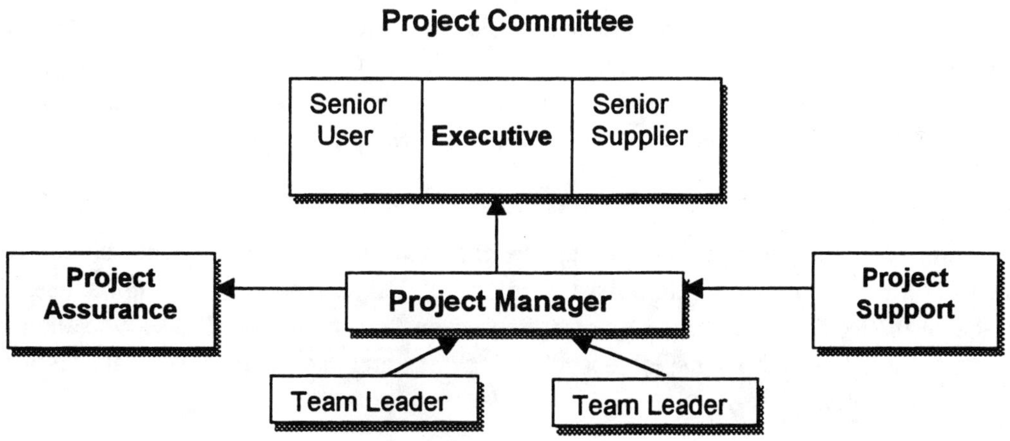

The basic PRINCE project organizational structure is illustrated in Figure 5. The PRINCE guidance specifies quite precisely the roles and responsibilities of each member of the project organization.

- *Project Committee* - Provides senior input to the management of the project. This committee carries overall responsibility for the success or failure of the project. Members of the Project Committee must be of sufficient seniority to be able to secure the resources needed by the Project Manager to manage the project.

- *Project Manager* - Is given authority, within certain tolerances, by the Project Committee to manage the project on a day-to-day level.

- *Team Leader* - Is not a mandatory role. There may be one or more Team Leaders involved in a project. The Project Manager delegates responsibility to Team Leaders to produce the project products. Team Leaders may be contractors not directly employed by the customer organization. Team Leaders receive Work Packages from the Project Manager.

- *Project Assurance* - Provides independent monitoring of the progress of the project on behalf of the Project Board. A Project Assurance Team, usually of three members, ensures that the Business User and Technical aspects of the project are continually monitored.

- *Project Support* - Is also an optional set of roles. A Project Support Office if provided undertakes administrative activities required to keep the project going. These activities will typically include arranging meetings, updating project plans on project planning software, and filing project documents. For smaller projects, existing administrative and clerical staff in the organization can fulfil this role.

B.2.2.5. Management of Risk

Risk is defined as "the chance of exposure to the adverse consequences of future events". Successful identification and management of risk can greatly improve the chances of project success. The PRINCE method offers quite detailed guidance on risk management. As with other elements of the method, organizations are able to select the level of detail they feel they require for each specific project. The more expensive or important projects are likely to require more effort to be expended on risk management. Risk Management is broken down into two phases: Risk Analysis and Risk Management.

- *Risk Analysis* - In the risk analysis phase the following processes take place: Risk Identification when a list of possible risks is compiled; Risk Estimation when an assessment is made of the likelihood of each risk occurring within the project; and Risk Evaluation, an assessment is made of the acceptable level of each risk and alternative actions are identified to avoid unacceptable risks.

- *Risk Management* - In the risk management phase the following processes take place:
    - Planning - the course of action most suited to managing each risk is agreed upon.
    - Resourcing - the resources required to handle the risk are identified and assigned.
    - Monitoring - the status of risks is monitored. Checks are made to ensure that countermeasures are working effectively.
    - Controlling - making sure that the risk management plan is being fully implemented as agreed.

The range of action that can be taken to help manage risk includes:

- *Prevention* - implementing measures to counteract or eliminate the risk.
- *Reduction* - taking steps to reduce the impact of identified risks.
- *Transference* - passing the risk onto a third party, e.g., a contractor or an insurance company.
- *Contingency* - actions that are planned to come into force if and when the identified risk occurs.
- *Acceptance* - of the possibility that identified risks might occur but the proposed countermeasures are too expensive to implement.

B.2.2.6. Quality in the Project Environment

The International Standards Organization defines quality as the "totality of features and characteristics of a product or service which bear on its ability to satisfy stated and implied needs" (ISO 8402). PRINCE offers a complete quality control method for projects including the following elements:

- A *quality system*, encompassing organization, procedures, and processes to ensure that quality assurance is taken care of throughout projects.

- *Quality planning*, which involves setting the quality targets for the project and ensuring that plans are in place to achieve them.

- *Quality control*, which involves installing mechanisms to inspect each product produced to ensure it meets agreed quality standards.

B.2.2.7. Configuration Management

Effective project management is a key component of procuring, developing, or implementing IT systems in health care. Many such health systems projects can be complex, expensive, and risky to implement. The use of a structured, scalable project management method like PRINCE can increase the odds of delivering a project on time, within budget, and to the right quality standard or, in a word, successfully. Configuration Management is about product control. It provides a mechanism, which can be used to track the evolution of project products and as such keeps track of product versions.

- *Change Control* - Change impacts on all projects. If change is not carefully managed then it can have a detrimental, sometimes devastating, effect on a project. An almost infinite range of changes can happen during projects, from changes of government to changes of project personnel. PRINCE manages change through the use of Project Issue Reports (PIR's) a simple paper-form based mechanism used to capture both general issues and change issues that arise throughout projects. Project Issues can be about anything to do with the project such as suggestions, questions, or requests for changes to be made. PIR's can be raised by anyone involved in the project. The Project Manager prioritizes each PIR and an impact analysis is carried out.

- *Prioritization of proposed changes* - Proposed issues can be can be categorized as follows:

  - changes which are a must; a final product will not work without this change
  - important changes; their absence would be very problematic though a workaround is possible for a while
  - changes which are nice to have but not vital
  - cosmetic changes of no importance
  - project issues which in fact do not involve a change.

- *Impact analysis* - The impact of each proposed change will involve consideration of the following questions:

  - what would have to change to accommodate this Project Issue Report?
  - what effort is needed to implement the change?
  - what impact will the change have on project risks?
  - will there be an impact on the project's Business Case?

B.3. Information Systems and Information Technology Planning Phases

- *Phase 0* – Establish context and scope for healthcare institution information systems plan

- *Phase 1* – Determine healthcare institution information and support needs

- *Phase 2* – Establish information architectures and options for solutions

- *Phase 3* – Determine strategic solutions

- *Phase 4* – Prepare and deliver the implementation plan

Phase 0 - Establish context and scope for healthcare institution information systems plan

Initiate the study

- Study context, scope, and terms of reference
- Prerequisites identified
- Essential parallel activities scoped and initiated
- Steering group set up and briefed
- Other key management members involved and briefed
- Initial interview schedule established

Phase 1 - Determine healthcare institution information and support needs

[a] Preparatory information collection
- Outputs being produced
- Inventory and assessment of all available information about:
    - Healthcare institution goals, directions, and plans
    - Current and planned application systems
    - IT assets and inventory, current and on order
    - Human resource/skills

[b] Determine healthcare institution information, support needs, and priorities
- Outputs desired
- Agreed statement of healthcare institution information, support needs, and priorities based on consensus
- Document showing supporting detail of needs

Phase 2 - Establish information architectures and options for solutions

[a] Assess current applications and IT technical status as well as match IT to needs
- Outputs being produced
- Full inventory of current application portfolio and IT assets
- Assessment of strengths and weaknesses
- Outline of action plan for each high-priority weak area
- Preliminary view of rapid development opportunities where appropriate

[b] Developing information architectures
- Draft architecture for healthcare institution structure
- Draft information architecture – application systems, databases, and technology requirements
- Identify key gaps/weaknesses in current status which will constrain the development of the architectures

[c] Establish initial options for strategic solutions
- Identify key gaps/weaknesses in current coverage which require applications solutions
- Provide overall IS strategic vision of the preferred means for meeting the healthcare institution needs
- In the case of high-priority needs, a preliminary set of options for application solutions
- Modifications to emerging information architectures

[d] Develop cost/benefit justification for meeting needs
- List of committed partners/stakeholders
- Present cases for meeting all key needs
- Action plan so that cases are carried forward through selection of solutions and implementation planning

Phase 3 - Determine strategic solutions

[a] Identify and initiate urgent actions
- Scope definition of a project to meet each appropriate need
- Completed developments
- Required healthcare institution outcome achieved

[b] Determine application and database solutions
- Selection of the most appropriate application solutions
- Definition of the most appropriate application and database structures to support the solutions
- Log of options considered and reasons for selection or rejection
- Updates to the emerging information architectures as appropriate

- Specification of workload volumes and other technology requirements to support the solutions
- Basis for development of migration strategy to the proposed solution

[c] Evaluate IT status and opportunities and set key IT directions
- Assessment of current IT status, especially the gaps and soft spots
- Assessment of key developments and vendors in so far as they are relevant to the healthcare institution needs
- Identification of options and opportunities for meeting healthcare institution and application needs
- Preliminary identification of technology support options

Phase 4 - Prepare and deliver the implementation plan

[a] Prepare applications and database projects plan
- Statement of preferred strategic application solutions
- Complete development and implementation plan for applications and databases, linked to the IT and HR plans

[b] Prepare IT technical projects plan
- Statement of preferred strategic technology solution
- Complete development plan for computer hardware, software, communications, workstations, and development environments which supports the applications and databases development plan

[c] Prepare organization and skills/resources development plan
- Statement of organization and skills/resources solutions
- Complete development plan for IS organization and human resource skills and resources which support the applications and IT development plans

[d] Integrate costs and case justification
- Provide justification for the application, IT, and human resource plans
- Results of negotiations with stakeholders to ensure that final recommended delivery rate and sequence are acceptable
- Integrate financial analysis to support the recommended strategic solutions

[e] Present plan and negotiate implementation
- Agreed plans
- Application
- Technology
- Skills/resources
- Budgetary commitments
- Implementation program
- Agreed basis for maintaining and re-assessing the plans when healthcare institution circumstances change

B.4. Defining a Successful Implementation

The most challenging part of an information system strategy is successfully implementing the plan. But what do we really mean by implementation and how does one knows if it is successful?

When we refer to implementation, we mean far more than merely plugging in the computer and peripherals and the communication hardware, and turning on the screen — implementation also involves the process of introducing an information system throughout the institution and ensuring that its full potential benefits are achieved. A successful implementation is one that promotes and supports the institution's ability to execute its plans and meet its goals. Organizations are discovering that successful information systems implementation in the health services institution requires a firm understanding of the organization's overall strategic plan. A health services information system has the purpose of improving the overall performance of the institution. The system being implemented must be recognized as a strategic tool and corporate asset that represents an investment in the organization's viability.

In the case of Latin America and the Caribbean, in particular, one must also consider the many different levels of technology available or currently in use in the region. All too often there exists the tendency to rush to the latest and most advanced technology, irrespective of the user's ability to absorb it, that is, to install, maintain, and make the best use of it. Different needs and capabilities co-exist in the same country, same political subdivision, and even inside the boundaries of the same organization.

A technology that is appropriate to an advanced, sophisticated user such as a large teaching institution in an urban area may not be appropriate for an emerging health services organization in a rural setting. The social and economic context must always be considered along with issues related to availability of resources and personnel, health information infrastructure, sustainability and continuity of the decisions, and appropriate flow of financial resources.

B.4.1. Processes and Roles

To respond to the customer needs, the institution must be able to execute key processes efficiently and effectively and provide adequate information support to critical roles. A process is essentially a set of activities, with a distinct beginning and end that results in the delivery of a product or service to customers. In general, health services institutions manage between twelve and fourteen critical processes:

- Planning services
- Coordinating services
- Delivering care
- Scheduling patients and resources

- Managing material
- Collecting revenue
- Developing staff
- Assessing patient care, planning, and outcomes
- Health services
- Reviewing care
- Documenting care managing costs
- Managing facilities
- Managing information
- Managerial decision making.

The identification of critical processes lays the foundation for defining key roles. Roles are defined as a set of job characteristics that describe how (tasks, events, responsibilities, and priorities), what (goals, objectives, and targets), and the enablers (skills, accountabilities, incentives, and ownership).

B.4.2. The Information Strategic Plan

One must emphasize that IS&T is a supportive tool available to the institution, not an end in itself. For IS&T to be successful, its functions and capabilities must properly address the goals of the institution. When a health services institution decides to proceed with a computerization process, an information systems plan in keeping with the institution's strategies becomes an essential element in guaranteeing that the technologies incorporated fully correspond to the institution's requirements and structure. Accordingly, IS&T plans should usually follow on the heels of similar organizational planning at the institutional level.

Whether the computerization process is being implemented through the acquisition of a standard market solution or by the development of custom-designed applications, the Information Strategic Plan is an unavoidable requirement.

The project plan should make it possible to understand the overall organization's mission and the position of IS&T within that mission; gain an understanding of the institution's policies and strategies; determine the management information that the each management level will require for operation and control; and determine the extent and level of satisfaction provided by the currently operating computer system.

A strategic plan entails the accomplishment of the following steps:

- Involve users in the determination of requirements, functions, design, and selection of solutions for application implementation.

- Incorporate all relevant applications into the plan, along with implementation timetables, resource requirements, critical assumptions, and dependencies (see Implementation Phases below).

- Provide tangible solutions to problems detected during the execution of the project.

- Develop appropriate mechanisms for measurement of implementation results and eventual adjustments to the IS&T plan.

The resulting Information Systems Plan should allow the Institution to understand its current position and in what direction it should head, with regard to information systems. Furthermore, it must contain an overall information strategy, with critical inputs that include users' needs, assessments, physical and technological infrastructure, organizational culture, human resources, and education as to the potential of IS&T to support the organization goals.

Part of the strategy may address regional networks, partners, the Internet, and other external influences that will need to be considered, such as government and crediting agencies (Figure 6).

Figure 6. Aligning IT Strategy to the Health Services Institution Strategy

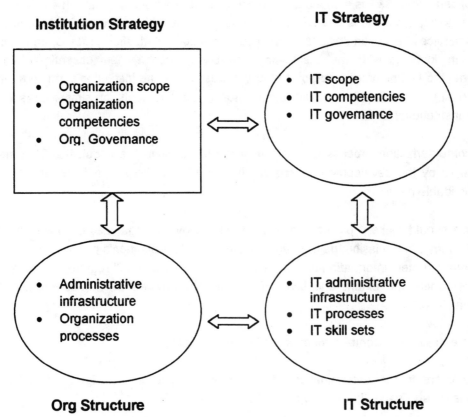

B.4.3.   Selecting a Systems Architecture

Building, implementing, and managing systems in an open and distributed environment is a very complex endeavor. As the user evaluates new solutions, the possible technological infrastructure options provide the backdrop for a consistent methodology for assessing the fit of a solution, from both a functional and an architectural perspective.

Such detailed evaluation of alternatives will permit reaching informed decisions regarding the balance of short-term needs against long term objectives. Of course, there will still be situations where short-term needs outweigh the desire to fully comply with the open architecture, resulting perhaps in the implementation of one or more proprietary systems. However, these decisions should also be informed decisions, with the pros and cons of these decisions clearly understood in advance, and plans for evolution over time set in place from the onset.

In developing countries, it is important to consider the technological infrastructure of the health services institution when evaluating systems architecture. Regional differences in technical infrastructure, telecommunications capabilities, and IS&T personnel resources bring an additional factor to bear on IS&T decisions. Also, it is important to consider the "life expectancy" of any system and the rapid growth and early maturity that characterize today's systems. Users must be especially careful to avoid investing in systems prone to early obsolescence.

B.4.4.   Alternatives for Application Software Acquisition

There are four basic options for acquiring software, and of course, any combination of these:

- In-house development
- Contract development
- Purchased package (Turn-key)
- Transported system.

B.4.4.1.   In-house Development

Under this option, the organization utilizes its own staff for the planning, definition, analysis, design, and implementation of the applications. New staff may be hired or existing personnel can be trained in information systems and computer technology.

In-house development of software offers the following advantages:

- Complete internal control over project staff and schedules.

- Lower per hour labor cost than contract development.

- System maintenance and modification ability retained within the organization.

Disadvantages of in-house development include:

- Hiring, supervision, and personnel management responsibilities.

- Long-term expense of maintaining a technical staff.

- No contractual (legal and financial) leverage over development, implementation, and maintenance.

- Possibly a lower level of productivity than with contractor personnel and thus higher development cost.

- Staff turnover and training requirements.

B.4.4.2. Contract Development

This alternative entails contracting with a software development organization for the design and implementation of the desired applications.

The advantages of contract development include:

- Tight control of development cost.

- Legal and financial leverage over contractor.

- Probably stronger technical talent than could be hired for an in-house team.

- Possibly specific applicable prior experience of contractor.

- Probably better adherence to development and implementation timetables.

- Less requirement for in-house technical staff.

Development of software by a contractor may involve the following disadvantages:

- Higher per hour labor cost than with in-house staff.

- Possible business instability of the contractor.

- Lack of assurance of long-term system maintenance without a continued contractual relationship.

- Additional time and expense for Request for Proposal preparation, proposal evaluation, negotiation, and contracting.

- Lack of understanding by contractor of actual and specific organizational requirements.

B.4.4.3. Purchased Package

The package option includes any arrangement whereby the organization acquires computer software, and frequently also associated installation requirements, from another organization under a purchase or license contract. This applies to either an in-house computer system or the contracted use of equipment off premises.

The advantages of a purchased package include:

- Proven and technically sound software.

- Generally shorter implementation time.

- Minimal development of new forms and procedures.

- Lower cost than custom development.

- Implementation experience usually available.

- User references usually available.

- Specific performance contract easier to define.

- Warranty and short-term support generally available.

The disadvantages of a purchased package may include:

- Incompatibility between packaged system capabilities and hospital's requirements.

- Possible reliance on vendor for long-term support, maintenance, and modification.

- Requirements for specific computer equipment.

- Restrictions regarding copyright, distribution, and utilization of the system and modifying the programs.

- Limited staff involvement at the contracting organization.

B.4.4.4. Transported System

This alternative involves acquiring a system on an "as is" basis from another organization where the system was developed and is in production. This option includes either implementation using in-house hardware or the sharing of the computer facilities and network with the originating organization.

This alternative offers the following advantages:

- Very low direct acquisition cost.

- Installation and use advice normally available.

Disadvantages of this acquisition method include:

- Minimal documentation generally available.

- Reliance on originating organization or internal personnel for support, maintenance, and modification.

- No extensive contractual recourse usually available.

- Possible inability of system to meet some specific organizational requirements.

- Possibility of inordinately high implementation cost due to policy differences, quality of documentation, and software difficulties.

- Limited contracting organization staff involvement.

B.4.5. Selecting an Acquisition Alternative

An objective comparison of options for the acquisition of software applications is rarely possible. A completely objective analysis can be done only if one assumes that absolutely equivalent systems would be acquired and only the manner of acquisition would differ. Table 1 compares the four software acquisition alternatives.

Table 1. Summary of Project Requirements and Application Software Acquisition Alternatives

Project Requirement	Acquisition Alternative			
	In-house Development	*Contract Development*	*Purchased Package (Turn-key)*	*Transported System*
Contract	Not applicable	Tight control of cost And schedules; recourse against contractor possible; may include warranty and support	Predefined cost and schedule; ease of specific performance statement; recourse against vendor well defined; should include warranty and support provisions	Not normally available
Development or Acquisition Cost	High	High	Moderate	Low
Implementation Cost	High to moderate	High to moderate	Moderate to low	High to low
Systems' Reliability	Moderate	Moderate to high	High	Moderate to low
Flexibility in Meeting User's Requirements	Excellent	Excellent	Moderate	Minimal
Maintenance and Ease of Modification	High with permanent in-house staff, difficult otherwise	High with support contract, low without	High if performed by vendor, probably extremely difficult otherwise	Limited to support available from original developer and quality of documentation
Confidence in Final Product's Operation (1-4) where 1 = low	2. (assuming competent staff)	3. (assuming competent contractor)	4. (assuming proven package)	1. (assuming no previous widespread distribution)
Planning and Analysis Requirement	Full conceptual plan Required; general Analysis completed; minimal detail design required	Full conceptual plan required; general analysis completed; full detail design defined; milestones defined; project management plan completed	Conceptual plan necessary for package selection; general analysis completed for adaptation; no detail design required	Conceptual plan necessary for package selection; general analysis completed for adaptation; no detail design required
Implementation Time/complexity (1-4) where 1 = best	3.	2.	1.	4. (generality and documentation problems)
Staffing Needed	Project management, administrative functions, systems analysis, systems design, programming	Project management, administrative functions, systems analysis	Administrative functions, minimal project management required	Project management, administrative functions, programming (if outside support is unavailable)
Major Potential Problems	Technical staffing, personnel management, project management, cost control, control of system scope	RFP preparation, contracting, project administration, contractor reliability, staff acceptance of system, long-term support	Package capabilities and adaptability, staff acceptance of system, maintenance, modifications, upgrading, long-term support	System capabilities and adaptability, reliability, implementation support and cost, documentation, long-term support, maintenance, upgrading, modification, staff acceptance

B

Although theoretically possible, this assumption is unlikely to be the case except possibly in a comparison of in-house development and contract development. The following assumptions about acquisition alternatives could reflect a more realistic set of circumstances:

- The in-house staff is competent, but not as experienced or technically strong overall as the staff a good contractor could provide, and there will be turnover in the in-house staff.

- The contractor has worked in the same or a closely related application area, will not be prone to miss schedules, and will not fully comprehend all aspects of the hospital's management requirements.

- The packaged system comes close to the actual requirement but will require modification, and the package has been successfully installed beyond its original development point.

- The transported system was originally developed to meet a very specific set of requirements for another facility and it is not well documented.

Each of the four alternatives offers inherent advantages and disadvantages. However, all the options share several basic requirements:

- Determination of minimum system requirements must precede any move to acquire an information system.

- Planning for the implementation process must be carefully developed and documented well in advance.

- Policies and procedures to support the systems must be established before implementation is complete.

- Management commitment to and support of the system must be very strong and evident.

In many situations, the best approach may well be a combination of the four options. For example, a reliable system might be available from another health organization or an independent software vendor that appears to meet the majority of the organization's needs. In this case, a contractor could be employed to make modifications to the software and assist in implementation planning and conversion. In-house staff could be hired to assist in the modification process, conduct staff training, provide conversion support, and provide long-range system maintenance.

B.4.6. Implementation Phases

One of the most crucial decisions faced by health services managers is the selection of applications for a phased implementation. In fact, the ingredients of each phase will almost certainly vary from one institution to the next, and therefore defy generalization. On the other hand, it is expected that the health services institutions deriving the most benefit from this manual are those still in the *early-to-*

intermediate stages of application automation. For this very reason, the focus herein is on providing information specific to these basic applications.

Regardless of the specific applications, each implementation should adhere to a number of well-defined and proved steps to maximize the opportunities for success. In general, implementation takes place in two phases: *pre-decision* and *post-decision.* As with other sections of this document, there is ample literature available that details implementation planning. A brief summary of key activities in these two phases includes, but is not limited to, the ones displayed in Table 2.

B

Table 2. Information Systems and Technology Implementation Phases

Pre-decision Phase	Post-decision Phase
Information systems plan	Human resource assignment
Education	Infrastructure installation
Assessment of user needs	Hardware/software installation
Request for information	Application installation
Obtain vendor information	User training
Link user needs to system specifications	System testing
Establish "make or buy" criteria	System phase-in / pilot
Determine need for process reengineering	System roll-out
Request for Proposals	Evaluation
Site visits	
Cost/Effectiveness-Benefit analysis	
System selection	

One of the most important instruments in IS&T systems design and selection is the *Request for Proposals* (RFP). For more detailed information and guidelines on the productive use of the RFP, refer to Section C.2.

Specific plans for application module implementation are extremely difficult to generalize. Variables include the number and complexity of planned applications, their source, the current state of readiness of the health services institution, and the relative amount of work to be performed by the vendor versus the user. For this reason no specific guidelines for timetables can be made. As always, users should plan carefully with the appropriate vendors, consultants, and internal management when planning implementation timetables.

B.4.7. Requirements for a Successful Health Services Information Systems Implementation

Health services institutions, when considering the implementation of information systems, must consider a number of system-wide implementation factors that cross application boundaries. These include:

- Organization mission, strategies, and scope of services

- Who are the customers and the targeted population

- Value of health and healthcare to the individual and community

- Current ways to assess individual and collective health problems (community health)

- Needs of the individual, community, and nation

- Institutional user needs and commitments

- Organization competencies.

By analyzing the strengths and weaknesses of the organization, the implementation team can determine the organization's core objectives, clients, and competencies in terms both of health service provision and information capabilities. The following areas must be closely examined:

Organization governance is the collection of rules and policies that control the organization operation. It is linked to the social, economic, political, and legal ownership choices made by the organization. The governance choices are directly related to the scope and competencies. It involves:

- Organization Structure

- Administrative Infrastructure and management structure, roles, responsibilities, and authority required to execute the defined business strategy

- Should the organization be centralized, with minimal authority and responsibility delegated to the local level?

- Organization Processes

- Which of the organization's processes are going to be affected?

- Employee Skills

- What are the new skills required to satisfy the organization strategy and structure?

- Can the existing employees be trained to perform the new activities?

Information Technology Strategy involves determining which information technology the organization needs to best support its organizational strategy:

- Does the organization require more IT to make it productive and effective?

- Does the organization have to significantly enhance the employees' skills?

- Can the organization use the existing IT to enhance its scope of business or competencies?

- How can IT be used to improve the organization processes?

- Should the organization get involved in the development of applications?

Information Technology Scope involves examining the array of available information technologies in the IT marketplace and choosing those that enhance the organization's strategy:

- What level of sophistication and range of IT (LAN, Internet, document processing) would provide the organization with the best support to meet its needs?

- Does it make sense to outsource IT services, given the level of IT required to support the organization strategy?

Information Technology Competencies enable the organization to use the information technology it has chosen to be productive in the sector. Rules and standards governing the IT operation must be set so that the technology meets everyone's expectations and delivers what was promised.

Information Technology Governance is the set of policies an organization must establish to control ownership decisions, set rules and standards for, and regulate the use of IT. The decisions made for IT scope and competencies affect these policies.

Information Technology Administrative Infrastructure determines the management structure, roles, responsibilities, authority, and technical considerations required to execute the defined IT strategy:

- What are the information and IT technical architectures required?

- What hardware and software should be installed?

- What level of decentralization should be adopted for the utilization of IT?

Focus on Standards - The Information Services organization needs to be customer oriented with a focus on standards. These include:

- Standards for technology selection (application and hardware)

B

- Standards for communication protocols for all systems

- Standard processes for requesting services

- Standard approaches to reporting problems

- A methodology for managing projects with a project team concept

- Standards for accomplishing various activities such as computer and telecommunications hardware installation.

Information Services Budget is a critical component of the administrative infrastructure. The budget needs to be developed and evaluated at three levels:

- Maintenance of current systems (hardware and applications)

- Information Services staff salaries

- Planned capital expenditure and operating budget.

Information Technology Processes - The set of activities required to analyze a healthcare institution system or process, design an IT-based solution, program and test the solution, develop user manuals, and maintain the system.

Information Technology Skills - Staff IS&T skills require strong communication and project planning skills. Given the institution's IT strategy and structure, what are the new skill sets required? It is important to evaluate the current skills of information services staff with a focus on their ability to learn and support new applications and technologies. It may be required to develop a human resource development plan to support the training existing information services staff on new technologies, or recruit additional staff with the specific skill sets in the new technologies. Employees must have knowledge of:

- Rapid application development tools

- Knowledge of networking and interface standards

B.4.8. Products from the IS&T Planning Process

[a] End products
- Statements of strategic solutions for IS and IT
- Phased development plans for:
  - Application systems and databases
  - IS&T development projects
  - Staff skills upgrade

- Basis for implementation
- Justification with financial plan
- Criteria and process for plan review, fine tuning, and maintenance

[b] Organization-oriented intermediate products
- Agreed report of hospital information, support needs, and priorities
- Indication of key areas of risk and uncertainty on which the viability of recommended solutions depend
- Assessment of current information systems in terms of the extent and quality of coverage of business needs
- Urgent action plan for interim "quick fixes"

[c] IS&T-oriented products
- Assessment of current IS and IT status:
  - Objective facts indicating what systems and technology there is
  - Judgmental statements indicating its quality as well as current and future relevance
- Target applications and database architecture
- Target IT architecture
- Skills and resource strategy

B.4.9. Criteria for Appraisal of the Financial Investment in IS&T Projects

When investing in IS&T, a number of key criteria for evaluating and approving the project must be considered. Investments in IS&T are no different to other significant investments in terms of the procedures they must follow and the need for rigorously constructed business plans. However, the mixture of technical and organizational issues raised by such investment demand that several questions must be raised by the decision-makers involved in the process of systems planing, design, and acquisition. They form the basis for criteria against which approval will be given. The criteria apply irrespective of the source of financing.

The discussion that follows is based on recommended criteria used by the U.K. National Health Services, developed by the NHS Management Executive, Information Management Group. Criteria which management should apply in assessing all IS&T investments, and against which approval will be given for those which are substantial, are:

1. The investment is part of an overall IS&T strategy based on the organization's business plan

Every IS&T investment must support the business and service objectives of the organization. These are usually detailed within the organization's business plan. It is also important that the total of all the IS&T systems within an organization provide consistent and coherent support to the business. It is, therefore, essential that every investment is part of an overall IS&T strategy based on the organization's business plan. Strategic horizons will generally be three to five years with an annual review.

2. There is a properly structured business plan based on good investment appraisal and realistic scheduling, with staged review points

When scrutinizing a business plan one must expect that the appropriate development of a Project Plan has been considered according to the criteria defined in Sections B.2.1. to B.2.8. above.

3. Account has been taken of achieving the same benefits from better use of existing assets

A range of IS&T options will usually exist, delivering differing levels of benefit but at differing costs and must be considered within the investment appraisal. The following options must be considered:

(a) *Status quo* - what would happen if the investment did not proceed? This must always be included for comparison purposes.

(b) *The non-IS&T solution* - is it possible to alter current practices to achieve increased benefits without implementing an IS&T solution?

(c) *Changing existing systems* - is it possible to increase the benefits from existing systems by changing the systems or the organization's working practices rather than implementing a new system?

4. The benefits (cash-releasing and noncash-releasing) have been properly and realistically identified and assessed with a commitment from the affected parties to their realization

In order for a benefit to be properly and realistically identified and achieved, it is necessary that:

(a) the benefit is accurately and precisely described;
(b) methods for measuring the benefit are outlined;
(c) the tasks required to achieve the benefit are identified; and
(d) a commitment to the achievement of the benefit is obtained from those affected.

If an investment in a provider organization is likely to result in increased costs to purchasers, then the continued viability of the provider's business plans should be considered. National demonstration projects may be of help in identifying the benefits that can be achieved.

B

5. Full assessment of the risks surrounding the investment is carried out at an early stage together with an evaluation, setting out how sensitive options are to change in the underlying assumptions that have been made

Options are often close together in terms of costs and benefits and the estimates used in the option appraisal can be uncertain. It is important to perform an analysis of these uncertainties and two essential elements — sensitivity analysis and risk analysis — must be addressed.

Sensitivity analysis will identify the assumptions made and consider the impact of varying the assumptions made on the options. Risk analysis considers the nature of the risks associated with the investment and their impact on the project. What measures can be introduced to minimize their impact?

6. There is a clear understanding of the procurement process

The procurement process will vary depending on the type, complexity, and size of the project being undertaken. In all cases the procurement process and the proposed contract will be expected to follow the guidelines explained in detail in Part C of this document. The contract must conform to all the necessary contractual safeguards.

7. The project will be handled in a structured manner

Each major project must be managed using a well-structured methodology. Guidelines can be found in a number of easily available general publications related to technology project management. A general introduction and recommendations are found in Sections B.2.1. to B.2.8. above. For large investments, consideration should be given to appointing a Project Supervisory Committee.

All participants in the project management structure must have an appropriate level of training and/or awareness of their roles. The Project Manager must be fully trained and experienced in information systems project management, and projects should not be started unless this can be demonstrated.

8. There is an unequivocal commitment from the Project Manager and Project Supervisory Committee and clear understanding of their roles, and of their senior staff, in the procurement, implementation, and benefits realization process

Implementation of a major IS&T investment can have a major impact on an organization. Senior members of the organization must be aware of all the potential internal and external impacts and be committed to the successful achievement of the investment.

9. There are sufficient and adequately skilled IS&T resources to manage successfully the specification, procurement, and implementation of the project

The IS&T human resources requirement must be identified. Where such resources are not available within the organization, the methods for obtaining the resources must be identified. When resources are obtained from outside the organization (outsourcing) it is important to ensure that the organization has sufficient skills to absorb their contribution and supervise those resources.

This will be an area of particular scrutiny. It can be difficult to recognize that in-house skills and experience may not be sufficient. However, this will be critical to a project's success. The larger the project the more skilled and experienced the project manager and internal IS&T staff need to be. It is the responsibility of the organization to make decisions on the suitability of their IS&T staff.

10. There is a resourced and structured training program

Implementing a major IS&T investment will mean training staff to operate the new procedures. A training need assessment should be performed and a structured training program produced to meet the needs identified. The plan for achieving benefits will normally be described within the business case. This will often be a substantial part of the investment — up to 15% of the capital costs.

11. There is a clear plan for benefits realization, including a commitment to assign responsibility for realizing benefits to an individual with sufficient authority and resources to deliver

In order to obtain benefits from an IS&T investment, changes to the organization and its work practices will often be required. To successfully implement the investment requires that an individual with sufficient authority and resources be prepared to commit to achieving the benefits outlined. To ensure that all parties play their role in achieving benefits, that authority should normally derive directly from the Project Manager.

As benefits are normally obtained within user departments or units, the managers of those departments, rather than IS&T specialists, will normally be responsible for the actual achievement of benefits. It is the responsibility of the Project Manager to ensure that they do so.

12. There is a commitment to post-implementation evaluation, the results of which will be made available to the authority approving the investment

It is essential to have a formal post-implementation review program whose prime purpose should be to identify problems and initiate appropriate remedial action. The process should not be regarded solely as a single exercise that occurs once the project has been implemented, but should be based on a continuing process which contributes to a final formal review at an appropriate point. This review should be aligned to a suitable milestone in the achievement of benefits, and should occur within two years of implementation. Plans for collecting monitoring and evaluating data should be set out in the preparation phase of the business case.

Where projects take a year or more to implement from the signing of the contract, or if there is no contract one should consider the start of implementation, the organization should identify a significant milestone in each year. At this milestone the Project Committee should review the project to ensure it is on schedule, within costs and that it should continue. A report should be submitted to the normal approval body. For projects where implementation will take a year or less, a post-implementation review report should also be submitted at the end of the scheduled implementation.

B.4.10. *Maintenance of Information Systems*

After the systems implementation phase, the maintenance phase takes over. Systems maintenance is the on-going maintenance of a system after it has been placed into operation.

When developing information strategy plans, organizations cannot afford to neglect the fact that systems maintenance is the longest and costliest phase of the systems life cycle. The implications of the maintenance workload upon the information strategy plans for an organization is a subject that deserves special attention. The organization structure needs flexibility to support the maintenance of existing systems concurrently with the implementation of new technologies.

It is important to consider the evaluation and monitoring of a system for needed maintenance and consequently, to lower or contain maintenance costs. Systems maintenance can be categorized into four groups. Each of these four categories can affect an organization's information strategy plan in different ways:

- *Corrective Maintenance*. Regardless of how well designed, developed, and tested a system or application may be, errors will inevitably occur. This type of maintenance deals with fixing or correcting problems with the system. This usually refers to problems that were not identified during the implementation phase. An example of remedial maintenance is the lack of a user-required feature or the improper functionality of it.

- *Customized Maintenance*. This type of maintenance refers to the creation of new features or adapting existing ones as required by changes in the organization or by the users, e.g., changes on the organization's tax code or internal regulations.

- *Enhancement Maintenance*. It deals with enhancing or improving the performance of the system either by adding new features or by changing existing ones. An example of this type of maintenance is the conversion of text-based systems to GUI (Graphical User Interface).

- *Preventive Maintenance.* This type of maintenance may be one of the most cost effective, since if performed timely and properly, it can avoid major problems with the system. An example of this maintenance is the correction for the year 2000.

SETTING UP HEALTHCARE SERVICES INFORMATION SYSTEMS

A DON'T LIST

1. Don't depend too much on one pioneering innovator, and do not leave any such innovator in charge — they will become too rigid and narrow-minded in their views, and stifle change and development.

2. Don't spend a large amount of time creating a detailed, rigid specification — it will be out of date before being designed, built, and implemented; rather, specify core principles and functionality together with a design-and-build or prototyping methodology.

3. Don't leave performance criteria, both in terms of functions provided and maximum percentage downtime to chance, but include them in the procurement contract.

4. Don't forget error correction and maintenance — write minimum standards into supply contracts, and ensure that there are sanctions, e.g., part of procurement payment held back until satisfactory functioning over a specified period; maintenance payments paid partly at the end of each period with reductions for loss of service.

5. Don't let the supplier determine needs or performance; instead, ensure that the customer remains in control.

6. Don't exploit your supplier — whilst the customer should lead, an aggrieved supplier provides a poor service and a bankrupted supplier disappears and leaves the customer stranded.

7. Don't impose "solutions" on end users and data suppliers; rather, ensure that they feel they are valued and want the system.

8. Don't automate today's paper processes — look at what new functions and methods automated Information Systems can undertake.

9. Don't specify too futuristically — there is a limit to how much people or an organization can change in one move; instead allow an evolutionary path.

(continues next page)

(continuation from the previous page)

10. Don't treat the organization or the specification as rigid structure, but instead allow for organizational and end-user learning, as well as technological and environmental change.

11. Don't stop evaluation at the point of installation testing — there will be ongoing organizational and personal behavioral change that must be identified and appropriate adjustments made.

12. Don't stop investing in a "successful" system — it will soon become out-of-date, and disillusionment will set in thus, to the dismay of users and paying parties, the "success" will soon evaporate.

13. Don't be complacent with a "successful" system — the very word of its success will increase usage, overload access, and degrade performance — this applies to all elements, including data networks and communications.

14. Don't confuse *Education* (concerned with changing professional practice and performance) with *Training* (about how to operate a system).

15. Don't change practice and switch on a system in one activity, but also don't computerize old practice — separate the two change processes, even though this will mean a short period of dysfunctional working, so as to ensure that the different changes are fully understood, and any problems can be traced to the correct source to facilitate rapid adjustment.

16. Don't rely on memory or suppliers — persons can forget, become ill, or leave; suppliers can go out of business or be taken over. Ensure that everything is properly documented, including performance agreements, and all systems specifications, functionalities, applications, and operational routines — the constant test must be "Could a new person take over that task tomorrow?".

17. Don't overlook the need for convincing answers on confidentiality — it will be a prime question from all health professionals before they use a system.

18. Don't think that removing names from records creates confidentiality — other factual combinations in records can effectively identify indirectly by implication or circumstance.

19. Don't assume that any types of data item are of low confidentiality — for some individuals any specific item may be very confidential because of personal circumstances, e.g., address or blood group.

20. Don't touch anything which does not run on open standards, is of a closed proprietary nature, or cannot accommodate modern recognized data and other standards — any short-term gain will be minimal compared with the cost of the dead end up which you are committing your organization.

21. Don't think that any Information System project is ever finished — if it successful, people will want more of it; if it unsuccessful, adjustments are clearly needed; and in any eventuality circumstances will change.

B

B.5. Health Informatics - Who Leads, Who Represents?

Information systems and particularly information technology are often seen negatively, and without a full appreciation of their essential role in healthcare delivery. Given that information is at the heart of healthcare and is essential for the management processes and the fact that science and technology are being harnessed widely by other segments of the society to improve upon paper-based methods, it is a matter of major concern that there is a lack of shared vision and leadership for IS&T in the health sector. There is a lack of focused research programs and structured evaluation, and many academic units are struggling for funding and little opportunity is taken to learn from overseas experience or developments. Even where there are national initiatives, such as in moves to support professional education and operations-support applications, projects and their development are generally uncoordinated and we are still far from common policies or standards. The losers are the public as consumers, health, and other professionals directly involved, and the informatics industry.

Meanwhile, the rapidly changing relationship between the functional capacity and price of modern technology is increasingly seen as the way to improve production processes while saving time and money, with wider benefits, including better quality of communication and thus, for the health sector, of care. Notwithstanding all the problems and constraints mentioned, Health Informatics is becoming an everyday part of healthcare practice, but often in a piecemeal and managerially led way. Consequently, those with a direct interest in constructive and ethical use of Health Informatics in clinical care and in advanced use of technology are less than happy with the current environment. To solve the major development and acceptance problems the following issues must be addressed by the health informatics community:

- Coordination amongst policy makers
- Poor use of IS&T by the health sector
- Patchy success in solving complex issues
- Leadership and cooperation
- Variety of stakeholders and their agendas
- Divergent priorities
- Need for independent associations.

1. Absent coordination amongst policy-makers

There is continual tension between policy-makers at the national and local levels, healthcare organizations, health professionals, and systems suppliers. Important initiatives to circumvent those problems exist, but are often felt not to achieve their full potential. Frequently each of the technical, administrative, and operational constituent parts of public, and sometimes also private, health organizations have their own information management and technology strategy, with little coordination on identification and agreement of underpinning common principles or priorities. Moreover, liaison with the academic, research, and industrial communities appears to be at arm's length rather than closely integrated.

2. Wide use, poor usefulness, of IS&T

Other service industries such as banking, commerce, and travel have already gone much further than healthcare in the widespread harnessing of information technology to provide better and cost-effective services. New patterns of communication and information are almost entirely dependent upon information technology, and the use of Internet and Intranet systems shows great promise, as do many health telematics applications. Nevertheless, many domestic households have more powerful computing and telecommunications infrastructure than many clinical departments. Although health informatics is becoming a part of healthcare practice and few diagnostic departments could function nowadays without computer technology, poor utilization of IS&T by the health sector poses a great challenge.

3. Patchy success in solving complex issues

Healthcare raises a greater range of more taxing issues than most other areas of information technology application. These issues range from the representation of illness and the clinical needs and treatment objectives of patients, through the maintenance of confidentiality and avoidance of abuse where large volumes of highly personal and potentially financially valuable information are concerned. Many countries, e.g., the United Kingdom, the United States, France, Sweden, Holland, and others, have been very active not just in pioneering and deepening the use of health IS&T, but also in tackling innovatively some of the core issues related to standards development and implementation and the representation of clinical concepts. Yet at the same time there is much to be done regarding practical implementation, quality control aspects, structured evaluation methodologies for IS&T, and the education of health professionals in informatics.

4. Need for leadership and cooperation

Health informatics offers major opportunities to support efficient and high-quality healthcare. It also has a potential to repeat past failures or introduce new risks. It is a surprising and worrying paradox that this fundamental area of healthcare science and policy has a limited number of leading organizations and very few common meeting points for debate. The major international technical cooperation organizations have approached the issue in a fragmented, uncoordinated, and technically deficient manner. Many projects sponsored, designed, or funded by such agencies have a narrow perspective, and some were technically unsound and failed to take advantage of the available technological opportunities. Exceptions to this sad state of affairs are the international and national health informatics scientific and technical associations of which the International Medical Informatics Association (IMIA) is a prime example — unfortunately they have limited influence over most decision-makers, who continue to be uninformed about IS&T.

This leadership vacuum has heightened the tension between leading individuals of the clinical professions, whose vision is on informatics as a tool for the clinician, one that may engender parochial approaches, and national policies aimed at providing an efficient informatics infrastructure, which can be perceived as being bureaucratic or having a hidden agenda.

5. Variety of stakeholders and their agendas

(a) The direct care professions

Many professional groups, including specialty societies, have established mechanisms to consider informatics issues in their own domains, and approaches taken have varied from objective reviews of data-related issues, standards, application systems, to the consideration of educational needs. However, there is a tendency towards medical computing special interest groups, which focus primarily upon practitioner-designed stand-alone systems, that undoubtedly have intrinsic value, but when developed in isolation are not conducive to integrated policies or standards. We have seen that each health professional body now has an interest group in informatics, but the majority are largely unfunded and with a restricted number of active associates. Perversely, in a supposed era of integrated and seamless healthcare there is no vehicle for these professional interests to come together to develop a common interprofessional view, or to explore common ground.

(b) Academic bodies

Academic units for health informatics undertake research as well as teach. Although well respected in their specialist areas, in general, they suffer difficulties in obtaining funds as a result of the generally low recognition of the importance of health informatics. Obtaining funding is particularly difficult as informatics falls right across the boundaries between medicine, physical science, economics, and social sciences. Therefore, most strategic research projects — those which would identify informatics solutions and evaluate their effects upon healthcare — have no natural prime funding source, no master vision, no overall control, and no coordination. This is in contrast to most other areas of healthcare development, where academic units and the clinical professions work in tandem, and routes to research funding are clear. Similarly, information and informatics do not feature high on the research and development agenda at the national or regional level in most countries.

Some progress on the professional education side is being made in determining informatics components of the medical undergraduate and postgraduate curricula but these are, in nearly all instances, quite separate from real project development and operation.

(c) IS&T professionals and the industry

Most professional associations for IS&T are active in seeking to raise the status and the education of IS&T professionals. They should develop much stronger links with health professional interests. The unhelpful perception by many health professionals of IS&T technical personnel being "administrative", in the pejorative healthcare interpretation of the term, needs to be broken. Health professionals must recognize the importance and contribution of the information specialist profession in ensuring the sound implementation and operation of informatics systems, whilst informaticians must be conspicuously in tune with the health professionals' requirements and understanding of their anxieties.

Finally, but importantly, the hardware and software supplier industry is active and innovative, and does have a trade association function. Unfortunately, in any free market situation, suppliers are nearly always seen as being motivated by self-interest to a greater degree than is actually the case, and there is a strong argument for strengthening links with health-focused supplier bodies over generic policy, standards, and development issues.

6. Divergent priorities

Examples abound to prove that healthcare informatics in most countries is fragmented and without leadership. Certainly, it is holding back the better and safer application of modern technology in the interests of good healthcare. It also creates destructive suspicion and tension when cooperation and coordination would be more appropriate. Because opportunities for discussion of divergent and sometimes outright conflicting priorities are few, there is no open objective forum for analysis, research, or debate, and above all there is a lack of patient representation. A coming together for the common good, and the creation of a shared vision and voice for health informatics development and use, are greatly needed.

One must focus on alliances between suppliers, academic units, and care providers, without overlooking the importance of splitting the commissioning of research, the pursuit of innovation, and independent evaluation, as in the pharmaceutical science model. Issues of common learning versus proprietary interests, and of balancing commercial confidence and published concepts, must be adequately considered, and the overall legal and ethical implications must be addressed.

7. Need for independent associations

What is missing throughout is the common ground, organizational and intellectual, where health professional health informaticians, suppliers, and other interested parties can come together in a noncompetitive and nonconfrontational setting to constructively advance the science and ethical principles of health informatics.

Healthcare computing conferences and related exhibitions are important contributions, but they have limitations as policy and developmental settings, particularly in a science-based field. The equivalent of the respected American Medical Informatics Association (AMIA) does not exist in most countries. Such professional and technical associations can provide an open and influential analysis and debating forum. In Latin America and the Caribbean there are active health informatics associations, particularly in Brazil, Argentina, Uruguay, Mexico, and Cuba, but the number of associates and representation across the stakeholders' spectrum is still rather limited.

At the international level, the International Medical Informatics Association (IMIA) is an effective organization that is addressing the key issues here discussed. Working groups cover not only the traditional interests such as nursing informatics and data security, but also the need for better evaluative methodologies, the impact of informatics upon healthcare organizations, and how appropriate expertise can be transferred from developed to developing countries.

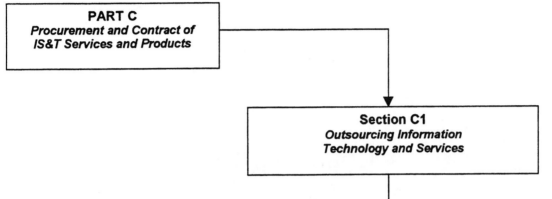

PART C
Procurement and Contract of IS&T Services and Products

Section C1
Outsourcing Information Technology and Services

Section C2
Request for Proposals and Contracting IS&T Service Providers

C

Part C. Procurement and Contract of IS&T Services and Products

C

Part C. Procurement and Contract of IS&T Services and Products

It is not the oath that makes us believe the man, but the man the oath.

Aeschylus (525–456 B.C.)

C.1. Outsourcing Information Technology and Services

Healthcare IS&T application development and implementation are expensive. Development, support, and operation are high-cost components and experienced personnel are mandatory. One of the major reasons for the high price tag is the complexity of healthcare systems, which requires the use of sophisticated technology and highly skilled support. While in other lines of business applications, technology may answer the user needs with off-the-shelf or relatively uncomplicated products, healthcare applications must focus on elaborate information technology that may require different vendors' solutions and platforms.

IS&T managers have no choice but to prepare for a future that includes outsourcing, and organizations of all sizes are seriously considering shifting some IS&T assets to a third party. To meet systems targets and bottom-line objectives, managers must deal with change, manage complexity, and find skilled workers. That is where outsourcing is seen to greatly improve the efficiency of development and operation of information systems. Firms that have opted to outsource cite several key goals:

- Reduce operating costs
- Share risks with outsourcing partners
- Access cutting-edge IS&T capabilities through vendors' expertise
- Improve focus on core competencies.

Outsourcing IS&T infrastructure tasks permits many companies to concentrate on core competencies, product development, and other concerns more directly related to service provision or revenue development. Indeed, IS&T operations are outsourced more than any other kind of business operation. IS&T outsourcing may be the best solution for many healthcare institutions as a way to solve these problems while increasing the on-time and on-budget performance and improving services.

C.1.1. Definition and Types

Outsourcing is a contractual relationship with a service provider to assume responsibility of one or more functions of an institution. *Outsourcing IS&T functions is becoming a common practice among many industries, including the health industry, driven by a shortage of skills and the need to concentrate efforts and energy in the core business of healthcare services.* Healthcare institutions are overwhelmed with the many applications that need to be developed, rewritten, converted, or re-engineered.

There is a large growth in outsourcing various types of services. Including the following:

- *Application Development* - New systems are being developed every day, either to replace old ones or to implement new applications.

- *Applications Maintenance* - Users have new demands and changing requirements and the rapid evolution of IS&T is characterized by new hardware and software platforms and existing applications must be ported to new environments. As an example, one of the major requirements for the end of this century is the fix of the so-called "Year 2000 Bug". Old systems did not account for the double "0" (zero) digit that can cause a chaotic situation in many legacy systems. The demand for this service is higher than the current supply of service providers available for the job.

- *Systems Integration* - It is a trend in almost all industries nowadays to implement and customize off-the-shelf applications for their needs, even for large integrated applications. In many instances, these off-the-shelf applications will have to be integrated with older systems and platforms, as well as custom-designed systems. Many institutions purchasing and installing packaged applications request the assistance of service providers to support the total implementation or the various steps in the process of integration across heterogeneous hardware platforms and networks.

- *Data Centers* - The healthcare sector, its institutions, and technology are all changing faster and faster. In-house data centers are either outsourced or not implemented because the costs of staffing and maintaining them are prohibitive to many institutions.

- *Networking Services* - Establishment and maintenance of Local Area Network (LAN) and Wide Area Network (WAN).

- *End-user Computing* - End-user computing establishes specific guidelines and quality services to be applied for the acquisition, utilization, and integration of hardware, software, and accessories to ensure an effective use of desktop technologies. The role of internal, external, or vendor consultants in facilitating and guiding end-user computing is to determine hardware and software selection procedures; troubleshooting end-user problems; development of training plans, procedures, handbooks, and instructional materials; and setup strategies for promoting technological change.

- *User Training* - User training is usually customized to the types of users and the needs of the organization. It can be performed by the same service provider used for implementation or, depending on the complexity of the systems developed and availability of training personnel, by another contractor.

"Outsourcing" has become a common word among institutions that are updating and/or developing IS&T solutions in the healthcare and other industries. In a recent article in Healthcare Informatics, a U.S.-based magazine, it was reported that the healthcare industry has been increasingly investing more money in outsourcing of IS&T solutions, mainly in the areas of implementation of information systems, processing services, and other IS&T-related operations. Worldwide corporate spending on outsourcing services reached US$86 billion in 1996 and is expected to surpass US$136 billion by 2001. The U.S. represented the strongest outsourcing market, comprising nearly fifty percent of all outsourcing spending. The growth in the outsourcing market is being driven by various factors including globalization, privatization, deregulation, and technological innovation.

Table 1. Outsourcing Areas in Health Information Technology (1996)

IS&T Areas Outsourced in Healthcare	Responses
Software development, implementation and support	21%
Network design and support	20%
PC/desktop maintenance and support	19%
Data center operation	14%
Consulting and contract programming	10%
Hardware maintenance and support	9%
Billing/financial system operation and support	8%
Telecommunications support	7%
Technical services	7%
PC/desktop acquisition and installation	6%
Help desk	6%
Management	5%
WAN design and support	4%
PC/desktop training	3%
Clinical system operation and support	2%
Base: 512 IS&T executives in the U.S. Source: College of Healthcare Information Management Executives (Healthcare Informatics, Feb '97)	

C

The IS&T and telecommunications industry have diversified immensely in the past decade. Outsourcing has become an answer to the fast growth of software and platforms. Information Technology can be compared to the field of medicine, in which specialization is essential for conducting the technical work and providing appropriate services. The pace of hardware and software development is so fast that training in-house personnel becomes a major challenge and a difficult task to be accomplished. Even established information service providers face the challenges of getting qualified staff.

Outsourcing can provide an institution with these "hard-to-find" professionals, but at a high cost. Nevertheless, outsourcing, if implemented correctly and with the full participation of in-house management and IS&T personnel, can be one way to track productivity, produce higher quality of services, and improve the information available to the users and the timeliness of information systems delivery. The widespread utilization of outsourcing can be judged by the Table 1, which presents information surveyed from 512 U.S. executives that were asked which were the top IS&T areas outsourced by their organizations.

C.1.2. Reasons for Outsourcing

Healthcare institutions outsource IS&T functions for a number of reasons:

- *Lack of qualified staff* - Because of such complexity and demands, most healthcare institutions have outrun the capability of their internal resources. Today's systems demand personnel skills that are new and may not be answered by the current IS&T staff. The result is constant training efforts and delayed progress, or increased cost through recruiting and the use of external consultants.

- *Allow healthcare institutions to focus on healthcare services rather than on IS&T development and implementation* - In the past, application development projects were usually kept in-house. Today, however, health organizations frequently find that they lack the necessary skills or ability to meet their requirements for releasing applications on time and must resort to outsourcing.

- *Establish new IS&T models and processes* - Healthcare institutions are under significant pressure to cut costs while improving quality and building and positioning technology to serve its payers better. Payers now demand more services and information from the healthcare industry. Through the availability of medical libraries, Internet services, decision support systems for physicians, and other IS&T services and systems, this challenge can be met.

- *Accommodate changing infrastructure* - Use of telecommunications, distributed systems, and networks in healthcare.

- *Extend reach of services* - Health promotion, distance learning, imaging transfer, telemedicine projects, etc.

- *Facilitate implementation* - Especially in the case of new and advanced applications.

- *Improve quality of healthcare services* - This can be achieved by organizing information and facilitating the use and dissemination of information for primary healthcare, health planning, and managing costs efficiently.

- *Stay on the leading edge of technology* - To take full advantage of the opportunities of IS&T requires qualified specialized staff and constant examination of new developments and products.

- *Convert old to new systems* - Outdated systems are often a barrier to support the changes of the healthcare systems because of costs involved and long cycle times to implement changes. Nevertheless, with the right methodology, these systems can be a springboard to reduce both the cost and cycle time of new development initiatives.

- *Optimize IS&T capabilities* - Outdated systems and procedures must be improved to cope with the actual demand of healthcare institutions.

- *Share implementation risk* - Outsourcing is an opportunity for splitting project risks with outsourcing service providers.

- *Gain control of difficult-to-manage functions and manage increased diversity and complexity* - Those require specialized knowledge and accumulated experience.

C.1.3. Success Factors in Outsourcing

Risks are always present when outsourcing is used. To avoid potential problems and to increase the chance for a successful outsourcing project, some important issues should be considered, including, but not limited to:

- *Select what to outsource* - Define, establish, and follow a planning process for the outsourcing project. Allow time for due diligence and select an internal multi-professional group to prepare an evaluation report on the institution's IS&T requirements, identifying which areas are going to be outsourced according to the institution's plans and priorities.

- *Selection of service provider* - The selection of a service provider for outsourcing is critical. Terms and conditions of contract must be carefully considered in advance of signing any agreement. The organization outsourcing IS&T must be prepared to supervise, measure, and manage the results of the outsourcing contract. The main goal of most service providers is to increase revenue, and the way to achieve this goal is to sell large new systems or extended services to customers, rather than building on existing customer applications. Vendors also offer services by seeking alliances with other vendors, which may not be in the best interest of the client. The issue of dealing with vendors is so important to outsourcing that we are dedicating one entire section to assist managers to reach appropriate decisions on this matter.

- *IS&T leadership* - IS&T leadership is a major issue for the successful delivery of IS&T, and the existence of a leader in the outsourcing organization with expertise in IS&T and in charge of the process of IS&T outsourcing is highly recommended. Continuity of in-house expertise may be a problem—although exceptions do exist, the tenure of a *Chief Information Officer (CIO)* or *Director for IS&T* in the U.S. is around three to four years, a much shorter time than it takes to deploy complex projects.

- *Choose a committed and competent implementation team* - A team to supervise the outsourcing project should be assembled early in the process and it should have the right mix of users and technical professionals. It is also important to get the promise of managers for these people to be assigned, sometimes full time, to the project team.

- *Establish progress report meetings and milestone analysis* - Frequent revisions of the project plan by interviews and participation of the implementation team during the selection process are indispensable. The channels of communication between the implementation team and management should always be open for discussion of unforeseeable issues during the implementation period. Managers should supervise the activities, ensure that the agreements and implementation timetable are being enforced, and provide the necessary resources for the team to conduct its affairs in the most proactive way.

- *Education of project management team and users* - Recognize the concerns and doubts that outsourcing brings and have a strategy for dealing with the complex "people issues" that arise during any implementation. Poor interpersonal communication and lack of user education in the issues related to IS&T can and will put a burden in outsourcing. It is important for the project team to get support from all users or customers of the system.

- *Management support of IS&T projects* - Management support is vital for the success of IS&T projects. Senior management must view IS&T implementation as a corporate process, essential for the healthcare institution, which integrates disparate information requirements and changes the managerial and day-to-day tasks and functions, with the objective of improving the operational performance.

- *Establishment of realistic goals for vendors* - Vendors that offer quick fixes to long-term problems should be avoided. Set up realistic time frames for the completion of complex tasks. It takes time for an outside entity to fully understand the business of an institution, to set up operations, and to put processes in place. Complex projects do take time.

- *Test frequently during the development or maintenance of an application* - Institutions should make sure that an internal team performs a meticulous testing of outsource applications. The outsourced system development or maintenance project should be free of errors and functionally complete. The parameters defined during the implementation phase must have been fully addressed, and the system must integrate effectively with other systems in the institution and must perform at satisfactory levels.

Outsourcing vendors face many of the same problems experienced by their customers. A shortage of skilled IS&T workers and an extremely competitive marketplace have caused some vendors to spread personnel too thin relative to the number and complexity of projects they have. This may make some prospective customers, especially those with adequate resources to focus on both IS&T and business operations, to opt for the relative security of in-house development or operations control. Some customers may also hesitate because of stories about overextended outsourcing vendors who demand full control of IS&T departments and communications breakdowns that hampered operations. A maturing market, though, means more customers know what they want and need, and more vendors are determined to help them meet their goals.

C.1.4. *Why Outsourcing Contracts May Fail*

Some of the reasons why outsourcing contracts may fail are the following:

- *Institutional objectives are not clearly communicated to the service provider* - The contract that is structured does not match the institution's objectives. This situation can happen when the members of the evaluation team have different objectives from each other or management, which sends the vendor mixed signals regarding the real goals.

- *Vendors control the contract* - Vendors have a tendency to offer customers more than what they really need as a way to increase revenue, while giving customers the impression that they are getting the best return on their investment. Institutions want to believe that outsourcing will solve all their problems. Consequently, frequently they gullibly accept many of the exaggerated claims made by the vendor sales team. The more organized and realistic the customers' plans are up front, the happier they tend to be with the contract.

- *Unanticipated changes in technology* - The pace in which technology is advancing is so fast that it is hard to predict if today's vendor will be able to deliver tomorrow's technology. The longer the term of the contract, the more likely that someday the contract will not adequately address the requirements of the institution.

- *Unanticipated changes in policies* - Changes in internal and/or external policies can happen anytime. These changes, even though they are difficult to avoid, can mangle decisions or delay outsourcing contracts.

- *Customers spend inadequate attention, time, and resources on managing the contract* - Institutions should not underestimate the time and effort needed to ensure success in an outsourcing contract. Outsourcing requires a number of highly skilled and talented staff. The quality, quantity, continuity, professionalism, and organizational structure of the institution's project management team are the most important factors in obtaining a successful outsourcing contract.

- *Most outsourcing contracts do not consider the impact of price shifts of the market* - Institutions want to negotiate a good price for a contract, but how can they be assured that this "good" price will still be a good price six months after the contract is signed? With the shift in the information technology market, pricing should be considered a very important aspect of the contract. Vendors and outsourcers should be able to renegotiate rates in long-term contracts or they may not meet their cost expectations. On the other hand, contracts should not be negotiated on prices alone.

- *Lack of skilled personnel* - One of the reasons why institutions outsource is to transfer the responsibility of recruiting, retraining, and retaining skilled staff to an external service provider. However, one must not forget that service providers are competing in the same labor market as their customers. When the service provider does not offer the best salaries and working conditions to employ "best-of-breed" personnel, inadequately skilled personnel come aboard to fill the gap and the outsourcing organization runs the risk of being supported by poorly qualified professionals.

C.1.5. How to Avoid Outsourcing Problems

Once a company sets the best allocation of internal IS&T resources, analysts urge caution in going forward with an outsourcing agreement. It is imperative to go to the negotiating table with definite requests for references from satisfied customers in hand. Outsourcing providers should be able to produce a track record of previous projects' on-time and on-budget performance. Also, managers should make clear to potential outsourcing partners exactly who will report to whom and when before signing a contract.

Service-level agreements, including quality benchmarks and the experience of staff members who will be working on the project, should also be spelled out. Many providers may begin a project with senior-level staff, only to pull them out for use on their next deal, leaving junior staff that cannot perform at the same level.

Service providers should be willing to take a financial hit if they cannot deliver their promises. Penalties should be associated with long-term underperformance. Do not negotiate a contract based on your existing processes and structure contracts looking out three to five years into the future. For managers who do not have experience in forecasting their needs, it is advisable to hire a reputable outsourcing consultant. Because the outsourcing company could merge with or acquire another firm and because technology advances could dictate new investments, it is recommended that the terms of contract renegotiation and the issues should be renegotiated. One must be aware of monopolistic pricing policies and of vendors who have demanded to have control of everything to achieve economy of scale.

Risks exist in almost any contract. Nevertheless, there are a few essential rules or principles that institutions can follow when structuring an outsourcing contract to avoid problems later. Some of them are as follows:

- *An outsourcing plan should be made in the context of the institution's IS&T general plan* - Research the real needs of the institutions and outsource only the projects that cannot be developed in-house. Service providers should be able to complete an outsourcing project faster and better than if done in-house.

- *Institutions should be selective when inviting service providers to bid for contracts* - Before writing a Request for Proposals (RFP), prepare a Request for Information (RFI) to investigate which vendors may have the appropriate experience, knowledge, and resources to handle an outsourcing contract for the institution. Only the most qualified vendors should then be invited to bid and receive an RFP.

- *Institutions should be wary of service providers that promise quick fixes to long-term problems* - The evaluation team should conduct a thorough evaluation of the vendor to avoid future problems.

- *Vendors, consultants, and service providers should not be selected because of price alone* - Recognize that IS&T providers who hire "best-of-breed" professionals and dedicate more resources to the contract may cost more than vendors that simply want to win a contract.

- *Choose multiple providers, if necessary* - Service providers, consultants, and IS&T suppliers specialize in different areas. A total contract with one vendor may be risky if the vendor is not in the leading edge of the service being required. Specialization helps customers get the most competent vendors for their needs.

- *Avoid signing long-term contracts* - Instead, healthcare institutions should write short-term contracts with extension clauses to avoid committing one entire contract to a vendor who, eventually, will be found to perform poorly.

- *Present a clear and comprehensive description of the scope of services required* - The clearer and more comprehensive the definition of scope of services is, the easier it will be for the vendor to understand and accomplish the tasks under a contract.

- *Establish effective and unencumbered communication channels between management, project team, and service provider* - Progress reports should be prepared periodically to report problems, solutions, and improvements and to make sure the proper schedule is being followed.

C

C.2. Request for Proposals and Contracting IS&T Service Providers

Use of suitable implementation processes and practices in the procurement of technology can result in significant better procurement routines and cost savings. Because of the fast changes in IS&T and the changing environment of the health sector, now more than ever, healthcare institutions must have timely and accurate information and comparative performance analysis concerning the best available products and services. An integral part of the procurement process is the *Request for Proposal* (RFP). The benefits of an effective RFP go far beyond cost savings. If done correctly, an RFP can help anticipate needs and resource requirements.

A Request for Proposals details to potential service providers the needs and requirements of a healthcare institution's information systems plan and priorities. It provides guidelines by which the organization can measure a vendor's ability to provide the required product and service. An effective RFP articulates the possible answers and solutions to the real problems and lays the foundation for assessing vendor capabilities. It is a tool to aid the institution in the selection of a provider for the purchase of equipment and products and for the delivery of services.

It is advisable for those institutions without a standard RFP format to review formats of RFPs of similar healthcare institutions to compare areas of concern. Vendors usually respond only to questions asked, and some healthcare institutions may not be aware of other concerns until they face an unforeseen expense or problem. Ideally, RFPs should include as great a degree of specification as possible and should only be prepared once the institution has clearly defined:

- The objectives of the implementation and the tasks the vendor is expected to perform or provide

- Short- and long-term plans for itself

- Which vendors may be the best candidates to perform the needed initiatives and therefore those that should be invited to submit a proposal.

Some institutions may not be fully prepared to issue an RFP, but instead a *Request for Information* (RFI). An RFI is a simple request for information regarding the vendor itself, its experience, products, financial stability, and projects, whereas an RFP requires detailed information regarding the requirements of the institution.

C.2.1. Preliminary Tasks

A comprehensive and specific Request for Proposals should be written, making sure to identify to all interested vendors what the needs of the institution are, and what are the expectations regarding the delivery of services or products. This process also helps to organize thoughts about which characteristics are most important.

Even though it may take a long time to write a detailed RFP, this is a task that should not be undertaken lightly. It is essential to transmit to the vendors as much information as possible about the institution, its mission, plans, services, systems requirements, hardware and software specifications, and any other type of information that could assist vendors to understand the objectives, operations, and clientele of the healthcare organization. Thus, in elaborating an RFP one should include as much specification for the IS&T as possible. This information is important to establish that the organization knows in advance exactly what it expects to get from the vendor or service provider.

It may be wise for health information managers to develop an RFP with enough specificity to realistically evaluate proposals and estimate costs of applications.

Necessary steps must be taken to ensure a competitive RFP and fairness in the selection of a provider. Through a detailed invitation letter, potential vendors should be requested to submit proposals. The letter should specify the date when the proposals are due and to whom they should be addressed. Both the letter and the accompanying RFP should state that all documentation submitted with the proposal will become the property of the healthcare institution. The following tasks must be accomplished before preparing the RFP:

- Document the need for a Health Services Information System;

- Define the institution's mission and work plans;

- Document the functional organization of the institution;

- Document the existing system;

- Identify clinical documents, clinical records, report formats, and other support documents necessary for data collection, input, and report preparation;

- Request staff participation in the project by inquiring about information and reporting needs;

- Identify problems with the existing system;

- Select qualified staff and a project manager for the project;

- Develop a comprehensive description of the user requirements;

- Obtain the commitment of top-level managers, administrators, and staff;

- Clarify and develop policies and procedures necessary to support the system development effort and successful implementation.

All systems specifications issues must be addressed within the framework established by the IS&T objectives of the health service, including the feasibility study recommendations and proposed timeframe. It is important to specify the types of vendor support and services needed, e.g., installation assistance, support services, program documentation, maintenance/modification support from vendor, user training program, etc.

If an RFP was never prepared before, the institution should, besides evaluating RFPs from similar types of institutions, consider hiring an outside consultant to assist in its preparation. A minimum of three proposals should be solicited, and the maximum number of proposals should be established in order to allow ample time for the review of all of them. When deciding which vendors to send an invitation to bid, the institution should expect that some vendors will not respond. Users and service providers must be always ready to accept changes in systems requirements and provider, if necessary.

C.2.2. Outlining a Request for Proposals

RFPs should be presented in clear language, comprehensive terminology, and standardized format to facilitate the understanding, by the vendors, of the systems objectives of the organization. A sample RFP outline for a healthcare institution is set forth below for reference. This is a sample outline that does not list all required information for all types of institutions:

- *Introduction/Statement of Purpose* - Brief history of the healthcare institution, institution's services and mission, procurement and contract administration, overall specifications, and service and/or equipment delivery.

- *Institution's Profile* - Physical configuration, patient/inpatient statistics, clinic statistics, services and department, etc.

- *Terms, Conditions, and Scope of the Outsourcing for Services.*

- *Information on Current Systems* - With details of existing applications, routines and procedures, and characteristics of the implementation environment.

- *Functional Systems Requirements* - Administration of patients, service scheduling, out-patient care, admissions, transfers, and discharge (census, patient information, patient tracking); support services management (materials management, inventory control); emergency services (registration, history and charting, order processing); finances (general ledger, accounts receivable, billing); medical records; nursing services; pharmacy; radiology; dietary services; clinical laboratory; laundry; maintenance and housekeeping; staffing; human resources; etc.

- *Technical Requirements* - Hardware (description, capacity, storage devices, response time, interfaces); development and basic software (operating system, programming languages, development tools, data security and integrity, documentation); and application software functionalities and data sets.

- *Training Requirements* - Skills required for the operation of systems and applications; training plan; determination of training end-points; expected recycling; training materials and timeframe.

- *Implementation Process* - How it is expected to be done, assumptions, and constraints.

- *Financial Considerations* - Capital and recurrent costs expectations.

- *Vendor Information* - Corporate history, financial status, client list, previous experience with similar projects.

- *Conditions of Bidding* - Acceptance, timetable, and withdraw clauses.

- *Evaluation Criteria* - To be used to evaluate vendors, proposals, and deliverables.

- *Decision Timetable* - Ranges of acceptable time for the decisions that must be made, from the search of service providers, preparation of detailed specifications, preparation of procurement documentation, and the selection and contract of services.

- *Responsibilities of the Institution and the Vendor* - Expectations of the organization regarding contract provisions.

- *Cost* - Range of expected disbursement over time.

C.2.3. Evaluation Process

The first step toward the decision of selecting one or other provider is to conduct an initial review and evaluation of all proposals to determine whether they satisfy the basic requirements. Relevant questions should be asked and the construction of a matrix of requirements versus offerings is a helpful tool in the comparison of proposals. After the initial review of the proposals, a second-level evaluation should be made.

C.2.3.1. Evaluation of Proposals

The submitted proposals may be very complex, in terms both of the application description and techniques to be used in the implementation. If the institution does not have qualified personnel to perform the evaluation of the proposals, it is advisable to again consider using an external consultant for the evaluation process. The consultant may be able to apply specific experience to the evaluation of techniques proposed, as well as provide an objective and credible point of view. A written report from the consultant regarding the proposals, the selection process, and recommendations for contracting can serve as a valuable starting point for approval and negotiation. If none of the proposals submitted are acceptable, or if the number of responses is too few to constitute a competitive bid, the healthcare institution may reject all proposals and submit another invitation letter to potential vendors. At the end of the evaluation process, the individual or group performing the review should select one vendor. Some suggested criteria to be used when evaluating proposals are:

- Suitability of software, hardware, telecommunications equipment, and services to meet the specified requirements;

- Does it offer proprietary authoring tools and programming languages or open systems?

- Degree of security, control, and auditability provided;

- Strength and quality of local support, particularly in:
  [a] Account management and customer liaison
  [b] Education, training, and implementation
  [c] Software and hardware maintenance;

- Timeframe for development and implementation of the proposed solution and the degree to which the proposed timeframe meets the dates which the purchaser has in mind;

- Cost/price-performance in terms of computing and communication equipment, maintenance, conversion of current system, training of processing and end-user staff, software, programming costs, other fixed and operating costs;

- Speed of data access, including the estimated healthcare institution needs compared to proposed system capabilities;

- Expandability in terms of the ability to handle applications growth and increase in processing volumes;

- Interconnectivity with other platforms (software and hardware) and systems;

- Reliability and Performance, including quality of system and hardware support);

- Hardware convenience (suitability to proposed applications, ease of maintenance and upgrading);

- Software convenience (ability to handle the necessary tasks effectively):
  [a] System benefits
  [b] Expected system lifetime.
  [c] Reputation and reliability of manufacturer/service provider.

C.2.3.2. Service Provider Evaluation and Selection

The proposal describing the apparently "ideal" information system will be the basis for a system that is only as good as the vendor installing it. It is advisable to develop a selection process that puts all vendors on the same level playing field. This process should quickly and easily identify which vendors have the necessary strengths. Therefore, once the proposals have been analyzed, the qualifications of the vendor become a critical evaluation criterion. When evaluating the qualifications of a vendor, a healthcare institution should consider the following criteria:

- *Record of success in the healthcare sector* - The outsourcing vendor must have proved experience in the healthcare industry in order to be able to support the provider organization's varied business objectives. It takes time, experience, and a dedicated group of experts to learn the complexities and nuances of healthcare services.

- *Access to all technological options* - Information technology in general has moved from single vendor turn-key application implementation, to an environment characterized by multiproduct, multivendor integration. In the healthcare industry, the presence of a great number of specialized products and vendors is even more evident. Since many vendors have agreements among themselves for the purchase of each other's hardware and software, the institution must avoid contracting with biased vendors and suppliers of information technology products.

- *Availability of references* - The best way to find out about vendors is to talk with their clients. Other users should be contacted regarding the vendor's ability to meet schedules, workability of the hardware and software, maintenance costs, accuracy and usability of manuals, and any problems encountered. References should be asked whether they would contract with the vendor again should the need arise.

- *Length of time in business* - It is important to know how long the vendor has been in business and working with health systems. The ability to manage complex projects comes with time and experience in each specific industry and service area.

- *Number and type of staff* - The degree of individual staff and corporate expertise in health information systems should be analyzed in a vendor. One of the most frequent reasons why institutions outsource is the lack of skilled staff to perform the necessary IS&T tasks. In these situations the vendor must be able to provide the necessary expertise in all aspects of project management, including size and cost estimation, project planning, tracking, development, and control.

- *Financial stability of business and warranties* - The financial resources required for hiring a vendor for the implementation of healthcare IS&T are usually very high. To avoid any financial loss it is important to hire a vendor with excellent financial stability and willing to offer warranties for any loss, damage, and unsatisfactory work.

- *Systems and equipment* - The availability of operating systems, application software, and hardware that are compatible with the client's own for the development of the project is another very important factor, mainly when the work will be conducted at the vendor's location. Outdated systems and equipment that are not compatible with the client's equipment can be catastrophic for project development and implementation.

C.2.4. Contracting Service Providers

Healthcare professionals are not formally prepared to make deals or to negotiate contracts, nor are they expected to know the intricacies of applicable law and legal aspects of the process, whereas vendors are, by nature, professional negotiators. Vendors usually have standard sales contracts that secure the maximum protection, while providing the healthcare institution with minimal legal protection. Before signing a contract, its terms and conditions must be thoroughly understood. A standard contract should be modified if necessary, but a combination of legal and technical expertise is essential for dealing with amendments and modifications.

To avoid problems and to examine the vendor's performance, contracts for services should be staged to avoid lock-in to a vendor that performs poorly. One should favor short-term contracts with extension clauses instead of long-term contracts with commitment to one vendor. Some of the steps to be taken before signing a contract are the following:

- Hire or assign in-house staff to be part of a contract management team,

- Resist vendor pressure for longer term contracts,

- Employ the "best-of-breed" approach when evaluating vendors,

- Ensure that the higher level management is in agreement with the outsourcing contract and is prepared to evaluate the expected results, limitations, products, and impact of the project.

C.2.4.1. The Negotiation Process

The negotiation process should clarify the purpose and limits of each item in the contract. When negotiating a contract, the team should explicitly list priority items that should be addressed. A checklist of items to be discussed should include major contract objectives such as acceptance criteria parameters, maintenance warranties, cost limits for vendor charges, and delivery standards in terms of time, quantity, and quality.

The checklist for contract negotiations should be closely followed to ensure proper consideration of all items. Items on the list must include documentation manuals, payment terms, performance standards, corrective tasks to software or hardware, placement of equipment and software under the contract in case the vendor goes out of business, and causes for a right to cancel the contract.

A number of important points should be clearly specified in any contract for off-the-shelf, custom-adapted, or custom-designed systems:

- *Changes* - The contract must specify whether the healthcare institution or the contractor may change system specifications, what authorizations are required to do this, the rates at which the contractor is reimbursed for additional authorized work, and the results of any impact on deadlines, dates, or schedules.

- *Disputes* - The contract should contain provisions resolving contract disputes, the mediation process, which person is legally authorized to resolve the issue, and the remedies available to each party.

- *Default* - The conditions that shall constitute default by either party should be carefully detailed, and the remedies available to the other party clearly stated. The statement should include specific liability for costs incurred as a result of the default.

- *Rights to technical data and development* - The contract should specify who retains rights to any technical data, products, documents, or developments arising from the contract performance. The healthcare institution can reasonably expect to retain some interest in such developments if it desires; the healthcare institution should not expect rights to technical data or developments used by contractors that were not developed during the contract. A statement should be included in the contract specifying whether the healthcare institution, the vendor, or both retain ownership of the system after completion.

- *Acceptance* - Perhaps the most important contractual statement for both parties is a clear delineation of what constitutes acceptance of intermediate and final results of the contract effort. This specification should include system capabilities, schedules, and formal conditions for acceptance.

- *Authorizations* - The contract should state who is authorized to commit each of the parties to the contract and who can authorize changes or additions.

- *Warranty, maintenance, and modification* - The contract should clearly specify whether the vendor provides any warranties on the system and its operation, the time limit on the warranty, and any limitations or exclusions. It should also include statements regarding provisions for maintenance and modification of the system during and after the warranty period.

C.2.4.2. Contract Negotiations

Contract negotiations should be carefully prepared, making sure that all relevant points will be taken into consideration. Some of the actions to be taken before contract negotiations are the following:

- Appoint contract negotiators (hospital administrators, managers, clinical and accounting technical staff, legal representative) and determine levels of authority and responsibility.

- If needed, contract outside expert to assist the organization to make the appropriate decision regarding this most crucial task.

- Determine type of contract to be negotiated (i.e., fixed price, cost reimbursement, time and materials, combination).

- Determine which areas to be negotiated are flexible and which must be rigidly defined.

- Clarify terminology used in the contract.

- Define healthcare institution and vendor responsibilities for assessment of requirements and systems design, development, and implementation.

- Determine and define components of contract:

  [a] Basic system specifications
  [b] Reliability and maintenance
  [c] Other vendor services
  [d] Terms of acceptance
  [e] Costs and terms of payment
  [f] Delivery
  [g] Rights of the user
  [h] User options
  [i] Price protection
  [j] Damages or penalties
  [k] Other provisions.

C.2.4.3. Components of an Information System Contract

- *Glossary of terms* - Listing and explanation of major technical terms.

- *Basic system specifications* - Hardware configuration, software configuration, component performance standards, system performance standards, component compatibility (interoperability) guarantees, alterations and attachments, security and confidentiality provisions.

- *Reliability and maintenance* - Parameters to be used, guarantees, replacement, replacement costs, malfunction reports, maintenance location, maintenance credit, unreliable equipment, emergency equipment, response times, continued availability.

- *Other vendor services* - Support and assistance including: software development or modification, database design, supporting documents, design, conversion, site planning, installation, public relations. Education and training (curriculum, allotment, guarantee of continuation, availability of instructors, materials, rights to future courses). Documentation (availability, reproduction rights, copyright and patent protection, future materials). Machine time for testing, development, and emergency use (amount, schedule, location).

- *Terms of acceptance* - Acceptance testing, deliverables, criteria for acceptance of each deliverable, sign-off.

- *Costs and terms of payment* - Terms of agreement by specific cost type, method of payment, conditions for nonpayment, taxes, charges and method of charging for overtime and holiday use, maintenance, transportation, relocation, insurance, supplies.

- *Delivery* - Dates of delivery, options for early delivery, delays, installation responsibility, site preparation responsibility, damages to hardware, software, and site during delivery, relocation, and return of equipment.

- *Rights of user* - Use and function of system, location of system, component cancellation, component substitution, changes and attachments, upgrading hardware or software, rights to technical data.

- *User options* - Purchase, rental, rental credit, trade-in, title passage, option to upgrade, availability of expansion units, alternative sources.

- *Price protection* - Prior to delivery, during term of contract, upgrading and expansion, maintenance, supplies, and services.

- *Damages or penalties* - Breach prior to delivery, after delivery, and during development, including damages, user costs, and breach with consent.

- *Other provisions.*

C

C.2.4.4. Checklist of Essential Contract Provisions

Contract provisions should necessarily include, but not be limited to, the following (Table 2):

Table 2. Checklist of Essential Contract Provisions

1.	Length of term
2.	Shared risk
3.	Performance
4.	Access to all of the vendor's capabilities
5.	Capital commitments to acquire facilities, equipment, or technology, including assets currently owned by the healthcare organization, as required
6.	Delivery
7.	Acceptance of the system
8.	Documentation
9.	Rights to the programs
10.	Training of personnel
11.	User physical facilities
12.	Back-up equipment
13.	Warranties
14.	Insurance
15.	Confidentiality and disclosure issues
16.	Access of vendor/provider to client's facilities and corporate documents
17.	Maintenance
18.	Arbitration
19.	Infringement protection
20.	Upgrades
21.	Special contract provisions
22.	Software warranties
23.	Maintenance support
24.	Reliability guarantee
25.	New release clause
26.	Renewal option
27.	Termination clause

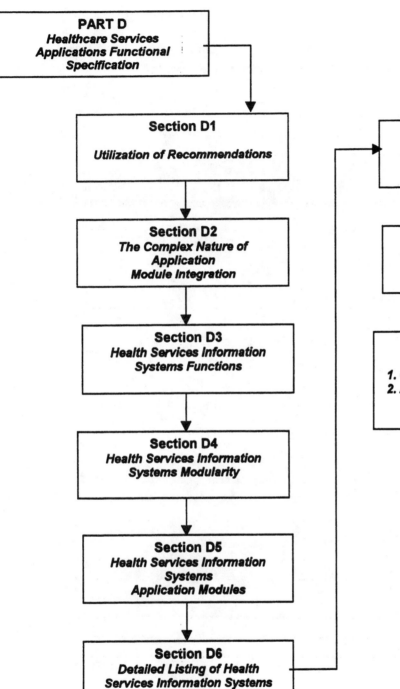

PART D
*Healthcare Services
Applications Functional
Specification*

Section D1

Utilization of Recommendations

Section D2
*The Complex Nature of
Application
Module Integration*

Section D3
*Health Services Information
Systems Functions*

Section D4
*Health Services Information
Systems Modularity*

Section D5
*Health Services Information
Systems
Application Modules*

Section D6
*Detailed Listing of Health
Services Information Systems
Functions*

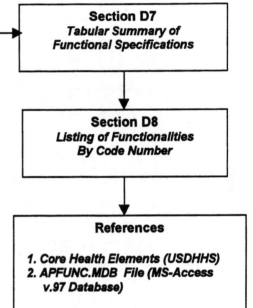

Section D7
*Tabular Summary of
Functional Specifications*

Section D8
*Listing of Functionalities
By Code Number*

References

*1. Core Health Elements (USDHHS)
2. APFUNC.MDB File (MS-Access
   v.97 Database)*

D

Part D. Health Services Applications Functional Specification

D

Part D. Health Services Applications Functional Specification

Success is counted sweetest
By those who ne'er succeed.
To comprehend a nectar
Requires sorest need.

Emily Dickinson (1830–1886)

This chapter contains detailed functional specifications for each of the basic application modules that are required for the operation and management of most health services and support units. The modules and functions here described are directed to support of the majority of the common tasks conducted in healthcare services and do not depict all possible particular applications that may be required by specialized services or administrative units.

Not every organization will have the desire, or the resources, for deploying all possible applications. The professionals responsible for the decisions regarding the implementation of information systems in a particular healthcare organization should base their decisions on careful deliberation with users and consideration of objectives, infrastructure, and resources. Smaller hospitals, for instance, may find that computerization of some departments may not be cost-effective.

To facilitate their usage, the functional specifications (*functionalities*) will be presented considering the following categories:

- **Generic Application Functionalities** - functions that are pertinent and common to all applications modules.

- **Generic Systems Functionalities** - technological functions, i.e., related to systems design, that are pertinent and common to all applications modules.

- **Application Specific Functionalities** - functions that are pertinent to each specific application module.

D.1. Utilization of Recommendations

The specifications described for each module are intended to be general guidelines, to be used as a departure point in developing a customized statement of requirements. They are a composite of features requested by users, offered commercially by healthcare IS&T vendors, or both.

To allow for the possibility that some of these applications may be implemented individually, there is some intentional overlap of features from one area to another. For example, Orders and Scheduling can be implemented as stand-alone applications or as components of integrated applications (e.g., Clinical Laboratory and Medical Imaging).

Healthcare organizations will need to apply rigorous due diligence in developing their own detailed system functional specification requirements. As part of such effort, the organization should have the initial listing of functional specifications reviewed by experts familiar with each of the specific application areas, either from within the organization or under an outsourcing contract.

D.2. The Complex Nature of Application Module Integration

The degree of integration and communication among the different modules will change according to each implementation environment's particular requirements; however, a categorization of the degree to which applications are integrated must be considered when defining the functionalities desired in each application area.

The following classes of systems are possible, considering the desired degree of application module integration:

- **Class A Systems** - Individual stand-alone applications that address specific requirements of single departments, specialties, or operational units (e.g., Current Accounts and Billing, Pharmacy, Materials Management, Clinical Laboratory, etc.)

- **Class B Systems** - Application use spans departmental or specialty boundaries and may include partial or full utilization of data elements from each individual application (e.g., Orders; Medical Records; Inpatient, Outpatient and Other Service Scheduling; Admissions / Discharge / Transfer; etc.)

- **Class C Systems** - Applications are integrated considering an orientation towards the patient and the medical record. These systems are similar to Class B Systems; the major difference lies in structure: while Class B Systems use administrative or financial applications as the basic link, Class C Systems by design include fully integrated ancillary subsystems modules.

The implementation of a fully integrated patient management information system (PMIS) is an extremely complex endeavor even in the best circumstances. The complex nature of the data interrelationships that must be maintained in a PMIS requires the ability to access and update individual module data in a controlled and consistent manner. However, current database technology provides the capability to maintain and access common data in any required sequence without regards to its physical location. Those capabilities set the stage for multiple concurrent use of data regardless of user location, function, or required procedure.

In the past decade the evolution of the health software market has been characterized by the proliferation of providers of departmental applications. Although there are many vendors that offer "integrated" products, the best applications frequently come from developers that are highly specialized and dedicated to a single line of product, such as laboratory, radiology, medical equipment maintenance, stock management, personnel management, etc. Their expertise and large number of clients allow their products to be regularly updated. The downside of this situation relates to the difficulty for the user in selecting the best provider for each specialized or departmental system and integrating products that may run in different hardware and software platforms. The most serious problem, for users, is that they must now deal with a number of vendors with application products developed in a variety of software platforms. The problem of integrating such applications and dealing with the technical aspects of a multi-vendor environment can be of frightening proportion. When selecting multiple-provider systems great care must be exercised regarding the identification of a single integrator responsible for the technical and managerial decisions and to act as a single line of contact with the vendors.

D.3. Health Services Information Systems Functions

There are many functions that can be incorporated into the technical (clinical) and the business (administrative) components of health services information systems. These fall into four types: transactional functions, control reporting, operational planning, and strategic planning.

- **Transactional Functions** - Handle the day-to-day operational and administrative tasks of the organization. Examples of transactional technical functions include: Order Entry; Consultation, Treatment and Service Scheduling; Nursing and other Health Personnel Staffing and Scheduling; Inpatient Census; Clinical Data Recording; Results Reporting; etc. Examples of transactional administrative functions include: Payroll; Current Accounts; Billing; Accounts Receivable and Payable; Laundry; Purchasing; Inventory Control; Maintenance Work Orders; etc.

- **Control Reporting Functions and Operational Planning Functions** - Provide summarized data about the operation of the organization to managers and healthcare professionals that will permit the monitoring of the various activities for which they are responsible. In addition, these systems provide executive management with resources to plan and control the organization. Examples of technical functions supported by these systems include: Medical Records Tracking; Medical Audit and Peer Review; Utilization Review; Medical Staff Education; Treatment Planning; Inpatient Occupancy, Patient Mix, and Discharge Planning; Drug Interactions; Infection Control; Drug Profiling; etc. Examples of administrative functions supported by these systems include: Materials Utilization; Supplier Analysis; Backorders and Stockouts; Contracted Services; Kitchen Planning; Preventive Maintenance; Personnel Benefits Administration; Personnel Absence and Turnover; Eligibility and Payment Delinquency; Cost Allocation; Patient Satisfaction; etc.

- **Strategic Planning Functions** - Provide a framework for decisions with long-range implications. Some issues in strategic planning requirements include: Patient Care

Strategy (levels of care, occupancy and service demand, requirements, and projected costs); Professional Staffing (forecasting, recruitment, community needs assessment and trend analysis); Facilities Planning; Budgeting; utilization of Contracted Services; Credit, Reimbursement, and Collection Policies; etc.

D.4. Health Services Information Systems Modularity

There are many possible ways to categorize applications into functional modules. For the objectives of this publication, a classification that would contemplate merely technical or administrative functions was not considered appropriate, as some functions have aspects of both, which led to a more operational approach being favored.

We elected to group all health services basic application modules in four groups: Logistics of Patient Care, Clinical Data Management, Technical Support Services Operation, and Administration and Resource Management. The Technical Support Services Operation group is further categorized into two subgroups: Diagnostic and Therapeutic, and Population and Environment Technical Support Services.

Any categorization must be, however, taken with caution. From a broader functional perspective, one should attempt to see all information related to patients comprehensively interconnected. This concept, sometimes referred to as a Patient Management Information System (PMIS), ideally consists of a fully integrated approach to maintaining patient-related administrative and clinical data considering the continuum of care, independent of site or provider. A PMIS provides the opportunity for enhancing communication between members of the healthcare team as is physically represented by a set of databases containing medical, financial, statistical, and other pertinent data. Typically, patient data would be captured directly from the day-to-day tasks associated with individual patient healthcare.

Each group (Logistics of Patient Care, Clinical Data Management, Technical Support Services Operation, and Administration and Resource Management) comprises a number of modules that are functionally related and, in many instances, modules can be independently implemented in a step-wise fashion. In these circumstances, a careful evaluation of the spectrum of functionalities of related modules must be done in order to verify if, how, and when they should be added to the ones selected for initial or subsequent implementation.

Although many application modules for healthcare services can be deployed in stand-alone mode, as for example in Class A systems, the degree of benefit to managers and decision-makers grows exponentially, as modules are progressively integrated and able to share their data.

The advantages of integrating application modules are evident. Case-related data can be used extensively in providing and managing present and future services to the patient and, in addition, a large number of data elements have multiple functions. For example, in a pharmacy the integrated PMIS would allow access to extensive pharmaceutical formulary data required to process medication orders; evaluation of prescribed drug interactivity with other drugs, dietary regimens, scheduled diagnostic or therapeutic procedures; check for eventual allergies and drug intolerance; cross-reference with individual drug usage pattern; processing and distribution of prescribed drugs; interactive stock control and product reorder; automatic billing to patient current account or third parties; etc. A fully functional PMIS requires, therefore, the implementation of all patient-related modules.

The content to follow will be presented as a general tool that includes basic specifications. The intent of this information is to provide the reader with an overview of some of the basic and necessary clinical and administrative information systems functions. The list of specifications is not exhaustive and some of them depend on the needs and wants of the institution that will be implementing the system. Furthermore, It is necessary to emphasize the advancement of technology, which will make other options available in the future.

D.5. Health Services Information Systems Application Modules

For the purpose of this document the four basic functional groups of applications are further categorized into modules. Each group of applications is made up of the following modules:

D

Health Services Information Systems Module Groups

A. Logistics of Patient Care

- Registration
- Outpatient Admission
- Inpatient Admission, Discharge, and Transfer
- Service Scheduling and Appointment Management
- Orders

B. Clinical Data Management

- Medical Records
- Nursing Care
- Clinical Audit

C. Diagnostic and Therapeutic Technical Support Services Operation

- Clinical Laboratory
- Medical Imaging: Diagnostic and Interventional
- Radiation Therapy
- Pharmacy
- Transfusion and Blood Bank
- Dietary Service

D. Population and Environment Technical Support Services Operation

- Environmental Health
- Immunization
- Clinical Surveillance and Databases

E. Administration and Resource Management

- Finance Management
  - *Billing / Accounts Receivable*
  - *Accounts Payable*
  - *General Accounting / Bookkeeping*
  - *Cost Accounting*
  - *General Ledger*
- Human Resources
  - *Payroll*
  - *Human Resource Management*
  - *Staffing*
  - *Benefits*
- Materials Management
  - *Purchasing*
  - *Inventory Control*
- Fixed Assets Management
- Medical Equipment Maintenance
- Physical Facilities Maintenance
- Laundry Services
- Transportation Services
- Budgeting and Executive Support

D.6. Detailed Listing of Health Services Information Systems Functions

D.6.1. Generic Application Functionalities

Generic Application Functionalities are those functions that are pertinent and common to all applications modules.

- Management reports. Provides reports for administration and upper management to direct, control and plan organizational business and clinical functions. (1)

- Forms management. Provides support for form design to ensure appropriate data collection, management of inventory, ordering, and stocking of paper forms. (2)

- Interdisciplinary progress notes or templates. The system should support multidisciplinary summary of clinical data from a specified patient. All direct care professionals should be able to view and enter information on-line, depending on access rights of each user. (3)

- Administrative policy development and retrieval. The system should have the ability to develop and quickly retrieve administrative, clinical, safety, and regulatory bodies' policies and procedures. It should have ability to cross-reference materials. (4)

- Fax or print notes. The system should allow the flexibility to customize the content of the reports/notes and also where they are printed. (5)

- Internal quality control. Provides reports to monitor and improve staff productivity, manage workload, and measure provider and user (i.e., medical staff, administration, patient, etc.) satisfaction level. (6)

- External quality control. Provides support for health care institution-wide quality control functions by providing reports and statistics requested by department, administration, and medical staff. (7)

- Client identification to be entered in a care unit site. An identifier must be used that will facilitate unique identification and client information data entry and retrieval. The Patient Index (PI) should be provided with a flexible screen builder capability that allows design and customization of a variety of possible registration screens. (8)

- Use-defined fields and tables. The health care institution should be able to define fields and tables for data that are not included in the vendor-supplied standard data set. The system should have a build facility that will provide an easy way for users to implement such definitions. (9)

D

- Required fields flexibility. User should be able to designate screen data fields as "required" or "not required" and to assign valid values, ranges, and other consistency checks. Required fields must have entry of valid data before the clerk can move forward to the next screen field. (10)

- Values edited to tables. Data entry to fields with system defined tables or profiles should be edited against the internal table values during data entry. (11)

- Help screen capability. Application should support extensive on-line help features. Descriptive text and examples should include the display of values from a table or valid profile linked to a data field. (12)

- Audit functions. System should provide audit trails of schedule events and results of scheduling activity. (13)

- Create patient labels and forms. Allows health care institutions to design formats for printing special forms and labels. Print functions should be accessible from registration screens. (14)

- Standard reports. The system should provide for standard and on-demand reporting capabilities in both on-line and batch modes. (15)

- Ad hoc reporting. Query facility support for generic reporting. Provide reports created based upon user-specified data fields as opposed to standard programmed reports. (16)

- User-definable reports. The system should have the capability to create programmable user-defined reports, with formatting and header construction capabilities, and permit saving and schedule these reports as standard reports. (17)

- Standard managerial reporting functions. Reports to enable decision makers at all levels to view integrated financial and statistical information from all departments, facilities, and corporations to make informed decisions and guide strategic plans. It should gather and assemble information from the following systems: admissions, nursing, laboratory, radiology, general ledger, payroll/personnel, Diagnostic Related Groups (DRGs) management, billings/accounts receivable, accounts payable, and materials management. Should provide for the assimilation of historical administrative, financial, and patient care information. Report generator should provide standard views of all data fields in place and have the ability to create extensive fields of the user's choosing. (18)

- Government-required codes. The system should be able to incorporate the government-required codes for the specific country, state, or municipality. (19)

- User-controlled posting. User-controlled sequence of posting reporting and closing, on-line review, free-text descriptions of each transaction, and edit of batch data available before posting to accounts. (20)

- Support for client-specific window customization. System should have capability to set required fields determined by department requirements and resource management characteristics. (21)

- Ability to enter comments. System should allow users to enter free-text comments related to specific data fields as determined by users during systems adaptation and implementation. (22)

D.6.2. Generic Systems Functionalities

Generic Systems Functionalities are those technological functions, i.e. related to systems design that are pertinent and common to all applications modules.

- Look up patient record using phonetic search. System should support phonetic searches when the name entered for search has phonetic equivalents. The system should support searches in multiple languages. (23)

- Menu driven screens. The system should have the ability to move back and forth through a set of screens using menu selections, ideally using a graphic user interface environment (GUI). (24)

- The system should have a flexible screen builder facility to allow design and customization of screens, determination of the sequence of screens, placement of fields on a screen, type of controllers used (button, pull-down, toggle, etc.) and the definition of field edits, labels, and echoes. (25)

- Edit capability for screens. Screen builder should allow definition of field edits and default data to allow data to be directly edited on entry. (26)

- Passwords, levels of access, and privilege facilities. System must have a transaction audit tract that maintains the identification and a record of authorization, utilization (transactions), and changes related to system's users. (27)

- Embosser and/or barcode card/labels print/reprint. Vendor should support interface to common embossing and barcoding machines so that patient cards for embossing and scanning can be created. (28)

- Dictation tracking - type, edit, review, etc. The system should allow the dictation to have several different formats. The users need a preliminary, final, duplicate, and addendum notification to print on the reports. The system should also provide error correction editing and also track before and after copies of any final report that is edited. (29)

- Integration with other modules. Integrated as appropriate or feasible with modules such as all nursing applications, general ledger, diagnostic and procedure categorization for payment

D

(e.g., DRG management), billings/accounts receivable, executive support system, and payroll/personnel systems. (30)

- Message communication. Allows the users to communicate with other units and departments though functions that create and transmit messages, such as e-mail systems. (31)

D.6.3. Application Specific Functionalities

Application Specific Functionalities are functions pertinent to each specific application module.

A. Logistics of Patient Care

The purpose of the applications of this group is to provide a fully integrated approach to maintaining data related to: client identification; financial and reimbursement; medical alert; scheduling and management of health-related contacts and services; inpatient and outpatient management; orders for therapeutic and diagnostic services. Typically such information is captured, validated, updated, and available at any time during the routine operation of the system at any "point of care" location. Different user may have different levels of access (what is displayed) and privileges (read only, read and change) at each implemented function.

Applications of this group include the following modules:

- Registration
- Outpatient Admission
- Inpatient Admission, Discharge and Transfer
- Service Scheduling and Appointment Management
- Orders

Registration

- Patient Index (PI). Should have multiple search capabilities. The PI should be able to qualify searches by name, date of birth, sex, national individual identifiers (such as National Registration Number, Social Security Number, Health Plan Number, etc.) The index should support a variety of possible internal identifiers such as medical record number, case number, multiple account numbers, etc., for each patient and be able to maintain cross-reference to other existing identifiers in each of the facilities used by the patient in the same site or in other locations. (32)

- System should support a Master Patient Index (MPI), at multi-site, multi-institutional, regional, or national levels that links existing Patient Indices together. (33)

- Ability to look up patient "also-known-as" (AKA). The MPI should support multiple names so that patients who change their names can still be located with an MPI search. MPI name searches should search both the name and the AKA files during name searches. (34)

- Link family members. The system should contain a cross-reference facility for linkage of records belonging to different family members. (35)

- Name alert search. Patients with same last name and same first name and initial should be flagged to alert users of possible conflict. (36)

- Enrollment program. Registration systems should support enrollment and cancellation of enrollment in roup or managed care programs. The system should support a posting program that should allow the member data to be downloaded from external insurance, group provider, or managed care organizations. (37)

- Inpatient / outpatient pre-admission. System should allow pre-admit or pre-registration of patients prior to their actual arrival. Pre-admission function should allow clerk to collect the standard registration data for patients with or without existing medical records, case number, etc. Patients pre-admitted without identifiers must have them assigned when admission to inpatient care or outpatient contact is activated. (38)

- Registration system should support different registration screens and data set requirements for Emergency Care Services, Outpatient Services (First and Return Contacts) and for Inpatient Admission. (39)

- Quick inpatient/outpatient/emergency services registration. The system should provide an alternate set of screens for quick registration, admission, or creation of a new record when patient information is incomplete or unavailable. The quick screens would allow an alternate set of entry screens for inpatient and outpatient care, emergency services, and diagnostic services. (40)

- Automatically assign billing number. A unique billing or account number is assigned for each patient visit, admission, or care cycle. Alternately, the health care institution should be able, for certain patient or visit types, to link multiple visits to a single number for serial or monthly billing. (41)

- Retrievable key fields values capable of bringing forward key field data from prior registrations and/or MPI. (42)

- Field updates from transactions in the Patient Registration module pass to MPI. On subsequent interactions the operator should be able to change and update registration fields were updating is allowed. Updated registration file should pass updated data to the MPI. (43)

- Cancel registration of ambulatory active visit. Cancel function should allow an active visit to be canceled. Canceled visits should be reflected correctly in usage statistics. (44)

- Face sheet print and reprint. System should allow client to define face sheets for registration and clinical management functions. System should support multiple sheets with automatically or manually selected print functions. System should support the Reprint function so that updates or corrections can be reprinted. (45)

- Front-end insurance capture. Allows insurance verification function and levels of benefits. (47)

- Update fields capability. Allows updates to previously recorded patient data provided field is unlocked for such updating and user is authorized to do so. (49)

- Check-in/check-out functionality. System should allow patients to be checked-in at point of service or in a central registration area. System should support entry of check-out times. (86)

Outpatient Admission

- Patient Index (PI). Should have multiple search capabilities. The PI should be able to qualify searches by name, date of birth, sex, national individual identifiers (such as National Registration Number, Social Security Number, Health Plan Number, etc.) The index should support a variety of possible internal identifiers such as medical record number, case number, multiple account numbers, etc., for each patient and be able to maintain cross-reference to other existing identifiers in each of the facilities used by the patient in the same site or in other locations. (32)

- System should support a Master Patient Index (MPI), at multi-site, multi-institutional, regional, or national levels that links existing Patient Indices together. (33)

- Ability to look up patient "also-known-as" (AKA). The MPI should support multiple names so that patients who change their names can still be located with an MPI search. MPI name searches should search both the name and the AKA files during name searches. (34)

- Link family members. The system should contain a cross-reference facility for linkage of records belonging to different family members. (35)

- Name alert search. Patients with same last name and same first name and initial should be flagged to alert users of possible conflict. (36)

- Enrollment program. Registration systems should support enrollment and cancellation of enrollment in group or managed care programs. The system should support a posting program that should allow the member data to be downloaded from external insurance, group provider, or managed care organizations. (37)

- Inpatient / outpatient pre-admission. System should allow pre-admit or pre-registration of patients prior to their actual arrival. Pre-admission function should allow clerk to collect the standard registration data for patients with or without existing medical records, case number, etc. Patients pre-admitted without identifiers must have them assigned when admission to inpatient care or outpatient contact is activated. (38)

- Registration system should support different registration screens and data set requirements for Emergency Care Services, Outpatient Services (First and Return Contacts) and for Inpatient Admission. (39)

- Quick inpatient/outpatient/emergency services registration. The system should provide an alternate set of screens for quick registration, admission, or creation of a new record when patient information is incomplete or unavailable. The quick screens would allow an alternate set of entry screens for inpatient and outpatient care, emergency services, and diagnostic services. (40)

- Automatically assign billing number. A unique billing or account number is assigned for each patient visit, admission, or care cycle. Alternately, the health care institution should be able, for certain patient or visit types, to link multiple visits to a single number for serial or monthly billing. (41)

- Retrievable key fields values capable of bringing forward key field data from prior registrations and/or MPI. (42)

- Field updates from transactions in the Patient Registration module pass to MPI. On subsequent interactions the operator should be able to change and update registration fields were updating is allowed. Updated registration file should pass updated data to the MPI. (43)

- Cancel registration of ambulatory active visit. Cancel function should allow an active visit to be canceled. Canceled visits should be reflected correctly in usage statistics. (44)

- Face sheet print and reprint. System should allow client to define face sheets for registration and clinical management functions. System should support multiple sheets with automatically or manually selected print functions. System should support the Reprint function so that updates or corrections can be reprinted. (45)

- Convert or activate pre-admission. On patient arrival to the care unit, allow clerk to activate and update data from pre-admission record. Also permits specifying purge parameters for holding pre-admission records beyond expected pre-admission date. (46)

- Front-end insurance capture. Allows insurance verification function and levels of benefits. (47)

- Retroactive admission. Allows back dating of admissions, with appropriate adjustments to billing, reporting, revenue, and usage statistics. (48)

- Update fields capability. Allows updates to previously recorded patient data provided field is unlocked for such updating and user is authorized to do so. (49)

D

- Outpatient discharge. The health care institution should have the option of entering the discharge date on emergency services and outpatient accounts, or profiling the system to change them to discharge status after a certain number of hours or days. (50)

- Allow change in patient status from emergency room or outpatient to inpatient, so that when patients are admitted the original registration data should be rolled over to the inpatient visit. (58)

- No limitation on facilities or departments. The system should support a large number of primary, specialty, and subspecialty clinics and departments. (78)

- Check-in/check-out functionality. System should allow patients to be checked-in at point of service or in a central registration area. System should support entry of check-out times. (86)

- Access to registration MPI (Master Patient Index) and pass updates. Be able to view MPI to lookup and identify patient by demographics or Medical Records number. (92)

- Ability to generate a "chart-pull" list for the Medical Records Department. System should create a list of charts needed for each clinic each day. The list may be electronically sent to the Medical Records Department or printed on demand in a department or in decentralized medical records storage facilities. (98)

Inpatient Admission, Discharge and Transfer

- Patient Index (PI). Should have multiple search capabilities. The PI should be able to qualify searches by name, date of birth, sex, national individual identifiers (such as National Registration Number, Social Security Number, Health Plan Number, etc.) The index should support a variety of possible internal identifiers such as medical record number, case number, multiple account numbers, etc., for each patient and be able to maintain cross-reference to other existing identifiers in each of the facilities used by the patient in the same site or in other locations. (32)

- System should support a Master Patient Index (MPI), at multi-site, multi-institutional, regional, or national levels that links existing Patient Indices together. (33)

- Ability to look up patient "also-known-as" (AKA). The MPI should support multiple names so that patients who change their names can still be located with an MPI search. MPI name searches should search both the name and the AKA files during name searches. (34)

- Link family members. The system should contain a cross-reference facility for linkage of records belonging to different family members. (35)

- Name alert search. Patients with same last name and same first name and initial should be flagged to alert users of possible conflict. (36)

- Enrollment program. Registration systems should support enrollment and cancellation of enrollment in group or managed care programs. The system should support a posting program that should allow the member data to be downloaded from external insurance, group provider, or managed care organizations. (37)

- Inpatient / outpatient pre-admission. System should allow pre-admit or pre-registration of patients prior to their actual arrival. Pre-admission function should allow clerk to collect the standard registration data for patients with or without existing medical records, case number, etc. Patients pre-admitted without identifiers must have them assigned when admission to inpatient care or outpatient contact is activated. (38)

- Registration system should support different registration screens and data set requirements for Emergency Care Services, Outpatient Services (First and Return Contacts) and for Inpatient Admission. (39)

- Quick inpatient/outpatient/emergency services registration. The system should provide an alternate set of screens for quick registration, admission, or creation of a new record when patient information is incomplete or unavailable. The quick screens would allow an alternate set of entry screens for inpatient and outpatient care, emergency services, and diagnostic services. (40)

- Automatically assign billing number. A unique billing or account number is assigned for each patient visit, admission, or care cycle. Alternately, the health care institution should be able, for certain patient or visit types, to link multiple visits to a single number for serial or monthly billing. (41)

- Retrievable key fields values capable of bringing forward key field data from prior registrations and/or MPI. (42)

- Field updates from transactions in the Patient Registration module pass to MPI. On subsequent interactions the operator should be able to change and update registration fields were updating is allowed. Updated registration file should pass updated data to the MPI. (43)

- Face sheet print and reprint. System should allow client to define face sheets for registration and clinical management functions. System should support multiple sheets with automatically or manually selected print functions. System should support the Reprint function so that updates or corrections can be reprinted. (45)

- Convert or activate pre-admission. On patient arrival to the care unit, allow clerk to activate and update data from pre-admission record. Also permits specifying purge parameters for holding pre-admission records beyond expected pre-admission date. (46)

- Front-end insurance capture. Allows insurance verification function and levels of benefits. (47)

- Retroactive admission. Allows back dating of admissions, with appropriate adjustments to billing, reporting, revenue, and usage statistics. (48)

- Update fields capability. Allows updates to previously recorded patient data provided field is unlocked for such updating and user is authorized to do so. (49)

- Bed reservation. Beds should be able to be reserved prior to admission. (51)

- Create patient identification wrist band. System should support formatting of data and print function for printing wrist bands. (52)

- Cancel inpatient admission or discharge. Cancel function should allow an active admission or discharge to be canceled. Canceled events should be reflected correctly in usage statistics and room charges should be adjusted retroactively to the beginning of a stay. (53)

- On-demand query of bed availability, status (vacant, blocked, active, planned discharge, planned transfer) and expected change of status. (54)

- Transfer emergency services to observation. System should support an observation status for patients admitted to Emergency Services. Observation patients should be able to be assigned to special observation beds and manually discharged. (55)

- On-demand census of beds. The census feature should support query by a variety of perspectives including patient identifiers, bed, unit, medical problem grouping, attending doctor, patient type, etc.. This function should also support a public information service to facilitate location of patients and to generate directions to visitors. (56)

- Support different admission screen sets and data requirements for emergency room and transfer admissions and discharge to outpatient clinic. (57)

- Allow change in patient status from emergency room or outpatient to inpatient, so that when patients are admitted the original registration data should be rolled over to the inpatient visit. (58)

- Leave of absence processing. Allow leave of absence processing on inpatient accounts so that account may remain active without generating room charges for a period of time. (59)

- Event notices. System should create "event notices" that can be routed to one or more printers based on the following events: pre-admit, admit or registration, transfer, reservation booked, discharge scheduled, discharge, financial class update, bed status (housekeeping) changed, new medical record number assigned. (60)

- Mother-newborn link. System should support the rollover of a mother's information to a "newborn" record, so that shared information from the mother's admission record should be shown on the baby's record. A permanent cross reference between the two systems should automatically be created (or manually entered when needed) to allow for an inquiry on the mother's or newborn's visit by reference to any visit number. (61)

- Newborn pre-admission. System should allow user to pre-admit a newborn with the mother's information. At the time of the birth the account should be activated and a medical record number assigned. (62)

- Housekeeping/maintenance. The system should identify beds for housekeeping when a patient is discharged. Housekeeping should be able to update bed status to "available" when the bed is made. (63)

- On-line view of census. Allow on-line review of census by nursing unit. User can choose to review all beds, all occupied beds, and all empty beds for display by nursing unit. Occupied beds would indicate the patient name and number, data of admission, and attending physician. (64)

- Nursing unit summary. System should provide a real-time display of nursing unit statistics. Display should give a summary for all units, including current summary of total beds, beds occupied, and the percentage of beds occupied. (65)

- No limitation on facilities or departments. The system should support a large number of primary, specialty, and subspecialty clinics and departments. (78)

- Check-in/check-out functionality. System should allow patients to be checked-in at point of service or in a central registration area. System should support entry of check-out times. (86)

- Access to registration MPI (Master Patient Index) and pass updates. Be able to view MPI to lookup and identify patient by demographics or Medical Records number. (92)

- Ability to generate a "chart-pull" list for the Medical Records Department. System should create a list of charts needed for each clinic each day. The list may be electronically sent to the Medical Records Department or printed on demand in a department or in decentralized medical records storage facilities. (98)

Service Scheduling and Appointment Management

- Patient Index (PI). Should have multiple search capabilities. The PI should be able to qualify searches by name, date of birth, sex, national individual identifiers (such as National Registration Number, Social Security Number, Health Plan Number, etc.) The index should support a variety of possible internal identifiers such as medical record number, case number, multiple account numbers, etc., for each patient and be able to maintain cross-reference to other existing identifiers in each of the facilities used by the patient in the same site or in other locations. (32)

- System should support a Master Patient Index (MPI), at multi-site, multi-institutional, regional, or national levels that links existing Patient Indices together. (33)

- Ability to look up patient "also-known-as" (AKA). The MPI should support multiple names so that patients who change their names can still be located with an MPI search. MPI name searches should search both the name and the AKA files during name searches. (34)

- Name alert search. Patients with same last name and same first name and initial should be flagged to alert users of possible conflict. (36)

- Quick inpatient/outpatient/emergency services registration. The system should provide an alternate set of screens for quick registration, admission, or creation of a new record when patient information is incomplete or unavailable. The quick screens would allow an alternate set of entry screens for inpatient and outpatient care, emergency services, and diagnostic services. (40)

- Retrievable key fields values capable of bringing forward key field data from prior registrations and/or MPI. (42)

- Field updates from transactions in the Patient Registration module pass to MPI. On subsequent interactions the operator should be able to change and update registration fields were updating is allowed. Updated registration file should pass updated data to the MPI. (43)

- Cancel registration of ambulatory active visit. Cancel function should allow an active visit to be canceled. Canceled visits should be reflected correctly in usage statistics. (44)

- Front-end insurance capture. Allows insurance verification function and levels of benefits. (47)

- Update fields capability. Allows updates to previously recorded patient data provided field is unlocked for such updating and user is authorized to do so. (49)

- Scheduling rules. The system should be based on flexible, powerful computer-driven "rules" which correspond to the processes of scheduling currently employed in healthcare institutions. (66)

- Support centralized and decentralized scheduling. The system should allow for either scheduling at a single point of control, or decentralized scheduling controlled by individual departments, or a combination. (67)

- Connection to and support of departmental scheduling. The system should be able to coexist with existing departmental scheduling systems (such as laboratory, diagnostic images, operating room), and be able to interface with those systems. (68)

- Conflict-free scheduling. The system should always return a conflict-free schedule to the administrator, or identify the conflicts if a conflict-free schedule is not possible. (69)

- Make/reschedule appointments. System should support the integrated scheduling of appointments and resources across all client entities. (70)

- Change/cancel appointment flexibility. System should support the cancellation, changing, or updating of appointments with minimal data entry. (71)

- Copy appointments for resources. Copy current appointment information forward for future appointments. (72)

- Reschedule resources. System should allow mass rescheduling of a physician's or service unit appointments to another date. (73)

- Print schedule using multiple types of sorts. Schedules should be printed by resources, department, provider, and for date ranges. (74)

- Print appointment notices. Users should be able to demand printed appointment notices for one or a group of patients. (75)

- Automatic patient notices/mailings. System should support data mailer appointment notices. The mail functions should be profile driven in order that that multiple providers can establish different parameters. (76)

- Flexibility to define multiple resources. System should define various resource types such as providers, locations, equipment, and staff. The system should be able to verify the availability of all defined resources in its determination of service/procedure availability. (77)

- No limitation on facilities or departments. The system should support a large number of primary, specialty, and subspecialty clinics and departments. (78)

- Schedule all patient type/time. System should support slotting of all types of patients for all times of day. (79)

- Flexibility of changing appointment type/time. System should allow for various service and procedure appointment types and the ability to use them at various times and to change an existing appointment type. (80)

- Capability of multiple schedule storage. Physicians or other resources may have different schedules for different days. (81)

- Flexible security/access to schedule. System should provide a security or control mechanism for restricting access to specific schedules. (82)

- Ease of loading and building schedules. System should have "copy" function for ease in building and loading schedules. (83)

D

- Overbooking flexibility. Systems should have capability to allow overbooking by resource or department. (84)

- View open time slots on-line. System should allow viewing open appointments by resource and/or department. (85)

- Check-in/check-out functionality. System should allow patients to be checked-in at point of service or in a central registration area. System should support entry of check-out times. (86)

- Waiting list capability. User should be able to wait-list patients when no appointment slots are available. (87)

- Ease of scheduling walk-ins. System should support walk-in processing so that these patients can be scheduled at the point of service. (88)

- Reserve block of appointments. Allow blocking of appointments by provider, resource, and date. (89)

- Collapse appointments. System should be able to modify appointment lengths, allowing alteration of appointment times. (90)

- On-line view of past/future appointments. System should have capability to view on-line all or a set of past, present and future appointments by range of dates, resource, and patient. (91)

- Access to registration MPI (Master Patient Index) and pass updates. Be able to view MPI to lookup and identify patient by demographics or Medical Records number. (92)

- Maintain record of canceled appointments. The system should have the capability to view canceled appointments for at least one year. (93)

- View/print reasons for appointments. The system should have a "reason for appointment" field that can be viewed on time as printed with schedule. (94)

- Comment/alert for appointment type. System should provide alert if identical appointment types are scheduled for the same patient. It should also warn if the patient is a chronic no-show type of user. (95)

- Print patient instructions/comments on appointment slip. Allow user to include special instructions or requirements on the appointment slips, such as preparation instructions, or directions from one department to another. (96)

- Revise appointment type. Allow changing an appointment type for a rescheduled appointment, and update department statistics correctly. (97)

- Ability to generate a "chart-pull" list for the Medical Records Department. System should create a list of charts needed for each clinic each day. The list may be electronically sent to the Medical Records Department or printed on demand in a department or in decentralized medical records storage facilities. (98)

- Chart reservation. Provide the ability to have a chart available on a particular date, for patient care, audit, reviews and physician studies, or release of information. The request may be generated by the scheduling system. (123)

- Immunization scheduling and management. (277)

Orders

- Patient Index (PI). Should have multiple search capabilities. The PI should be able to qualify searches by name, date of birth, sex, national individual identifiers (such as National Registration Number, Social Security Number, Health Plan Number, etc.) The index should support a variety of possible internal identifiers such as medical record number, case number, multiple account numbers, etc., for each patient and be able to maintain cross-reference to other existing identifiers in each of the facilities used by the patient in the same site or in other locations. (32)

- System should support a Master Patient Index (MPI), at multi-site, multi-institutional, regional, or national levels that links existing Patient Indices together. (33)

- Ability to look up patient "also-known-as" (AKA). The MPI should support multiple names so that patients who change their names can still be located with an MPI search. MPI name searches should search both the name and the AKA files during name searches. (34)

- Name alert search. Patients with same last name and same first name and initial should be flagged to alert users of possible conflict. (36)

- Retrievable key fields values capable of bringing forward key field data from prior registrations and/or MPI. (42)

- Field updates from transactions in the Patient Registration module pass to MPI. On subsequent interactions the operator should be able to change and update registration fields were updating is allowed. Updated registration file should pass updated data to the MPI. (43)

- Face sheet print and reprint. System should allow client to define face sheets for registration and clinical management functions. System should support multiple sheets with automatically or manually selected print functions. System should support the Reprint function so that updates or corrections can be reprinted. (45)

- Front-end insurance capture. Allows insurance verification function and levels of benefits. (47)

- Update fields capability. Allows updates to previously recorded patient data provided field is unlocked for such updating and user is authorized to do so. (49)

- Access to registration MPI (Master Patient Index) and pass updates. Be able to view MPI to lookup and identify patient by demographics or Medical Records number. (92)

- Order entry. Allow for on-line entry of orders along with all of the information necessary to complete the order in an efficient and accurate manner. (99)

- Verified and unverified orders. Allow for entry of orders as either unverified (not approved) or verified (approved and activated), depending upon the security level of the user. (100)

- Order verification. Allows for personnel with proper access authorization to either verify (approve) orders or void the orders if appropriate. (101)

- Order cancellation. Allow for cancellation of orders, either verified or unverified, and allow for inclusion of reason for cancellation. (102)

- Occurrences. Generate performance-related occurrences of the order each time the service is to be done within the active period of the order. Allow for additional occurrences to be appended to existing orders. (103)

- Ordering logistics. Allow for automatic scheduling of orders according to guidelines customized to fit the needs of the institution or technical constraints. (104)

- Profile orders. Allow for generation of a set of medically or administratively grouped orders using profiles, such as a battery of tests, or coupled orders such as dietary and pharmacy preparations associated with radiology exams. (105)

- Renewal of expiring orders. Allows for renewal of expiring orders, with the ability to bring forward information from the original order to create a new order, possibly with an extended duration. (106)

- Print requisitions. Provide ability to print requisitions, if necessary, in the performing departments where the orders will be filled, as well as the ability to display the orders on computer screens. (107)

- Order processing. Allow for personnel in the performing departments to process orders using the information forwarded by the orders system. (108)

- Order progress recording. Provides the ability to automatically schedule the date and time of performance for each occurrence of an order, to schedule a performance manually after order entry, and to reschedule one that has been previously scheduled. (109)

- Order tracking. Provides the ability to track and record the status of an order, if necessary identifying related information at specific stages (ordered, accessioned, partial, and completed). Allow for recording of reasons for an incomplete (outstanding) order. (110)

- Order activities. Allow for recording of related activities associated with an order, such as patient preparation and follow-up activities associated with a procedure, and provide the ability to update these activities and record their status of completion. (111)

- Verified and unverified results. Allows entry of verified (values confirmed or checked) or unverified results. (112)

- Results transmission. Provides the ability to transmit verified results back to the ordering station, for viewing or printing, as specified by the user, with storage of results in the patient's physical (paper) or electronic record. (113)

- Order display. Provide on-line order information necessary for patient care and department management, including lists and details of orders, occurrences, and results for each patient. (114)

- Work lists. Allow patient treatment units and department personnel to view lists of work to be done. Permit organization by scheduled performance time within department or location sequence. Allow display of details for specific occurrences and results upon request. (115)

- Audit trails. Provide necessary audit trail information for access by authorized users. Include functions performed for each order, occurrence, and result, along with the identification of the user that is making the change, and the date and time of entry. When results are modified, the previous data should be maintained in the database for display on demand. (116)

- Patient medical data retrieval. Allows for retrieval of pertinent data recorded on the registration module and additional patient medical data required by patient care personnel, including, but not limited to, pre-existing conditions, allergies, blood type, and visit-related data such as height and weight. (117)

- Observations. Allow on-line charting by nurses, therapists, and other healthcare professionals of observations, if not already provided by nursing care management module. (118)

- Orders system maintenance. Provides on-line maintenance of the order file, tailored according to the needs of the individual users and departments. Allows definition of characteristics for all items, tasks, and services that can be ordered. (119)

- Diagnostic order management. The system should allow order entry for nursing interventions, medication, ancillary services, social work, transportation, physiotherapy, and other therapies. (140)

- Provide Web-based linkage to clinical references. The system should have the ability to link electronically (Web) to external medical reference sources, such as Medline. (143)

D

- Drug utilization/usage review. Ability to set up specific parameters for the review of orders, review of historical data. Outpatient prescriptions to be tracked by patients on specific drugs, patients on a given drug for a given diagnosis, patients on a given drug for a given diagnosis for a given provider, and most frequently dispensed drugs by provider. (249)

B. Clinical Data Management

The purpose of the applications of this group is to support the clinical needs of care providers including maintaining accurate medical records. Ideally, a clinical data management system should provide a fully integrated approach to maintaining clinical data with appropriate linkages to the patient care logistics modules and data should be captured, validated, updated, and available at any time during the routine operation of the system at any "point of care" location.

Maintenance of medical records (nowadays more often called "health records" to accentuate the promotion of the continuum of care) is usually the responsibility of a dedicated department. Functions include abstracting, diagnosis and procedure update, and monitoring to ensure document and signature completion. Medical record also monitors and assists in defining quality outcomes and research, and diagnosis coding. Different user may have different levels of access (what is displayed) and privileges (read only, read and change) at each implemented function.

Applications of this group include the following modules:

- Medical Records
- Nursing Care
- Clinical Audit

Medical Records

- Patient Index (PI). Should have multiple search capabilities. The PI should be able to qualify searches by name, date of birth, sex, national individual identifiers (such as National Registration Number, Social Security Number, Health Plan Number, etc.) The index should support a variety of possible internal identifiers such as medical record number, case number, multiple account numbers, etc., for each patient and be able to maintain cross-reference to other existing identifiers in each of the facilities used by the patient in the same site or in other locations. (32)

- System should support a Master Patient Index (MPI), at multi-site, multi-institutional, regional, or national levels that links existing Patient Indices together. (33)

- Ability to look up patient "also-known-as" (AKA). The MPI should support multiple names so that patients who change their names can still be located with an MPI search. MPI name searches should search both the name and the AKA files during name searches. (34)

- Link family members. The system should contain a cross-reference facility for linkage of records belonging to different family members. (35)

- Name alert search. Patients with same last name and same first name and initial should be flagged to alert users of possible conflict. (36)

- Retrievable key fields values capable of bringing forward key field data from prior registrations and/or MPI. (42)

- Field updates from transactions in the Patient Registration module pass to MPI. On subsequent interactions the operator should be able to change and update registration fields were updating is allowed. Updated registration file should pass updated data to the MPI. (43)

- Face sheet print and reprint. System should allow client to define face sheets for registration and clinical management functions. System should support multiple sheets with automatically or manually selected print functions. System should support the Reprint function so that updates or corrections can be reprinted. (45)

- Convert or activate pre-admission. On patient arrival to the care unit, allow clerk to activate and update data from pre-admission record. Also permits specifying purge parameters for holding pre-admission records beyond expected pre-admission date. (46)

- Front-end insurance capture. Allows insurance verification function and levels of benefits. (47)

- Retroactive admission. Allows back dating of admissions, with appropriate adjustments to billing, reporting, revenue, and usage statistics. (48)

- Update fields capability. Allows updates to previously recorded patient data provided field is unlocked for such updating and user is authorized to do so. (49)

- No limitation on facilities or departments. The system should support a large number of primary, specialty, and subspecialty clinics and departments. (78)

- Access to registration MPI (Master Patient Index) and pass updates. Be able to view MPI to lookup and identify patient by demographics or Medical Records number. (92)

- Ability to generate a "chart-pull" list for the Medical Records Department. System should create a list of charts needed for each clinic each day. The list may be electronically sent to the Medical Records Department or printed on demand in a department or in decentralized medical records storage facilities. (98)

- Chart tracking. Provide ability to print out written guides, requests, location of charts, pull lists, and derelict returns. (120)

D

- Chart deficiency/incomplete record processing. Provide capability to automatically review the chart to ensure that necessary forms are present, entries are properly authenticated, informed consent forms are present, and good documentation procedures have been employed. The review identifies obvious areas that are incomplete and deficient. (121)

- Chart storage and retrieval. Provide the ability for chart storage and retrieval, including the type of filing system, filing equipment used, record purging capability, transportation management, and chart tracking management. (122)

- Chart reservation. Provide the ability to have a chart available on a particular date, for patient care, audit, reviews and physician studies, or release of information. The request may be generated by the scheduling system. (123)

- Transcription management. Provides the ability to include dictated reports or notes typed directly into the system (history, physical examination, provider observations, and case evolution notes) with transcription done in-house or outsourced. (124)

- Clinical coding for statistics and billing. Provides for the assignment of International Classification of Diseases and/or any other coding scheme/s to classify episodes of inpatient and outpatient care. (125)

- Clinical data abstracting. Provides the ability to extract certain patient data from records over and above the basic demographic data (e.g., weeks of gestation, usual living arrangements, allergies, images, photographs, etc.) (126)

- Release of information and correspondence. Provides for the management of requests for the release of patient information to various parties (e.g., other physicians, the patient, third-party payers, attorneys, etc.), including the correspondence involved with such requests. (127)

- Utilization management. Provides the ability to include a review of medical appropriateness and an analysis of the facility's efficiency in providing necessary services in the most cost-effective manner possible. (128)

- Maintain indices. Provide the ability to maintain a medical record index, a guide (manual, hard copy, or computerized) that points out or facilitates reference to patient information. Some examples of indices: service, diagnosis, diagnosis-related groups (DRGs), provider, procedure, length of stay, etc. (129)

- Archive management. Provide the ability to track patient records converted from hardcopy to another medium (e.g., microfilm, microfiche, optical disk, etc.) (130)

- Risk management. Provides reporting designed to protect an organization against potential liability through appropriate insurance coverage, reducing liability when compensable events occur, and prevention of events that are likely to lead to liabilities. Supports the review of accidents, injuries, and patient safety organization-wide. (131)

- Legal case file management. Supports the maintenance of patient records involved in legal actions and the correspondence associated with it. (132)

- Clinical data recording. Allows the recording of signs, symptoms, findings, treatment, and procedures, etc. The system should support a variety of documentation methodologies, for events such as assessments, signs and symptoms, treatments, procedures, etc. The user should be able to select from popular methodologies such as precoded options, charting by exception, narrative notes, free text, etc. (134)

- Review of historical patient information. Inpatient and outpatient history should be supported for documentation and on-line retrieval. (135)

- Referral management. Tracking of the follow-up care both internal and external to the institution should be supported. (136)

- Track outcomes. The system should be able to capture and manage data in a way that enables the caregivers to determine whether the patient is progressing toward a favorable outcome, or if not, what are the variances. (137)

- Provide Web-based linkage to clinical references. The system should have the ability to link electronically (Web) to external medical reference sources, such as Medline. (143)

- Flowsheet completion. The system should support posting of the patient's medical data in typical flowsheet formats, including graphically, over long periods of time, and across multiple episodes of care. It should support acquisition of information from medical devices and posting it in a flowsheet. (145)

- Critical pathway development tracking. The system should provide a comprehensive, multidisciplinary approach for developing activities and tasks for patient care over a specified timeline. It should be usable in both inpatient and outpatient settings. (146)

- Critical pathways with variance monitoring. The system should support documentation of the actual tasks completed and tracking reasons for straying from the established critical pathway. (147)

- Focused, problem-oriented charting. Quantitative data should be able to be displayed as trends in flowsheet format with focused and problem-oriented documentation in the progress notes. (148)

- Insurance. The system should have the ability to view or ascertain insurance and coverage information to assist clinical decision-making. (149)

- Capture of positive biopsy results. The system needs to provide the tools to capture the new data that are required for clinical management of patients with positive biopsy results. (207)

D

Nursing Care

- Patient Index (PI). Should have multiple search capabilities. The PI should be able to qualify searches by name, date of birth, sex, national individual identifiers (such as National Registration Number, Social Security Number, Health Plan Number, etc.) The index should support a variety of possible internal identifiers such as medical record number, case number, multiple account numbers, etc., for each patient and be able to maintain cross-reference to other existing identifiers in each of the facilities used by the patient in the same site or in other locations. (32)

- System should support a Master Patient Index (MPI), at multi-site, multi-institutional, regional, or national levels that links existing Patient Indices together. (33)

- Ability to look up patient "also-known-as" (AKA). The MPI should support multiple names so that patients who change their names can still be located with an MPI search. MPI name searches should search both the name and the AKA files during name searches. (34)

- Name alert search. Patients with same last name and same first name and initial should be flagged to alert users of possible conflict. (36)

- Retrievable key fields values capable of bringing forward key field data from prior registrations and/or MPI. (42)

- Field updates from transactions in the Patient Registration module pass to MPI. On subsequent interactions the operator should be able to change and update registration fields were updating is allowed. Updated registration file should pass updated data to the MPI. (43)

- Face sheet print and reprint. System should allow client to define face sheets for registration and clinical management functions. System should support multiple sheets with automatically or manually selected print functions. System should support the Reprint function so that updates or corrections can be reprinted. (45)

- Convert or activate pre-admission. On patient arrival to the care unit, allow clerk to activate and update data from pre-admission record. Also permits specifying purge parameters for holding pre-admission records beyond expected pre-admission date. (46)

- Front-end insurance capture. Allows insurance verification function and levels of benefits. (47)

- Retroactive admission. Allows back dating of admissions, with appropriate adjustments to billing, reporting, revenue, and usage statistics. (48)

- Update fields capability. Allows updates to previously recorded patient data provided field is unlocked for such updating and user is authorized to do so. (49)

- On-demand census of beds. The census feature should support query by a variety of perspectives including patient identifiers, bed, unit, medical problem grouping, attending doctor, patient type, etc.. This function should also support a public information service to facilitate location of patients and to generate directions to visitors. (56)

- On-line view of census. Allow on-line review of census by nursing unit. User can choose to review all beds, all occupied beds, and all empty beds for display by nursing unit. Occupied beds would indicate the patient name and number, data of admission, and attending physician. (64)

- No limitation on facilities or departments. The system should support a large number of primary, specialty, and subspecialty clinics and departments. (78)

- Access to registration MPI (Master Patient Index) and pass updates. Be able to view MPI to lookup and identify patient by demographics or Medical Records number. (92)

- Patient medical data retrieval. Allows for retrieval of pertinent data recorded on the registration module and additional patient medical data required by patient care personnel, including, but not limited to, pre-existing conditions, allergies, blood type, and visit-related data such as height and weight. (117)

- Risk management. Provides reporting designed to protect an organization against potential liability through appropriate insurance coverage, reducing liability when compensable events occur, and prevention of events that are likely to lead to liabilities. Supports the review of accidents, injuries, and patient safety organization-wide. (131)

- Patient/family assessment reporting. System should support a clinical, cognitive, environmental, psychosocial, subjective and objective nursing assessment observation reporting of patient, parent(s), legal guardian(s), and/or significant other. (133)

- Clinical data recording. Allows the recording of signs, symptoms, findings, treatment, and procedures, etc. The system should support a variety of documentation methodologies, for events such as assessments, signs and symptoms, treatments, procedures, etc. The user should be able to select from popular methodologies such as precoded options, charting by exception, narrative notes, free text, etc. (134)

- Review of historical patient information. Inpatient and outpatient history should be supported for documentation and on-line retrieval. (135)

- Referral management. Tracking of the follow-up care both internal and external to the institution should be supported. (136)

- Track outcomes. The system should be able to capture and manage data in a way that enables the caregivers to determine whether the patient is progressing toward a favorable outcome, or if not, what are the variances. (137)

D

- Generate patient care plan. System should allow the caregiver to develop a problem list and corrective interventions and timelines, ascertain expected outcomes and measure results based on assessments. Individualized plans of care should have ability to evaluate patient outcomes. (138)

- Provide patient education/instructional material. System should provide facilities for the production and generation of customized diagnosis-driven patient education materials based on the care plan. (139)

- Diagnostic order management. The system should allow order entry for nursing interventions, medication, ancillary services, social work, transportation, physiotherapy, and other therapies. (140)

- Medication management. The system should provide drug interaction/adverse reaction and possible resolution information; dosage calculation based on weight; dispensing tracking by time intervals; and warnings for clinically contraindicated medication or inappropriate dosage. (141)

- Patient classification system. The system should support a validated patient classification system based on clinical variables. It should be able to calculate the acuity level of the patient and determine required nursing resources needed as a result. It should provide expected productivity targets and suggest staffing patterns. (142)

- Provide Web-based linkage to clinical references. The system should have the ability to link electronically (Web) to external medical reference sources, such as Medline. (143)

- Record point-of-care nursing activities. System should be able to chart point-of-care activities/bedside diagnostics at the time when care is being delivered. Typical examples include vital signs, blood pressure, order entry, results retrieval, etc. Provide for flexible options regarding point-of-care devices. (144)

- Flowsheet completion. The system should support posting of the patient's medical data in typical flowsheet formats, including graphically, over long periods of time, and across multiple episodes of care. It should support acquisition of information from medical devices and posting it in a flowsheet. (145)

- Critical pathway development tracking. The system should provide a comprehensive, multidisciplinary approach for developing activities and tasks for patient care over a specified timeline. It should be usable in both inpatient and outpatient settings. (146)

- Critical pathways with variance monitoring. The system should support documentation of the actual tasks completed and tracking reasons for straying from the established critical pathway. (147)

- Focused, problem-oriented charting. Quantitative data should be able to be displayed as trends in flowsheet format with focused and problem-oriented documentation in the progress notes. (148)

- Insurance. The system should have the ability to view or ascertain insurance and coverage information to assist clinical decision-making. (149)

- Nursing practice and utilization. Provide the ability to determine if the assigned staffing level/skill mix meet the need(s) specified by the critical pathway/acuity level. (150)

Clinical Audit

- Patient Index (PI). Should have multiple search capabilities. The PI should be able to qualify searches by name, date of birth, sex, national individual identifiers (such as National Registration Number, Social Security Number, Health Plan Number, etc.) The index should support a variety of possible internal identifiers such as medical record number, case number, multiple account numbers, etc., for each patient and be able to maintain cross-reference to other existing identifiers in each of the facilities used by the patient in the same site or in other locations. (32)

- System should support a Master Patient Index (MPI), at multi-site, multi-institutional, regional, or national levels that links existing Patient Indices together. (33)

- Ability to look up patient "also-known-as" (AKA). The MPI should support multiple names so that patients who change their names can still be located with an MPI search. MPI name searches should search both the name and the AKA files during name searches. (34)

- Link family members. The system should contain a cross-reference facility for linkage of records belonging to different family members. (35)

- Name alert search. Patients with same last name and same first name and initial should be flagged to alert users of possible conflict. (36)

- Enrollment program. Registration systems should support enrollment and cancellation of enrollment in group or managed care programs. The system should support a posting program that should allow the member data to be downloaded from external insurance, group provider, or managed care organizations. (37)

- On-demand census of beds. The census feature should support query by a variety of perspectives including patient identifiers, bed, unit, medical problem grouping, attending doctor, patient type, etc.. This function should also support a public information service to facilitate location of patients and to generate directions to visitors. (56)

- Ability to generate a "chart-pull" list for the Medical Records Department. System should create a list of charts needed for each clinic each day. The list may be electronically sent to the Medical Records Department or printed on demand in a department or in decentralized medical records storage facilities. (98)

- Audit trails. Provide necessary audit trail information for access by authorized users. Include functions performed for each order, occurrence, and result, along with the identification of the user that is making the change, and the date and time of entry. When results are modified, the previous data should be maintained in the database for display on demand. (116)

- Chart deficiency/incomplete record processing. Provide capability to automatically review the chart to ensure that necessary forms are present, entries are properly authenticated, informed consent forms are present, and good documentation procedures have been employed. The review identifies obvious areas that are incomplete and deficient. (121)

- Utilization management. Provides the ability to include a review of medical appropriateness and an analysis of the facility's efficiency in providing necessary services in the most cost-effective manner possible. (128)

- Risk management. Provides reporting designed to protect an organization against potential liability through appropriate insurance coverage, reducing liability when compensable events occur, and prevention of events that are likely to lead to liabilities. Supports the review of accidents, injuries, and patient safety organization-wide. (131)

- Capture of positive biopsy results. The system needs to provide the tools to capture the new data that are required for clinical management of patients with positive biopsy results. (207)

- Drug utilization/usage review. Ability to set up specific parameters for the review of orders, review of historical data. Outpatient prescriptions to be tracked by patients on specific drugs, patients on a given drug for a given diagnosis, patients on a given drug for a given diagnosis for a given provider, and most frequently dispensed drugs by provider. (249)

C. Diagnostic and Therapeutic Technical Support Services Operation

The modules of this group have the objective of supporting the day-to-day operation and management of vital diagnostic and therapeutic services. These services are high-volume activity areas often using manual methods to internally process tests and procedures. A minimum level of automation includes linkage with the Registration, Admissions, Scheduling, Orders, and the processing of test requisitions, prescriptions, and procedure results. Because of the volume of data involved and the heavy interdepartmental communications, each module must provide information to support the improvement of the corresponding area workflow, the determination at any time of the exact status of all technical work currently being carried out, and provide quality control routines. Many modern diagnostic and therapeutic equipment have analog or digital output channels that can provide data directly to a PMIS.

Applications of this group include the following modules:

- Clinical Laboratory
- Medical Imaging: Diagnostic and Interventional
- Radiation Therapy
- Pharmacy
- Transfusion and Blood Bank
- Dietary Service

Clinical Laboratory

- Patient Index (PI). Should have multiple search capabilities. The PI should be able to qualify searches by name, date of birth, sex, national individual identifiers (such as National Registration Number, Social Security Number, Health Plan Number, etc.) The index should support a variety of possible internal identifiers such as medical record number, case number, multiple account numbers, etc., for each patient and be able to maintain cross-reference to other existing identifiers in each of the facilities used by the patient in the same site or in other locations. (32)

- System should support a Master Patient Index (MPI), at multi-site, multi-institutional, regional, or national levels that links existing Patient Indices together. (33)

- Ability to look up patient "also-known-as" (AKA). The MPI should support multiple names so that patients who change their names can still be located with an MPI search. MPI name searches should search both the name and the AKA files during name searches. (34)

- Name alert search. Patients with same last name and same first name and initial should be flagged to alert users of possible conflict. (36)

- Quick inpatient/outpatient/emergency services registration. The system should provide an alternate set of screens for quick registration, admission, or creation of a new record when patient information is incomplete or unavailable. The quick screens would allow an alternate set of entry screens for inpatient and outpatient care, emergency services, and diagnostic services. (40)

- Automatically assign billing number. A unique billing or account number is assigned for each patient visit, admission, or care cycle. Alternately, the health care institution should be able, for certain patient or visit types, to link multiple visits to a single number for serial or monthly billing. (41)

- Retrievable key fields values capable of bringing forward key field data from prior registrations and/or MPI. (42)

- Field updates from transactions in the Patient Registration module pass to MPI. On subsequent interactions the operator should be able to change and update registration fields were updating is allowed. Updated registration file should pass updated data to the MPI. (43)

- Cancel registration of ambulatory active visit. Cancel function should allow an active visit to be canceled. Canceled visits should be reflected correctly in usage statistics. (44)

- Face sheet print and reprint. System should allow client to define face sheets for registration and clinical management functions. System should support multiple sheets with automatically or manually selected print functions. System should support the Reprint function so that updates or corrections can be reprinted. (45)

- Front-end insurance capture. Allows insurance verification function and levels of benefits. (47)

- Update fields capability. Allows updates to previously recorded patient data provided field is unlocked for such updating and user is authorized to do so. (49)

- On-line view of census. Allow on-line review of census by nursing unit. User can choose to review all beds, all occupied beds, and all empty beds for display by nursing unit. Occupied beds would indicate the patient name and number, data of admission, and attending physician. (64)

- Scheduling rules. The system should be based on flexible, powerful computer-driven "rules" which correspond to the processes of scheduling currently employed in healthcare institutions. (66)

- Support centralized and decentralized scheduling. The system should allow for either scheduling at a single point of control, or decentralized scheduling controlled by individual departments, or a combination. (67)

- Connection to and support of departmental scheduling. The system should be able to coexist with existing departmental scheduling systems (such as laboratory, diagnostic images, operating room), and be able to interface with those systems. (68)

- Conflict-free scheduling. The system should always return a conflict-free schedule to the administrator, or identify the conflicts if a conflict-free schedule is not possible. (69)

- Make/reschedule appointments. System should support the integrated scheduling of appointments and resources across all client entities. (70)

- Change/cancel appointment flexibility. System should support the cancellation, changing, or updating of appointments with minimal data entry. (71)

- Copy appointments for resources. Copy current appointment information forward for future appointments. (72)

- Print schedule using multiple types of sorts. Schedules should be printed by resources, department, provider, and for date ranges. (74)

- Print appointment notices. Users should be able to demand printed appointment notices for one or a group of patients. (75)

- Automatic patient notices/mailings. System should support data mailer appointment notices. The mail functions should be profile driven in order that that multiple providers can establish different parameters. (76)

- Flexibility to define multiple resources. System should define various resource types such as providers, locations, equipment, and staff. The system should be able to verify the availability of all defined resources in its determination of service/procedure availability. (77)

- No limitation on facilities or departments. The system should support a large number of primary, specialty, and subspecialty clinics and departments. (78)

- Schedule all patient type/time. System should support slotting of all types of patients for all times of day. (79)

- Flexibility of changing appointment type/time. System should allow for various service and procedure appointment types and the ability to use them at various times and to change an existing appointment type. (80)

- Capability of multiple schedule storage. Physicians or other resources may have different schedules for different days. (81)

- Flexible security/access to schedule. System should provide a security or control mechanism for restricting access to specific schedules. (82)

- Ease of loading and building schedules. System should have "copy" function for ease in building and loading schedules. (83)

- Overbooking flexibility. Systems should have capability to allow overbooking by resource or department. (84)

- View open time slots on-line. System should allow viewing open appointments by resource and/or department. (85)

- Check-in/check-out functionality. System should allow patients to be checked-in at point of service or in a central registration area. System should support entry of check-out times. (86)

- Waiting list capability. User should be able to wait-list patients when no appointment slots are available. (87)

- Ease of scheduling walk-ins. System should support walk-in processing so that these patients can be scheduled at the point of service. (88)

D

- Reserve block of appointments. Allow blocking of appointments by provider, resource, and date. (89)

- Collapse appointments. System should be able to modify appointment lengths, allowing alteration of appointment times. (90)

- On-line view of past/future appointments. System should have capability to view on-line all or a set of past, present and future appointments by range of dates, resource, and patient. (91)

- Access to registration MPI (Master Patient Index) and pass updates. Be able to view MPI to lookup and identify patient by demographics or Medical Records number. (92)

- Maintain record of canceled appointments. The system should have the capability to view canceled appointments for at least one year. (93)

- View/print reasons for appointments. The system should have a "reason for appointment" field that can be viewed on time as printed with schedule. (94)

- Comment/alert for appointment type. System should provide alert if identical appointment types are scheduled for the same patient. It should also warn if the patient is a chronic no-show type of user. (95)

- Print patient instructions/comments on appointment slip. Allow user to include special instructions or requirements on the appointment slips, such as preparation instructions, or directions from one department to another. (96)

- Revise appointment type. Allow changing an appointment type for a rescheduled appointment, and update department statistics correctly. (97)

- Profile orders. Allow for generation of a set of medically or administratively grouped orders using profiles, such as a battery of tests, or coupled orders such as dietary and pharmacy preparations associated with radiology exams. (105)

- Order processing. Allow for personnel in the performing departments to process orders using the information forwarded by the orders system. (108)

- Order progress recording. Provides the ability to automatically schedule the date and time of performance for each occurrence of an order, to schedule a performance manually after order entry, and to reschedule one that has been previously scheduled. (109)

- Order tracking. Provides the ability to track and record the status of an order, if necessary identifying related information at specific stages (ordered, accessioned, partial, and completed). Allow for recording of reasons for an incomplete (outstanding) order. (110)

- Order activities. Allow for recording of related activities associated with an order, such as patient preparation and follow-up activities associated with a procedure, and provide the ability to update these activities and record their status of completion. (111)

- Verified and unverified results. Allows entry of verified (values confirmed or checked) or unverified results. (112)

- Results transmission. Provides the ability to transmit verified results back to the ordering station, for viewing or printing, as specified by the user, with storage of results in the patient's physical (paper) or electronic record. (113)

- Order display. Provide on-line order information necessary for patient care and department management, including lists and details of orders, occurrences, and results for each patient. (114)

- Work lists. Allow patient treatment units and department personnel to view lists of work to be done. Permit organization by scheduled performance time within department or location sequence. Allow display of details for specific occurrences and results upon request. (115)

- Audit trails. Provide necessary audit trail information for access by authorized users. Include functions performed for each order, occurrence, and result, along with the identification of the user that is making the change, and the date and time of entry. When results are modified, the previous data should be maintained in the database for display on demand. (116)

- Patient medical data retrieval. Allows for retrieval of pertinent data recorded on the registration module and additional patient medical data required by patient care personnel, including, but not limited to, pre-existing conditions, allergies, blood type, and visit-related data such as height and weight. (117)

- Observations. Allow on-line charting by nurses, therapists, and other healthcare professionals of observations, if not already provided by nursing care management module. (118)

- Orders system maintenance. Provides on-line maintenance of the order file, tailored according to the needs of the individual users and departments. Allows definition of characteristics for all items, tasks, and services that can be ordered. (119)

- Provide Web-based linkage to clinical references. The system should have the ability to link electronically (Web) to external medical reference sources, such as Medline. (143)

- Flowsheet completion. The system should support posting of the patient's medical data in typical flowsheet formats, including graphically, over long periods of time, and across multiple episodes of care. It should support acquisition of information from medical devices and posting it in a flowsheet. (145)

D

- Laboratory order entry. Provides the ability to enter orders for laboratory services from nursing stations, doctors' offices, or other points of care. (151)

- Unique order number. Assigns a unique order number to each lab order for identifying both specimen and order throughout processing cycle. Duplicate order checking provides control at the test component level with the option of manual override. (152)

- Add/cancel/credit orders. Provide the ability to add, cancel, and credit orders to existing order(s), including rescheduling of tests. (153)

- Charge capture. Provides the ability to capture charges at time of order, accession or test completion, depending on user requirements. (154)

- Group orders/work list. Provide the ability to group orders for collection purposes and accessions/orders in the batch. Automatically create order batches at designated times and sort orders by various categories to produce collection work lists of tests ordered for each analytical area/section/bay. (155)

- Label printing. Produces labels at accession time (alphanumeric, barcode) and ability to print labels automatically and on demand. Produce batch collection labels by collector or location; other options may include patient account number. (156)

- Specimen rejection. Provides for specimen rejection, including statement for reason and generation of lists for repeat collection. (157)

- Order priorities. Provide for lab order priorities: stat, routine, timed, etc. (158)

- Batch processing. Provides for batch processing of manually generated results or via analog-digital conversion of results generated by auto-analyzers. (159)

- Results entry. Provides for both manual and automated methods of results entry. (160)

- Incomplete work. Provides a listing of pending or incomplete work including reason/s. (161)

- Standardized results. Provide table-driven user defined "standardized results". Provide for high/low ranges comparison and display. (162)

- Textual results. Provide ability to include textual results entry and storage. (163)

- Supervisor review. Provides a method for supervisor review and approval of each test result and for eventual corrections. Based on supervisor approval, release test result for general reviewing, displaying, and reporting. (164)

- Produce sets of labels for each order, including master specimen container, isolation, and instructions. (165)

- Remote site label printing. Ability to redirect the printing of labels to various locations. (166)

- Printouts. Provide for order entry-driven, test-specific printout to hard copy or screen of detailed patient pretesting or laboratory instructions. (167)

- Results reporting. Provides ability for reporting test results and for immediate printing of emergency (stat) reports. Provides also ability for reporting on demand (patient-specific inquiry) or an interim basis. Users should be able to selectively choose the data they want to view, using a variety of selection options. (168)

- Summary reports. Provide summary reports (outpatients.) Provide the ability to produce and sort test results by attending physician within location. (169)

- Cumulative trends. Provide abiity for cumulative trend reporting. (170)

- Deviations. Provide necessary reporting for results deviating from normal ranges and corrected results. (171)

- Cross links. Provide a method to cross-link equivalent components of test results across different test codes and instruments. (172)

- Quality control (internal.) Capture quality control data and monitor conditions established by the laboratory. (173)

- Automatic notification. Provides automatic notification of product/reagent expiration dates. (174)

- Reporting statistics. Provide reporting statistics and workload to assist in staff and equipment budgeting and productivity. Provide appropriate administrative/management reports by capturing data from the lab system. (175)

- Results storage. Provides ability for storage of patient lab results based on user-defined data retention parameters. (176)

- Inventory. Provides for the management of inventory items. (177)

- Transcription interface. Provides a transcription system to be part of or interfaced with the Pathology Laboratory Information System. Provides ability to attend the unique needs of histology, cytology, autopsy, and other pathology areas. (178)

- Contracts. Provide the laboratory manager with reference to laboratory contract information to assist in analyzing performance and monitor adherence to contractual agreements. (179)

- Vendor tracking. Provides information to track vendor maintenance, training, supplies, equipment support, and maintenance. (180)

D

- System integration. Providers must have access to laboratory and pharmacy results. The system requirements are that the system should integrate with other diagnostic and therapeutic systems. There are certain exams where it is required to record and report data from other ancillary services on a final report. (200)

- Multiple exam "turnaround" time tracking. Captures multiple exam/test/procedure data that can be queried for exam or procedure timing information. (201)

- On-call exam/procedure data recording. Exam/procedure data entry or patient check-in feature should provide technically required fields for recording exams/procedures performed by all on-call personnel. (206)

- Capture of positive biopsy results. The system needs to provide the tools to capture the new data that are required for clinical management of patients with positive biopsy results. (207)

Medical Imaging: Diagnostic and Interventional

- Patient Index (PI). Should have multiple search capabilities. The PI should be able to qualify searches by name, date of birth, sex, national individual identifiers (such as National Registration Number, Social Security Number, Health Plan Number, etc.) The index should support a variety of possible internal identifiers such as medical record number, case number, multiple account numbers, etc., for each patient and be able to maintain cross-reference to other existing identifiers in each of the facilities used by the patient in the same site or in other locations. (32)

- System should support a Master Patient Index (MPI), at multi-site, multi-institutional, regional, or national levels that links existing Patient Indices together. (33)

- Ability to look up patient "also-known-as" (AKA). The MPI should support multiple names so that patients who change their names can still be located with an MPI search. MPI name searches should search both the name and the AKA files during name searches. (34)

- Name alert search. Patients with same last name and same first name and initial should be flagged to alert users of possible conflict. (36)

- Quick inpatient/outpatient/emergency services registration. The system should provide an alternate set of screens for quick registration, admission, or creation of a new record when patient information is incomplete or unavailable. The quick screens would allow an alternate set of entry screens for inpatient and outpatient care, emergency services, and diagnostic services. (40)

- Automatically assign billing number. A unique billing or account number is assigned for each patient visit, admission, or care cycle. Alternately, the health care institution should be able, for certain patient or visit types, to link multiple visits to a single number for serial or monthly billing. (41)

- Retrievable key fields values capable of bringing forward key field data from prior registrations and/or MPI. (42)

- Field updates from transactions in the Patient Registration module pass to MPI. On subsequent interactions the operator should be able to change and update registration fields were updating is allowed. Updated registration file should pass updated data to the MPI. (43)

- Cancel registration of ambulatory active visit. Cancel function should allow an active visit to be canceled. Canceled visits should be reflected correctly in usage statistics. (44)

- Face sheet print and reprint. System should allow client to define face sheets for registration and clinical management functions. System should support multiple sheets with automatically or manually selected print functions. System should support the Reprint function so that updates or corrections can be reprinted. (45)

- Front-end insurance capture. Allows insurance verification function and levels of benefits. (47)

- Update fields capability. Allows updates to previously recorded patient data provided field is unlocked for such updating and user is authorized to do so. (49)

- On-line view of census. Allow on-line review of census by nursing unit. User can choose to review all beds, all occupied beds, and all empty beds for display by nursing unit. Occupied beds would indicate the patient name and number, data of admission, and attending physician. (64)

- Scheduling rules. The system should be based on flexible, powerful computer-driven "rules" which correspond to the processes of scheduling currently employed in healthcare institutions. (66)

- Support centralized and decentralized scheduling. The system should allow for either scheduling at a single point of control, or decentralized scheduling controlled by individual departments, or a combination. (67)

- Connection to and support of departmental scheduling. The system should be able to coexist with existing departmental scheduling systems (such as laboratory, diagnostic images, operating room), and be able to interface with those systems. (68)

- Conflict-free scheduling. The system should always return a conflict-free schedule to the administrator, or identify the conflicts if a conflict-free schedule is not possible. (69)

- Make/reschedule appointments. System should support the integrated scheduling of appointments and resources across all client entities. (70)

D

- Change/cancel appointment flexibility. System should support the cancellation, changing, or updating of appointments with minimal data entry. (71)

- Copy appointments for resources. Copy current appointment information forward for future appointments. (72)

- Print schedule using multiple types of sorts. Schedules should be printed by resources, department, provider, and for date ranges. (74)

- Print appointment notices. Users should be able to demand printed appointment notices for one or a group of patients. (75)

- Automatic patient notices/mailings. System should support data mailer appointment notices. The mail functions should be profile driven in order that that multiple providers can establish different parameters. (76)

- Flexibility to define multiple resources. System should define various resource types such as providers, locations, equipment, and staff. The system should be able to verify the availability of all defined resources in its determination of service/procedure availability. (77)

- No limitation on facilities or departments. The system should support a large number of primary, specialty, and subspecialty clinics and departments. (78)

- Schedule all patient type/time. System should support slotting of all types of patients for all times of day. (79)

- Flexibility of changing appointment type/time. System should allow for various service and procedure appointment types and the ability to use them at various times and to change an existing appointment type. (80)

- Capability of multiple schedule storage. Physicians or other resources may have different schedules for different days. (81)

- Flexible security/access to schedule. System should provide a security or control mechanism for restricting access to specific schedules. (82)

- Ease of loading and building schedules. System should have "copy" function for ease in building and loading schedules. (83)

- Overbooking flexibility. Systems should have capability to allow overbooking by resource or department. (84)

- View open time slots on-line. System should allow viewing open appointments by resource and/or department. (85)

- Check-in/check-out functionality. System should allow patients to be checked-in at point of service or in a central registration area. System should support entry of check-out times. (86)

- Waiting list capability. User should be able to wait-list patients when no appointment slots are available. (87)

- Ease of scheduling walk-ins. System should support walk-in processing so that these patients can be scheduled at the point of service. (88)

- Reserve block of appointments. Allow blocking of appointments by provider, resource, and date. (89)

- Collapse appointments. System should be able to modify appointment lengths, allowing alteration of appointment times. (90)

- On-line view of past/future appointments. System should have capability to view on-line all or a set of past, present and future appointments by range of dates, resource, and patient. (91)

- Access to registration MPI (Master Patient Index) and pass updates. Be able to view MPI to lookup and identify patient by demographics or Medical Records number. (92)

- Maintain record of canceled appointments. The system should have the capability to view canceled appointments for at least one year. (93)

- View/print reasons for appointments. The system should have a "reason for appointment" field that can be viewed on time as printed with schedule. (94)

- Comment/alert for appointment type. System should provide alert if identical appointment types are scheduled for the same patient. It should also warn if the patient is a chronic no-show type of user. (95)

- Print patient instructions/comments on appointment slip. Allow user to include special instructions or requirements on the appointment slips, such as preparation instructions, or directions from one department to another. (96)

- Revise appointment type. Allow changing an appointment type for a rescheduled appointment, and update department statistics correctly. (97)

- Profile orders. Allow for generation of a set of medically or administratively grouped orders using profiles, such as a battery of tests, or coupled orders such as dietary and pharmacy preparations associated with radiology exams. (105)

- Order processing. Allow for personnel in the performing departments to process orders using the information forwarded by the orders system. (108)

D

- Order progress recording. Provides the ability to automatically schedule the date and time of performance for each occurrence of an order, to schedule a performance manually after order entry, and to reschedule one that has been previously scheduled. (109)

- Order tracking. Provides the ability to track and record the status of an order, if necessary identifying related information at specific stages (ordered, accessioned, partial, and completed). Allow for recording of reasons for an incomplete (outstanding) order. (110)

- Order activities. Allow for recording of related activities associated with an order, such as patient preparation and follow-up activities associated with a procedure, and provide the ability to update these activities and record their status of completion. (111)

- Verified and unverified results. Allows entry of verified (values confirmed or checked) or unverified results. (112)

- Results transmission. Provides the ability to transmit verified results back to the ordering station, for viewing or printing, as specified by the user, with storage of results in the patient's physical (paper) or electronic record. (113)

- Order display. Provide on-line order information necessary for patient care and department management, including lists and details of orders, occurrences, and results for each patient. (114)

- Work lists. Allow patient treatment units and department personnel to view lists of work to be done. Permit organization by scheduled performance time within department or location sequence. Allow display of details for specific occurrences and results upon request. (115)

- Audit trails. Provide necessary audit trail information for access by authorized users. Include functions performed for each order, occurrence, and result, along with the identification of the user that is making the change, and the date and time of entry. When results are modified, the previous data should be maintained in the database for display on demand. (116)

- Patient medical data retrieval. Allows for retrieval of pertinent data recorded on the registration module and additional patient medical data required by patient care personnel, including, but not limited to, pre-existing conditions, allergies, blood type, and visit-related data such as height and weight. (117)

- Observations. Allow on-line charting by nurses, therapists, and other healthcare professionals of observations, if not already provided by nursing care management module. (118)

- Orders system maintenance. Provides on-line maintenance of the order file, tailored according to the needs of the individual users and departments. Allows definition of characteristics for all items, tasks, and services that can be ordered. (119)

- Provide Web-based linkage to clinical references. The system should have the ability to link electronically (Web) to external medical reference sources, such as Medline. (143)

- Reporting statistics. Provide reporting statistics and workload to assist in staff and equipment budgeting and productivity. Provide appropriate administrative/management reports by capturing data from the lab system. (175)

- Exam data entry. The exam data entry module should cover all of the functions used to enter processing information and results for an examination. Exam data entry should capture the following data: exam events; user-defined result entry fields; specialized exams (mammography, intravenous urography, ultrasound, tomography, etc.) tracking and reporting; report archive functionality; on-call exams tracking; and pregnancy and shielded/unshielded. (182)

- Film room management. Film room management required to log and track the movement of films inside the institution. Film management should perform the following: film tracking for physician or department sign-out; film room tracking functions; film archive management. (183)

- Administration. Provides all the managerial and personnel functions and management reporting, including the following: productivity functions and reporting; work projections; quality control reports; and utilization statistics for equipment and facilities. (184)

- Activity tracking. This module is required to track information about patient utilization of the medical imaging facilities. (185)

- Imaging equipment maintenance. The system needs to provide a module that will allow collection and capture of data elements in order to generate equipment maintenance monitoring reports and alerts. Options for maintaining all aspects of the imaging equipment. The system must support user-defined help text. Remote accessibility to the system is a critical priority. The system should support ad hoc reporting capability for all modules. Include flexible parameters for screens and menus based on institutional, facility, or user-defined criteria. (186)

- Exam and result turnaround time tracking. The system needs to capture exam data that can be queried for exam and exam result turnaround times. (187)

- Transcription management and productivity transcription. The system needs to provide incomplete work reports and views. Capture keystroke average and turnaround time average for report completion. (188)

- Quality control data collection/reports. Provide the ability to track repeat exams and film utilization with related reasons to facilitate problem pattern identification. (189)

- Contrast reaction record and report. Provide ability to record and report on contrast reactions. The system should provide ease of capture of this information. (191)

D

- Technologist productivity functions and reporting. The system needs to capture data on technologists' exam performance and provide reporting tools. (192)

- Report review. Report review functionality is the ability to review transcribed reports. This function should allow the responsible professional to electronically sign the reports and release them. Report review should also allow for auto-fax. Auto-fax is the ability to send final reports via fax to clinic destinations after they have been released by the radiologist. The report review module should support auto-dictation upload and download. Remote access to report review is also a functional requirement. (193)

- Outside film management. Logs and tracks movement of films loaned or borrowed from other institutions. (194)

- Activity tracking. This module is required to track scheduling and utilization information related to each patient visit to the department. (195)

- Historical patient management. This is needed to purge information from the radiology system. The system should also contain tools to manage film archiving or destruction. On-line imaging interface or compatibility is also required. (196)

- Patient inquiry. This is used to review all current, previous, and historical data by authorized staff. (197)

- Physician activity report. This is required where electronic signature or any information related to the physicians involved in the exam, from ordering to the result completion, can be tracked and managed. This module should have reporting capability. (198)

- System integration. Providers must have access to laboratory and pharmacy results. The system requirements are that the system should integrate with other diagnostic and therapeutic systems. There are certain exams where it is required to record and report data from other ancillary services on a final report. (200)

- Multiple exam "turnaround" time tracking. Captures multiple exam/test/procedure data that can be queried for exam or procedure timing information. (201)

- Radiologist tracking and productivity. Track and provide reports on the reporting, assisting, and consulting Radiologists. (203)

- On-call exam/procedure data recording. Exam/procedure data entry or patient check-in feature should provide technically required fields for recording exams/procedures performed by all on-call personnel. (206)

- Capture of positive biopsy results. The system needs to provide the tools to capture the new data that are required for clinical management of patients with positive biopsy results. (207)

- Mammography tracking/reporting. Positive exams must link to report biopsy findings and must generate doctor notification and follow-up letters. (208)

- Film archive management. Radiology departments archive their film from active film rooms to inactive film rooms. The system needs to track films through the cycle. (209)

- Tuberculosis screening data capture/report. Provide ability to track positive chest X-Rays. Record the room, equipment, and personnel exposed to the infected patient. (210)

- Ad hoc reporting. The system should provide an ad hoc or system query function. It should be able to access all specialized data elements for query purposes. (211)

- Specialized report requirements. The system should provide for standard, ad hoc, and on-demand reporting capabilities in both on-line and batch modes that consider the special needs related to clinical imaging and radiotherapy. (212)

- Digital filmless imaging. Image can be electronically transmitted. (213)

Radiation Therapy

- Patient Index (PI). Should have multiple search capabilities. The PI should be able to qualify searches by name, date of birth, sex, national individual identifiers (such as National Registration Number, Social Security Number, Health Plan Number, etc.) The index should support a variety of possible internal identifiers such as medical record number, case number, multiple account numbers, etc., for each patient and be able to maintain cross-reference to other existing identifiers in each of the facilities used by the patient in the same site or in other locations. (32)

- System should support a Master Patient Index (MPI), at multi-site, multi-institutional, regional, or national levels that links existing Patient Indices together. (33)

- Ability to look up patient "also-known-as" (AKA). The MPI should support multiple names so that patients who change their names can still be located with an MPI search. MPI name searches should search both the name and the AKA files during name searches. (34)

- Name alert search. Patients with same last name and same first name and initial should be flagged to alert users of possible conflict. (36)

- Automatically assign billing number. A unique billing or account number is assigned for each patient visit, admission, or care cycle. Alternately, the health care institution should be able, for certain patient or visit types, to link multiple visits to a single number for serial or monthly billing. (41)

- Retrievable key fields values capable of bringing forward key field data from prior registrations and/or MPI. (42)

- Field updates from transactions in the Patient Registration module pass to MPI. On subsequent interactions the operator should be able to change and update registration fields were updating is allowed. Updated registration file should pass updated data to the MPI. (43)

- Cancel registration of ambulatory active visit. Cancel function should allow an active visit to be canceled. Canceled visits should be reflected correctly in usage statistics. (44)

- Face sheet print and reprint. System should allow client to define face sheets for registration and clinical management functions. System should support multiple sheets with automatically or manually selected print functions. System should support the Reprint function so that updates or corrections can be reprinted. (45)

- Front-end insurance capture. Allows insurance verification function and levels of benefits. (47)

- Update fields capability. Allows updates to previously recorded patient data provided field is unlocked for such updating and user is authorized to do so. (49)

- On-line view of census. Allow on-line review of census by nursing unit. User can choose to review all beds, all occupied beds, and all empty beds for display by nursing unit. Occupied beds would indicate the patient name and number, data of admission, and attending physician. (64)

- Scheduling rules. The system should be based on flexible, powerful computer-driven "rules" which correspond to the processes of scheduling currently employed in healthcare institutions. (66)

- Support centralized and decentralized scheduling. The system should allow for either scheduling at a single point of control, or decentralized scheduling controlled by individual departments, or a combination. (67)

- Connection to and support of departmental scheduling. The system should be able to coexist with existing departmental scheduling systems (such as laboratory, diagnostic images, operating room), and be able to interface with those systems. (68)

- Conflict-free scheduling. The system should always return a conflict-free schedule to the administrator, or identify the conflicts if a conflict-free schedule is not possible. (69)

- Make/reschedule appointments. System should support the integrated scheduling of appointments and resources across all client entities. (70)

- Change/cancel appointment flexibility. System should support the cancellation, changing, or updating of appointments with minimal data entry. (71)

- Copy appointments for resources. Copy current appointment information forward for future appointments. (72)

- Print schedule using multiple types of sorts. Schedules should be printed by resources, department, provider, and for date ranges. (74)

- Print appointment notices. Users should be able to demand printed appointment notices for one or a group of patients. (75)

- Automatic patient notices/mailings. System should support data mailer appointment notices. The mail functions should be profile driven in order that that multiple providers can establish different parameters. (76)

- Flexibility to define multiple resources. System should define various resource types such as providers, locations, equipment, and staff. The system should be able to verify the availability of all defined resources in its determination of service/procedure availability. (77)

- No limitation on facilities or departments. The system should support a large number of primary, specialty, and subspecialty clinics and departments. (78)

- Schedule all patient type/time. System should support slotting of all types of patients for all times of day. (79)

- Flexibility of changing appointment type/time. System should allow for various service and procedure appointment types and the ability to use them at various times and to change an existing appointment type. (80)

- Capability of multiple schedule storage. Physicians or other resources may have different schedules for different days. (81)

- Flexible security/access to schedule. System should provide a security or control mechanism for restricting access to specific schedules. (82)

- Ease of loading and building schedules. System should have "copy" function for ease in building and loading schedules. (83)

- Overbooking flexibility. Systems should have capability to allow overbooking by resource or department. (84)

- View open time slots on-line. System should allow viewing open appointments by resource and/or department. (85)

- Check-in/check-out functionality. System should allow patients to be checked-in at point of service or in a central registration area. System should support entry of check-out times. (86)

D

- Waiting list capability. User should be able to wait-list patients when no appointment slots are available. (87)

- Ease of scheduling walk-ins. System should support walk-in processing so that these patients can be scheduled at the point of service. (88)

- Reserve block of appointments. Allow blocking of appointments by provider, resource, and date. (89)

- Collapse appointments. System should be able to modify appointment lengths, allowing alteration of appointment times. (90)

- On-line view of past/future appointments. System should have capability to view on-line all or a set of past, present and future appointments by range of dates, resource, and patient. (91)

- Access to registration MPI (Master Patient Index) and pass updates. Be able to view MPI to lookup and identify patient by demographics or Medical Records number. (92)

- Maintain record of canceled appointments. The system should have the capability to view canceled appointments for at least one year. (93)

- View/print reasons for appointments. The system should have a "reason for appointment" field that can be viewed on time as printed with schedule. (94)

- Comment/alert for appointment type. System should provide alert if identical appointment types are scheduled for the same patient. It should also warn if the patient is a chronic no-show type of user. (95)

- Print patient instructions/comments on appointment slip. Allow user to include special instructions or requirements on the appointment slips, such as preparation instructions, or directions from one department to another. (96)

- Revise appointment type. Allow changing an appointment type for a rescheduled appointment, and update department statistics correctly. (97)

- Profile orders. Allow for generation of a set of medically or administratively grouped orders using profiles, such as a battery of tests, or coupled orders such as dietary and pharmacy preparations associated with radiology exams. (105)

- Order processing. Allow for personnel in the performing departments to process orders using the information forwarded by the orders system. (108)

- Order progress recording. Provides the ability to automatically schedule the date and time of performance for each occurrence of an order, to schedule a performance manually after order entry, and to reschedule one that has been previously scheduled. (109)

- Order tracking. Provides the ability to track and record the status of an order, if necessary identifying related information at specific stages (ordered, accessioned, partial, and completed). Allow for recording of reasons for an incomplete (outstanding) order. (110)

- Order activities. Allow for recording of related activities associated with an order, such as patient preparation and follow-up activities associated with a procedure, and provide the ability to update these activities and record their status of completion. (111)

- Results transmission. Provides the ability to transmit verified results back to the ordering station, for viewing or printing, as specified by the user, with storage of results in the patient's physical (paper) or electronic record. (113)

- Order display. Provide on-line order information necessary for patient care and department management, including lists and details of orders, occurrences, and results for each patient. (114)

- Work lists. Allow patient treatment units and department personnel to view lists of work to be done. Permit organization by scheduled performance time within department or location sequence. Allow display of details for specific occurrences and results upon request. (115)

- Audit trails. Provide necessary audit trail information for access by authorized users. Include functions performed for each order, occurrence, and result, along with the identification of the user that is making the change, and the date and time of entry. When results are modified, the previous data should be maintained in the database for display on demand. (116)

- Patient medical data retrieval. Allows for retrieval of pertinent data recorded on the registration module and additional patient medical data required by patient care personnel, including, but not limited to, pre-existing conditions, allergies, blood type, and visit-related data such as height and weight. (117)

- Observations. Allow on-line charting by nurses, therapists, and other healthcare professionals of observations, if not already provided by nursing care management module. (118)

- Orders system maintenance. Provides on-line maintenance of the order file, tailored according to the needs of the individual users and departments. Allows definition of characteristics for all items, tasks, and services that can be ordered. (119)

- Clinical data recording. Allows the recording of signs, symptoms, findings, treatment, and procedures, etc. The system should support a variety of documentation methodologies, for events such as assessments, signs and symptoms, treatments, procedures, etc. The user should be able to select from popular methodologies such as precoded options, charting by exception, narrative notes, free text, etc. (134)

- Provide Web-based linkage to clinical references. The system should have the ability to link electronically (Web) to external medical reference sources, such as Medline. (143)

D

- Transcription management and productivity transcription. The system needs to provide incomplete work reports and views. Capture keystroke average and turnaround time average for report completion. (188)

- Quality control data collection/reports. Provide the ability to track repeat exams and film utilization with related reasons to facilitate problem pattern identification. (189)

- Equipment maintenance. The system needs to provide a module that will allow collection and capture of data elements in order to generate equipment maintenance monitoring reports and alerts. Options for maintaining all aspects of the radiation therapy equipment. The system must support user-defined help text. Remote accessibility to the system is a critical priority. The system should support ad hoc reporting capability for all modules. Include flexible parameters for screens and menus based on institutional, facility, or user-defined criteria. (190)

- Technologist productivity functions and reporting. The system needs to capture data on technologists' exam performance and provide reporting tools. (192)

- Report review. Report review functionality is the ability to review transcribed reports. This function should allow the responsible professional to electronically sign the reports and release them. Report review should also allow for auto-fax. Auto-fax is the ability to send final reports via fax to clinic destinations after they have been released by the radiologist. The report review module should support auto-dictation upload and download. Remote access to report review is also a functional requirement. (193)

- Activity tracking. This module is required to track scheduling and utilization information related to each patient visit to the department. (195)

- Patient inquiry. This is used to review all current, previous, and historical data by authorized staff. (197)

- Physician activity report. This is required where electronic signature or any information related to the physicians involved in the exam, from ordering to the result completion, can be tracked and managed. This module should have reporting capability. (198)

- Procedure turnaround time tracking. The system needs to capture procedure data that can be queried for procedure turnaround timing. (199)

- System integration. Providers must have access to laboratory and pharmacy results. The system requirements are that the system should integrate with other diagnostic and therapeutic systems. There are certain exams where it is required to record and report data from other ancillary services on a final report. (200)

- Multiple exam "turnaround" time tracking. Captures multiple exam/test/procedure data that can be queried for exam or procedure timing information. (201)

- Result turnaround time tracking. The system needs to capture exam data that can be queried for exam result complete turnaround information. (202)

- Report archive management (microfiche). The system should provide archive management to help users track archived reports in the system. (204)

- Procedure data recording. The system needs to provide flexible, user-defined, facility-driven data entry screens. They should be able to be pulled into the final report if needed. (205)

- On-call exam/procedure data recording. Exam/procedure data entry or patient check-in feature should provide technically required fields for recording exams/procedures performed by all on-call personnel. (206)

- Capture of positive biopsy results. The system needs to provide the tools to capture the new data that are required for clinical management of patients with positive biopsy results. (207)

- Mammography tracking/reporting. Positive exams must link to report biopsy findings and must generate doctor notification and follow-up letters. (208)

- Ad hoc reporting. The system should provide an ad hoc or system query function. It should be able to access all specialized data elements for query purposes. (211)

- Specialized report requirements. The system should provide for standard, ad hoc, and on-demand reporting capabilities in both on-line and batch modes that consider the special needs related to clinical imaging and radiotherapy. (212)

- Radiotherapist tracking and productivity. Track and provide reports on the reporting, assisting, and consulting Radiotherapist. (303)

Pharmacy

- Patient Index (PI). Should have multiple search capabilities. The PI should be able to qualify searches by name, date of birth, sex, national individual identifiers (such as National Registration Number, Social Security Number, Health Plan Number, etc.) The index should support a variety of possible internal identifiers such as medical record number, case number, multiple account numbers, etc., for each patient and be able to maintain cross-reference to other existing identifiers in each of the facilities used by the patient in the same site or in other locations. (32)

- System should support a Master Patient Index (MPI), at multi-site, multi-institutional, regional, or national levels that links existing Patient Indices together. (33)

- Ability to look up patient "also-known-as" (AKA). The MPI should support multiple names so that patients who change their names can still be located with an MPI search. MPI name searches should search both the name and the AKA files during name searches. (34)

- Name alert search. Patients with same last name and same first name and initial should be flagged to alert users of possible conflict. (36)

- Quick inpatient/outpatient/emergency services registration. The system should provide an alternate set of screens for quick registration, admission, or creation of a new record when patient information is incomplete or unavailable. The quick screens would allow an alternate set of entry screens for inpatient and outpatient care, emergency services, and diagnostic services. (40)

- Automatically assign billing number. A unique billing or account number is assigned for each patient visit, admission, or care cycle. Alternately, the health care institution should be able, for certain patient or visit types, to link multiple visits to a single number for serial or monthly billing. (41)

- Retrievable key fields values capable of bringing forward key field data from prior registrations and/or MPI. (42)

- Field updates from transactions in the Patient Registration module pass to MPI. On subsequent interactions the operator should be able to change and update registration fields were updating is allowed. Updated registration file should pass updated data to the MPI. (43)

- Front-end insurance capture. Allows insurance verification function and levels of benefits. (47)

- Update fields capability. Allows updates to previously recorded patient data provided field is unlocked for such updating and user is authorized to do so. (49)

- On-line view of census. Allow on-line review of census by nursing unit. User can choose to review all beds, all occupied beds, and all empty beds for display by nursing unit. Occupied beds would indicate the patient name and number, data of admission, and attending physician. (64)

- No limitation on facilities or departments. The system should support a large number of primary, specialty, and subspecialty clinics and departments. (78)

- Access to registration MPI (Master Patient Index) and pass updates. Be able to view MPI to lookup and identify patient by demographics or Medical Records number. (92)

- Profile orders. Allow for generation of a set of medically or administratively grouped orders using profiles, such as a battery of tests, or coupled orders such as dietary and pharmacy preparations associated with radiology exams. (105)

- Order processing. Allow for personnel in the performing departments to process orders using the information forwarded by the orders system. (108)

- Order progress recording. Provides the ability to automatically schedule the date and time of performance for each occurrence of an order, to schedule a performance manually after order entry, and to reschedule one that has been previously scheduled. (109)

- Order tracking. Provides the ability to track and record the status of an order, if necessary identifying related information at specific stages (ordered, accessioned, partial, and completed). Allow for recording of reasons for an incomplete (outstanding) order. (110)

- Order activities. Allow for recording of related activities associated with an order, such as patient preparation and follow-up activities associated with a procedure, and provide the ability to update these activities and record their status of completion. (111)

- Results transmission. Provides the ability to transmit verified results back to the ordering station, for viewing or printing, as specified by the user, with storage of results in the patient's physical (paper) or electronic record. (113)

- Order display. Provide on-line order information necessary for patient care and department management, including lists and details of orders, occurrences, and results for each patient. (114)

- Work lists. Allow patient treatment units and department personnel to view lists of work to be done. Permit organization by scheduled performance time within department or location sequence. Allow display of details for specific occurrences and results upon request. (115)

- Audit trails. Provide necessary audit trail information for access by authorized users. Include functions performed for each order, occurrence, and result, along with the identification of the user that is making the change, and the date and time of entry. When results are modified, the previous data should be maintained in the database for display on demand. (116)

- Patient medical data retrieval. Allows for retrieval of pertinent data recorded on the registration module and additional patient medical data required by patient care personnel, including, but not limited to, pre-existing conditions, allergies, blood type, and visit-related data such as height and weight. (117)

- Observations. Allow on-line charting by nurses, therapists, and other healthcare professionals of observations, if not already provided by nursing care management module. (118)

- Orders system maintenance. Provides on-line maintenance of the order file, tailored according to the needs of the individual users and departments. Allows definition of characteristics for all items, tasks, and services that can be ordered. (119)

- Medication management. The system should provide drug interaction/adverse reaction and possible resolution information; dosage calculation based on weight; dispensing tracking by time intervals; and warnings for clinically contraindicated medication or inappropriate dosage. (141)

- Provide Web-based linkage to clinical references. The system should have the ability to link electronically (Web) to external medical reference sources, such as Medline. (143)

- Alpha access. Ability to create alphabetized file used during inventory alpha access functions. (181)

- Medication/solution order entry/review. Allow entering, modifying, and reviewing of medication and parenteral solution orders. The system should allow: pharmacists to confirm order entry and pharmacy technician conditional order entry (which requires pharmacist's approval before the orders are fully processed for dispensing and charging to patient's account.) (215)

- On-screen patient profile review. Ability to review a patient's medication utilization profile and drug sensibility information on the screen. Should provide checking for drug duplication and alert for drug interactions. (216)

- Charge/credit medication/solution orders. Facility that allows transfer of all charges to patient account. (217)

- PRN (Pro Re Nata = if needed) order update. Display ordered medications to be used if the clinical situation demands, or PRN schedule, for dispensing and charge to patient by nurse. (218)

- Drug/food allergy interactions. Ability to query on-line database of drug-drug and drug-food interactions, and therapeutic overlap. Provide the user with procedures for regular updating. (219)

- Medication label printing. Ability to print labels for dispensed medication. (220)

- Auxiliary label function. Allows the printing of auxiliary label codes for designated medications (221)

- Physician dispensing. Allows for record keeping and labels needed for prescription dispensing directly by physicians from local stores at ambulatory facilities. (222)

- Help prompts and messages. Allow the requesting of on-screen help messages. (223)

- Medication/solution distribution. Allows the production of fill lists for unit dose systems labels, solution preparation, processing of charges for scheduled medication and solution orders, and the printing of administration records for nurses. (224)

- Medication preparation (unit dose.) Ability to produce fill lists and update fill lists for cart filling with unit dose systems. Ability to interface with automatic dispensing machines. (225)

- Solution preparation labels. Ability to produce labels and update labels for solution orders. Produce labels for each hour dose is due for specified time entered. (226)

- Medication/solution dose timing control. Ability to advance the internal charging clocks accumulating charges and administer doses for scheduled, unit dose orders; discontinued orders having reached their stop times and date. (227)

- Medication/solution administration reports. Ability to produce medication and solution administration reports indicating all current orders on each patient, with times doses are due on scheduled orders. Ability to produce medication reports for 24-hours, seven-day and 31-day intervals. (228)

- Mail order distribution. Allows for the processing of outpatient prescriptions for mail order distribution. (229)

- Add new items. Ability to enter new items into pharmacy stock inventory file. (230)

- Modify/delete items. Ability to modify or delete an existing item from the master pharmacy stock inventory file. (231)

- Reports. Ability to produce various defined reports on records in the inventory file. (232)

- Stock movement. Ability to receive, issue, and write-off stock from inventory, perform interdepartmental transfers, return to stock, issue control substances, and set up ward stock items. (233)

- Update orders from inventory. Ability to update orders and predefined formulas with attribute and/or cost changes made to base inventory item. (234)

- Purchase orders. Ability to set up a purchasing inventory; create, modify, and print purchase orders, receive stock from purchase orders; and maintain purchase order statistics. (235)

- Global order cost update. Ability to update active orders, medication order groups, solution formulas, and inventory items with most recent prices. (236)

- Controlled/narcotic drugs. Allow the tracking of controlled/narcotic medications products stocked and dispensed. (237)

- Medication utilization profile report. Provides listing of patient medication and/or solution orders with pertinent order data indicated, including professional prescribing, organizational unit, and related clinical data. (238)

- Medication/solution renewal lists. Provide listing of patient's medications and/or solution orders which are scheduled to be stoppedor renewed in a specified time. (239)

- Update profiles. Provide listing of a patient's medication/solution profile indicating whether orders were updated in given periods. (240)

D

- PRN (if situation required) medication report. Provide listing of medication given on a PRN schedule and details of order including timing, dosage, prescribing, and dispensing professional. (241)

- Pharmacy database report generator. Allows for the creation of operator-designed reports displayed on screen, sent to printer or file from existing data files, or operator-created data files. (242)

- Special medication summary. Provides printing of designated data for minimum data setup dating (such as number of medications, patient on list for seven days or more, number of injections, any new medications in the last 90 days including antibiotics, tranquilizers, psychotropic, diuretics, hormones, and other). (243)

- Drug utilization information sheets. Ability to generate inpatient medication utilization information sheets, in multiple languages as required by the client population. (244)

- Psychotropic consent renewal list. Ability to print listing of existing psychotropic patient consent orders, if applicable. (245)

- Prescription reporting groups. Ability to generate reports for controlled/narcotic drugs, prescription refill summary, and new prescriptions for a specified period. (246)

- Compliance reporting. Produce reports to monitor specific medications against patient health problems, perform computer check between number of days supply and date of last refill. (247)

- Statistics. Ability to produce statistical reports and modify or purge statistical records. (248)

- Drug utilization/usage review. Ability to set up specific parameters for the review of orders, review of historical data. Outpatient prescriptions to be tracked by patients on specific drugs, patients on a given drug for a given diagnosis, patients on a given drug for a given diagnosis for a given provider, and most frequently dispensed drugs by provider. (249)

- Physician information maintenance. Allow for the logging of basic physician information (name, phone, etc.). (250)

- Prescription directions management. Ability to predefine the standard directions used in prescriptions and modify these directions, provide multiple language capability. (251)

- Pharmacokinetics. The calculation of medication dose based on specific patient parameters, such as age and weight. (252)

- Intervention log. Allows the logging and reporting of pharmacist clinical interventions. (253)

- Intervention cost analysis. Ability to calculate cost savings of clinical interventions. (254)

- Laboratory results access. Provide access to patient laboratory data files. (255)

- Support and store data for all facilities on-line for up to two years for inpatients and outpatients; archive records for historical retrieval on-line for all drugs up to five years; controlled substances for seven years; and thereafter purge records on retrievable media. Periods indicated may vary according to local legislation. (256)

- Capability to broadcast reports and schedules on-site to nursing stations and other healthcare provision sites. (257)

- Capability to generate custom/ad hoc trends and graphs to track patient prescription history. (258)

- Support for standard, ad hoc, and on-demand reporting capabilities in both on-line and batch modes. (259)

- Capability to create user-defined reports. Ability to save and schedule them as standard reports. (260)

- Validate technician medication/solution orders. Ability to review pharmacy technician orders and interactive approval facility. Log of transactions. (304)

D

Transfusion and Blood Bank

- Patient Index (PI). Should have multiple search capabilities. The PI should be able to qualify searches by name, date of birth, sex, national individual identifiers (such as National Registration Number, Social Security Number, Health Plan Number, etc.) The index should support a variety of possible internal identifiers such as medical record number, case number, multiple account numbers, etc., for each patient and be able to maintain cross-reference to other existing identifiers in each of the facilities used by the patient in the same site or in other locations. (32)

- System should support a Master Patient Index (MPI), at multi-site, multi-institutional, regional, or national levels that links existing Patient Indices together. (33)

- Ability to look up patient "also-known-as" (AKA). The MPI should support multiple names so that patients who change their names can still be located with an MPI search. MPI name searches should search both the name and the AKA files during name searches. (34)

- Name alert search. Patients with same last name and same first name and initial should be flagged to alert users of possible conflict. (36)

- Quick inpatient/outpatient/emergency services registration. The system should provide an alternate set of screens for quick registration, admission, or creation of a new record when patient information is incomplete or unavailable. The quick screens would allow an alternate set of entry screens for inpatient and outpatient care, emergency services, and diagnostic services. (40)

- Automatically assign billing number. A unique billing or account number is assigned for each patient visit, admission, or care cycle. Alternately, the health care institution should be able, for certain patient or visit types, to link multiple visits to a single number for serial or monthly billing. (41)

- Retrievable key fields values capable of bringing forward key field data from prior registrations and/or MPI. (42)

- Field updates from transactions in the Patient Registration module pass to MPI. On subsequent interactions the operator should be able to change and update registration fields were updating is allowed. Updated registration file should pass updated data to the MPI. (43)

- Cancel registration of ambulatory active visit. Cancel function should allow an active visit to be canceled. Canceled visits should be reflected correctly in usage statistics. (44)

- Face sheet print and reprint. System should allow client to define face sheets for registration and clinical management functions. System should support multiple sheets with automatically or manually selected print functions. System should support the Reprint function so that updates or corrections can be reprinted. (45)

- Front-end insurance capture. Allows insurance verification function and levels of benefits. (47)

- Update fields capability. Allows updates to previously recorded patient data provided field is unlocked for such updating and user is authorized to do so. (49)

- On-line view of census. Allow on-line review of census by nursing unit. User can choose to review all beds, all occupied beds, and all empty beds for display by nursing unit. Occupied beds would indicate the patient name and number, data of admission, and attending physician. (64)

- Support centralized and decentralized scheduling. The system should allow for either scheduling at a single point of control, or decentralized scheduling controlled by individual departments, or a combination. (67)

- Connection to and support of departmental scheduling. The system should be able to coexist with existing departmental scheduling systems (such as laboratory, diagnostic images, operating room), and be able to interface with those systems. (68)

- Conflict-free scheduling. The system should always return a conflict-free schedule to the administrator, or identify the conflicts if a conflict-free schedule is not possible. (69)

- Make/reschedule appointments. System should support the integrated scheduling of appointments and resources across all client entities. (70)

- Change/cancel appointment flexibility. System should support the cancellation, changing, or updating of appointments with minimal data entry. (71)

- Copy appointments for resources. Copy current appointment information forward for future appointments. (72)

- Print schedule using multiple types of sorts. Schedules should be printed by resources, department, provider, and for date ranges. (74)

- Print appointment notices. Users should be able to demand printed appointment notices for one or a group of patients. (75)

- Automatic patient notices/mailings. System should support data mailer appointment notices. The mail functions should be profile driven in order that that multiple providers can establish different parameters. (76)

- No limitation on facilities or departments. The system should support a large number of primary, specialty, and subspecialty clinics and departments. (78)

- Schedule all patient type/time. System should support slotting of all types of patients for all times of day. (79)

- Flexibility of changing appointment type/time. System should allow for various service and procedure appointment types and the ability to use them at various times and to change an existing appointment type. (80)

- Capability of multiple schedule storage. Physicians or other resources may have different schedules for different days. (81)

- Flexible security/access to schedule. System should provide a security or control mechanism for restricting access to specific schedules. (82)

- Ease of loading and building schedules. System should have "copy" function for ease in building and loading schedules. (83)

- Overbooking flexibility. Systems should have capability to allow overbooking by resource or department. (84)

- View open time slots on-line. System should allow viewing open appointments by resource and/or department. (85)

- Check-in/check-out functionality. System should allow patients to be checked-in at point of service or in a central registration area. System should support entry of check-out times. (86)

D

- Waiting list capability. User should be able to wait-list patients when no appointment slots are available. (87)

- Ease of scheduling walk-ins. System should support walk-in processing so that these patients can be scheduled at the point of service. (88)

- Reserve block of appointments. Allow blocking of appointments by provider, resource, and date. (89)

- Collapse appointments. System should be able to modify appointment lengths, allowing alteration of appointment times. (90)

- On-line view of past/future appointments. System should have capability to view on-line all or a set of past, present and future appointments by range of dates, resource, and patient. (91)

- Access to registration MPI (Master Patient Index) and pass updates. Be able to view MPI to lookup and identify patient by demographics or Medical Records number. (92)

- Maintain record of canceled appointments. The system should have the capability to view canceled appointments for at least one year. (93)

- View/print reasons for appointments. The system should have a "reason for appointment" field that can be viewed on time as printed with schedule. (94)

- Comment/alert for appointment type. System should provide alert if identical appointment types are scheduled for the same patient. It should also warn if the patient is a chronic no-show type of user. (95)

- Print patient instructions/comments on appointment slip. Allow user to include special instructions or requirements on the appointment slips, such as preparation instructions, or directions from one department to another. (96)

- Revise appointment type. Allow changing an appointment type for a rescheduled appointment, and update department statistics correctly. (97)

- Order processing. Allow for personnel in the performing departments to process orders using the information forwarded by the orders system. (108)

- Order progress recording. Provides the ability to automatically schedule the date and time of performance for each occurrence of an order, to schedule a performance manually after order entry, and to reschedule one that has been previously scheduled. (109)

- Order tracking. Provides the ability to track and record the status of an order, if necessary identifying related information at specific stages (ordered, accessioned, partial, and completed). Allow for recording of reasons for an incomplete (outstanding) order. (110)

- Order activities. Allow for recording of related activities associated with an order, such as patient preparation and follow-up activities associated with a procedure, and provide the ability to update these activities and record their status of completion. (111)

- Results transmission. Provides the ability to transmit verified results back to the ordering station, for viewing or printing, as specified by the user, with storage of results in the patient's physical (paper) or electronic record. (113)

- Order display. Provide on-line order information necessary for patient care and department management, including lists and details of orders, occurrences, and results for each patient. (114)

- Work lists. Allow patient treatment units and department personnel to view lists of work to be done. Permit organization by scheduled performance time within department or location sequence. Allow display of details for specific occurrences and results upon request. (115)

- Audit trails. Provide necessary audit trail information for access by authorized users. Include functions performed for each order, occurrence, and result, along with the identification of the user that is making the change, and the date and time of entry. When results are modified, the previous data should be maintained in the database for display on demand. (116)

- Patient medical data retrieval. Allows for retrieval of pertinent data recorded on the registration module and additional patient medical data required by patient care personnel, including, but not limited to, pre-existing conditions, allergies, blood type, and visit-related data such as height and weight. (117)

- Observations. Allow on-line charting by nurses, therapists, and other healthcare professionals of observations, if not already provided by nursing care management module. (118)

- Orders system maintenance. Provides on-line maintenance of the order file, tailored according to the needs of the individual users and departments. Allows definition of characteristics for all items, tasks, and services that can be ordered. (119)

- Clinical data recording. Allows the recording of signs, symptoms, findings, treatment, and procedures, etc. The system should support a variety of documentation methodologies, for events such as assessments, signs and symptoms, treatments, procedures, etc. The user should be able to select from popular methodologies such as precoded options, charting by exception, narrative notes, free text, etc. (134)

- Provide Web-based linkage to clinical references. The system should have the ability to link electronically (Web) to external medical reference sources, such as Medline. (143)

- Activity tracking. This module is required to track scheduling and utilization information related to each patient visit to the department. (195)

D

- Multiple exam "turnaround" time tracking. Captures multiple exam/test/procedure data that can be queried for exam or procedure timing information. (201)

- On-call exam/procedure data recording. Exam/procedure data entry or patient check-in feature should provide technically required fields for recording exams/procedures performed by all on-call personnel. (206)

- Technical audit trail. Provides a method to maintain a technical audit trail of blood bank sample and component processing. (214)

- Automated interfaces. Provide an automated interface between the clinical laboratory system and the healthcare institution's blood bank system. (261)

- Lab system/blood bank transfer. Provides for passing blood orders and patient admission/transfer/discharge (ADT) information from the clinical laboratory system to the blood bank system. (262)

- Technologist observation. Provide a method for the technologist to record observations and results and pass the information to the system. (263)

- Blood type screening. Provide for ABO, Rh, and antibody screening on general result reports. (264)

- Preferred terminology. Accommodates blood bank "preferred" terminology for recording observations. (265)

- Information product validity. Maintains and provides reports on expiration date for stored blood and blood components. (266)

Dietary Service

- Patient Index (PI). Should have multiple search capabilities. The PI should be able to qualify searches by name, date of birth, sex, national individual identifiers (such as National Registration Number, Social Security Number, Health Plan Number, etc.) The index should support a variety of possible internal identifiers such as medical record number, case number, multiple account numbers, etc., for each patient and be able to maintain cross-reference to other existing identifiers in each of the facilities used by the patient in the same site or in other locations. (32)

- System should support a Master Patient Index (MPI), at multi-site, multi-institutional, regional, or national levels that links existing Patient Indices together. (33)

- Ability to look up patient "also-known-as" (AKA). The MPI should support multiple names so that patients who change their names can still be located with an MPI search. MPI name searches should search both the name and the AKA files during name searches. (34)

- Name alert search. Patients with same last name and same first name and initial should be flagged to alert users of possible conflict. (36)

- Automatically assign billing number. A unique billing or account number is assigned for each patient visit, admission, or care cycle. Alternately, the health care institution should be able, for certain patient or visit types, to link multiple visits to a single number for serial or monthly billing. (41)

- Field updates from transactions in the Patient Registration module pass to MPI. On subsequent interactions the operator should be able to change and update registration fields were updating is allowed. Updated registration file should pass updated data to the MPI. (43)

- Front-end insurance capture. Allows insurance verification function and levels of benefits. (47)

- Update fields capability. Allows updates to previously recorded patient data provided field is unlocked for such updating and user is authorized to do so. (49)

- On-line view of census. Allow on-line review of census by nursing unit. User can choose to review all beds, all occupied beds, and all empty beds for display by nursing unit. Occupied beds would indicate the patient name and number, data of admission, and attending physician. (64)

- Scheduling rules. The system should be based on flexible, powerful computer-driven "rules" which correspond to the processes of scheduling currently employed in healthcare institutions. (66)

- Support centralized and decentralized scheduling. The system should allow for either scheduling at a single point of control, or decentralized scheduling controlled by individual departments, or a combination. (67)

- Connection to and support of departmental scheduling. The system should be able to coexist with existing departmental scheduling systems (such as laboratory, diagnostic images, operating room), and be able to interface with those systems. (68)

- Conflict-free scheduling. The system should always return a conflict-free schedule to the administrator, or identify the conflicts if a conflict-free schedule is not possible. (69)

- No limitation on facilities or departments. The system should support a large number of primary, specialty, and subspecialty clinics and departments. (78)

- Access to registration MPI (Master Patient Index) and pass updates. Be able to view MPI to lookup and identify patient by demographics or Medical Records number. (92)

D

- Profile orders. Allow for generation of a set of medically or administratively grouped orders using profiles, such as a battery of tests, or coupled orders such as dietary and pharmacy preparations associated with radiology exams. (105)

- Order processing. Allow for personnel in the performing departments to process orders using the information forwarded by the orders system. (108)

- Order progress recording. Provides the ability to automatically schedule the date and time of performance for each occurrence of an order, to schedule a performance manually after order entry, and to reschedule one that has been previously scheduled. (109)

- Order tracking. Provides the ability to track and record the status of an order, if necessary identifying related information at specific stages (ordered, accessioned, partial, and completed). Allow for recording of reasons for an incomplete (outstanding) order. (110)

- Order activities. Allow for recording of related activities associated with an order, such as patient preparation and follow-up activities associated with a procedure, and provide the ability to update these activities and record their status of completion. (111)

- Order display. Provide on-line order information necessary for patient care and department management, including lists and details of orders, occurrences, and results for each patient. (114)

- Work lists. Allow patient treatment units and department personnel to view lists of work to be done. Permit organization by scheduled performance time within department or location sequence. Allow display of details for specific occurrences and results upon request. (115)

- Audit trails. Provide necessary audit trail information for access by authorized users. Include functions performed for each order, occurrence, and result, along with the identification of the user that is making the change, and the date and time of entry. When results are modified, the previous data should be maintained in the database for display on demand. (116)

- Patient medical data retrieval. Allows for retrieval of pertinent data recorded on the registration module and additional patient medical data required by patient care personnel, including, but not limited to, pre-existing conditions, allergies, blood type, and visit-related data such as height and weight. (117)

- Observations. Allow on-line charting by nurses, therapists, and other healthcare professionals of observations, if not already provided by nursing care management module. (118)

- Orders system maintenance. Provides on-line maintenance of the order file, tailored according to the needs of the individual users and departments. Allows definition of characteristics for all items, tasks, and services that can be ordered. (119)

- Provide Web-based linkage to clinical references. The system should have the ability to link electronically (Web) to external medical reference sources, such as Medline. (143)

- Essential nutrient analysis. Conducts nutrient/cost analysis and calorie count tracking. (267)

- Nutrition assessment forms. Provide patient tracking reports and basic individual patient nutrient analysis, NPO (Nihil Per Os = fasting) and clear liquid reports, tube feeding reports, printing of tube feeding labels, and matrix analysis reports for special groups (e.g., restrition on specific food or nutrient, diabetic, renal patients). (268)

- Print tally sheets and print tray line tickets and nourishment labels. To accompany meal distribution for double-checking at distribution points. (269)

- Patient profile. Provides on-line patient profile which includes preferences, personal dietary restrictions, diet types, supplements, nourishmens, medications, and food allergies. (270)

- Production scheduling and management. Support to cook/chill, cook/freeze, and conventional cooking methods. Management of recipes, purchasing reports, forecast production needs, provide ingredient pick lists, manage freezer and overall inventory, schedule kitchen equipment, and provide production logistics worksheets. (271)

- Production/utilization forecasting. Generates forecasts based on patient census and historical usage. (272)

- Event management. Capability to manage one-of-a kind situations such as catering for event. (273)

D

D. Population and Environment Technical Support Services Operation

The modules of this group have the objective of supporting the day-to-day operation and management of population-related interventions and actions directed to the environment. These services are usually provided in the context of public community health services where frequently lies the responsibility for primary care preventive care and environmental health. Because of the volume of data involved, and the need for interdepartmental and interinstitutional communications, each module must provide information to support the improvement of the corresponding area workflow, the determination at any time of the exact status of all technical work currently being carried out, and provide quality control routines.

- Environmental Health
- Immunization
- Clinical Surveillance and Databases

Environmental Health

- Patient profile. Provides on-line patient profilewhich includes previous vaccinations, immunization schemes, contra-indications, and allergies. (276)

Immunization

- Patient Index (PI). Should have multiple search capabilities. The PI should be able to qualify searches by name, date of birth, sex, national individual identifiers (such as National Registration Number, Social Security Number, Health Plan Number, etc.) The index should support a variety of possible internal identifiers such as medical record number, case number, multiple account numbers, etc., for each patient and be able to maintain cross-reference to other existing identifiers in each of the facilities used by the patient in the same site or in other locations. (32)

- System should support a Master Patient Index (MPI), at multi-site, multi-institutional, regional, or national levels that links existing Patient Indices together. (33)

- Ability to look up patient "also-known-as" (AKA). The MPI should support multiple names so that patients who change their names can still be located with an MPI search. MPI name searches should search both the name and the AKA files during name searches. (34)

- Link family members. The system should contain a cross-reference facility for linkage of records belonging to different family members. (35)

- Name alert search. Patients with same last name and same first name and initial should be flagged to alert users of possible conflict. (36)

- Enrollment program. Registration systems should support enrollment and cancellation of enrollment in group or managed care programs. The system should support a posting program that should allow the member data to be downloaded from external insurance, group provider, or managed care organizations. (37)

- Automatically assign billing number. A unique billing or account number is assigned for each patient visit, admission, or care cycle. Alternately, the health care institution should be able, for certain patient or visit types, to link multiple visits to a single number for serial or monthly billing. (41)

- Retrievable key fields values capable of bringing forward key field data from prior registrations and/or MPI. (42)

- Field updates from transactions in the Patient Registration module pass to MPI. On subsequent interactions the operator should be able to change and update registration fields were updating is allowed. Updated registration file should pass updated data to the MPI. (43)

- Cancel registration of ambulatory active visit. Cancel function should allow an active visit to be canceled. Canceled visits should be reflected correctly in usage statistics. (44)

- Convert or activate pre-admission. On patient arrival to the care unit, allow clerk to activate and update data from pre-admission record. Also permits specifying purge parameters for holding pre-admission records beyond expected pre-admission date. (46)

- Front-end insurance capture. Allows insurance verification function and levels of benefits. (47)

- Retroactive admission. Allows back dating of admissions, with appropriate adjustments to billing, reporting, revenue, and usage statistics. (48)

- Update fields capability. Allows updates to previously recorded patient data provided field is unlocked for such updating and user is authorized to do so. (49)

- Scheduling rules. The system should be based on flexible, powerful computer-driven "rules" which correspond to the processes of scheduling currently employed in healthcare institutions. (66)

- Support centralized and decentralized scheduling. The system should allow for either scheduling at a single point of control, or decentralized scheduling controlled by individual departments, or a combination. (67)

- Connection to and support of departmental scheduling. The system should be able to coexist with existing departmental scheduling systems (such as laboratory, diagnostic images, operating room), and be able to interface with those systems. (68)

- Conflict-free scheduling. The system should always return a conflict-free schedule to the administrator, or identify the conflicts if a conflict-free schedule is not possible. (69)

- Make/reschedule appointments. System should support the integrated scheduling of appointments and resources across all client entities. (70)

- Change/cancel appointment flexibility. System should support the cancellation, changing, or updating of appointments with minimal data entry. (71)

- Copy appointments for resources. Copy current appointment information forward for future appointments. (72)

- Print schedule using multiple types of sorts. Schedules should be printed by resources, department, provider, and for date ranges. (74)

- Print appointment notices. Users should be able to demand printed appointment notices for one or a group of patients. (75)

D

- Automatic patient notices/mailings. System should support data mailer appointment notices. The mail functions should be profile driven in order that that multiple providers can establish different parameters. (76)

- Schedule all patient type/time. System should support slotting of all types of patients for all times of day. (79)

- Flexibility of changing appointment type/time. System should allow for various service and procedure appointment types and the ability to use them at various times and to change an existing appointment type. (80)

- Capability of multiple schedule storage. Physicians or other resources may have different schedules for different days. (81)

- Flexible security/access to schedule. System should provide a security or control mechanism for restricting access to specific schedules. (82)

- Ease of loading and building schedules. System should have "copy" function for ease in building and loading schedules. (83)

- Overbooking flexibility. Systems should have capability to allow overbooking by resource or department. (84)

- View open time slots on-line. System should allow viewing open appointments by resource and/or department. (85)

- Check-in/check-out functionality. System should allow patients to be checked-in at point of service or in a central registration area. System should support entry of check-out times. (86)

- Waiting list capability. User should be able to wait-list patients when no appointment slots are available. (87)

- Ease of scheduling walk-ins. System should support walk-in processing so that these patients can be scheduled at the point of service. (88)

- Reserve block of appointments. Allow blocking of appointments by provider, resource, and date. (89)

- Collapse appointments. System should be able to modify appointment lengths, allowing alteration of appointment times. (90)

- On-line view of past/future appointments. System should have capability to view on-line all or a set of past, present and future appointments by range of dates, resource, and patient. (91)

- Access to registration MPI (Master Patient Index) and pass updates. Be able to view MPI to lookup and identify patient by demographics or Medical Records number. (92)

- Maintain record of canceled appointments. The system should have the capability to view canceled appointments for at least one year. (93)

- Comment/alert for appointment type. System should provide alert if identical appointment types are scheduled for the same patient. It should also warn if the patient is a chronic no-show type of user. (95)

- Print patient instructions/comments on appointment slip. Allow user to include special instructions or requirements on the appointment slips, such as preparation instructions, or directions from one department to another. (96)

- Revise appointment type. Allow changing an appointment type for a rescheduled appointment, and update department statistics correctly. (97)

- Ability to generate a "chart-pull" list for the Medical Records Department. System should create a list of charts needed for each clinic each day. The list may be electronically sent to the Medical Records Department or printed on demand in a department or in decentralized medical records storage facilities. (98)

- Patient medical data retrieval. Allows for retrieval of pertinent data recorded on the registration module and additional patient medical data required by patient care personnel, including, but not limited to, pre-existing conditions, allergies, blood type, and visit-related data such as height and weight. (117)

- Enrollment program. Registration systems should support enrollment and cancellation of enrollment in the immunization scheme. (274)

- Create patient or system selected menus. Allows clinical personnel to create individual menus or pick from systems-based list and permit automatic updates of scheduled prescribed immunization changes. (275)

- Patient profile. Provides on-line patient profile which includes previous vaccinations, immunization schemes, contra-indications, and allergies. (276)

- Immunization scheduling and management. (277)

- Vaccine utilization doses and equipment requirement forecasting. (278)

D

Clinical Surveillance

- Patient Index (PI). Should have multiple search capabilities. The PI should be able to qualify searches by name, date of birth, sex, national individual identifiers (such as National Registration Number, Social Security Number, Health Plan Number, etc.) The index should support a variety of possible internal identifiers such as medical record number, case number, multiple account numbers, etc., for each patient and be able to maintain cross-reference to other existing identifiers in each of the facilities used by the patient in the same site or in other locations. (32)

- System should support a Master Patient Index (MPI), at multi-site, multi-institutional, regional, or national levels that links existing Patient Indices together. (33)

- Ability to look up patient "also-known-as" (AKA). The MPI should support multiple names so that patients who change their names can still be located with an MPI search. MPI name searches should search both the name and the AKA files during name searches. (34)

- Link family members. The system should contain a cross-reference facility for linkage of records belonging to different family members. (35)

- Name alert search. Patients with same last name and same first name and initial should be flagged to alert users of possible conflict. (36)

- Enrollment program. Registration systems should support enrollment and cancellation of enrollment in group or managed care programs. The system should support a posting program that should allow the member data to be downloaded from external insurance, group provider, or managed care organizations. (37)

- Convert or activate pre-admission. On patient arrival to the care unit, allow clerk to activate and update data from pre-admission record. Also permits specifying purge parameters for holding pre-admission records beyond expected pre-admission date. (46)

- Retroactive admission. Allows back dating of admissions, with appropriate adjustments to billing, reporting, revenue, and usage statistics. (48)

- Update fields capability. Allows updates to previously recorded patient data provided field is unlocked for such updating and user is authorized to do so. (49)

- Ability to generate a "chart-pull" list for the Medical Records Department. System should create a list of charts needed for each clinic each day. The list may be electronically sent to the Medical Records Department or printed on demand in a department or in decentralized medical records storage facilities. (98)

- Results entry. Provides for both manual and automated methods of results entry. (160)

- Standardized results. Provide table-driven user defined "standardized results". Provide for high/low ranges comparison and display. (162)

- Textual results. Provide ability to include textual results entry and storage. (163)

- Supervisor review. Provides a method for supervisor review and approval of each test result and for eventual corrections. Based on supervisor approval, release test result for general reviewing, displaying, and reporting. (164)

- Results reporting. Provides ability for reporting test results and for immediate printing of emergency (stat) reports. Provides also ability for reporting on demand (patient-specific inquiry) or an interim basis. Users should be able to selectively choose the data they want to view, using a variety of selection options. (168)

- Summary reports. Provide summary reports (outpatients.) Provide the ability to produce and sort test results by attending physician within location. (169)

- Cumulative trends. Provide abity for cumulative trend reporting. (170)

- Deviations. Provide necessary reporting for results deviating from normal ranges and corrected results. (171)

- Cross links. Provide a method to cross-link equivalent components of test results across different test codes and instruments. (172)

- Results storage. Provides ability for storage of patient lab results based on user-defined data retention parameters. (176)

- Transcription interface. Provides a transcription system to be part of or interfaced with the clinical laboratory information system. Provides for the unique needs of laboratory, histology, cytology, autopsy, and pathology. (279)

E. Administration and Resource Management

Because, in many instances, administrative and resource management requirements of health organizations are very similar or even identical to the needs of other organizations, applications of this group were historically the first to be implemented in the health sector.

There are, however, major differences in the way organizations manage their resources in different countries and in the public and private sector. In contrast to the technical applications (logistics of patient care, clinical data management, diagnostic and therapeutic support, and population and environment applications), in administrative and resource management area of applications, legal regulations and other constraints play a fundamental role in the definition of desired functionalities.

Applications of this group include the following modules:

- Finance Management
    - (a) *Billing / Accounts Receivable*
    - (b) *Accounts Payable*
    - (c) *General Accounting / Bookkeeping*
    - (d) *Cost Accounting*
    - (e) *General Ledger*
- Human Resources
    - (a) *Payroll*
    - (b) *Human Resource Management*
    - (c) *Staffing*
    - (d) *Benefits*
- Materials Management
    - (a) *Purchasing*
    - (b) *Inventory Control*
- Fixed Assets Management
- Medical Equipment Maintenance
- Physical Facilities Maintenance
- Laundry Services
- Transportation Services
- Budgeting and Executive Support

Billing / Accounts Receivable

- Patient Index (PI). Should have multiple search capabilities. The PI should be able to qualify searches by name, date of birth, sex, national individual identifiers (such as National Registration Number, Social Security Number, Health Plan Number, etc.) The index should support a variety of possible internal identifiers such as medical record number, case number, multiple account numbers, etc., for each patient and be able to maintain cross-reference to other existing identifiers in each of the facilities used by the patient in the same site or in other locations. (32)

- System should support a Master Patient Index (MPI), at multi-site, multi-institutional, regional, or national levels that links existing Patient Indices together. (33)

- Ability to look up patient "also-known-as" (AKA). The MPI should support multiple names so that patients who change their names can still be located with an MPI search. MPI name searches should search both the name and the AKA files during name searches. (34)

- Link family members. The system should contain a cross-reference facility for linkage of records belonging to different family members. (35)

- Name alert search. Patients with same last name and same first name and initial should be flagged to alert users of possible conflict. (36)

- Enrollment program. Registration systems should support enrollment and cancellation of enrollment in group or managed care programs. The system should support a posting program that should allow the member data to be downloaded from external insurance, group provider, or managed care organizations. (37)

- Automatically assign billing number. A unique billing or account number is assigned for each patient visit, admission, or care cycle. Alternately, the health care institution should be able, for certain patient or visit types, to link multiple visits to a single number for serial or monthly billing. (41)

- Field updates from transactions in the Patient Registration module pass to MPI. On subsequent interactions the operator should be able to change and update registration fields were updating is allowed. Updated registration file should pass updated data to the MPI. (43)

- Front-end insurance capture. Allows insurance verification function and levels of benefits. (47)

- Outpatient discharge. The health care institution should have the option of entering the discharge date on emergency services and outpatient accounts, or profiling the system to change them to discharge status after a certain number of hours or days. (50)

- Allow change in patient status from emergency room or outpatient to inpatient, so that when patients are admitted the original registration data should be rolled over to the inpatient visit. (58)

- Leave of absence processing. Allow leave of absence processing on inpatient accounts so that account may remain active without generating room charges for a period of time. (59)

- Event notices. System should create "event notices" that can be routed to one or more printers based on the following events: pre-admit, admit or registration, transfer, reservation booked, discharge scheduled, discharge, financial class update, bed status (housekeeping) changed, new medical record number assigned. (60)

- Access to registration MPI (Master Patient Index) and pass updates. Be able to view MPI to lookup and identify patient by demographics or Medical Records number. (92)

- Real-time, interactive module. Should also be able to meet managed care requirements, contract management, interim billing, and late charge billing. Up-to-the-minute information, complete account details, and current account detailed history. (305)

- Integration with other financial functions. This module must be integrated with General Ledger, Accounts Payable, and Cost Accounting Systems. Must automatically transfer patient data to/from the admissions system and maintain guarantor, insurance, disease, and

D

procedure categorization for payment purposes (e.g., DRGs), and archive account data. (306)

- Account search and retrieval. There should be quick account identification by patient name, number, unit number, or guarantor number. (307)

- View patient account information on-line/comments. Provides comprehensive view of account information available on-line. Includes visit and demographic, insurance verification, level of benefits, patient admission/discharge/transfer (ADT) information, current charges and payments, previous charges and payments. Also include summary of charges by department, billing and accounts receivable status information and diagnosis. The system should allow posting and review of account comments. (308)

- Determine source of payments by payer. System should be able to review payment transactions on-line and determine source of payment. Should be able to write summary and detail reports that will identify payment sources. System should allow for daily cash payments by payer. (309)

- Contract benefits. The system must provide the organization the ability to control group or managed care agreements and assist in the monitoring of contracts with third-party payers. (310)

- Benefit plans predetermined billing. Standard or common insurance benefit plans should be defined in a master file and loaded into accounts at time of verification. Plans may be modified at any time for individual accounts. (311)

- User-defined insurance verification screens. System should support healthcare institution defined verification screens, so that major payer groups can have customized screens to capture critical elements for each group. Screens should allow the healthcare institution to define required fields for payer and benefit information. (312)

- Central charge master. System should support a charge master file for each facility within the enterprise. (313)

- Charges and credit entry. System should have ability to manually post charges and credits for both room and ancillary charges. Claims data entry system should have ability to post claims data not otherwise captured in registration or abstracting functions. Examples include value codes, occurrence codes, and dates. (314)

- Auto room charge posting, auto charge. System should allow for posting room charges based on nightly census. Should support multiple accommodation types and rates. System should post corrected charges and credits when changes or cancellations are made to admit or discharge dates. (315)

- Ability for "series bill" or "specific visit bill". For ambulatory processing the system should be able to support both "visit" and "series" billing. Series billing would include the ability to bill for stated time periods or for a particular type of treatment for the duration of a treatment plan. (316)

- Ability to post charges at the level of pre-admission. Allow posting to accounts prior to actual admission for pre-admission events. (317)

- Prorate benefits by multiple payers. System should have ability to identify and support insurance proration for basic and major medical insurance charging any number of possible payers. Should be able to support excluded charges, specific charge rates for contract payers, and contractuals amounts. (318)

- Log system/view on-line. System should allow on-line maintenance and inquiry to logs account data, and on-line request of standard reports. (319)

- Automated account follow-up. Automated systems should support follow-up by payer, patient name, account balance ranges, account age, and status (if there are pending payments in Accounts Receivable or bad debt history). System should include past account history and previous follow-up activity. (320)

- Sliding fee scales for private pay billing. System should support patient billing discounts based on family income and size. (321)

- Values and codes edited against tables. Common data elements should be table or profile driven with on-line editing during data entry. (322)

- Electronic claims submission. Provide ability to bill third-party payers. (323)

- Produce hard-copy bills. Produce bills for payers not accepting electronic claims. (324)

- Electronic remittance processing. System should retrieve remittance advice form from third-party payers, and support posting of payments, contracts, and adjustments to Accounts Receivable. (325)

- Batch charges posting (automated.) System should support batch posting routines for ancillary charges generated in order entry systems. (326)

- Payments adjustments. System should support manual payments, adjustments, and contractuals for insurance and self-pay. Should be able to transfer pro-rated balances in posting function. (327)

- Reclassify revenue by payer. System should support manual reclassification of revenue by insurance payer, financial class, patient type when accounts are rebilled or insurance information is transferred or prorated to another payer after initial billing. (328)

D

- Bill hold capability (parameter-driven.) System should be able to delay billing until all required fields are complete. Health care institution can define different bill hold requirements by patient type (inpatient, outpatient, emergency services) and insurance type. (329)

- Ability to produce demand bills (all forms.) System should be able to demand printing of a bill with current charges for non-discharged accounts or accounts on hold. (330)

- Ability to force bill patients. System should be able to allow users to manually force an account into billed status even though it may not have met all bill hold criteria. (331)

- Ability to cycle bills. System should allow for generation of cycle bills for inpatients based on payer, length of stay, and/or balance. (332)

- Rebill accounts. System should allow for re-bill of accounts following changes in payers, charges, length of stay, and benefits. (333)

- Accounts receivable bad debt write-off capability. System should have ability to manually transfer accounts from active receivable to a bad debt status. Bad debt accounts should remain on-line for review, reporting, posting payments, etc. Transfer should generate all of the accounting and revenue transactions associated with write-off and recovery of bad debt. (334)

- Bad debt to accounts receivable reinstatement. System should allow manual transfer from bad debt to receivable if account was written in error. This transaction should generate the appropriate accounting and revenue transactions. (335)

- Auto accounts receivable processing (parameter-driven.) System should be able to rebill, write-off small balances and bad debts, purge zero balances, and change accounts from insurance to self-pay without manual intervention if accounts meet auto-processing criteria. Those criteria would include account age, balance, financial class, number of payments received, patient type, etc. The system should allow healthcare institution to write and maintain rules to automate this process. (336)

- Purging capability (parameter-driven). System should have ability to purge accounts from active patient master and accounts receivable or bad debt files. Purge criteria should be healthcare institution-defined, based on number of days since account reached zero balance. (337)

- Financial logs. System should include financial logs to allow summary review of charges, payment, diagnosis, diagnostic or procedure categorization for payment (DRGs), revenue and utilization data for cost reporting, and contract analysis. Logs data should be able to be automatically collected and posted to the logs data base from other systems modules. Should include both standard reports and report writer capability. (338)

- Ability to transfer balances to different payers. System should allow the transfer of prorated balances between payers for billing or accounts receivable purposes. (339)

- Support revenue and usage statistics. Maintain statistics for revenues and services by patient type, medical service, financial class or payer, healthcare institution, department, clinic, and location. (340)

- Process collection agency tapes. System should be able to create an extract of account information for submittal to collection agencies. The tape should be created automatically based on write-off activity to collection agencies. (341)

- Pass billed data to automated collection system. System should provide an on-line collection system with health care institution tickler files for account follow-up. Information from billing and payment activity should pass to the collection system to provide collectors with current account data. (342)

- Produce parameter-driven data mailers. System should support production of data mailers and collection letters with healthcare institution-defined cycles. (343)

- Automated collection assignments and statistics. Automated system should support distribution of accounts to collectors and maintain work statistics for each collector indicating the number of accounts assigned, worked, backlogged, etc. (344)

- Integrated registration/billing/collection letter. Automated collections system should be integrated to registration and billing systems so that data entered in one will be noted in the others. Comments or field updates performed in one system will update in each database. (345)

- Electronic denial reasons posted to billed account. System should allow for denial reasons to be posted to accounts with electronic remittance processing. Denial information should be available for on-line review. (346)

- Physician/healthcare institution charges on same bill. System should have ability to include physician and healthcare institution charges on the same bill where permitted/required by payer. (347)

- Archiving/restoring. System should have ability to purge billing and account data and restore it at some later time. (348)

Accounts Payable

- Common accounts payable features/functions. Provides the ability to handle the common features and functions of Accounts Payable, including expense allocation, one-time vendors, payment plan management, price adjustments and variances, discounts, and suspended invoice processing. (349)

- Provider management. Provides the flexibility of handling a variety of vendor documents, including single payment invoices, recurring invoices, and credit memos. Ability to alter vendor arrangements to accommodate changes as to discount specifications, address changes, and payment from different bank accounts. (350)

- Purchase order interface. Provides the ability to access details of acquisition and payment information by purchase order number. (351)

- Materials management interface. Provides the ability to interface automatically to the materials management applications (pharmacy, inventory control, etc.), when necessary. (352)

- Automatic or manual payment. Permits the vouching process to handle either automatic or manual payment period/cycle and bank account. (353)

- Invoices. Provide the ability to produce invoices. (354)

- Vouchers/checks. Provide the ability to produce vouchers or requests for checks. (355)

- Payment cycles. Provide for payment cycles to be defined by the user. (356)

- One-time processing. Provides for the ability to process ad hoc payments for vendors not included in the vendor master file, on a one-time basis. (357)

- Check clearing. Provides for the ability to clear checks within the system. (358)

- Liability posting. Provides for the ability to automatically post liabilities. (359)

- Credit invoices. Provide for the ability to handle credit invoices. (360)

- Audit trail. Maintains a comprehensive audit trail and general ledger interface in accordance to legal requirements. (361)

- Tax reporting. Provide for automatic production of tax reports, as required by specific country and local governments. (362)

General Accounting / Bookkeeping

- Accounting functions. Compatible with the legal requirements of each case, including the following general functions: automatic transfer of transactions from all financial modules, transfer of transactions between different organizations in multi-organization environment. (363)

- User-defined accounting lines. User-defined systems of allocating expenses and revenues. (364)

- Transaction facilities. No limit to length of time detail and summary data are retained; must allow prior and future period transactions, master log report that displays all batch transactions, and immediate update of account balances upon posting. (365)

- On-line look-up. On-line account inquiries to allow authorized users to view up-to-the-minute account balances or activity on demand. These inquiries must provide an audit trail indicating the transaction sources. Entry lists available in order of entry or in account number sequence. (366)

Cost Accounting

- Cost determination. Determine the cost of a cost/service unit, which corresponds to procedure codes in billing utilizing allocation methodology of user choice. Must map procedure codes to individual and multiple service units and store past, present, and future average rates for resources such as labor and materials and prorated general costs. (367)

- Cost distribution. Generates detailed reports on comparisons of actual and standard costs, fixed and variable costs, budgets, variance analysis, service profitability, and departmental responsibility. (368)

- Cost reporting. Application should provide users with multiple profitability reports based on various selection criteria as well as standard cost and service usage by cost unit. These reports should allow for budget comparison and variance analysis by managers throughout the organization. (369)

General Ledger

- Chart of accounts. User-controlled chart of accounts with unlimited number of defined accounts should be available. Permit organizational hierarchy that allows reports to be defined for any level of management. (370)

Payroll

- Standard payroll features. Provide the ability to perform typical payroll calculations, such as gross-to-net salary on a table-driven basis. Payroll information, including base rate, effective date, step, current benefit plans, withholdings, and automatic start/stop dates. (371)

- Rollback function. Provides retroactive calculations and computes earnings, taxes, and deductions and must be capable of mass edit routines to employee withholdings and benefits and provide a payroll summary by department, payroll register, tax, and deduction registers. Facility for posting to general ledger. (372)

D

- Special payroll features/functions. Provide the ability to handle the common features and functions of payroll, including on-line, real-time data entry and editing, batch balancing, overtime calculations, salaries of employees working in multiple positions at multiple pay rates, and payroll history. The system should provide for real-time inquiry of employee earnings and compensation as well as year-to-date inquiry routines and compute multiple payrolls with different schedules, list employee pay information, and post payroll data in general ledger. (373)

- Special compensation. Provide the ability to handle compensation, including wage and salary analysis and job evaluation and the ability to handle situations that depart from regular compensation, including common items such as stock options, and deferred payment and bonuses. (374)

- Salaries funded by multiple sources. Provide the ability to track salaries funded by multiple sources. (375)

- Direct deposit. Provide the ability to forward employee salary checks directly to their banks, in addition to providing traditional paper checks. (376)

- Retroactive pay. Provides the ability to calculate pay on a retroactive basis. (377)

- Deduction arrears and recovery. Provide the ability to calculate and report deduction arrears and recovery. (378)

- Automated check reversal. Provides for reversing checks automatically, based on user-defined criteria. (379)

- Date sensitivity. Provides the ability to automatically produce payroll checks based on specific dates, or conditions, such as "the last working date before the last day of the month", or "every Friday". (380)

- Audit and transaction reports. Provide comprehensive audit and transaction reports that are available for review before producing checks. (381)

- Labor distribution. Distribute payroll amounts among the appropriate labor departments as established by the user. (382)

- Government reporting. Provides reporting for applicable federal, state, and local governments, as well as deductions for applicable taxes. (383)

- Budget management. Provides the ability to monitor expense versus budget data, and make on-line changes where appropriate. (384)

- Integration with human resources and benefits systems. Provides interface to institution's human resources and benefits systems, where applicable. (385)

Human Resources Management

- Position and staffing. Provide the ability to control details of staffing, including positions, employee skills, and resource allocation. The on-line database should provide instant access to employee detailed personal record and history. Minimum data in the employee file should include: applicant tracking through recruiting, interviewing, and selection process, demographics, qualifications, training history, dependents, payroll status, hire date, next evaluation date, attendance template, position number, department, and job code. (386)

- Training and development. Provide the ability to track and manage training of employees, including course crediting, where applicable. (387)

- Performance tracking. Provides the ability to record, track, and manage employee performance, on a regular basis. Include the ability to have multiple inputs to evaluation, by the employee, by the employee's peers, and by management. (388)

- Career planning. Provides the ability to record and track career plans by employee, allowing input from both the employee and management. Includes ability to modify and update career plans dynamically. (389)

- Labor relations. Provide the ability to track and manage common elements of labor relations, including the status of collective bargaining agreements and union contract details. (390)

- Job applicant tracking. Provides the ability to enter and track the status of applicants through the recruiting, interviewing, and selection process. (391)

Staffing

- On-line scheduling. Department managers should be able to create templates to allow diverse groups with varying needs to set their own scheduling criteria. It will also process special requests on-line, e.g., days off, vacation, planned sick days, or jury duty. Specialized skills of individual staff should be viewable on-line and provide ad hoc scheduling reports of staff whose certification will expire shortly. (392)

- Schedule-makers should be able to experiment with draft schedules before creating a final schedule. Productive/nonproductive time data will provide the ability to track productivity based on real hours of work. (393)

- Expected attendance. Forecast of attendance data will be stored on a template for the employee and may be edited as necessary for the pay period. There will be on-line entry of summary time card data and the ability to accommodate daily time card entry. (394)

- Staffing planning. Provide recommended staff schedules to work a shift which also identifies problems of over- or under-staffing. Patient load, degree of patient dependency, and case type also will be factored in scheduling of nursing staff. Information modeling provides the ability to model future human resource scenarios and make analyses. (395)

- Cost impact modeling. Budget capabilities will be inherent in this system to help managers evaluate the cost effectiveness of their proposed schedules with funds available in their budget. The budget dollars will be prorated by specific time frames to match past experience of high census and degree of patient dependency status and severity of illness. (396)

- Timecards. Generation of timecards for employees for the use of payroll/personnel system. These will support any combination of job codes and shifts. (397)

Benefits

- Labor relations. Provide the ability to track and manage common elements of labor relations, including the status of collective bargaining agreements and union contract details. (390)

- General functions. Provide the ability to manage and track benefits, including medical and dental benefits, retirement, sick leave, and vacations. (398)

- Complex tax support. Provides the ability to handle complex taxes, including federal, state, and local taxes. (399)

- Periodic/nonperiodic payments. Provide the ability to handle both periodic and nonperiodic benefit payments. (400)

- Sources/deductions. Provide the ability to handle an unlimited number of sources and deductions per account. (401)

- Disbursements. Provide the ability to handle third-party disbursement processing. (402)

- Payment/deductions history. Provide the ability to have on-line benefits payment/deductions history. (403)

Purchasing

- Vendor information. Provide for on-line retrieval of detailed vendor information. (404)

- Vendor revalidation/invalidation. Provides the ability to invalidate or revalidate vendor for future purchases. (405)

- Vendor accounts payable. Links to Provide vendor accounts payable data and the ability to update it on-line. (406)

- Stock/nonstock requisition. Provides ability to handle on-line requisition of items, whether normal stock items or not. (407)

- Standard purchase order. Provides ability to support all standard purchase order processing types, e.g., standard, blanket, and consignment, as well as flexibility to support other, user-defined purchase order types. Provide ability to modify existing purchase orders. It will generate "standing" and blanket purchase orders at user-defined intervals. (408)

- Order status tracking. It will provide the status of any purchase order, accommodate multi-facility environments, and generate automatic purchase orders for items at or below their minimum reorder points and nonstock items ordered via department purchase requisitions. (409)

- Contract/open market items. Provide the ability to monitor on-line contract or acquisition of open market items. (410)

- Back-order processing. Allow for handling of back-ordered items. (411)

- Blanket/standing order receipts. Provide the ability to handle blanket or standing order receipts. (412)

- Shipment tolerances. Permit the user to define shipment acceptable tolerances. (413)

- Management and statistical reporting. Vendor performance, cost change, and buyer activity reports. (414)

D

Inventory Control

- Item database. Provide the ability to capture and maintain all purchased items code and description. Ability to search the database for items easily, by any combination of search arguments. (415)

- Item classification. Allows for classification of database items by product type or by group, and for on-line maintenance of the database. (416)

- Nonstock Items. Allow for capture of nonstock items. (417)

- Receiving functions. Produce receiving documents to record receipts of items with purchase order, and also handle blind receiving and receiving by exception. It should automatically match invoiced amounts to received values. There will be automatic update of quantity on-hand (stock control function) upon posting receipts of inventoried items. On-line inquiry of any purchase order and receipt information as well as providing on-line invoice reconciliation of purchase orders and accounts payable invoices. (418)

- Stock control. Permits recording of descriptive data,commercial brand name, manufacturer, supplier, purchase date, acquisition cost, warranties, and exclusions. Provides real-time updating of on-hand quantities. There will be inventory control features to supply a record of inventory activity such as issues, returns, adjustments, transfers, and purchase order history and provide both report and inquiry capabilities to help users monitor current stock levels. Will be able to support unlimited number of inventories. (419)

- Just in time inventory. Provides ability to support JIT or stockless inventory management techniques. (420)

- Order book. Be able to set up an order book of user-defined item requisition forms. (421)

- Requisitioning. Provides simultaneous order and issue functionality. (422)

- Remote location. Provides the ability to requisition inventory items from a remote location of the health care institution. (423)

- Automatic requisitioning. Supports automatic requisitioning for the purchase of items that fall below user-defined thresholds. (424)

- Delivery tickets. Provide the ability to produce customized delivery ticket, along with stocking instructions. (425)

- Consignment items. Provide the ability to manage items taken from vendors on consignment. (426)

- Inventory report. Provides the ability to produce a complete report of all inventory items, department usage report, stock status reports by type of item, most frequently used, and physical inventory worksheet and comparison reports. (427)

- Multiple units of issue. Support multiple issue of item from any inventory location. (428)

Fixed Assets Management

- Fixed assets database. Permits recording of descriptive data,commercial brand name, manufacturer, supplier, purchase date, acquisition cost, warranties, exclusions, maintenance data. Should be able to use international coding schemes. Provides the ability to update the location and condition of the item. Provides a complete audit trail of transactions affecting each fixed asset item, including disposal (removal from active inventory.) Ability to assign equipment to specific locations. Linkage to Medical Equipment Maintenance or Physical Facility Maintenance Module when they exist. (280)

- Depreciation categories. Provide the ability to assign a depreciation category to the item within the fixed asset schedule. Permit entering data regarding final disposition. (281)

- Asset depreciation. Permits automatic depreciation for all capital purchases and forecast future depreciation. (282)

- Depreciation status. Allows the user access to pertinent statistical data regarding these capital items, as well as appropriate reports to identify the status of purchases within the fixed asset schedule. (283)

- Predated items. Allow for entry of items that predate the introduction of the asset management system to be entered into the system. (284)

- Materials management interface. Provides the ability to interface automatically to the materials management applications (pharmacy, inventory control, etc.), when necessary. (352)

Medical Equipment Maintenance

- Equipment inventory. The equipment inventory should identify the commercial name (brand), manufacturer, size, model number, serial number, acquisition date, price, expected life cycle, warranties, maintenance contracts (including dates), physical location of the equipment in the institution, and any other information needed for maintaining or repairing equipment. (285)

- Order/service database. Provides entry of service requests, scheduled maintenance actions, and scheduling of staff for all preventative maintenance actions and work orders. (287)

- Order execution. Compiles and archives maintenance history, including date work performed, person performing, time to perform procedure, equipment/facility serviced, and any condition evaluation required by the maintenance action along with parts and consumables used in performance of the maintenance or repair action. Provide reports on service realized, labor costs, operating costs (costs of energy, procurement costs, life expectancy, salvage value, and training costs). (288)

- Fixed asset linkage. This should be linked to the Fixed Assets Management Module if it exists. When feasible should be integrated with asset management to provide budget information; life cycle cost analysis, replacement and repair evaluation, energy alternatives, and system effectiveness. (289)

- Parts inventory link. There should be data links to repair parts inventory to determine safe stocking levels as well as providing accurate part number, description, and supplier. (290)

- Manufacturer/supplier information. Data about name, address, telephone, fax, e-mail, and technical support contact of manufacturer, importer, supplier, technical support services. This should be linked to the equipment inventory database. (291)

D

Physical Facilities Maintenance

- General facility/equipment inventory. The equipment inventory should identify the commercial name (brand), manufacturer, size, model number, serial number, acquisition date, price, expected life cycle, warranties, maintenance contracts (including dates), physical location of the equipment in the institution, and any other information needed for maintaining or repairing equipment. (286)

- Order/service database. Provides entry of service requests, scheduled maintenance actions, and scheduling of staff for all preventative maintenance actions and work orders. (287)

- Order execution. Compiles and archives maintenance history, including date work performed, person performing, time to perform procedure, equipment/facility serviced, and any condition evaluation required by the maintenance action along with parts and consumables used in performance of the maintenance or repair action. Provide reports on service realized, labor costs, operating costs (costs of energy, procurement costs, life expectancy, salvage value, and training costs). (288)

- Fixed asset linkage. This should be linked to the Fixed Assets Management Module if it exists. When feasible should be integrated with asset management to provide budget information; life cycle cost analysis, replacement and repair evaluation, energy alternatives, and system effectiveness. (289)

- Parts inventory link. There should be data links to repair parts inventory to determine safe stocking levels as well as providing accurate part number, description, and supplier. (290)

- Manufacturer/supplier information. Data about name, address, telephone, fax, e-mail, and technical support contact of manufacturer, importer, supplier, technical support services. This should be linked to the equipment inventory database. (291)

Laundry Services

- Linen warehouse locations. Provide the ability to accommodate both linen warehouse locations and circulating linen locations. (292)

- Linen accounting. Provides the ability to account for linen issues/returns by cost center and expense code. The linen analysis system should provide accurate linen usage by linen type and linen items or by ward unit. Ability to track and monitor uniform usage as well as providing accurate billing and credits directly to ward and end users. (293)

- Pick lists. Provide the ability to handle issues or returns of linen based on pick list, or on-line, on demand. (294)

- Linen weights. Provide the ability to record and monitor linen weights to verify laundering expense. (295)

- Laundry orders/receipts. Provide the ability to record laundry orders and receipts by weight. (296)

Transportation Services

- Ability to manage the transport services information including number of kilometers driven, consumption of gas and oil, and other inputs. (297)

- Ability to generate transportation notification through order management. (298)

- Ability to generate an efficiency report on why patient was not brought to the institution. (299)

Budgeting and Executive Support

- Depreciation status. Allows the user access to pertinent statistical data regarding these capital items, as well as appropriate reports to identify the status of purchases within the fixed asset schedule. (283)

- General budgeting functions. Control entry of budget and statistical account data, including: supporting multiple files for current or future periods and department level access for budget development and analysis. It should provide for payroll budget information by department, job code, and earning type (for hours and dollars.) It must generate budget variance reports and comparison reports providing payroll information on hours and dollar amounts. (300)

- Budget transactions. Allow users to initialize budget data for accounts from current or previous budgets, actual data, and annualizations of current year's actual data. Allow users to update budget data for accounts by entering amounts for each period, or yearly amount, or by applying a percentage increase or decrease. (301)

- Payroll and fixed assets linkage. Automatic entry of budget files created in payroll and in fixed asset accounting modules. (302)

- Support revenue and usage statistics. Maintain statistics for revenues and services by patient type, medical service, financial class or payer, healthcare institution, department, clinic, and location. (340)

- Audit trail. Maintains a comprehensive audit trail and general ledger interface in accordance to legal requirements. (361)

D

- Tax reporting. Provide for automatic production of tax reports, as required by specific country and local governments. (362)

- On-line look-up. On-line account inquiries to allow authorized users to view up-to-the-minute account balances or activity on demand. These inquiries must provide an audit trail indicating the transaction sources. Entry lists available in order of entry or in account number sequence. (366)

- Cost determination. Determine the cost of a cost/service unit, which corresponds to procedure codes in billing utilizing allocation methodology of user choice. Must map procedure codes to individual and multiple service units and store past, present, and future average rates for resources such as labor and materials and prorated general costs. (367)

- Cost distribution. Generates detailed reports on comparisons of actual and standard costs, fixed and variable costs, budgets, variance analysis, service profitability, and departmental responsibility. (368)

- Cost reporting. Application should provide users with multiple profitability reports based on various selection criteria as well as standard cost and service usage by cost unit. These reports should allow for budget comparison and variance analysis by managers throughout the organization. (369)

- Chart of accounts. User-controlled chart of accounts with unlimited number of defined accounts should be available. Permit organizational hierarchy that allows reports to be defined for any level of management. (370)

- Budget management. Provides the ability to monitor expense versus budget data, and make on-line changes where appropriate. (384)

- Position and staffing. Provide the ability to control details of staffing, including positions, employee skills, and resource allocation. The on-line database should provide instant access to employee detailed personal record and history. Minimum data in the employee file should include: applicant tracking through recruiting, interviewing, and selection process, demographics, qualifications, training history, dependents, payroll status, hire date, next evaluation date, attendance template, position number, department, and job code. (386)

- Labor relations. Provide the ability to track and manage common elements of labor relations, including the status of collective bargaining agreements and union contract details. (390)

- Cost impact modeling. Budget capabilities will be inherent in this system to help managers evaluate the cost effectiveness of their proposed schedules with funds available in their budget. The budget dollars will be prorated by specific time frames to match past experience of high census and degree of patient dependency status and severity of illness. (396)

- Management and statistical reporting. Vendor performance, cost change, and buyer activity reports. (414)

- Inventory report. Provides the ability to produce a complete report of all inventory items, department usage report, stock status reports by type of item, most frequently used, and physical inventory worksheet and comparison reports. (427)

D

D.7. Tabular Summary of Functional Specifications

To facilitate identification of recommended functionalities for each module, an alphabetical listing of modules is presented with the corresponding pertinent specific functionalities. *The listing does not include the generic or systemic functions, common to all modules.*

Module	*Specific Functionality Code*
Accounts Payable	349, 350, 351, 352, 353, 354, 355, 356, 357, 358, 359, 360, 361, 362
Benefits (Staff)	390, 398, 399, 400, 401, 402, 403
Billing/Accounts Receivable	32, 33, 34, 35, 36, 37, 41, 43, 47, 50, 58, 59, 60, 92, 305, 306, 307, 308, 309, 310, 311, 312, 313, 314, 315, 316, 317, 318, 319, 320, 321, 322, 323, 324, 325, 326, 327, 328, 329, 330, 331, 332, 331, 334, 335, 336, 337, 338, 339, 340, 341, 342, 343, 344, 345, 346, 347, 348
Budget and Executive Support	283, 300, 301, 302, 340, 361, 362, 366, 367, 368, 369, 370, 384, 386, 390, 396, 414, 427
Clinical Audit	32, 33, 34, 35, 36, 37, 56, 98, 116, 121, 128, 131, 207, 249
Clinical Laboratory	32, 33, 34, 36, 40, 41, 42, 43, 44, 45, 47, 49, 64, 66, 67, 68, 69, 70, 71, 72, 74, 75, 76, 77, 78, 79, 80, 81, 82, 83, 84, 85, 86, 87, 88, 89, 90, 91, 92, 93, 94, 95, 96, 97, 105, 108, 109, 110, 111, 112, 113, 114, 115, 116, 117, 118, 119, 143, 145, 151, 152, 153, 154, 155, 156, 157, 158, 159, 160, 161, 162, 163, 164, 165, 166, 167, 168, 169, 170, 171, 172, 173, 174, 175, 176, 177, 178, 179, 180, 200, 201, 206, 207
Clinical Surveillance	32, 33, 34, 35, 36, 37, 46, 48, 49, 98, 160, 162, 163, 164, 168, 169, 170, 171, 172, 176, 279
Cost Accounting	367, 368, 369
Dietary Services	32, 33, 34, 36, 41, 43, 47, 49, 64, 66, 67, 68, 69, 78, 92, 105, 108, 109, 110, 111, 114, 115, 116, 117, 118, 119, 143, 267, 268, 269, 270, 271, 272, 273
Environmental Health	276
Fixed Assets Management	280, 281, 282, 283, 284, 352
General Accounting/Bookkeeping Functions	363, 364, 365, 366
General Ledger	370
Human Resources	386, 387, 388, 389, 390, 391
Immunization	32, 33, 34, 35, 36, 37, 41, 42, 43, 44, 46, 47, 48, 49, 66, 67, 68, 69, 70, 71, 72, 74, 75, 76, 79, 80, 81, 82, 83, 84, 85, 86, 87, 88, 89, 90, 91, 92, 93, 95, 96, 97, 98, 117, 274, 275, 276, 277, 278
Inpatient Admissions, Discharge and Transfer (ADT)	32, 33, 34, 35, 36, 37, 38, 39, 40, 41, 42, 43, 45, 46, 47, 48, 49, 51, 52, 53, 54, 55, 56, 57, 58, 59, 60, 61, 62, 63, 64, 65, 78, 86, 92, 98
Inventory Control	415, 416, 417, 418, 419, 420, 421, 422, 423, 424, 425, 426, 427, 428

Laundry Services	292, 293, 294, 295, 296
Medical Equipment Maintenance	285, 287, 288, 289, 290, 291
Medical Imaging	32, 33, 34, 36, 40, 41, 42, 43, 44, 45, 47, 49, 64, 66, 67, 68, 69, 70, 71, 72, 74, 75, 76, 77, 78, 79, 80, 81, 82, 83, 84, 85, 86, 87, 88, 89, 90, 91, 92, 93, 94, 95, 96, 97, 105, 108, 109, 110, 111, 112, 113, 114, 115, 116, 117, 118, 119, 143, 175, 182, 183, 184, 185, 186, 187, 188, 189, 191, 192, 193, 194, 195, 196, 197, 198, 200, 201, 203, 206, 207, 208, 209, 210, 211, 212, 213
Medical Records	32, 33, 34, 35, 36, 42, 43, 45, 46, 47, 48, 49, 78, 92, 98, 120, 121, 122, 123, 124, 125, 126, 127, 128, 129, 130, 131, 132, 134, 135, 136, 137, 143, 145, 146, 147, 148, 149, 207
Nursing Care	32, 33, 34, 36, 42, 43, 45, 46, 47, 48, 49, 56, 64, 78, 92, 117, 131, 133, 134, 135, 136, 137, 138, 139, 140, 141, 142, 143, 144, 145, 146, 147, 148, 149, 150
Orders	32, 33, 34, 36, 42, 43, 45, 47, 49, 92, 99, 100, 101, 102, 103, 104, 105, 106, 107, 108, 109, 110, 111, 112, 113, 114, 115, 116, 117, 118, 119, 140, 143, 249
Outpatient Admission	32, 33, 34, 35, 36, 37, 38, 39, 40, 41, 42, 43, 44, 45, 46, 47, 48, 49, 50, 58, 78, 86, 92, 98
Patient Registration	32, 33, 34, 35, 36, 37, 38, 39, 40, 41, 42, 43, 44, 45, 47, 49, 86
Payroll	371, 372, 373, 374, 375, 376, 377, 378, 379, 380, 381, 382, 383, 384, 385
Pharmacy	32, 33, 34, 36, 40, 41, 42, 43, 47, 49, 64, 78, 92, 105, 108, 109, 110, 111, 113, 114, 115, 116, 117, 118, 119, 141, 143, 181, 215, 216, 217, 218, 219, 220, 221, 222, 223, 224, 225, 226, 227, 228, 229, 230, 231, 232, 233, 234, 235, 236, 237, 238, 239, 240, 241, 242, 243, 244, 245, 246, 247, 248, 249, 250, 251, 252, 253, 254, 255, 256, 257, 258, 259, 260, 304
Physical Facilities Maintenance	286, 287, 288, 289, 290, 291
Purchasing	404, 405, 406, 407, 408, 409, 410, 411, 412, 413, 414
Radiation Therapy	32, 33, 34, 36, 41, 42, 43, 44, 45, 47, 49, 64, 66, 67, 68, 69, 70, 71, 72, 74, 75, 76, 77, 78, 79, 80, 81, 82, 83, 84, 85, 86, 87, 88, 89, 90, 91, 92, 93, 94, 95, 96, 97, 105, 108, 109, 110, 111, 113, 114, 115, 116, 117, 118, 119, 134, 143, 188, 189, 190, 192, 193, 195, 197, 198, 199, 200, 201, 202, 204, 205, 206, 207, 208, 211, 212, 303
Service Scheduling and Appointment Manager	32, 33, 34, 36, 40, 42, 43, 44, 47, 49, 66, 67, 68, 69, 70, 71, 72, 73, 74, 75, 76, 77, 78, 79, 80, 81, 82, 83, 84, 85, 86, 87, 88, 89, 90, 91, 92, 93, 94, 95, 96, 97, 98, 123, 277
Staffing	392, 393, 394, 395, 396, 397
Transfusion and Blood Bank	32, 33, 34, 36, 40, 41, 42, 43, 44, 45, 47, 49, 64, 67, 68, 69, 70, 71, 72, 74, 75, 76, 78, 79, 80, 81, 82, 83, 84, 85, 86, 87, 88, 89, 90, 91, 92, 93, 94, 95, 96, 97, 108, 109, 110, 111, 113, 114, 115, 116, 117, 118, 119, 134, 143, 195, 201, 206, 214, 261, 262, 263, 264, 265, 266
Transportation Services	297, 298, 299

D

D.8. Listing of Functionalities by Code Number

For reference purpose, follows a descriptive listing of functionalities sorted by the function identifying number used in the previous sections.

1. Management reports. Provides reports for administration and upper management to direct, control and plan organizational business and clinical functions.

2. Forms management. Provides support for forms design to ensure appropriate data collection, management of inventory, ordering, and stocking of paper forms.

3. Interdisciplinary progress notes or templates. The system should support multidisciplinary summary of clinical data from a specified patient. All direct care professionals should be able to view and enter information on-line, depending on access rights of each user.

4. Administrative policy development and retrieval. The system should have the ability to develop and quickly retrieve administrative, clinical, safety, and regulatory bodies' policies and procedures. It should have ability to cross-reference materials.

5. Fax or print notes. The system should allow the flexibility to customize the content of the reports/notes and also where they are printed.

6. Internal quality control. Provides reports to monitor and improve staff productivity, manage workload, and measure providera and user (i.e., medical staff, administration, patient, etc.) satisfaction level.

7. External quality control. Provides support for health care institution-wide quality control functions by providing reports and statistics requested by department, administration, and medical staff.

8. Client identification to be entered in a care unit site. An identifier must be used that will facilitate unique idemtification and client information data entry and retrieval. The Patient Index (PI) should be provided with a flexible screen builder capability that allows design and customization of a variety of possible registration screens.

9. Use-defined fields and tables. The health care institution should be able to define fields and tables for data that are not included in the vendor-supplied standard data set.The system should have a build facility that will provide an easy way for users to implement such definitions.

10. Required fields flexibility. User should be able to designate screen data fields as "required" or "not required" and to assign valid values, ranges, and other consistency checks. Required fields must have entry of valid data before the clerk can move forward to the next screen field.

11. Values edited to tables. Data entry to fields with system defined tables or profiles should be edited against the internal table values during data entry.

12. Help screen capability. Application should support extensive on-line help features. Descriptive text and examples should include the display of values from a table or valid profile linked to a data field.

13. Audit functions. System should provide audit trails of schedule events and results of scheduling activity.

14. Create patient labels and forms. Allows health care institutions to design formats for printing special forms and labels. Print functions should be accessible from registration screens.

15. Standard reports. The system should provide for standard and on-demand reporting capabilities in both on-line and batch modes.

16. Ad hoc reporting. Query facility support for generic reporting. Provide reports created based upon user-specified data fields as opposed to standard programmed reports.

17. User-definable reports. The system should have the capability to create programmable user-defined reports, with formatting and header construction capabilities, and permit saving and schedule these reports as standard reports.

18. Standard managerial reporting functions. Reports to enable decision makers at all levels to view integrated financial and statistical information from all departments, facilities, and corporations to make informed decisions and guide strategic plans. It should gather and assemble information from the following systems: admissions, nursing, laboratory, radiology, general ledger, payroll/personnel, Diagnostic Related Groups (DRGs) management, billings/accounts receivable, accounts payable, and materials management. Should provide for the assimilation of historical administrative, financial, and patient care information. Report generator should provide standard views of all data fields in place and have the ability to create extensive fields of the user's choosing.

19. Government-required codes. The system should be able to incorporate the government-required codes for the specific country, state, or municipality.

20. User-controlled posting. User-controlled sequence of posting reporting and closing, on-line review, free-text descriptions of each transaction, and edit of batch data available before posting to accounts.

21. Support for client-specific window customization. System should have capability to set required fields determined by department requirements and resource management characteristics.

22. Ability to enter comments. System should allow users to enter free-text comments related to specific data fields as determined by users during systems adaptation and implementation.

D

23. Look up patient record using phonetic search. System should support phonetic searches when the name entered for search has phonetic equivalents. The system should support searches in multiple languages.

24. Menu driven screens. The system should have the ability to move back and forth through a set of screens using menu selections, ideally using a graphic user interface environment (GUI).

25. The system should have a flexible screen builder facility to allow design and customization of screens, determination of the sequence of screens, placement of fields on a screen, type of controllers used (button, pull-down, toggle, etc.) and the definition of field edits, labels, and echoes.

26. Edit capability for screens. Screen builder should allow definition of field edits and default data to allow data to be directly edited on entry.

27. Passwords, levels of access, and privilege facilities. System must have a transaction audit tract that maintains the identification and a record of authorization, utilization (transactions), and changes related to system's users.

28. Embosser and/or barcode card/labels print/reprint. Vendor should support interface to common embossing and barcoding machines so that patient cards for embossing and scanning can be created.

29. Dictation tracking - type, edit, review, etc. The system should allow the dictation to have several different formats. The users need a preliminary, final, duplicate, and addendum notification to print on the reports. The system should also provide error correction editing and also track before and after copies of any final report that is edited.

30. Integration with other modules. Integrated as appropriate or feasible with modules such as all nursing applications, general ledger, diagnostic and procedure categorization for payment (e.g., DRG management), billings/accounts receivable, executive support system, and payroll/personnel systems.

31. Message communication. Allows the users to communicate with other units and departments though functions that create and transmit messages, such as e-mail systems.

32. Patient Index (PI). Should have multiple search capabilities. The PI should be able to qualify searches by name, date of birth, sex, national individual identifiers (such as National Registration Number, Social Security Number, Health Plan Number, etc.) The index should support a variety of possible internal identifiers such as medical record number, case number, multiple account numbers, etc., for each patient and be able to maintain cross-reference to other existing identifiers in each of the facilities used by the patient in the same site or in other locations.

33. System should support a Master Patient Index (MPI), at multi-site, multi-institutional, regional, or national levels that links existing Patient Indices together.

34. Ability to look up patient "also-known-as" (AKA). The MPI should support multiple names so that patients who change their names can still be located with an MPI search. MPI name searches should search both the name and the AKA files during name searches.

35. Link family members. The system should contain a cross-reference facility for linkage of records belonging to different family members.

36. Name alert search. Patients with same last name and same first name and initial should be flagged to alert users of possible conflict.

37. Enrollment program. Registration systems should support enrollment and cancellation of enrollment in group or managed care programs. The system should support a posting program that should allow the member data to be downloaded from external insurance, group provider, or managed care organizations.

38. Inpatient / outpatient pre-admission. System should allow pre-admit or pre-registration of patients prior to their actual arrival. Pre-admission function should allow clerk to collect the standard registration data for patients with or without existing medical records, case number, etc. Patients pre-admitted without identifiers must have them assigned when admission to inpatient care or outpatient contact is activated.

39. Registration system should support different registration screens and data set requirements for Emergency Care Services, Outpatient Services (First and Return Contacts) and for Inpatient Admission.

40. Quick inpatient/outpatient/emergency services registration. The system should provide an alternate set of screens for quick registration, admission, or creation of a new record when patient information is incomplete or unavailable. The quick screens would allow an alternate set of entry screens for inpatient and outpatient care, emergency services, and diagnostic services.

41. Automatically assign billing number. A unique billing or account number is assigned for each patient visit, admission, or care cycle. Alternately, the health care institution should be able, for certain patient or visit types, to link multiple visits to a single number for serial or monthly billing.

42. Retrievable key fields values capable of bringing forward key field data from prior registrations and/or MPI.

43. Field updates from transactions in the Patient Registration module pass to MPI. On subsequent interactions the operator should be able to change and update registration fields were updating is allowed. Updated registration file should pass updated data to the MPI.

44. Cancel registration of ambulatory active visit. Cancel function should allow an active visit to be canceled. Canceled visits should be reflected correctly in usage statistics.

D

45. Face sheet print and reprint. System should allow client to define face sheets for registration and clinical management functions. System should support multiple sheets with automatically or manually selected print functions. System should support the Reprint function so that updates or corrections can be reprinted.

46. Convert or activate pre-admission. On patient arrival to the care unit, allow clerk to activate and update data from pre-admission record. Also permits specifying purge parameters for holding pre-admission records beyond expected pre-admission date.

47. Front-end insurance capture. Allows insurance verification function and levels of benefits.

48. Retroactive admission. Allows back dating of admissions, with appropriate adjustments to billing, reporting, revenue, and usage statistics.

49. Update fields capability. Allows updates to previously recorded patient data provided field is unlocked for such updating and user is authorized to do so.

50. Outpatient discharge. The health care institution should have the option of entering the discharge date on emergency services and outpatient accounts, or profiling the system to change them to discharge status after a certain number of hours or days.

51. Bed reservation. Beds should be able to be reserved prior to admission.

52. Create patient identification wrist band. System should support formatting of data and print function for printing wrist bands.

53. Cancel inpatient admission or discharge. Cancel function should allow an active admission or discharge to be canceled. Canceled events should be reflected correctly in usage statistics and room charges should be adjusted retroactively to the beginning of a stay.

54. On-demand query of bed availability, status (vacant, blocked, active, planned discharge, planned transfer) and expected change of status.

55. Transfer emergency services to observation. System should support an observation status for patients admitted to Emergency Services. Observation patients should be able to be assigned to special observation beds and manually discharged.

56. On-demand census of beds. The census feature should support query by a variety of perspectives including patient identifiers, bed, unit, medical problem grouping, attending doctor, patient type, etc.. This function should also support a public information service to facilitate location of patients and to generate directions to visitors.

57. Support different admission screen sets and data requirements for emergency room and transfer admissions and discharge to outpatient clinic.

58. Allow change in patient status from emergency room or outpatient to inpatient, so that when patients are admitted the original registration data should be rolled over to the inpatient visit.

59. Leave of absence processing. Allow leave of absence processing on inpatient accounts so that account may remain active without generating room charges for a period of time.

60. Event notices. System should create "event notices" that can be routed to one or more printers based on the following events: pre-admit, admit or registration, transfer, reservation booked, discharge scheduled, discharge, financial class update, bed status (housekeeping) changed, new medical record number assigned.

61. Mother-newborn link. System should support the rollover of a mother's information to a "newborn" record, so that shared information from the mother's admission record should be shown on the baby's record. A permanent cross reference between the two systems should automatically be created (or manually entered when needed) to allow for an inquiry on the mother's or newborn's visit by reference to any visit number.

62. Newborn pre-admission. System should allow user to pre-admit a newborn with the mother's information. At the time of the birth the account should be activated and a medical record number assigned.

63. Housekeeping/maintenance. The system should identify beds for housekeeping when a patient is discharged. Housekeeping should be able to update bed status to "available" when the bed is made.

64. On-line view of census. Allow on-line review of census by nursing unit. User can choose to review all beds, all occupied beds, and all empty beds for display by nursing unit. Occupied beds would indicate the patient name and number, data of admission, and attending physician.

65. Nursing unit summary. System should provide a real-time display of nursing unit statistics. Display should give a summary for all units, including current summary of total beds, beds occupied, and the percentage of beds occupied.

66. Scheduling rules. The system should be based on flexible, powerful computer-driven "rules" which correspond to the processes of scheduling currently employed in healthcare institutions.

67. Support centralized and decentralized scheduling. The system should allow for either scheduling at a single point of control, or decentralized scheduling controlled by individual departments, or a combination.

68. Connection to and support of departmental scheduling. The system should be able to coexist with existing departmental scheduling systems (such as laboratory, diagnostic images, operating room), and be able to interface with those systems.

69. Conflict-free scheduling. The system should always return a conflict-free schedule to the administrator, or identify the conflicts if a conflict-free schedule is not possible.

D

70. Make/reschedule appointments. System should support the integrated scheduling of appointments and resources across all client entities.

71. Change/cancel appointment flexibility. System should support the cancellation, changing, or updating of appointments with minimal data entry.

72. Copy appointments for resources. Copy current appointment information forward for future appointments.

73. Reschedule resources. System should allow mass rescheduling of a physician's or service unit appointments to another date.

74. Print schedule using multiple types of sorts. Schedules should be printed by resources, department, provider, and for date ranges.

75. Print appointment notices. Users should be able to demand printed appointment notices for one or a group of patients.

76. Automatic patient notices/mailings. System should support data mailer appointment notices. The mail functions should be profile driven in order that that multiple providers can establish different parameters.

77. Flexibility to define multiple resources. System should define various resource types such as providers, locations, equipment, and staff. The system should be able to verify the availability of all defined resources in its determination of service/procedure availability.

78. No limitation on facilities or departments. The system should support a large number of primary, specialty, and subspecialty clinics and departments.

79. Schedule all patient type/time. System should support slotting of all types of patients for all times of day.

80. Flexibility of changing appointment type/time. System should allow for various service and procedure appointment types and the ability to use them at various times and to change an existing appointment type.

81. Capability of multiple schedule storage. Physicians or other resources may have different schedules for different days.

82. Flexible security/access to schedule. System should provide a security or control mechanism for restricting access to specific schedules.

83. Ease of loading and building schedules. System should have "copy" function for ease in building and loading schedules.

84. Overbooking flexibility. Systems should have capability to allow overbooking by resource or department.

85. View open time slots on-line. System should allow viewing open appointments by resource and/or department.

86. Check-in/check-out functionality. System should allow patients to be checked-in at point of service or in a central registration area. System should support entry of check-out times.

87. Waiting list capability. User should be able to wait-list patients when no appointment slots are available.

88. Ease of scheduling walk-ins. System should support walk-in processing so that these patients can be scheduled at the point of service.

89. Reserve block of appointments. Allow blocking of appointments by provider, resource, and date.

90. Collapse appointments. System should be able to modify appointment lengths, allowing alteration of appointment times.

91. On-line view of past/future appointments. System should have capability to view on-line all or a set of past, present and future appointments by range of dates, resource, and patient.

D

92. Access to registration MPI (Master Patient Index) and pass updates. Be able to view MPI to lookup and identify patient by demographics or Medical Records number.

93. Maintain record of canceled appointments. The system should have the capability to view canceled appointments for at least one year.

94. View/print reasons for appointments. The system should have a "reason for appointment" field that can be viewed on time as printed with schedule.

95. Comment/alert for appointment type. System should provide alert if identical appointment types are scheduled for the same patient. It should also warn if the patient is a chronic no-show type of user.

96. Print patient instructions/comments on appointment slip. Allow user to include special instructions or requirements on the appointment slips, such as preparation instructions, or directions from one department to another.

97. Revise appointment type. Allow changing an appointment type for a rescheduled appointment, and update department statistics correctly.

98. Ability to generate a "chart-pull" list for the Medical Records Department. System should create a list of charts needed for each clinic each day. The list may be electronically sent to the Medical Records Department or printed on demand in a department or in decentralized medical records storage facilities.

99. Order entry. Allow for on-line entry of orders along with all of the information necessary to complete the order in an efficient and accurate manner.

100. Verified and unverified orders. Allow for entry of orders as either unverified (not approved) or verified (approved and activated), depending upon the security level of the user.

101. Order verification. Allows for personnel with proper access authorization to either verify (approve) orders or void the orders if appropriate.

102. Order cancellation. Allow for cancellation of orders, either verified or unverified, and allow for inclusion of reason for cancellation.

103. Occurrences. Generate performance-related occurrences of the order each time the service is to be done within the active period of the order. Allow for additional occurrences to be appended to existing orders.

104. Ordering logistics. Allow for automatic scheduling of orders according to guidelines customized to fit the needs of the institution or technical constraints.

105. Profile orders. Allow for generation of a set of medically or administratively grouped orders using profiles, such as a battery of tests, or coupled orders such as dietary and pharmacy preparations associated with radiology exams.

106. Renewal of expiring orders. Allows for renewal of expiring orders, with the ability to bring forward information from the original order to create a new order, possibly with an extended duration.

107. Print requisitions. Provide ability to print requisitions, if necessary, in the performing departments where the orders will be filled, as well as the ability to display the orders on computer screens.

108. Order processing. Allow for personnel in the performing departments to process orders using the information forwarded by the orders system.

109. Order progress recording. Provides the ability to automatically schedule the date and time of performance for each occurrence of an order, to schedule a performance manually after order entry, and to reschedule one that has been previously scheduled.

110. Order tracking. Provides the ability to track and record the status of an order, if necessary identifying related information at specific stages (ordered, accessioned, partial, and completed). Allow for recording of reasons for an incomplete (outstanding) order.

111. Order activities. Allow for recording of related activities associated with an order, such as patient preparation and follow-up activities associated with a procedure, and provide the ability to update these activities and record their status of completion.

112. Verified and unverified results. Allows entry of verified (values confirmed or checked) or unverified

113. Results transmission. Provides the ability to transmit verified results back to the ordering station, for viewing or printing, as specified by the user, with storage of results in the patient's physical (paper) or electronic record.

114. Order display. Provide on-line order information necessary for patient care and department management, including lists and details of orders, occurrences, and results for each patient.

115. Work lists. Allow patient treatment units and department personnel to view lists of work to be done. Permit organization by scheduled performance time within department or location sequence. Allow display of details for specific occurrences and results upon request.

116. Audit trails. Provide necessary audit trail information for access by authorized users. Include functions performed for each order, occurrence, and result, along with the identification of the user that is making the change, and the date and time of entry. When results are modified, the previous data should be maintained in the database for display on demand.

117. Patient medical data retrieval. Allows for retrieval of pertinent data recorded on the registration module and additional patient medical data required by patient care personnel, including, but not limited to, pre-existing conditions, allergies, blood type, and visit-related data such as height and weight.

118. Observations. Allow on-line charting by nurses, therapists, and other healthcare professionals of observations, if not already provided by nursing care management module.

119. Orders system maintenance. Provides on-line maintenance of the order file, tailored according to the needs of the individual users and departments. Allows definition of characteristics for all items, tasks, and services that can be ordered.

120. Chart tracking. Provide ability to print out written guides, requests, location of charts, pull lists, and derelict returns.

121. Chart deficiency/incomplete record processing. Provide capability to automatically review the chart to ensure that necessary forms are present, entries are properly authenticated, informed consent forms are present, and good documentation procedures have been employed. The review identifies obvious areas that are incomplete and deficient.

122. Chart storage and retrieval. Provide the ability for chart storage and retrieval, including the type of filing system, filing equipment used, record purging capability, transportation management, and chart tracking management.

123. Chart reservation. Provide the ability to have a chart available on a particular date, for patient care, audit, reviews and physician studies, or release of information. The request may be generated by the scheduling system.

124. Transcription management. Provides the ability to include dictated reports or notes typed directly into the system (history, physical examination, provider observations, and case evolution notes) with transcription done in-house or outsourced.

125. Clinical coding for statistics and billing. Provides for the assignment of International Classification of Diseases and/or any other coding scheme/s to classify episodes of inpatient and outpatient care.

126. Clinical data abstracting. Provides the ability to extract certain patient data from records over and above the basic demographic data (e.g., weeks of gestation, usual living arrangements, allergies, images, photographs, etc.)

127. Release of information and correspondence. Provides for the management of requests for the release of patient information to various parties (e.g., other physicians, the patient, third-party payers, attorneys, etc.), including the correspondence involved with such requests.

128. Utilization management. Provides the ability to include a review of medical appropriateness and an analysis of the facility's efficiency in providing necessary services in the most cost-effective manner possible.

129. Maintain indices. Provide the ability to maintain a medical record index, a guide (manual, hard copy, or computerized) that points out or facilitates reference to patient information. Some examples of indices: service, diagnosis, diagnosis-related groups (DRGs), provider, procedure, length of stay, etc.

130. Archive management. Provide the ability to track patient records converted from hardcopy to another medium (e.g., microfilm, microfiche, optical disk, etc.)

131. Risk management. Provides reporting designed to protect an organization against potential liability through appropriate insurance coverage, reducing liability when compensable events occur, and prevention of events that are likely to lead to liabilities. Supports the review of accidents, injuries, and patient safety organization-wide.

132. Legal case file management. Supports the maintenance of patient records involved in legal actions and the correspondence associated with it.

133. **Patient/family assessment reporting.** System should support a clinical, cognitive, environmental, psychosocial, subjective and objective nursing assessment observation reporting of patient, parent(s), legal guardian(s), and/or significant other.

134. **Clinical data recording.** Allows the recording of signs, symptoms, findings, treatment, and procedures, etc. The system should support a variety of documentation methodologies, for events such as assessments, signs and symptoms, treatments, procedures, etc. The user should be able to select from popular methodologies such as precoded options, charting by exception, narrative notes, free text, etc.

135. **Review of historical patient information.** Inpatient and outpatient history should be supported for documentation and on-line retrieval.

136. **Referral management.** Tracking of the follow-up care both internal and external to the institution should be supported.

137. **Track outcomes.** The system should be able to capture and manage data in a way that enables the caregivers to determine whether the patient is progressing toward a favorable outcome, or if not, what are the variances.

138. **Generate patient care plan.** System should allow the caregiver to develop a problem list and corrective interventions and timelines, ascertain expected outcomes and measure results based on assessments. Individualized plans of care should have ability to evaluate patient outcomes.

139. **Provide patient education/instructional material.** System should provide facilities for the production and generation of customized diagnosis-driven patient education materials based on the care plan.

140. **Diagnostic order management.** The system should allow order entry for nursing interventions, medication, ancillary services, social work, transportation, physiotherapy, and other therapies.

141. **Medication management.** The system should provide drug interaction/adverse reaction and possible resolution information; dosage calculation based on weight; dispensing tracking by time intervals; and warnings for clinically contraindicated medication or inappropriate dosage.

142. **Patient classification system.** The system should support a validated patient classification system based on clinical variables. It should be able to calculate the acuity level of the patient and determine required nursing resources needed as a result. It should provide expected productivity targets and suggest staffing patterns.

143. **Provide Web-based linkage to clinical references.** The system should have the ability to link electronically (Web) to external medical reference sources, such as Medline.

D

144. Record point-of-care nursing activities. System should be able to chart point-of-care activities/bedside diagnostics at the time when care is being delivered. Typical examples include vital signs, blood pressure, order entry, results retrieval, etc. Provide for flexible options regarding point-of-care devices.

145. Flowsheet completion. The system should support posting of the patient's medical data in typical flowsheet formats, including graphically, over long periods of time, and across multiple episodes of care. It should support acquisition of information from medical devices and posting it in a flowsheet.

146. Critical pathway development tracking. The system should provide a comprehensive, multidisciplinary approach for developing activities and tasks for patient care over a specified timeline. It should be usable in both inpatient and outpatient settings.

147. Critical pathways with variance monitoring. The system should support documentation of the actual tasks completed and tracking reasons for straying from the established critical pathway.

148. Focused, problem-oriented charting. Quantitative data should be able to be displayed as trends in flowsheet format with focused and problem-oriented documentation in the progress notes.

149. Insurance. The system should have the ability to view or ascertain insurance and coverage information to assist clinical decision-making.

150. Nursing practice and utilization. Provide the ability to determine if the assigned staffing level/skill mix meet the need(s) specified by the critical pathway/acuity level.

151. Laboratory order entry. Provides the ability to enter orders for laboratory services from nursing stations, doctors' offices, or other points of care.

152. Unique order number. Assigns a unique order number to each lab order for identifying both specimen and order throughout processing cycle. Duplicate order checking provides control at the test component level with the option of manual override.

153. Add/cancel/credit orders. Provide the ability to add, cancel, and credit orders to existing order(s), including rescheduling of tests.

154. Charge capture. Provides the ability to capture charges at time of order, accession or test completion, depending on user requirements.

155. Group orders/work list. Provide the ability to group orders for collection purposes and accessions/orders in the batch. Automatically create order batches at designated times and sort orders by various categories to produce collection work lists of tests ordered for each analytical area/section/bay.

156. Label printing. Produces labels at accession time (alphanumeric, barcode) and ability to print labels automatically and on demand. Produce batch collection labels by collector or location; other options may include patient account number.

157. Specimen rejection. Provides for specimen rejection, including statement for reason and generation of lists for repeat collection.

158. Order priorities. Provide for lab order priorities: stat, routine, timed, etc.

159. Batch processing. Provides for batch processing of manually generated results or via analog-digital conversion of results generated by auto-analyzers.

160. Results entry. Provides for both manual and automated methods of results entry.

161. Incomplete work. Provides a listing of pending or incomplete work including reason/s.

162. Standardized results. Provide table-driven user defined "standardized results". Provide for high/low ranges comparison and display.

163. Textual results. Provide ability to include textual results entry and storage.

164. Supervisor review. Provides a method for supervisor review and approval of each test result and for eventual corrections. Based on supervisor approval, release test result for general reviewing, displaying, and reporting.

165. Produce sets of labels for each order, including master specimen container, isolation, and instructions.

166. Remote site label printing. Ability to redirect the printing of labels to various locations.

167. Printouts. Provide for order entry-driven, test-specific printout to hard copy or screen of detailed patient pretesting or laboratory instructions.

168. Results reporting. Provides ability for reporting test results and for immediate printing of emergency (stat) reports. Provides also ability for reporting on demand (patient-specific inquiry) or an interim basis. Users should be able to selectively choose the data they want to view, using a variety of selection options.

169. Summary reports. Provide summary reports (outpatients.) Provide the ability to produce and sort test results by attending physician within location.

170. Cumulative trends. Provide abiity for cumulative trend reporting.

171. Deviations. Provide necessary reporting for results deviating from normal ranges and corrected results.

D

172. Cross links. Provide a method to cross-link equivalent components of test results across different test codes and instruments.

173. Quality control (internal.) Capture quality control data and monitor conditions established by the laboratory.

174. Automatic notification. Provides automatic notification of product/reagent expiration dates.

175. Reporting statistics. Provide reporting statistics and workload to assist in staff and equipment budgeting and productivity. Provide appropriate administrative/management reports by capturing data from the lab system.

176. Results storage. Provides ability for storage of patient lab results based on user-defined data retention parameters.

177. Inventory. Provides for the management of inventory items.

178. Transcription interface. Provides a transcription system to be part of or interfaced with the Pathology Laboratory Information System. Provides ability to attend the unique needs of histology, cytology, autopsy, and other pathology areas.

179. Contracts. Provide the laboratory manager with reference to laboratory contract information to assist in analyzing performance and monitor adherence to contractual agreements.

180. Vendor tracking. Provides information to track vendor maintenance, training, supplies, equipment support, and maintenance.

181. Alpha access. Ability to create alphabetized file used during inventory alpha access functions.

182. Exam data entry. The exam data entry module should cover all of the functions used to enter processing information and results for an examination. Exam data entry should capture the following data: exam events; user-defined result entry fields; specialized exams (mammography, intravenous urography, ultrasound, tomography, etc.) tracking and reporting; report archive functionality; on-call exams tracking; and pregnancy and shielded/unshielded.

183. Film room management. Film room management required to log and track the movement of films inside the institution. Film management should perform the following: film tracking for physician or department sign-out; film room tracking functions; film archive management.

184. Administration. Provides all the managerial and personnel functions and management reporting, including the following: productivity functions and reporting; work projections; quality control reports; and utilization statistics for equipment and facilities.

185. Activity tracking. This module is required to track information about patient utilization of the medical imaging facilities.

186. Imaging equipment maintenance. The system needs to provide a module that will allow collection and capture of data elements in order to generate equipment maintenance monitoring reports and alerts. Options for maintaining all aspects of the imaging equipment. The system must support user-defined help text. Remote accessibility to the system is a critical priority. The system should support ad hoc reporting capability for all modules. Include flexible parameters for screens and menus based on institutional, facility, or user-defined criteria.

187. Exam and result turnaround time tracking. The system needs to capture exam data that can be queried for exam and exam result turnaround times.

188. Transcription management and productivity transcription. The system needs to provide incomplete work reports and views. Capture keystroke average and turnaround time average for report completion.

189. Quality control data collection/reports. Provide the ability to track repeat exams and film utilization with related reasons to facilitate problem pattern identification.

190. Equipment maintenance. The system needs to provide a module that will allow collection and capture of data elements in order to generate equipment maintenance monitoring reports and alerts. Options for maintaining all aspects of the radiation therapy equipment. The system must support user-defined help text. Remote accessibility to the system is a critical priority. The system should support ad hoc reporting capability for all modules. Include flexible parameters for screens and menus based on institutional, facility, or user-defined criteria.

191. Contrast reaction record and report. Provide ability to record and report on contrast reactions. The system should provide ease of capture of this information.

192. Technologist productivity functions and reporting. The system needs to capture data on technologists' exam performance and provide reporting tools.

193. Report review. Report review functionality is the ability to review transcribed reports. This function should allow the responsible professional to electronically sign the reports and release them. Report review should also allow for auto-fax. Auto-fax is the ability to send final reports via fax to clinic destinations after they have been released by the radiologist. The report review module should support auto-dictation upload and download. Remote access to report review is also a functional requirement.

194. Outside film management. Logs and tracks movement of films loaned or borrowed from other institutions.

195. Activity tracking. This module is required to track scheduling and utilization information related to each patient visit to the department.

196. Historical patient management. This is needed to purge information from the radiology system. The system should also contain tools to manage film archiving or destruction. On-line imaging interface or compatibility is also required.

197. Patient inquiry. This is used to review all current, previous, and historical data by authorized staff.

198. Physician activity report. This is required where electronic signature or any information related to the physicians involved in the exam, from ordering to the result completion, can be tracked and managed. This module should have reporting capability.

199. Procedure turnaround time tracking. The system needs to capture procedure data that can be queried for procedure turnaround timing.

200. System integration. Providers must have access to laboratory and pharmacy results. The system requirements are that the system should integrate with other diagnostic and therapeutic systems. There are certain exams where it is required to record and report data from other ancillary services on a final report.

201. Multiple exam "turnaround" time tracking. Captures multiple exam/test/procedure data that can be queried for exam or procedure timing information.

202. Result turnaround time tracking. The system needs to capture exam data that can be queried for exam result complete turnaround information.

203. Radiologist tracking and productivity. Track and provide reports on the reporting, assisting, and consulting Radiologists.

204. Report archive management (microfiche). The system should provide archive management to help users track archived reports in the system.

205. Procedure data recording. The system needs to provide flexible, user-defined, facility-driven data entry screens. They should be able to be pulled into the final report if needed.

206. On-call exam/procedure data recording. Exam/procedure data entry or patient check-in feature should provide technically required fields for recording exams/procedures performed by all on-call personnel.

207. Capture of positive biopsy results. The system needs to provide the tools to capture the new data that are required for clinical management of patients with positive biopsy results.

208. Mammography tracking/reporting. Positive exams must link to report biopsy findings and must generate doctor notification and follow-up letters.

209. Film archive management. Radiology departments archive their film from active film rooms to inactive film rooms. The system needs to track films through the cycle.

210. Tuberculosis screening data capture/report. Provide ability to track positive chest X-Rays. Record the room, equipment, and personnel exposed to the infected patient.

211. Ad hoc reporting. The system should provide an ad hoc or system query function. It should be able to access all specialized data elements for query purposes.

212. Specialized report requirements. The system should provide for standard, ad hoc, and on-demand reporting capabilities in both on-line and batch modes that consider the special needs related to clinical imaging and radiotherapy.

213. Digital filmless imaging. Image can be electronically transmitted.

214. Technical audit trail. Provides a method to maintain a technical audit trail of blood bank sample and component processing.

215. Medication/solution order entry/review. Allow entering, modifying, and reviewing of medication and parenteral solution orders. The system should allow: pharmacists to confirm order entry and pharmacy technician conditional order entry (which requires pharmacist's approval before the orders are fully processed for dispensing and charging to patient's account.)

216. On-screen patient profile review. Ability to review a patient's medication utilization profile and drug sensibility information on the screen. Should provide checking for drug duplication and alert for drug interactions.

217. Charge/credit medication/solution orders. Facility that allows transfer of all charges to patient account.

218. PRN (Pro Re Nata = if needed) order update. Display ordered medications to be used if the clinical situation demands, or PRN schedule, for dispensing and charge to patient by nurse.

219. Drug/food allergy interactions. Ability to query on-line database of drug-drug and drug-food interactions, and therapeutic overlap. Provide the user with procedures for regular updating.

220. Medication label printing. Ability to print labels for dispensed medication.

221. Auxiliary label function. Allows the printing of auxiliary label codes for designated medications

222. Physician dispensing. Allows for record keeping and labels needed for prescription dispensing directly by physicians from local stores at ambulatory facilities.

223. Help prompts and messages. Allow the requesting of on-screen help messages.

D

224. Medication/solution distribution. Allows the production of fill lists for unit dose systems labels, solution preparation, processing of charges for scheduled medication and solution orders, and the printing of administration records for nurses.

225. Medication preparation (unit dose.) Ability to produce fill lists and update fill lists for cart filling with unit dose systems. Ability to interface with automatic dispensing machines.

226. Solution preparation labels. Ability to produce labels and update labels for solution orders. Produce labels for each hour dose is due for specified time entered.

227. Medication/solution dose timing control. Ability to advance the internal charging clocks accumulating charges and administer doses for scheduled, unit dose orders; discontinued orders having reached their stop times and date.

228. Medication/solution administration reports. Ability to produce medication and solution administration reports indicating all current orders on each patient, with times doses are due on scheduled orders. Ability to produce medication reports for 24-hours, seven-day and 31-day intervals.

229. Mail order distribution. Allows for the processing of outpatient prescriptions for mail order distribution.

230. Add new items. Ability to enter new items into pharmacy stock inventory file.

231. Modify/delete items. Ability to modify or delete an existing item from the master pharmacy stock inventory file.

232. Reports. Ability to produce various defined reports on records in the inventory file.

233. Stock movement. Ability to receive, issue, and write-off stock from inventory, perform interdepartmental transfers, return to stock, issue control substances, and set up ward stock items.

234. Update orders from inventory. Ability to update orders and predefined formulas with attribute and/or cost changes made to base inventory item.

235. Purchase orders. Ability to set up a purchasing inventory; create, modify, and print purchase orders, receive stock from purchase orders; and maintain purchase order statistics.

236. Global order cost update. Ability to update active orders, medication order groups, solution formulas, and inventory items with most recent prices.

237. Controlled/narcotic drugs. Allow the tracking of controlled/narcotic medications products stocked and dispensed.

238. Medication utilization profile report. Provides listing of patient medication and/or solution orders with pertinent order data indicated, including professional prescribing, organizational unit, and related clinical data.

239. Medication/solution renewal lists. Provide listing of patient's medications and/or solution orders which are scheduled to be stoppedor renewed in a specified time.

240. Update profiles. Provide listing of a patient's medication/solution profile indicating whether orders were updated in given periods.

241. PRN (if situation required) medication report. Provide listing of medication given on a PRN schedule and details of order including timing, dosage, prescribing, and dispensing professional.

242. Pharmacy database report generator. Allows for the creation of operator-designed reports displayed on screen, sent to printer or file from existing data files, or operator-created data files.

243. Special medication summary. Provides printing of designated data for minimum data setup dating (such as number of medications, patient on list for seven days or more, number of injections, any new medications in the last 90 days including antibiotics, tranquilizers, psychotropic, diuretics, hormones, and other).

244. Drug utilization information sheets. Ability to generate inpatient medication utilization information sheets, in multiple languages as required by the client population.

245. Psychotropic consent renewal list. Ability to print listing of existing psychotropic patient consent orders, if applicable.

246. Prescription reporting groups. Ability to generate reports for controlled/narcotic drugs, prescription refill summary, and new prescriptions for a specified period.

247. Compliance reporting. Produce reports to monitor specific medications against patient health problems, perform computer check between number of days supply and date of last refill.

248. Statistics. Ability to produce statistical reports and modify or purge statistical records.

249. Drug utilization/usage review. Ability to set up specific parameters for the review of orders, review of historical data. Outpatient prescriptions to be tracked by patients on specific drugs, patients on a given drug for a given diagnosis, patients on a given drug for a given diagnosis for a given provider, and most frequently dispensed drugs by provider.

250. Physician information maintenance. Allow for the logging of basic physician information (name, phone, etc.).

251. Prescription directions management. Ability to predefine the standard directions used in prescriptions and modify these directions, provide multiple language capability.

D

252. Pharmacokinetics. The calculation of medication dose based on specific patient parameters, such as age and weight.

253. Intervention log. Allows the logging and reporting of pharmacist clinical interventions.

254. Intervention cost analysis. Ability to calculate cost savings of clinical interventions.

255. Laboratory results access. Provide access to patient laboratory data files.

256. Support and store data for all facilities on-line for up to two years for inpatients and outpatients; archive records for historical retrieval on-line for all drugs up to five years; controlled substances for seven years; and thereafter purge records on retrievable media. Periods indicated may vary according to local legislation.

257. Capability to broadcast reports and schedules on-site to nursing stations and other healthcare provision sites.

258. Capability to generate custom/ad hoc trends and graphs to track patient prescription history.

259. Support for standard, ad hoc, and on-demand reporting capabilities in both on-line and batch modes.

260. Capability to create user-defined reports. Ability to save and schedule them as standard reports.

261. Automated interfaces. Provide an automated interface between the clinical laboratory system and the healthcare institution's blood bank system.

262. Lab system/blood bank transfer. Provides for passing blood orders and patient admission/transfer/discharge (ADT) information from the clinical laboratory system to the blood bank system.

263. Technologist observation. Provide a method for the technologist to record observations and results and pass the information to the system.

264. Blood type screening. Provide for ABO, Rh, and antibody screening on general result reports.

265. Preferred terminology. Accommodates blood bank "preferred" terminology for recording observations.

266. Information product validity. Maintains and provides reports on expiration date for stored blood and blood components.

267. Essential nutrient analysis. Conducts nutrient/cost analysis and calorie count tracking.

268. Nutrition assessment forms. Provide patient tracking reports and basic individual patient nutrient analysis, NPO (Nihil Per Os = fasting) and clear liquid reports, tube feeding reports, printing of tube feeding labels, and matrix analysis reports for special groups (e.g., restrition on specific food or nutrient, diabetic, renal patients).

269. Print tally sheets and print tray line tickets and nourishment labels. To accompany meal distribution for double-checking at distribution points.

270. Patient profile. Provides on-line patient profile which includes preferences, personal dietary restrictions, diet types, supplements, nourishmens, medications, and food allergies.

271. Production scheduling and management. Support to cook/chill, cook/freeze, and conventional cooking methods. Management of recipes, purchasing reports, forecast production needs, provide ingredient pick lists, manage freezer and overall inventory, schedule kitchen equipment, and provide production logistics worksheets.

272. Production/utilization forecasting. Generates forecasts based on patient census and historical usage.

273. Event management. Capability to manage one-of-a kind situations such as catering for event.

274. Enrollment program. Registration systems should support enrollment and cancellation of enrollment in the immunization scheme.

275. Create patient or system selected menus. Allows clinical personnel to create individual menus or pick from systems-based list and permit automatic updates of scheduled prescribed immunization changes.

276. Patient profile. Provides on-line patient profile which includes previous vaccinations, immunization schemes, contra-indications, and allergies.

277. Immunization scheduling and management.

278. Vaccine utilization doses and equipment requirement forecasting.

279. Transcription interface. Provides a transcription system to be part of or interfaced with the clinical laboratory information system. Provides for the unique needs of laboratory, histology, cytology, autopsy, and pathology.

280. Fixed assets database. Permits recording of descriptive data,commercial brand name, manufacturer, supplier, purchase date, acquisition cost, warranties, exclusions, maintenance data. Should be able to use international coding schemes. Provides the ability to update the location and condition of the item. Provides a complete audit trail of transactions affecting each fixed asset item, including disposal (removal from active inventory.) Ability to assign equipment to

specific locations. Linkage to Medical Equipment Maintenance or Physical Facility Maintenance Module when they exist.

281. Depreciation categories. Provide the ability to assign a depreciation category to the item within the fixed asset schedule. Permit entering data regarding final disposition.

282. Asset depreciation. Permits automatic depreciation for all capital purchases and forecast future depreciation.

283. Depreciation status. Allows the user access to pertinent statistical data regarding these capital items, as well as appropriate reports to identify the status of purchases within the fixed asset schedule.

284. Predated items. Allow for entry of items that predate the introduction of the asset management system to be entered into the system.

285. Equipment inventory. The equipment inventory should identify the commercial name (brand), manufacturer, size, model number, serial number, acquisition date, price, expected life cycle, warranties, maintenance contracts (including dates), physical location of the equipment in the institution, and any other information needed for maintaining or repairing equipment.

286. General facility/equipment inventory. The equipment inventory should identify the commercial name (brand), manufacturer, size, model number, serial number, acquisition date, price, expected life cycle, warranties, maintenance contracts (including dates), physical location of the equipment in the institution,and any other information needed for maintaining or repairing equipment.

287. Order/service database. Provides entry of service requests, scheduled maintenance actions, and scheduling of staff for all preventative maintenance actions and work orders.

288. Order execution. Compiles and archives maintenance history, including date work performed, person performing, time to perform procedure, equipment/facility serviced, and any condition evaluation required by the maintenance action along with parts and consumables used in performance of the maintenance or repair action. Provide reports on service realized, labor costs, operating costs (costs of energy, procurement costs, life expectancy, salvage value, and training costs).

289. Fixed asset linkage. This should be linked to the Fixed Assets Management Module if it exists. When feasible should be integrated with asset management to provide budget information; life cycle cost analysis, replacement and repair evaluation, energy alternatives, and system effectiveness.

290. Parts inventory link. There should be data links to repair parts inventory to determine safe stocking levels as well as providing accurate part number, description, and supplier.

291. Manufacturer/supplier information. Data about name, address, telephone, fax, e-mail, and technical support contact of manufacturer, importer, supplier, technical support services. This should be linked to the equipment inventory database.

292. Linen warehouse locations. Provide the ability to accommodate both linen warehouse locations and circulating linen locations.

293. Linen accounting. Provides the ability to account for linen issues/returns by cost center and expense code. The linen analysis system should provide accurate linen usage by linen type and linen items or by ward unit. Ability to track and monitor uniform usage as well as providing accurate billing and credits directly to ward and end users.

294. Pick lists. Provide the ability to handle issues or returns of linen based on pick list, or on-line, on demand.

295. Linen weights. Provide the ability to record and monitor linen weights to verify laundering expense.

296. Laundry orders/receipts. Provide the ability to record laundry orders and receipts by weight.

297. Ability to manage the transport services information including number of kilometers driven, consumption of gas and oil, and other inputs.

298. Ability to generate transportation notification through order management.

299. Ability to generate an efficiency report on why patient was not brought to the institution.

300. General budgeting functions. Control entry of budget and statistical account data, including: supporting multiple files for current or future periods and department level access for budget development and analysis. It should provide for payroll budget information by department, job code, and earning type (for hours and dollars.) It must generate budget variance reports and comparison reports providing payroll information on hours and dollar amounts.

301. Budget transactions. Allow users to initialize budget data for accounts from current or previous budgets, actual data, and annualizations of current year's actual data. Allow users to update budget data for accounts by entering amounts for each period, or yearly amount, or by applying a percentage increase or decrease.

302. Payroll and fixed assets linkage. Automatic entry of budget files created in payroll and in fixed asset accounting modules.

303. Radiotherapist tracking and productivity. Track and provide reports on the reporting, assisting, and consulting Radiotherapist.

304. Validate technician medication/solution orders. Ability to review pharmacy technician orders and interactive approval facility. Log of transactions.

305. Real-time, interactive module. Should also be able to meet managed care requirements, contract management, interim billing, and late charge billing. Up-to-the-minute information, complete account details, and current account detailed history.

306. Integration with other financial functions. This module must be integrated with General Ledger, Accounts Payable, and Cost Accounting Systems. Must automatically transfer patient data to/from the admissions system and maintain guarantor, insurance, disease, and procedure categorization for payment purposes (e.g., DRGs), and archive account data.

307. Account search and retrieval. There should be quick account identification by patient name, number, unit number, or guarantor number.

308. View patient account information on-line/comments. Provides comprehensive view of account information available on-line. Includes visit and demographic, insurance verification, level of benefits, patient admission/discharge/transfer (ADT) information, current charges and payments, previous charges and payments. Also include summary of charges by department, billing and accounts receivable status information and diagnosis. The system should allow posting and review of account comments.

309. Determine source of payments by payer. System should be able to review payment transactions on-line and determine source of payment. Should be able to write summary and detail reports that will identify payment sources. System should allow for daily cash payments by payer.

310. Contract benefits. The system must provide the organization the ability to control group or managed care agreements and assist in the monitoring of contracts with third-party payers.

311. Benefit plans predetermined billing. Standard or common insurance benefit plans should be defined in a master file and loaded into accounts at time of verification. Plans may be modified at any time for individual accounts.

312. User-defined insurance verification screens. System should support healthcare institution defined verification screens, so that major payer groups can have customized screens to capture critical elements for each group. Screens should allow the healthcare institution to define required fields for payer and benefit information.

313. Central charge master. System should support a charge master file for each facility within the enterprise.

314. Charges and credit entry. System should have ability to manually post charges and credits for both room and ancillary charges. Claims data entry system should have ability to post claims data not otherwise captured in registration or abstracting functions. Examples include value codes, occurrence codes, and dates.

315. Auto room charge posting, auto charge. System should allow for posting room charges based on nightly census. Should support multiple accommodation types and rates. System should post corrected charges and credits when changes or cancellations are made to admit or discharge dates.

316. Ability for "series bill" or "specific visit bill". For ambulatory processing the system should be able to support both "visit" and "series" billing. Series billing would include the ability to bill for stated time periods or for a particular type of treatment for the duration of a treatment plan.

317. Ability to post charges at the level of pre-admission. Allow posting to accounts prior to actual admission for pre-admission events.

318. Prorate benefits by multiple payers. System should have ability to identify and support insurance proration for basic and major medical insurance charging any number of possible payers. Should be able to support excluded charges, specific charge rates for contract payers, and contractuals amounts.

319. Log system/view on-line. System should allow on-line maintenance and inquiry to logs account data, and on-line request of standard reports.

320. Automated account follow-up. Automated systems should support follow-up by payer, patient name, account balance ranges, account age, and status (if there are pending payments in Accounts Receivable or bad debt history). System should include past account history and previous follow-up activity.

321. Sliding fee scales for private pay billing. System should support patient billing discounts based on family income and size.

322. Values and codes edited against tables. Common data elements should be table or profile driven with on-line editing during data entry.

323. Electronic claims submission. Provide ability to bill third-party payers.

324. Produce hard-copy bills. Produce bills for payers not accepting electronic claims.

325. Electronic remittance processing. System should retrieve remittance advice form from third-party payers, and support posting of payments, contracts, and adjustments to Accounts Receivable.

326. Batch charges posting (automated.) System should support batch posting routines for ancillary charges generated in order entry systems.

327. Payments adjustments. System should support manual payments, adjustments, and contractuals for insurance and self-pay. Should be able to transfer pro-rated balances in posting function.

D

328. Reclassify revenue by payer. System should support manual reclassification of revenue by insurance payer, financial class, patient type when accounts are rebilled or insurance information is transferred or prorated to another payer after initial billing.

329. Bill hold capability (parameter-driven.) System should be able to delay billing until all required fields are complete. Health care institution can define different bill hold requirements by patient type (inpatient, outpatient, emergency services) and insurance type.

330. Ability to produce demand bills (all forms.) System should be able to demand printing of a bill with current charges for non-discharged accounts or accounts on hold.

331. Ability to force bill patients. System should be able to allow users to manually force an account into billed status even though it may not have met all bill hold criteria.

332. Ability to cycle bills. System should allow for generation of cycle bills for inpatients based on payer, length of stay, and/or balance.

333. Rebill accounts. System should allow for re-bill of accounts following changes in payers, charges, length of stay, and benefits.

334. Accounts receivable bad debt write-off capability. System should have ability to manually transfer accounts from active receivable to a bad debt status. Bad debt accounts should remain on-line for review, reporting, posting payments, etc. Transfer should generate all of the accounting and revenue transactions associated with write-off and recovery of bad debt.

335. Bad debt to accounts receivable reinstatement. System should allow manual transfer from bad debt to receivable if account was written in error. This transaction should generate the appropriate accounting and revenue transactions.

336. Auto accounts receivable processing (parameter-driven.) System should be able to rebill, write-off small balances and bad debts, purge zero balances, and change accounts from insurance to self-pay without manual intervention if accounts meet auto-processing criteria. Those criteria would include account age, balance, financial class, number of payments received, patient type, etc. The system should allow healthcare institution to write and maintain rules to automate this process.

337. Purging capability (parameter-driven). System should have ability to purge accounts from active patient master and accounts receivable or bad debt files. Purge criteria should be healthcare institution-defined, based on number of days since account reached zero balance.

338. Financial logs. System should include financial logs to allow summary review of charges, payment, diagnosis, diagnostic or procedure categorization for payment (DRGs), revenue and utilization data for cost reporting, and contract analysis. Logs data should be able to be automatically collected and posted to the logs data base from other systems modules. Should include both standard reports and report writer capability.

339. Ability to transfer balances to different payers. System should allow the transfer of prorated balances between payers for billing or accounts receivable purposes.

340. Support revenue and usage statistics. Maintain statistics for revenues and services by patient type, medical service, financial class or payer, healthcare institution, department, clinic, and location.

341. Process collection agency tapes. System should be able to create an extract of account information for submittal to collection agencies. The tape should be created automatically based on write-off activity to collection agencies.

342. Pass billed data to automated collection system. System should provide an on-line collection system with health care institution tickler files for account follow-up. Information from billing and payment activity should pass to the collection system to provide collectors with current account data.

343. Produce parameter-driven data mailers. System should support production of data mailers and collection letters with healthcare institution-defined cycles.

344. Automated collection assignments and statistics. Automated system should support distribution of accounts to collectors and maintain work statistics for each collector indicating the number of accounts assigned, worked, backlogged, etc.

345. Integrated registration/billing/collection letter. Automated collections system should be integrated to registration and billing systems so that data entered in one will be noted in the others. Comments or field updates performed in one system will update in each database.

346. Electronic denial reasons posted to billed account. System should allow for denial reasons to be posted to accounts with electronic remittance processing. Denial information should be available for on-line review.

347. Physician/healthcare institution charges on same bill. System should have ability to include physician and healthcare institution charges on the same bill where permitted/required by payer.

348. Archiving/restoring. System should have ability to purge billing and account data and restore it at some later time.

349. Common accounts payable features/functions. Provides the ability to handle the common features and functions of Accounts Payable, including expense allocation, one-time vendors, payment plan management, price adjustments and variances, discounts, and suspended invoice processing.

350. Provider management. Provides the flexibility of handling a variety of vendor documents, including single payment invoices, recurring invoices, and credit memos. Ability to alter vendor arrangements to accommodate changes as to discount specifications, address changes, and payment from different bank accounts.

D

351. Purchase order interface. Provides the ability to access details of acquisition and payment information by purchase order number.

352. Materials management interface. Provides the ability to interface automatically to the materials management applications (pharmacy, inventory control, etc.), when necessary.

353. Automatic or manual payment. Permits the vouching process to handle either automatic or manual payment period/cycle and bank account.

354. Invoices. Provide the ability to produce invoices.

355. Vouchers/checks. Provide the ability to produce vouchers or requests for checks.

356. Payment cycles. Provide for payment cycles to be defined by the user.

357. One-time processing. Provides for the ability to process ad hoc payments for vendors not included in the vendor master file, on a one-time basis.

358. Check clearing. Provides for the ability to clear checks within the system.

359. Liability posting. Provides for the ability to automatically post liabilities.

360. Credit invoices. Provide for the ability to handle credit invoices.

361. Audit trail. Maintains a comprehensive audit trail and general ledger interface in accordance to legal requirements.

362. Tax reporting. Provide for automatic production of tax reports, as required by specific country and local governments.

363. Accounting functions. Compatible with the legal requirements of each case, including the following general functions: automatic transfer of transactions from all financial modules, transfer of transactions between different organizations in multi-organization environment.

364. User-defined accounting lines. User-defined systems of allocating expenses and revenues.

365. Transaction facilities. No limit to length of time detail and summary data are retained; must allow prior and future period transactions, master log report that displays all batch transactions, and immediate update of account balances upon posting.

366. On-line look-up. On-line account inquiries to allow authorized users to view up-to-the-minute account balances or activity on demand. These inquiries must provide an audit trail indicating the transaction sources. Entry lists available in order of entry or in account number sequence.

367. Cost determination. Determine the cost of a cost/service unit, which corresponds to procedure codes in billing utilizing allocation methodology of user choice. Must map procedure codes to individual and multiple service units and store past, present, and future average rates for resources such as labor and materials and prorated general costs.

368. Cost distribution. Generates detailed reports on comparisons of actual and standard costs, fixed and variable costs, budgets, variance analysis, service profitability, and departmental responsibility.

369. Cost reporting. Application should provide users with multiple profitability reports based on various selection criteria as well as standard cost and service usage by cost unit. These reports should allow for budget comparison and variance analysis by managers throughout the organization.

370. Chart of accounts. User-controlled chart of accounts with unlimited number of defined accounts should be available. Permit organizational hierarchy that allows reports to be defined for any level of management.

371. Standard payroll features. Provide the ability to perform typical payroll calculations, such as gross-to-net salary on a table-driven basis. Payroll information, including base rate, effective date, step, current benefit plans, withholdings, and automatic start/stop dates.

372. Rollback function. Provides retroactive calculations and computes earnings, taxes, and deductions and must be capable of mass edit routines to employee withholdings and benefits and provide a payroll summary by department, payroll register, tax, and deduction registers. Facility for posting to general ledger.

373. Special payroll features/functions. Provide the ability to handle the common features and functions of payroll, including on-line, real-time data entry and editing, batch balancing, overtime calculations, salaries of employees working in multiple positions at multiple pay rates, and payroll history. The system should provide for real-time inquiry of employee earnings and compensation as well as year-to-date inquiry routines and compute multiple payrolls with different schedules, list employee pay information, and post payroll data in general ledger.

374. Special compensation. Provide the ability to handle compensation, including wage and salary analysis and job evaluation and the ability to handle situations that depart from regular compensation, including common items such as stock options, and deferred payment and bonuses.

375. Salaries funded by multiple sources. Provide the ability to track salaries funded by multiple sources.

376. Direct deposit. Provide the ability to forward employee salary checks directly to their banks, in addition to providing traditional paper checks.

377. Retroactive pay. Provides the ability to calculate pay on a retroactive basis.

378. Deduction arrears and recovery. Provide the ability to calculate and report deduction arrears and

379. Automated check reversal. Provides for reversing checks automatically, based on user-defined criteria.

380. Date sensitivity. Provides the ability to automatically produce payroll checks based on specific dates, or conditions, such as "the last working date before the last day of the month", or "every Friday".

381. Audit and transaction reports. Provide comprehensive audit and transaction reports that are available for review before producing checks.

382. Labor distribution. Distribute payroll amounts among the appropriate labor departments as established by the user.

383. Government reporting. Provides reporting for applicable federal, state, and local governments, as well as deductions for applicable taxes.

384. Budget management. Provides the ability to monitor expense versus budget data, and make on-line changes where appropriate.

385. Integration with human resources and benefits systems. Provides interface to institution's human resources and benefits systems, where applicable.

386. Position and staffing. Provide the ability to control details of staffing, including positions, employee skills, and resource allocation. The on-line database should provide instant access to employee detailed personal record and history. Minimum data in the employee file should include: applicant tracking through recruiting, interviewing, and selection process, demographics, qualifications, training history, dependents, payroll status, hire date, next evaluation date, attendance template, position number, department, and job code.

387. Training and development. Provide the ability to track and manage training of employees, including course crediting, where applicable.

388. Performance tracking. Provides the ability to record, track, and manage employee performance, on a regular basis. Include the ability to have multiple inputs to evaluation, by the employee, by the employee's peers, and by management.

389. Career planning. Provides the ability to record and track career plans by employee, allowing input from both the employee and management. Includes ability to modify and update career plans dynamically.

390. Labor relations. Provide the ability to track and manage common elements of labor relations, including the status of collective bargaining agreements and union contract details.

391. Job applicant tracking. Provides the ability to enter and track the status of applicants through the recruiting, interviewing, and selection process.

392. On-line scheduling. Department managers should be able to create templates to allow diverse groups with varying needs to set their own scheduling criteria. It will also process special requests on-line, e.g., days off, vacation, planned sick days, or jury duty. Specialized skills of individual staff should be viewable on-line and provide ad hoc scheduling reports of staff whose certification will expire shortly.

393. Schedule-makers should be able to experiment with draft schedules before creating a final schedule. Productive/nonproductive time data will provide the ability to track productivity based on real hours of work.

394. Expected attendance. Forecast of attendance data will be stored on a template for the employee and may be edited as necessary for the pay period. There will be on-line entry of summary time card data and the ability to accommodate daily time card entry.

395. Staffing planning. Provide recommended staff schedules to work a shift which also identifies problems of over- or under-staffing. Patient load, degree of patient dependency, and case type also will be factored in scheduling of nursing staff. Information modeling provides the ability to model future human resource scenarios and make analyses.

396. Cost impact modeling. Budget capabilities will be inherent in this system to help managers evaluate the cost effectiveness of their proposed schedules with funds available in their budget. The budget dollars will be prorated by specific time frames to match past experience of high census and degree of patient dependency status and severity of illness.

397. Timecards. Generation of timecards for employees for the use of payroll/personnel system. These will support any combination of job codes and shifts.

398. General functions. Provide the ability to manage and track benefits, including medical and dental benefits, retirement, sick leave, and vacations.

399. Complex tax support. Provides the ability to handle complex taxes, including federal, state, and local taxes.

400. Periodic/nonperiodic payments. Provide the ability to handle both periodic and nonperiodic benefit payments.

401. Sources/deductions. Provide the ability to handle an unlimited number of sources and deductions per account.

402. Disbursements. Provide the ability to handle third-party disbursement processing.

D

403. Payment/deductions history. Provide the ability to have on-line benefits payment/deductions history.

404. Vendor information. Provide for on-line retrieval of detailed vendor information.

405. Vendor revalidation/invalidation. Provides the ability to invalidate or revalidate vendor for future purchases.

406. Vendor accounts payable. Links to Provide vendor accounts payable data and the ability to update it on-line.

407. Stock/nonstock requisition. Provides ability to handle on-line requisition of items, whether normal stock items or not.

408. Standard purchase order. Provides ability to support all standard purchase order processing types, e.g., standard, blanket, and consignment, as well as flexibility to support other, user-defined purchase order types. Provide ability to modify existing purchase orders. It will generate "standing" and blanket purchase orders at user-defined intervals.

409. Order status tracking. It will provide the status of any purchase order, accommodate multi-facility environments, and generate automatic purchase orders for items at or below their minimum reorder points and nonstock items ordered via department purchase requisitions.

410. Contract/open market items. Provide the ability to monitor on-line contract or acquisition of open market items.

411. Back-order processing. Allow for handling of back-ordered items.

412. Blanket/standing order receipts. Provide the ability to handle blanket or standing order receipts.

413. Shipment tolerances. Permit the user to define shipment acceptable tolerances.

414. Management and statistical reporting. Vendor performance, cost change, and buyer activity reports.

415. Item database. Provide the ability to capture and maintain all purchased items code and description. Ability to search the database for items easily, by any combination of search arguments.

416. Item classification. Allows for classification of database items by product type or by group, and for on-line maintenance of the database.

417. Nonstock Items. Allow for capture of nonstock items.

418. Receiving functions. Produce receiving documents to record receipts of items with purchase order, and also handle blind receiving and receiving by exception. It should automatically match invoiced amounts to received values. There will be automatic update of quantity on-hand (stock control function) upon posting receipts of inventoried items. On-line inquiry of any purchase order and receipt information as well as providing on-line invoice reconciliation of purchase orders and accounts payable invoices.

419. Stock control. Permits recording of descriptive data, commercial brand name, manufacturer, supplier, purchase date, acquisition cost, warranties, and exclusions. Provides real-time updating of on-hand quantities. There will be inventory control features to supply a record of inventory activity such as issues, returns, adjustments, transfers, and purchase order history and provide both report and inquiry capabilities to help users monitor current stock levels. Will be able to support unlimited number of inventories.

420. Just in time inventory. Provides ability to support JIT or stockless inventory management techniques.

421. Order book. Be able to set up an order book of user-defined item requisition forms.

422. Requisitioning. Provides simultaneous order and issue functionality.

423. Remote location. Provides the ability to requisition inventory items from a remote location of the health care institution.

424. Automatic requisitioning. Supports automatic requisitioning for the purchase of items that fall below user-defined thresholds.

425. Delivery tickets. Provide the ability to produce customized delivery ticket, along with stocking instructions.

426. Consignment items. Provide the ability to manage items taken from vendors on consignment.

427. Inventory report. Provides the ability to produce a complete report of all inventory items, department usage report, stock status reports by type of item, most frequently used, and physical inventory worksheet and comparison reports.

428. Multiple units of issue. Support multiple issue of item from any inventory location.

D

REFERENCE 1

Core Health Data Elements

Edited Version of the Report of the National Committee
on Vital and Health Statistics
U.S. Department of Health and Human Services
August 1996

Table of Contents

1. Executive Summary

Introduction

The identification, definition, and implementation of standardized data in the health care and health care information fields are long overdue. The increasing use of electronic data, the evolving managed care field, and the growing requirement for performance monitoring and outcomes research have made it imperative that all health data collection activities, where possible, utilize standardized data elements and definitions.

The National Committee on Vital and Health Statistics (NCVHS) has undertaken a first step in bringing together leaders in the field to seek consensus on a small set of data elements that are often considered the core of many data collection efforts. The Committee's goal has been to develop a set of data elements with agreed-upon standardized definitions that, when needed in a data collection effort, can be used to collect and produce standardized data. The intent is not to specify a data set for mandated external reporting; the list of recommended data elements is by no means exhaustive, and, unlike earlier activities, is not a "data set" to be used in a specific setting.

It is the expectation of the Committee that the health care field will find these recommended data elements to be fundamentally important for any collection of person and health care encounter data and will consider these elements and standardized definitions for inclusion in their data collection efforts wherever possible. Favorable input has been received from a wide range of experts, and these elements should be compellingly useful both to states and to provider organizations.

D

Background

In August 1994, the Department of Health and Human Services asked the Committee to provide information and advice that will help maximize the utility of core person and encounter data for meeting the Department's responsibilities. Specifically, the Department charged the Committee to:

- Review state-of-the-art of widely-used core data sets in the United States and other countries (including coding and formatting features that allow for flexibility);

- Obtain input, through hearings and other means, from the diverse parties who will report and use standardized data sets;

- Interact closely with recognized standards-setting groups; and

- Promote consensus by identifying areas of agreement on data elements and data sets among different stakeholders and areas that will require further research and development before consensus can be reached.

In developing a strategy for accomplishing these tasks, the Committee described a context in which the project would be undertaken that included the following issues:

- Why such data sets are needed in the current and evolving health care arena;

- What multiple functions they might accomplish for a variety of different users;

- What data elements (including definitions, vocabularies and coding structures) they might contain; and

- What potential problems, such as assuring data quality and preserving confidentiality of identifiable records, can be expected and what approaches might be used to address these problems.

The Core Health Data Elements

The following list of data elements contains those elements selected for the first iteration of this process. Consensus has been reached on definitions for some of these elements; for others, there is much agreement, but definitions must still be finalized; and for a third group, additional study and testing are needed.

These elements apply to persons seen in both ambulatory and inpatient settings, unless otherwise specified. For the first 12 elements, with the exception of unique identifier, information may not need to be collected at each encounter. Standard electronic formats are recommended to the extent that they have been developed.

CORE HEALTH DATA ELEMENTS PROPOSED FOR STANDARDIZATION

1. **Personal/Unique Identifier 2/**
2. **Date of Birth**
3. **Gender**
4. **Race and Ethnicity**
5. **Residence**
6. **Marital Status**
7. **Living/Residential Arrangement 1/**
8. **Self-Reported Health Status 2/**
9. **Functional Status 2/**
10. **Years of Schooling**
11. **Patient's Relationship to Subscriber/Person Eligible for Entitlement**
12. **Current or Most Recent Occupation and Industry 2/**
13. **Type of Encounter 2/**
14. **Admission Date (inpatient)**
15. **Discharge Date (inpatient)**
16. **Date of Encounter (outpatient and physician services)**
17. **Facility Identification 1/**
18. **Type of Facility/Place of Encounter 1/**
19. **Health Care Practitioner Identification (outpatient) 1/**
20. **Location or Address of Encounter (outpatient)**
21. **Attending Physician Identification (inpatient) 1/**
22. **Operating Clinician Identification (inpatient) 1/**
23. **Health Care Practitioner Specialty 1/**
24. **Principal Diagnosis (inpatient)**

25. Primary Diagnosis (inpatient)
26. Other Diagnoses (inpatient)
27. Qualifier for Other Diagnoses (inpatient)
28. Patient's Stated Reason for Visit or Chief Complaint (outpatient) 2/
29. Diagnosis Chiefly Responsible for Services Provided (outpatient)
30. Other Diagnoses (outpatient)
31. External Cause of Injury
32. Birth Weight of Newborn
33. Principal Procedure (inpatient)
34. Other Procedures (inpatient)
35. Dates of Procedures (inpatient)
36. Procedures and Services (outpatient)
37. Medications Prescribed
38. Disposition of Patient (inpatient) 1/
39. Disposition (outpatient)
40. Patient's Expected Sources of Payment 1/
41. Injury Related to Employment
42. Total Billed Charges 1/

Footnotes: 1/ element for which substantial agreement has been reached but for which some amount of additional work is needed; 2/ element which has been recognized as significant but for which considerable work remains to be undertaken. A lack of footnote indicates that the element is ready for implementation.

Additional Data Items

While reviewing the draft list of data elements, respondents indicated a number of additional data elements that they felt were important core elements. Examples include information on health behaviors, such as smoking and alcohol consumption; information on preventive services; language ability; severity of illness indicators; provider certainty of diagnostic information; information to link a mother's and infant's charts; information on readmissions and complications. Future projects may undertake to seek consensus among some of these items.

Conclusions

As a result of the process followed in the conduct of this project and based on careful analysis by its members, the Committee has reached the following conclusions:

- The response to the Committee's activities through both participation in meetings and written comments indicates that the health care information field is solidly in favor of the identification and use of standardized data elements and definitions.

- The number of standards-setting organizations is growing; however, all that addressed the Committee are actively seeking participation by a 'recognized' leader/group who can forge consensus for the health care information field. But time is short; decisions are being made by organizations now.

- Response was significant and positive to the Committee's request to review a set of core data elements that were identified after a series of hearings and other information- gathering efforts were completed. Most organizations were supportive in wanting to 'get on board' with standardized data elements.

D

- There is already consensus, among data collectors and users for a significant number of data elements, especially elements related to person descriptors and to selected information on inpatient and ambulatory encounters.

- There is less agreement on data definitions, even for data items that have been in the field for years. Definitions must be refined and made available in standardized formats to data collectors.

- There are data items, such as health status and functional status, that are considered crucial elements, but for which substantial additional evaluation and testing must be undertaken to reach consensus on standardized content and definition.

- Because they recognize the significance of this project, respondents also recommended a number of additional items that they would like evaluated and possibly included in a core set of standardized data elements.

Recommendations to the Department

1. The Committee recommends that the HHS Data Council:

- Circulate the report within the Department for review and constructive criticism.

- Investigate the formation of leadership sites within the Department for each of the standards-setting organizations.

- Refer the core health data elements recommendations to the National Uniform Claim Committee for their consideration as they study the issue of uniform data elements for paper and electronic collection in Fall 1996.

- Provide stable resources to the project to establish an interagency work group, with DHSS taking the lead, to work with the key standards-setting organizations in the area of core health data elements.

2. The Committee recommends the following actions specifically related to the core data elements:

- For those elements that the Committee recommends as being ready to standardize, request each of the data collection entities within the Department to review the set of data elements and to match data contents and definitions with similar items that they are currently collecting or plan to collect. Report to the HHS Data Council on the viability of these elements and definitions being adopted in their program. If a reporting entity is using a different element or definition, explain why their current usage is preferable.

- Support implementation and testing activities for those data elements for which agreement on definitions has been reached and those for which minimal additional work is needed on definitional agreement. Public and private participants have indicated a willingness to work together to disseminate information, test data elements, and utilize electronic means to ensure the widest dissemination of these activities.

- For those data elements, which have been recognized as significant core elements, but for which there is not consensus on definition, support the formation of a public-private working group to conduct or coordinate additional study or research and to further refine definitions.

This group, or a separate group, could also be the focus for evaluating additions to the list of core data elements and for setting up methods for testing and promulgating the final products.

- Place the Committee's report, elements and definitions on an appropriate departmental Home Page as guidance to the field and as a means of encouraging use and soliciting further comments and suggestions while the report is under review within the Department.

3. Because agreement on a unique personal identifier has been recognized as a key element to the successful establishment of core data elements, and their use, support the formation of a public-private working group to study and provide recommendations in this area.

4. Support the NCVHS in continuing its work in this area, especially using its expertise to discuss research issues, to assist in consensus building, and to participate with the Data Council in the implementation of the core health data element project recommendations.

Core Health Data Elements Report

2. Introduction

The identification, definition, and implementation of standardized data in the health care and health care information fields are long overdue. Information is collected by a wide range of users and in a myriad of different formats. Work has been undertaken in the past to try to bring some semblance of order to selected areas of health data collection, especially in the areas of hospital inpatients and physician office visits.

The ever-expanding sites of care, combined with the increasing use of electronic data, make it imperative that all health data collection activities, where possible, utilize standardized data elements and definitions. Standardized data elements will be vitally important in the evolving managed care field, where there is a need to follow individuals through a continuum of care and at multiple sites. Performance monitoring and outcomes research are two additional areas that are currently hampered by the inability to link data sets from various sources due to varying data elements and definitions.

The National Committee on Vital and Health Statistics has completed a two-year project requested by the Department of Health and Human Services to review the current state of health-related core data sets; obtain input on their collection and use; interact with data standards-setting groups; and, most importantly, promote consensus by identifying areas of agreement on core health data elements and definitions. The Committee's goal has been to develop a set of data elements with agreed-upon standardized definitions that, when needed in a data collection effort, can be used to collect and produce standardized data. The intent is not to specify a data set for mandated external reporting; the list of recommended data elements is by no means exhaustive, and, unlike earlier activities, is not a "data set" to be used in a specific setting.

It is the expectation of the Committee that the health care field will find these recommended data elements to be fundamentally important for any collection of person and health care encounter data and will consider these elements and standardized definitions for inclusion in their data collection efforts wherever possible. Favorable input has been received from a wide range of experts, and these elements should be compellingly useful both to states and to provider organizations.

D

3. Background

The National Committee on Vital and Health Statistics (NCVHS) and the Department of Health and Human Services, which it advises, have initiated and completed the first iteration of a process to identify a set of core health data elements on persons and encounters or events that can serve multiple purposes and would benefit from standardization. In August 1994, the Department recognized the National Committee's unique history in promoting standardization of health information when it asked the Committee to provide information and advice that will help maximize the utility of core person and encounter data for meeting the Department's responsibilities. More recently, the Department has been asked by the Vice President to play a leadership role, working with the Committee, in accelerating evolution of public and private health information systems toward more uniform, shared data standards.

Charge and Context

Specifically, the Department charged the Committee to:

- Review state-of-the-art of widely used core data sets in the United States and other countries (including coding and formatting features that allow for flexibility);
- Obtain input, through hearings and other means, from the diverse parties who will report and use standardized data sets;
- Interact closely with recognized standards-setting groups; and
- Promote consensus by identifying areas of agreement on data elements and data sets among different stakeholders and areas that will require further research and development before consensus can be reached.

In developing a strategy for accomplishing these tasks, the Committee described a context in which the project would be undertaken that included the following issues:

- Why such data sets are needed in the current and evolving health care arena;
- What multiple functions they might accomplish for a variety of different users;
- What data elements (including definitions, vocabularies and coding structures) they might contain; and
- What potential problems, such as assuring data quality and preserving confidentiality of identifiable records, can be expected and what approaches might be used to address these problems.

In accepting these challenges, the Committee seeks to facilitate consensus development and incorporate the concepts of multiple use, continued change, and long-term evolution of core data elements into general thinking and practice. The goal is to see what commonalties already exist and to what extent there can be further movement toward greater commonality of terms and consistency of definition.

Uniform Data Set Development

The National Committee on Vital and Health Statistics has been a sentinel organization in the area of uniform data efforts. Promoting the standardization of health information has been a consistent and defining Committee activity for 25 years. The Committee's efforts, first in the area of inpatient hospital data (the Uniform Hospital Discharge Data Set or UHDDS) and later in the area of ambulatory care (the Uniform Ambulatory Care Data Set or UACDS) have moved the country in the direction of achieving comparability in the health data collected by federal agencies, states, localities and the private sector, as well as in the international community. The Committee recognizes the need for uniform, comparable standards across geographic areas, populations, systems, institutions and sites of care to maximize the effectiveness of health promotion and care and minimize the burden on those responsible for generating the data. To this end, the Committee has advised the Department on such matters as Federal-state relationships, nomenclatures and classification systems, core data sets, and access and confidentiality issues.

The data sets promulgated by the NCVHS have become *de facto* standards in their areas for data collection by Federal and state agencies, as well as public and private data abstracting organizations. They have influenced the claim forms on which Medicare and Medicaid data sets are based. Both the UHDDS and UACDS have been reviewed and updated by the NCVHS and the Department in recent years. In addition, the Committee and Department have been involved in activities related to standardizing the collection of data in the long-term care setting.

The UHDDS currently in use was promulgated by the Department in 1985; the NCVHS recommended and circulated a revision in 1992, with additional recommendations from an Interagency Task Force in 1993. The UACDS has never been officially promulgated by the Department, but a 1989 revision by the NCVHS and an Interagency Task Force has been widely circulated, as has a further refinement by the NCVHS in 1994. No decisions have been made by the Department on any of these recommended revisions of either the UHDDS or the UACDS.

Standardization and Confidentiality

In recent years, the Committee has recognized the importance of electronic standardization efforts, which are taking place in the business community. The Committee has appointed a liaison to participate in selected meetings of the American National Standards Institute (ANSI) Accredited Standards Committee (ASC) X-12, a private sector coalition that is developing transmission standards for health data. The focus of the NCVHS effort has been on the content of the data to be transmitted, rather than the method of transmission.

The Committee has recognized that data confidentiality is a major concern in the collection of health data from an increasing number of sites, and the Committee has long been concerned with personal privacy and data confidentiality issues. In the early 1990's, it formed an Ad Hoc Work Group on Confidentiality to study issues related to confidentiality, unique personal identifiers and data linkage across time and systems. Thus, the NCVHS was the natural locus of the continuing efforts of DHHS to investigate the further standardization of health data.

D

4. Process Followed by the Committee

4.1. Review State-of-the-Art of Widely-used Core Data Sets

4.1.1. Background

Standardized data sets can serve many purposes in the current and future health care arena. In the evolving managed care field, the need to follow individuals through a continuum of care and at multiple sites will become increasingly necessary. Performance monitoring and outcomes research are two areas that are currently hampered by the inability to link data sets from various sources.

Standardized data sets, starting with the UHDDS developed by the NCVHS, have been in use for more than two decades. There has been substantial agreement on data elements in these sets, but less agreement on data definitions. In addition, these efforts have concentrated on individual sites of care, ie., hospital inpatient, physician office, and nursing home, which, until recently, were the traditional sites of most care. In recent years, the focus of health care has been shifting to hospital outpatient and other outpatient care, including clinic, hospice and home care, sites for which standardized data collection had not been developed.

The transference of data sets from the traditional sources has not fully met the needs of these sites. Additionally the move in the health care payment system to managed care has increased the need to be able to link data sets and individual records across time, facility, and broader geographic locations. Thus to meet the needs for standardized data, movement must be made toward standardized definitions for those data sets that are already in use, and for an increased use of standardized data elements and definitions by those data collection efforts for which no current standardized data sets exist.

The data sets that are currently standardized are prime examples of satisfying multiple purposes with a single data set. With the use of UHDDS-defined data, for example, state and private abstracting systems have been providing comparable state and local data for health planners for many years. These same data bases are being used to provide input to Federal surveys such as the National Hospital Discharge Survey (NCHS) and the Hospital Cost and Utilization Project (AHCPR). However, AHCPR is in the process of publishing findings indicating definitional discrepancies even within the organizations collecting the UHDDS.

4.1.2. Current Activities

The National Committee is well aware of the numerous efforts currently underway in both the public and private sectors to standardize health data, especially the progress made during the past 10-15 years in developing uniform data sets (Uniform Hospital Discharge Data Set and the Uniform Ambulatory Care Data Set) as well as common claim forms (Uniform Bill 82 and its successor UB 92 and HCFA 1500). To document the current status of activities in the field, the Committee awarded a contract to produce a Compendium of Core Data Elements. In addition, information was solicited by the NCVHS through two large-scale mailings, and public meetings were held with agencies and organizations which are currently collecting health data sets.

4.1.3. Compendium of Core Data Elements

To measure the current state of the use of various data sets, the Committee contracted with the Center for Health Policy Studies (CHPS) in Columbia, MD to begin identifying major data sets already in existence, especially in the private field. A range of organizations was contacted including health plans/insurers, trade or professional associations, employers, data standards organizations, and Government. Although 61 requests were made regarding data sets, almost one-third of respondents indicated that they did not have a set of health data items that they collected. Of 18 trade or professional associations contacted, only four submitted data sets. Half of the ten major employers who were asked to participate declined; only four actually sent in a data set. However, in the three remaining areas of health plans/insurers, government, and data standards organizations, the vast majority supplied data sets. A total of 31 responses were received.

Data sets received were assessed for their consistency with other data sets, particularly minimum data sets such as the UHDDS and the UACDS, the HCFA 1500 and the UB 92 data sets, and also with other current and future data sets under development by data standards organizations (ANSI). These comparisons also included consideration of the general availability, reliability, validity, and utility of data elements. A series of matrices were prepared that arrayed individual data elements in use or proposed for use by different organizations with the type of organization.

Producing the compendium was a much more involved effort than was originally envisioned, and probably is representative of problems to be overcome in the future when standardization implementation is planned. Just trying to obtain data from some large organizations was quite difficult; responses were not received in a timely fashion, and when received, the data layouts often were computerized lists rather than lists of data items with their definitions. In some instances, lists of items were received with many basic data items not included. In these cases, it is possible that the data items, such as person characteristics, are part of a more basic file kept by the organization, and the information for that file was not included.

In a number of instances, lists of data items were obtained, but without definitions. Previous experience indicates that at least some, if not many, of these data items have differing definitions. The Committee recognizes the importance of having both data items and identical definitions in order to compare and analyze data elements.

One problem that was encountered was that of requesting what the private organizations consider proprietary information. It was thought that this was one of the reasons why some organizations, especially private employers, declined to participate.

From the respondents, a total of 138 different data elements were obtained. A large number were collected by only a few of the data sets. Also, although different data sets may include the same data element, in most cases it was not possible to verify that the data collection instructions and definitions were the same.

Based on the compendium effort, a working list of 47 data elements frequently collected or proposed for collection regarding eligibility, enrollment, encounters and claims in the United States was prepared.

4.1.4. Other Widely-used Data Sets

The Committee works closely with the National Center for Health Statistics, the Agency for Health Care Policy and Research, and the Health Care Financing Administration (HCFA). Updates of activities in each of the agencies are presented to the Committee on a regular basis. HCFA has also provided information on its efforts to define a core data set for states and managed health care plans (McData), which is undergoing review at this time. At the October 1995 meeting of the NCVHS, a session was held at which the Department of Veterans Affairs, the Georgia State Department of Health, and others, demonstrated their institutions' integrated financial, clinical, consumer, and public health information systems that are currently in place or being tested.

During the October 1995 and March 1996 NCVHS meetings, Dr. Don Detmer, University of Virginia, updated the Committee on international progress in data standardization and computerized patient records. He had visited a number of western European countries speaking with experts in health information infrastructure, and reported that several countries now have a national policy of support for the computerized patient record. Dr. Detmer identified four overarching issues: privacy and confidentiality, computerized patient records, standards and classification, and knowledge-based management. Also in March, a consultant to the NCVHS updated the World Health Organization on the core data element activity and returned with input to the process.

4.2. Obtain Input, through Hearings and other Means

Armed with the extensive listing of potential data elements culled from the Compendium, in September 1995, the NCVHS contacted approximately 2,000 individuals and organizations in the health care utilization and data fields to seek their input in identifying those basic elements most in need of collection and/or in need of uniform definitions. In addition to requesting a written response from these experts, they were invited to participate in one of two special meetings organized by the Committee to discuss the project and to seek input. In order to have as wide a participation at the meeting as possible, both East and West coast meetings were held in Oakland, CA, in early November, and in Washington, DC, in early December.

Both meetings were successful at bringing together experts in the field and expanding the knowledge base of the Committee. Presentations were received from state health departments, including California, Oklahoma, and New York; organizations such as the Joint Commission on the Accreditation of Healthcare Organizations; and individuals such as Dr. James Cooney, Associate Director, Georgia Center for Health Policy, who had participated in earlier Committee efforts to define uniform data sets.

4.3. Progress, Issues, and Problems Raised

Several major issues were raised that were broader than the discussions of specific data elements. Virtually all saw the need for uniform data items and definitions, and the issue of a unique identifier was a frequent topic. This issue represents more than just what item or set of items the identifier will include; it opens up the whole issue of data linkage, privacy, and data confidentiality with its relevant benefits and risks. Another issue was the role of the National Committee itself as the source of information on common data elements. Most participants eagerly supported an independent committee, such as this, to gather input and advise the public health and health care communities. However, the activities envisioned by many participants go much farther than an advisory committee can handle. These discussions led to the issue of needing DHHS staff dedicated to participating in the meetings of numerous data standards committees, advising the Department, and producing further iterations of data elements as future agreement is reached. Currently, such a staff does not exist.

Some states and organizations are on the cutting edge of multiple use of standardized data. For example, the State of California, in testimony to the NCVHS, described its efforts in improving health and health care delivery by linking data collected through medical facilities, school-based health and educational data bases, as well as need-based data bases such as eligibility listings for the Special Supplemental Nutrition Program for Women, Infants and Children (WIC) or reduced school-lunch programs. This project has brought together efforts from several state agencies, including education (for the school data), agriculture (the source of WIC data in some states), as well as health departments. Consensus building on data elements and definitions was, as always, a complex issue. Data quality is a perennial issue. Although the UHDDS has been in the field for two decades and its data items are widely used by government and private organizations, issues of quality and comparability remain. A presentation by AHCPR reported on a study of 10 state data organizations and two statewide hospital associations participating in the Healthcare Cost and Utilization Project (HCUP-3). (Currently approximately 40 states collect health data on inpatient hospital stays.) AHCPR compared the 12 systems with the UB-92 and monitored deviations at 3 levels - easy, moderately difficult, and difficult to correct problems.

A detailed report of these findings is in the process of publication by AHCPR, but findings have shown that even well-recognized standards are not consistently followed. Any new data items, as well as the old, must be produced with clear instruction on data collection and coding.

Confidentiality of identifiable records is another critical issue. Currently, data are often shared within a facility in an identifiable format. However, identifiers are commonly removed when a data set is provided outside of a facility, such as to a state health data organization. And now, with movement toward HMO's, PPO's, and other types of managed care, there may be a greater need to share identifiable data. States have varying laws to protect the confidentiality of these data, and often the laws do not protect data that have crossed state lines. Sufficient penalties for breach of confidentiality either do not exist or are not enforced. There have been several proposals for Federal legislation in recent years; however, to date, no Federal legislation protecting the confidentiality of health records exists.

Several states, including California, Oklahoma, and New York presented findings on using a combination of key data items to perform probabilistic matches. Using items such as first name of mother; first digits of last name; date of birth; place of birth, etc., matches could be obtained without identifying the individual. It appeared that some types of data linkage could be obtained in states with smaller populations, but might not work nationwide. New York, using the last 4 digits of the Social Security Number, with other characteristics (such as date of birth), indicated a match rate exceeding 99 percent.

Problems could arise from adding and modifying data items and definitions too frequently. James Cooney, Ph.D., former member, NCVHS, described the burden to organizations from the addition of a single data item. Each item that is recommended must be considered carefully. Additionally, too frequent modification of items or definitions will cause confusion, overlapping data definitions in a single data year, and add to the burden of the facility or organization.

In addition to the presentations at the meetings, more than 100 written responses to the solicitation letter were reviewed and considered. Of these, approximately 70 percent provided information about their data elements. Approximately 30 percent of respondents were from state and local governments, followed by professional associations and the Federal Government with 18 Percent and 17 percent respectively. Providers, Insurers, and universities represented about 7 percent each.

The Committee reviewed all of the input received from the hearings, meetings, letters and other communications. In addition, the historical knowledge of the NCVHS and its earlier decisions in the area of data standardization played a role in the preparation of a listing of core data elements and, where possible, recommended definitions. The draft listing was again disseminated in early April

D

1996 to the original mailing list and especially to those who had provided earlier assistance. To assure the widest possible distribution, the document was also placed on the DHHS and NCHS Home Pages in an electronic format. More than 150 responses to this second request were received, including responses from the leaders in the health care and health care information fields.

4.4. Interact Closely with Recognized Standards-setting Groups

The importance of participating in meetings of the various standard-setting groups has been recognized by the Committee. Members of the Committee and DHHS staff participate when possible, however, the increasing numbers of groups and meetings is problematic from a staff and budget point of view. To identify the large number of organizations involved in various aspects of health data standards, staff at NCHS produced a report describing the various groups by type of organization. The report provides important background information on coordinators and promoters of standards development; lead standards-development organizations; organizations developing performance measures indicators; departmental organizations; international organizations; and others.

To obtain the latest plans, at its October 1995 meeting, the NCVHS held a session focused on Standards Development Organizations and related organizations. Participating organizations included:

- ANSI (American National Standards Institute)
- ANSI HISPP (Health Informatics Standards Planning Panel),
- ANSI ASC X-12 (Accredited Standards Committee),
- HL-7 (Health Level 7)
- WEDI (WorkGroup on Electronic Data Interchange)
- ASTM (American Society for Testing and Materials),
- NUBC (National Uniform Billing Committee),
- NUCC (National Uniform Claim Committee), and
- NCQA (National Committee for Quality Assurance).

Although Committee members were aware in a general way of ongoing standards developments activities, this session focused on the need for action being required now and in the near future if the health care community is to obtain and maintain a presence as data standards are developed and finalized. At the very minimum, there need to be "place holders" provided to standards organizations to inform them that certain data elements are critical elements, even when the specific format of the items is currently undecided. It became obvious that staff dedicated to participating in and monitoring the activities of these organizations is crucial if all relevant voices (including public health and epidemiology) are to be heard. At the March 1996 NCVHS meeting, many of the same standards-setting groups were present and indicated their support of the Committee's efforts.

4.5. Promote Consensus by Identifying Areas of Agreement on Data Elements

The major output of this project to date has been the recommendation of core data elements, definitions, vocabulary and classifications. This effort, described below, is the culmination of input from the historical knowledge and work of the Committee, including the uniform basic data sets already developed; and information provided in meetings, hearings, and through correspondence with Federal, state and local health agencies, private organizations, universities, etc.

The goal has been to develop a set of data elements with agreed-upon standardized definitions that, when needed in a data collection effort, can be used to collect and produce standardized data. The Committee's intent is not to specify a data set for mandated external reporting; not every element may be needed in a specific collection effort, and these data elements do not represent all of the important data items that are collected in the field or needed for specific applications. They do represent those items that are routinely collected in many efforts, such as basic person information, as well as items specific to inpatient or ambulatory care settings, such as provider information, diagnoses, and services.

It is hoped that, as data collection evolves, certain data items, such as personal data, (i.e., date of birth, race, occupation) will only need to be collected at time of entry into a health care plan or to be updated on an annual basis, to reduce the burden of data collection. Other data items are related to a specific episode of care and will be provided at each encounter.

4.5.1. The Core Health Data Elements

The following list of data elements contains those elements selected for the first iteration of this process. Consensus has been reached on definitions for the majority of these elements; for others, there is much agreement, but definitions must still be finalized; and for a third group, additional study and testing are needed. These elements apply to persons seen in both ambulatory and inpatient settings, unless otherwise specified. For the first 12 elements, with the exception of unique identifier, information may not need to be collected at each encounter. Standard electronic formats are recommended to the extent that they have been developed.

The Committee recognizes that this is an iterative process and has included in these recommendations several elements that have been proposed for standardization, even though no consensus currently exists concerning appropriate or feasible definitions. The description of the element indicates this present lack of agreement. The Committee has chosen to include these elements because it believes that the need for the type of information they contain will continue to increase. The Committee encourages the Department and its partners to give high priority to conducting evaluation and testing on such elements and also seeks to alert organizations developing standards or data sets to leave place holders for their inclusion. In addition, a number of elements for which consensus is close, must be field tested to confirm their definitions and collectibility. A listing of the Core Health Data Elements grouped by level of readiness for implementation is provided after the section with the definitions of each data element.

The NCVHS has undertaken parallel efforts to identify elements specific to mental health, substance abuse, disability and long-term care settings. Some recommendations in the area of mental health and substance abuse are included here. Other recommendations will be circulated for comment at a future time.

D

TABLE OF CORE HEALTH DATA ELEMENTS

1. **Personal/Unique Identifier 2/**
2. **Date of Birth**
3. **Gender**
4. **Race and Ethnicity**
5. **Residence**
6. **Marital Status**
7. **Living/Residential Arrangement 1/**
8. **Self-Reported Health Status 2/**
9. **Functional Status 2/**
10. **Years of Schooling**
11. **Patient's Relationship to Subscriber/Person Eligible for Entitlement**
12. **Current or Most Recent Occupation and Industry 2/**
13. **Type of Encounter 2/**
14. **Admission Date (inpatient)**
15. **Discharge Date (inpatient)**
16. **Date of Encounter (outpatient and physician services)**
17. **Facility Identification 1/**
18. **Type of Facility/Place of Encounter 1/**
19. **Health Care Practitioner Identification (outpatient) 1/**
20. **Provider Location or Address of Encounter (outpatient)**
21. **Attending Physician Identification (inpatient) 1/**
22. **Operating Clinician identification 1/**
23. **Health Care Practitioner Specialty 1/**
24. **Principal Diagnosis (inpatient)**
25. **Primary Diagnosis (inpatient)**
26. **Other Diagnoses (inpatient)**
27. **Qualifier for Other Diagnoses (inpatient)**
28. **Patient's Stated Reason for Visit or Chief Complaint (outpatient) 2/**
29. **Diagnosis Chiefly Responsible for Services Provided (outpatient)**
30. **Other Diagnoses (outpatient)**
31. **External Cause of Injury**
32. **Birth Weight of Newborn**
33. **Principal Procedure (inpatient)**
34. **Other Procedures (inpatient)**
35. **Dates of Procedures (inpatient)**
36. **Procedures and Services (outpatient)**
37. **Medications Prescribed**
38. **Disposition of Patient (inpatient) 1/**
39. **Disposition (outpatient)**
40. **Patient's Expected Sources of Payment 1/**
41. **Injury Related to Employment**
42. **Total Billed Charges 1/**

   Footnotes: 1/ element for which substantial agreement has been reached but for which some amount of additional work is needed; 2/ element which has been recognized as significant but for which considerable work remains to be undertaken. A lack of footnote indicates that these elements are ready for implementation.

Person/Enrollment Data

The elements described in this section refer to information collected on enrollment or at an initial visit to a health care provider or institution. It is anticipated that these elements will be collected on a one-time basis or updated on an annual basis. With the exception of the personal/unique identifier, they do not need to be collected at each encounter.

1. Personal/Unique Identifier - the unique name or numeric identifier that will set apart information for an individual person for research and administrative purposes.

A. Name - Last name, first name, middle initial, suffix (e.g., Jr., III, etc.)

B. Numerical identifier

The personal/unique identifier is the element that is the most critical element to be collected uniformly. The NCVHS recommends the use of Social Security Number with a check item such as date of birth, while at the same time undertaking the study and evaluation needed to confirm this use or the recommendation of another identifier. More emphasis on the confidential use of SSN is essential. Standards groups should be consulted regarding setting criteria for recording of names.

Rationale and discussion

Without a universal unique identifier or a set of data items that can form a unique identifier, it will be impossible to link data across the myriad of healthcare locations and arrangements. In the 1992 revision of the Uniform Hospital Discharge Data Set (UHDDS), the NCVHS recommended "using the Social Security Number (SSN), with a modifier as necessary, as the best option currently available for this unique and universal patient identifier." However, recent testimony has led the Committee to investigate this issue further, in light of perceived inadequacies of the SSN (e.g., lack of a check digit, multiple SSN's, etc.), particularly when used alone, and impediments (legal and otherwise) to its use. Other potential problems include lack of numbers for newborns, legal and illegal non-citizens and persons who wish to hide their identity, as well as a recommendation that a system would need to be established to assign and track dummy numbers.

New York State presented testimony that indicated that the last four digits of the SSN combined with the birth date were capable of linking data to a very high degree of probability. The State of California has tested the use of a series of data items that are readily known by individuals and which can be combined to link data. By January 1998, all California State Department of Health data bases will contain five data items to facilitate linkage. These data items include birth name, date of birth, place of birth, gender, and mother's first name. Seven confirmatory data items (including SSN) should also be collected when possible.

Those present at the November and December 1995 NCVHS regional meetings agreed that the establishment of a unique identifier is the most important core data item. A unique identifier such as the SSN in conjunction with at least one other data item or, alternatively, an identifier drawn from another distinct set of data items routinely collected presently would seem the most viable. Whichever number is chosen, attention must be paid to which data linkages will be permitted and for what purposes.

Development of a unique identifier does not necessarily mean that the individual is identifiable to users. The NCVHS recognizes the vital importance of maintaining confidentiality and emphasizes that any public use of a unique identifier should be in an encrypted form. The unique identifier must be developed and protected in such a way that the American public is assured that their privacy will be protected.

2. Date of Birth - Year, month and day - As recommended by the UHDDS and the Uniform Ambulatory Care Data Set (UACDS). It is recommended that the year of birth be recorded in four digits to make the data element more reliable for the increasing number of persons of 100 years and older. It will also serve as a quality check as the date of birth approaches the new century mark.

3. Gender - As recommended by the UHDDS and the UACDS.
1. Male
2. Female
3. Unknown/not stated

4. Race and Ethnicity - The collection of race and ethnicity have been recommended by the UHDDS and the UACDS, and these elements have a required definition for Federal data collection in Office of Management and Budget (OMB) Directive 15. The definition has been expanded slightly from the OMB requirement:

4A. Race
1. American Indian/Eskimo/Aleut
2. Asian or Pacific Islander (specify)
3. Black
4. White
5. Other (specify)
6. Unknown/not stated

4B. Ethnicity
1. Hispanic Origin (specify)
2. Other (specify)
3. Unknown/not stated

It is recommended that this item be self-reported, not based on visual judgment or surnames. Whenever possible, the Committee and participants recommended collecting more detailed information on Asian and Pacific Islanders, as well as persons of Hispanic Origin.

Rationale and discussion

The collection of this element allows for the investigation of issues surrounding health and health care by a person's race and ethnic background. Although it is best understood in conjunction with a socioeconomic indicator, researchers may gain a better understanding of the trends and impact of care on racial/ethnic minorities in the U.S. It remains unclear whether the modest health gains seen in low-income and racial/ethnic minority populations in the last thirty years will continue, considering the changes in the U.S. health care system. These data assist in the examination of disparities in stage of illness, care, and outcome, some of which have been documented in the past among racial and ethnic groups.

OMB is currently investigating the possibility of changes to this classification, and the Committee will await the OMB recommendations. The Committee is concerned about the possible inclusion of a "multiracial" category, without an additional element requesting specific racial detail and/or primary racial identification, because of its anticipated impact on trend data and loss of specificity.

The National Association of Health Data Organizations has also opposed such an inclusion. A recent Bureau of Labor Statistics study found that only 1.5 percent of respondents will choose the multiracial category. The study also found that with the multiracial option there was a considerable decline in percentage terms (approximately 29 percent) of respondents choosing American Indian, Eskimo or Aleut. However, there is some evidence that the number of interracial marriages is accelerating.

5. Residence - Full address and ZIP code (nine digit ZIP code, if available) of the individual's usual residence.

Rationale and discussion

This recommendation is in accord with the 1992 UHDDS and the UACDS, as well as recommendations by the NCVHS Subcommittee on State and Community Health Statistics. The Subcommittee determined that residential street address has the advantage of enabling researchers to aggregate the data to any level of geographic detail (block, census tract, ZIP code, county, etc.) and is the best alternative to insure the availability of small area data. In addition, home address will allow the application of GIS (Geographic Information Systems) technology to the analysis of health issues. Some thought needs to be given to completing this item for persons with no known residence or persons whose residence is outside of the United States. Because the full residential address could serve as a proxy personal identifier, confidentiality of the complete information must be safeguarded in public use of the data.

6. Marital Status - The following definitions, as recommended by the NCVHS, should be used.

1. Married - A person currently married. Classify common law marriage as married.
A) living together
B) not living together

2. Never married - A person who has never been married or whose only marriages have been annulled.

3. Widowed - A person widowed and not remarried.

4. Divorced - A person divorced and not remarried.

5. Separated - A person legally separated.

6. Unknown/not stated

Rationale and discussion

The Committee recognizes that a person's social support system can be an important determinant of his or her health status, access to health care services, and use of services. Marital status is one element that is sometimes used as a surrogate for the social support system available to an individual and can be important for program design, targeting of services, utilization and outcome studies, or other research and development purposes. It also may be required to verify benefits.

7. Living/Residential Arrangement - The following definitions are recommended by the NCVHS:

7A. Living Arrangement
1. Alone
2. With spouse
3. With significant other/life partner
4. With children
5. With parent or guardian
6. With relatives other than spouse, children, or parents
7. With nonrelatives
8. Unknown/not stated

Multiple responses to this item are possible. This element refers to living arrangements only. Marital status is discussed in element 6.

7B. Residential Arrangement
1. Own home or apartment
2. Residence where health, disability, or aging related services or supervision are available
3. Other residential setting where no services are provided
4. Nursing home or other health facility
5. Other institutional setting (e.g. prison)
6. Homeless or homeless shelter
7. Unknown/not stated

Rationale and discussion

The usual living/residential arrangement of an individual is important for understanding the health status of the person as well as the person's follow-up needs when seen in a health care setting. Together with marital status, this element provides a picture of potential formal/informal resources available to the person. The element also provides information on patient origin for health resource planning, and for use as an indirect measure of socioeconomic status.

A key distinction to be ascertained in "residential arrangement" is whether organized care- giving services are being provided where the patient lives. The Committee encourages the use of the above definition, while continuing to study and evaluate other residential categories, such as those used by the Bureau of the Census.

8. Self-Reported Health Status - There was much interest in documenting health status, one element that can precipitate the demand for health care and help determine the prognosis, although there was no consensus on how its definition should be standardized. A commonly used measure is the person's rating of his or her own general health, as in the five-category classification, "excellent, very good, good, fair, or poor."

Used in the National Health Interview Survey and many other studies, this item has been shown to be predictive of morbidity, mortality, and future health care use, when collected in a general interview type of setting. This item would be collected at first clinical visit and periodically updated, at least annually. Additional evaluation and testing are needed on standardizing the health status element. At the present time, standards- setting organizations should assign place holder(s) for this element.

9. Functional Status - The functional status of a person is an increasingly important health measure that has been shown to be strongly related to medical care utilization rates. A number of scales have been developed that include both a) self-report measures, such as the listings of limitations of Activities of Daily Living (ADL) and Instrumental Activities of Daily Living (IADL) and the National Health Interview Survey age-specific summary evaluation of activity limitations, and b) clinical assessments, such as the International Classification of Impairments, Disabilities and Handicaps (ICIDH) and the Resident Assessment Instrument (RAI) (widely used in nursing homes). In addition, there are some disabilities, such as severe mental illness or blindness, where ADLs and IADLs are not sufficient measures. Self-report and clinician measurements are each valuable, and having both available is especially informative. Whichever method is used should be designated. Particular scales are more appropriate for measuring different functions or disabilities and should be selected on the basis of the needs of the patient population (such as, use of social functioning scales for those with mental disorders and substance abuse). Functional assessment scales must also be age-appropriate. At present, there is no widely recognized instrument for measuring the functional status of children. Periodicity of assessment also is an issue.

Consideration of these various issues and additional study and evaluation are needed before recommendations can be made for standardizing functional status measurement. Work on this topic is currently ongoing in the NCVHS Disability and Long-Term Care Statistics Subcommittee. It is possible that the description of functional status may entail more than a single measure, thus needing space for more than one measure and/or an additional element to document the scale used. At the current time, however, it is crucial that standards-settings organizations set aside place holder(s) for this element.

10. Years of Schooling - Highest grade of schooling completed by the enrollee/patient. For children under the age of 18, the mother's highest grade of schooling completed should be obtained.

Rationale and discussion

Collection of years of schooling has been recommended by the NCVHS and others as a proxy for socioeconomic status (SES). Years of schooling has been found to be highly predictive of health status and health care use.

Ideally, one would also collect income to more fully define socioeconomic status. However, income questions are often considered intrusive, whereas years of schooling are more acceptable to respondents. The NCVHS Subcommittee on Ambulatory and Hospital Care Statistics commented in the 1994 UACDS revision that years of schooling completed is the most feasible socioeconomic element to collect in the UACDS.

11. Patient's Relationship to Subscriber/person eligible for entitlement -

A. Self
B. Spouse
C. Child
D. Other (specify)

Rationale and discussion

This relationship (i.e., self, spouse or child of subscriber) is often obtained and can be of importance for payment and research purposes.

12. Current or Most Recent Occupation and Industry - This data item is very useful to track occupational diseases as well as to better define socioeconomic status. Standardized coding schemes, such as the Census Bureau's Alphabetical Listing of Occupation and Industry and the Standardized Occupation and Industry Coding (SOIC) software developed by the National Institute for Occupational Safety and Health, should be reviewed. In some situations, it is possible that a free-form narrative will be collected in place of the codes, to be coded at a later point. The Committee feels that, over time, there will be increasing attention focused on this item and reaffirms its recommendations in the 1994 revisions to the UACDS that additional study and evaluation be conducted on the feasibility and utility of collecting and periodically updating information on a person's occupation and industry. In addition, the usefulness of both current/most recent occupation and industry as well as the addition of usual or longest held occupation and industry must be evaluated. All have significant value and could result in the collection of four separate data elements.

Encounter Data

The elements described in this section refer to information related to a specific health care encounter and are collected at the time of each encounter.

13. Type of Encounter - This element is critical to the placement of an encounter of care within its correct location, i.e., hospital inpatient , outpatient, emergency department, observation, etc. However, there was no clear-cut listing of mutually exclusive encounter locations or definitions to draw upon. This term is one that needs study and evaluation before it can be implemented. However, a place holder for this element is recommended to the standards-setting organizations.

14. Admission Date (inpatient)- Year, month, and day of admission as currently recommended in the UHDDS and by ANSI ASC X12. An inpatient admission begins with the formal acceptance by a hospital of a patient who is to receive health care practitioner or other services while receiving room, board, and continuous nursing services. It is recommended that the year of admission contain 4 digits to accommodate problems surrounding the turn of the century.

15. Discharge Date (inpatient) - Year, month, and day of discharge as currently recommended in the UHDDS and by ANSI ASC X12. An inpatient discharge occurs with the termination of the room, board, and continuous nursing services, and the formal release of an inpatient by the hospital. Four digits are recommended for the discharge year.

16. Date of Encounter (outpatient and physician services) - Year, month, and day of encounter, visit, or other health care encounter, as recommended by the UACDS and ANSI ASC X12. Each encounter generates a date of service that can be used to link encounters for the same patient over time. Grouping of similar services provided on different dates,

as is often the case under batch billing, can be problematic if specificity of data elements is lost; the objective is to encourage identifying a unique date of record for each encounter. However, for services billed on a batch basis, two dates would be required to encompass the range of dates from the beginning of all treatments included under the batch (global) code to the end, with a check box to indicate that this is a batch-based encounter.

Health Care Facility and Practitioner Identifiers

Each provider should have a universal unique number across data systems. The National Provider Identifier and National Provider File (NPI/NPF), currently under development by the Health Care Financing Administration (HCFA) and intended for implementation in 1997, could and should meet this need, if all providers are included. The NPI/NPF will provide a common means of uniquely identifying health care providers, including institutions, individuals, and group practices, both Medicare providers and those in other programs. Participation in the system will be voluntary for non-HCFA providers at first. Currently some states are using state facility identifiers, but the Committee recommends that these identifiers be superseded by the NPI/NPF.

The immediate goal of the NPI/NPF project is to support HCFA's Medicare Transaction System initiative by providing a single, universal method for enumerating the providers who serve Medicare beneficiaries. It will do so by assigning a unique identifier to each provider. In the future, the system will integrate non-HCFA subscribers. It is planned that enumeration of Medicare providers will begin in calendar year 1996. The draft systems requirement definition was issued in January, 1995. It is recommended that the NPF be the source of all unique provider identifiers, for institutions and individuals. Systems may also choose to collect other identifiers (e.g., tax number), which they can link to the NPI. Items shown below with an asterisk (*) indicate that this type of information can be obtained from linking the NPI with the National Provider File and may not need separate collection. The Committee recognizes that all practitioners may not be included initially in this system, but ultimately all should be included.

D

17. Facility Identification - The unique HCFA identifier as described above. This identifier includes hospitals, ambulatory surgery centers, nursing homes, hospices, etc. If the HCFA system does not have separate identification numbers for parts of a hospital (i.e., Emergency Department, Outpatient Department), an additional element (such as element 13) will need to be collected along with the facility ID to differentiate these settings. The Committee recommends that the HCFA identifier be adopted when completed.

18. Type of Facility/Place of Encounter - As part of the NPI/NPF system, described above, HCFA is defining a taxonomy for type of facility. This taxonomy builds on previous NCVHS and departmental work and should be reviewed by the NCVHS and standards organizations. The Committee encourages the development of one taxonomy and will monitor progress.

19. Health Care Practitioner Identification (outpatient) - The unique national identification number assigned to the health care practitioner of record for each encounter. There may be more than one health care provider identified:

A. The health care practitioner professionally responsible for the services, including ambulatory procedures, delivered to the patient (health care practitioner of record)
B. The health care practitioner for each clinical service received by the patient, including ambulatory procedures

Initial enumeration by HCFA will focus on individual providers covered by Medicare and Medicaid; however, the system will enable enumeration of other health care practitioners, as identified by system users. The Committee recommends that the HCFA identifier be adopted when completed.

20. Location or Address of Encounter (outpatient) - The full address and Zip Code (nine digits preferred) for the location at which care was received from the health care practitioner of record (see 19A.). As recommended by the UACDS, address should be in sufficient detail (street name and number, city or town, county, State, and Zip Code) to allow for the computation of county and metropolitan statistical area.

21. Attending Physician Identification (inpatient) - The unique national identification number assigned to the clinician of record at discharge who is responsible for the discharge summary, as recommended by the 1992 UHDDS.

22. Operating Clinician Identification - The unique national identification number assigned to the clinician who performed the principal procedure, as recommended by the UHDDS.

23. Health Care Practitioner Specialty - As part of the NPI/NPF system, HCFA has identified a very detailed list of specialties for health care practitioners. This listing should be reviewed by the NCVHS and standards organizations and, if found acceptable, recommended for use.

24. Principal Diagnosis (inpatient) - As recommended by the UHDDS, the condition established after study to be chiefly responsible for occasioning the admission of the patient to the hospital or nursing home for care. The currently recommended coding instrument is the ICD-9-CM.

Rationale and discussion

Principal diagnosis is required by most systems for inpatient reporting. The Committee acknowledges that there are differences in coding guidelines for reporting diagnosis in inpatient and outpatient settings, and this may result in a lack of comparability in data between the two settings. It is recommended that convergence of these guidelines be investigated.

25. Primary Diagnosis (inpatient) - The diagnosis that is responsible for the majority of the care given to the patient or resources used in the care of the patient. The currently recommended coding instrument is the ICD-9-CM.

Rationale and discussion

The primary diagnosis is not part of the UHDDS, and in most diagnostic situations, the principal and primary diagnoses will be identical. Respondents have indicated a mixed use of this item for inpatients. There is also concern that medical personnel may be confusing the definitions/uses of principal versus primary diagnosis. Some respondents incorrectly interpreted this item as a means of classifying primary site for cancer, utilizing ICD-O (oncology). The NCVHS notes that the Department of Veterans Affairs routinely collects this element, and thus approves the continued inclusion in this core list, pending a review of uses and users of this element.

26. Other Diagnoses (inpatient) - As recommended by the UHDDS, all conditions that coexist at the time of admission, or develop subsequently, which affect the treatment received and/or the length of stay. Diagnoses that refer to an earlier episode that have no bearing on the current hospital or nursing home stay are to be excluded. Conditions should be coded that affect patient care in terms of requiring clinical evaluation; therapeutic treatment; diagnostic procedures; extended length of hospital or nursing home stay; or increased nursing care and/or monitoring. The currently recommended coding instrument is the ICD-9-CM.

27. Qualifier for Other Diagnoses (inpatient) - The following qualifier should be applied to each diagnosis coded under "other diagnoses," as was recommended in the 1992 revision of the UHDDS:
Onset prior to admission

1.Yes
2.No

Rationale and discussion

This element is currently being collected by California and New York hospital discharge data systems; there is an indication that use of this qualifier can contribute significantly to quality assurance monitoring, risk-adjusted outcome studies, and reimbursement strategies.

Ambulatory Conditions

The elements for ambulatory conditions contain information on the Patient's Stated Reason for Visit and the Problems, Diagnosis, or Assessment, both of which were recommended by the UACDS. The latter element, which describes all conditions requiring evaluation and/or treatment or management at the time of the encounter as designated by the health care practitioner, has been divided into two elements: 1) the diagnosis chiefly responsible for services provided, and 2) other diagnoses.

28. Patient's Stated Reason for Visit or Chief Complaint (outpatient) - Includes the patient's stated reason at the time of the encounter for seeking attention or care. This item attempts to define what actually motivated the patient to seek care and has utility for analyzing the demand for health care services, evaluating quality of care and performing risk adjustment. The NCVHS recommended this as an optional item in the UACDS but that high priority should be given to conducting additional study as to the feasibility, ease and practical utility of collecting the patient's reason for encounter, in as close to the patient's words as possible. There is not one agreed-upon coding system for this item; the International Classification of Primary Care, and the Reason For Visit Classification used by the National Ambulatory Medical Care Survey are two such systems. Additional evaluation and testing are warranted for this important information.

29. Diagnosis Chiefly Responsible for Services Provided (outpatient) - The diagnosis, condition, problem, or the reason for encounter/visit chiefly responsible for the services provided. Condition should be recorded to the highest documented level of specificity, such as symptoms, signs, abnormal test results, or other reason for visit, if a definitive diagnosis has not been established at the end of the visit/encounter. The currently recommended coding instrument is the ICD-9-CM.

Rationale and discussion

Information on all patient problems and diagnoses requiring attention at the encounter are needed to assess the quality of care delivered, to determine what types of health problems are being seen and treated in the different types of ambulatory care facilities, and for assessing the appropriateness of the setting used to perform the services. During the NCVHS review of core health data elements, discussion arose regarding the specificity of diagnoses reported The official national outpatient/physician coding and reporting guidelines provide instruction that a suspected or rule out condition not be reported as though it is a confirmed diagnosis.

The instruction clarifies that only what is known to the highest level of specificity should be reported. In some instances this may be a symptom or an abnormal finding. Medicare and many other payers adhere to these guidelines. Some third party payers, however, have ignored the guidelines and required facilities and health care practitioners to report a diagnosis that justifies the performance of services being provided. This has resulted in inconsistent data found in many outpatient databases and has skewed patient outcome studies. It is anticipated that the introduction of ICD-10 will alleviate this problem. The NCVHS recommends continued monitoring of provider practices with regard to coding and revision of these recommendations if current guidelines continue to be ignored.

30. Other Diagnoses (outpatient) - The additional code(s) that describes any coexisting conditions (chronic conditions or all documented conditions that coexist at the time of the encounter/visit, and require or affect patient management). Condition(s) should be recorded to the highest documented level of specificity. The ICD-9-CM is the recommended coding convention.

Rationale and discussion

Information on multiple diagnoses is important for developing severity indexes and assessing resource requirements and use.

31. External Cause of Injury - This item should be completed whenever there is a diagnosis of an injury, poisoning, or adverse effect. The currently recommended coding instrument is the ICD- 9-CM. The priorities for recording an External Cause-of-Injury code (E-code) are:

1. Principal diagnosis of an injury or poisoning
2. Other diagnosis of an injury, poisoning, or adverse effect directly related to the principal diagnosis.
3. Other diagnosis with an external cause.

Rationale and discussion

The collection of this element has been recommended by the UHDDS and the UACDS, and a separate element for its collection is included on the UB 92. The information that this element provides on the causes of patients' injuries or adverse effects is considered essential for the development of intervention, prevention and control strategies. Compelling evidence presented by the Indian Health Service, states and nonprofit organizations demonstrates that effective intervention strategies can be implemented in response to available data on external causes of injury.

Procedures

All significant procedures, and dates performed, are to be reported. A significant procedure is one that is:

1. Surgical in nature, or
2. Carries a procedural risk, or
3. Carries an anesthetic risk, or
4. Requires specialized training.

Surgery includes incision, excision, amputation, introduction, endoscopy, repair, destruction, suture, and manipulation. A qualifier element is recommended to indicate the type of coding structure used, i.e., ICD, CPT, etc.

32. Birth Weight of Newborn (inpatient) - The specific birth weight of the newborn, recorded in grams.

Rationale and discussion

Birth weight of newborn is readily available in the medical record and has singular importance for risk-adjustment outcome studies and health policy development related to maternal and infant health.

33. Principal Procedure (inpatient)- As recommended by the UHDDS, the principal procedure is one that was performed for definitive treatment, rather than one performed for diagnostic or exploratory purposes, or was necessary to take care of a complication. If there appear to be two procedures that are principal, then the one most related to the principal diagnosis should be selected as the principal procedure. ICD-9-CM Vol. 3 is required; however NCVHS strongly advocates a single procedure classification for inpatient and ambulatory care.

34. Other Procedures (inpatient) - All other procedures that meet the criteria described in element 33.

35. Dates of Procedures (inpatient) - Year, month, and day, as recommended in the UHDDS and by ANSI ASC X12, of each significant procedure.

36. Procedures and Services (outpatient) - As recommended by the UACDS, describe all diagnostic procedures and services of any type including history, physical

examination, laboratory, x-ray or radiograph, and others that are performed pertinent to the patient's reasons for the encounter; all therapeutic services performed at the time of the encounter; and all preventive services and procedures performed at the time of the encounter. Also, describe, to the extent possible, the provision of drugs and biologicals, supplies, appliances and equipment. The HCFA Common Procedure Coding System (HCPCS), based on CPT-4, is required for physician (ambulatory and inpatient), hospital outpatient department, and free-standing ambulatory surgical facility bills; however, NCVHS strongly advocates a single procedure classification for inpatient and ambulatory care. The Committee recognizes the importance and desirability of linking services with diagnoses, wherever feasible.

37. Medications Prescribed - Describe all medications prescribed or provided by the health care practitioner at the encounter (for outpatients) or given on discharge to the patient (for inpatients), including, where possible, National Drug Code, dosage, strength, and total amount prescribed.

Rationale and discussion

The collection of information on medications is crucial to understanding the health care encounter and the services provided to a patient. The Committee recognizes that not all providers are obtaining this detail, but it is anticipated that these data will be more frequently collected in the near future with the growth of computerized prescription information.

38. Disposition of Patient (inpatient) - As recommended by the UB 92 and as an expansion of the 1992-93 UHDDS data element:

1. Discharged Alive
    A. Discharged to home or self care (routine discharge)
    B. Discharged/transferred to another short term general hospital for inpatient care
    C. Discharged/transferred to skilled nursing facility (SNF)
    D. Discharged/transferred to an intermediate care facility (ICF)
    E. Discharged/transferred to another type of institution for inpatient care or referred for outpatient services to another institution
    F. Discharged/transferred to home under care of organized home health service organization
    G. Discharged/transferred to home under care of a Home IV provider
    H. Left against medical advice or discontinued care
2. Expired
3. Status not stated

Rationale and discussion
In addition to documenting whether the patient was discharged alive or died during the hospitalization, the patient disposition is an indicator of the patient's health status at the time of discharge and need for additional services.

39. Disposition (outpatient) - The health care practitioner's statement of the next step(s) in the care of the patient. Multiple responses are possible. At a minimum, the following classification is suggested:

1. No follow-up planned (return if needed, PRN)
2. Follow-up planned or scheduled

3. Referred elsewhere (including to hospital)
4. Expired

Rationale and discussion

The critical distinction here is whether follow-up is planned or scheduled, as an indicator of continuing health problems and continuity of care. Expired has been added because the outpatient setting includes a wide range of sites, including Emergency Departments and ambulatory surgery centers.

40. Patient's Expected Sources of Payment - The following categories are recommended for primary and secondary sources of payment:

40A. Primary Source - The primary source that is expected to be responsible for the largest percentage of the patient's current bill.

40B. Secondary Source - The secondary source, if any, that will be responsible for the next largest percentage of the patient's current bill.
Self-pay
Worker's Compensation
Medicare
Medicaid
Maternal and Child Health
Other government payments
Blue Cross
Insurance companies
No charge (free, charity, special research, or teaching)
Other
Unknown/not stated

D

Rationale and discussion

The categories in this element were recommended by the UHDDS for primary and secondary sources of payment. The Committee recognizes the ongoing discussion of discrepancies between 'expected' and 'actual' sources of payment. Source of payment categories, as recommended in the past, are no longer sufficient. The continuing expansion of types of payments and the combination of payments within groups is ever changing. However, the information is still considered useful to collect for trend purposes and for some indication of patients' coverage by third-party payers.

HCFA is developing a new system, called the HCFA PAYERID project, which will assign a unique identifier to every payer of health care claims in the United States. Participation is voluntary, and HCFA, which is funding its development, has been working to get consensus about the kind of system that would be useful. The database will contain payer names, billing addresses and business information. The information, which is already in the public domain, will be accessible by names and ID numbers, and available in several formats. Who will have access to the database for research purposes, and to what data, has yet to be determined. "Payers" are defined as public and private entities that have contract responsibility for health care payment.

Medicare decided a PAYERID was needed because of the difficulty its contractors were having in transferring claims to other insurance companies, due to incomplete information or multiple names for payers. It is hoped that the system will improve the coordination of benefits, as well as providing access to information about health insurance and making it easier to track third party liability situations. HCFA, however, has estimated that there are approximately 30,000 individual payers in the U.S. They currently are not developing a system of categories to accompany the IDs. Such a system would be helpful to the extent that it is feasible in the current highly dynamic market.

Because the PAYERID system is still being developed, and because HCFA currently has no plans to categorize payers, the Committee recommends the current UHDDS categories while encouraging continued study and evaluation of categories used by other data collectors.

41. Injury Related to Employment

Rationale and discussion

Whether an injury is work related or not can be of significant importance both in the area of injury prevention and in medical care payment. During the discussion on including External Cause of Injury in the 1994 revision to the UACDS, CDC and labor and business groups urged collection of whether or not an injury occurred at work or was work-related. This element is currently collected on the HCFA 1500 form.

42. Total Billed Charges - All charges for procedures and services rendered to the patient during a hospitalization or encounter.

Rationale and discussion

The UHDDS and UACDS have recommended the collection of all charges for procedures and services rendered to the patient during a hospitalization or encounter. This item already is collected by most state health data organizations collecting hospital discharge information and offers the only readily available information on the fiscal dimensions of care and the relative costs of different types of care. Although there is agreement that "payments" or "costs" are needed, most participants agreed that it is virtually impossible to collect these items consistently across time and locations. Moreover, in the electronic format, in most instances, payments would not be available at the time that patient and medical data are entered. It might not be feasible to expect the record to be updated to include payment data when it becomes available. Therefore, billed charges should be collected, at a minimum.

4.5.2. Core Data Elements Listed by Readiness for Implementation

<u>Elements Ready for Implementation:</u>

2. Date of Birth
3. Gender
4. Race and Ethnicity
5. Residence
6. Marital Status
10. Years of Schooling
11. Patient's Relationship to Subscriber/Person Eligible for Entitlement
14. Admission Date (inpatient)
15. Discharge Date (inpatient)
16. Date of Encounter (outpatient and physician services)
20. Location or Address of Encounter (outpatient)

24. Principal Diagnosis (inpatient)
25. Primary Diagnosis (inpatient)
26. Other Diagnoses (inpatient)
27. Qualifier for Other Diagnoses (inpatient)
29. Diagnosis Chiefly Responsible for Services Provided (outpatient)
30. Other Diagnoses (outpatient)
31. External Cause of Injury
32. Birth Weight of Newborn
33. Principal Procedure (inpatient)
34. Other Procedures (inpatient)
35. Dates of Procedures (inpatient)
36. Procedures and Services (outpatient)
37. Medications Prescribed
39. Disposition (outpatient)
41. Injury Related to Employment

Elements Substantially Ready for Implementation, but need some added work:

7. Living/Residential Arrangement
17. Facility Identification
18. Type of Facility/Place of Encounter
19. Health Care Practitioner Identification (outpatient)
21. Attending Physician Identification (inpatient)
22. Operating Clinician Identification (inpatient)
23. Health Care Practitioner Specialty
38. Disposition of Patient (inpatient)
40. Patient's Expected Sources of Payment
42. Total Billed Charges

Elements which require a substantial amount of study and evaluation:

1. Personal/Unique Identifier
8. Self-Reported Health Status
9. Functional Status
12. Current or Most Recent Occupation and Industry
13. Type of Encounter
28. Patient's Stated Reason for Visit or Chief Complaint (outpatient)

4.5.3. Additional data items

While reviewing the draft list of data elements, respondents indicated a number of additional data elements that they felt were important core elements. Some of these included information on health behaviors, such as smoking and alcohol consumption; information on preventive services; language ability; severity of illness indicators; provider certainty of diagnostic information; information to link a mother's and infant's charts; information on readmissions and complications, to mention a few. Future projects may undertake to seek consensus among some of these items.

4.5.4. Related Data Set Activities

Concurrent with these activities being undertaken by the full Committee, there are two related projects undertaken by the Subcommittee on Mental Health Statistics and the Subcommittee on Disability and Long Term Care Statistics. With the assistance of the Center for Mental Health Services, SAMHSA, and a contractor, Webman Associates, a study was undertaken to identify and survey a representative sample of mental health, managed care, substance abuse, disabilities and long term care experts who would be willing to offer recommendations about the content of an ideal minimal data set for a health care record that is inclusive of the relevant information. Over three dozen data sets were studied, among them two nationally approved data sets, the Mental Health Statistics Improvement Program Data Set MHSIP) and The Adoption and Foster Care Analysis and Reporting System (AFCARS) data set. After review of the data elements collected, the subcommittees decided to study in-depth six data clusters:

1. Disability
2. Mental Health and Substance Use History of Consumer and of Consumer's Family Members
3. Guardianship/Caregiver
4. Living Situation
5. Categorization and Coding of Wrap Around Services (including community-based services, housing assistance, job training, etc.)
6. Functional Assessment Criteria

The preliminary results of this project have been prepared. The process for these specialized areas is ongoing and final recommendations for specific elements have not yet been submitted to the full Committee. Respondents to this project welcomed the notion of a core data set and standardized forms in this area. It is important to note for this report, however, that the two subcommittees are in agreement with the core data elements that are described herein. Their continuing study is involved with more detailed data elements that relate specifically to the areas of mental heath, substance abuse, and long term care.

A second study is currently underway, one which will investigate core data elements in common use in data sets on persons with disability and/or persons receiving long term care. The major objectives of this project include the production of a report assessing existing data for care provided to persons with disabilities in institutional and community long term care settings, as well as in rehabilitation. Common data elements and areas for standardization will be considered as well as criteria for selection of data elements. Recommendations and linkage with the current project will be discussed.

5. Conclusions

As a result of the process followed in the conduct of this project and based on careful analysis by its members, the Committee has reached the following conclusions:

- The response to the Committee's activities both through participation in meetings and written comments indicates that the health care information field is solidly in favor of the identification and use of standardized data elements and definitions.

- The number of standards-setting organizations is growing; however, all who addressed the Committee are actively seeking participation by a 'recognized' leader/group who can forge consensus for the health care information field. But time is short; decisions are being made by organizations now.

- Response was significant and positive to the Committee's request to review a set of core data elements that were identified after a series of hearings and other information- gathering efforts were completed. Most organizations were supportive in wanting to 'get on board' with standardized data elements.

- There is already consensus among data collectors and users for a significant number of data elements, especially elements related to person descriptors and to selected information on inpatient and ambulatory encounters.

- There is less agreement on data definitions, even for data items that have been in the field for years. Definitions must be refined and made available in standardized formats to data collectors.

- There are data items, such as health status and functional status, that are considered crucial elements, but for which substantial additional study and evaluation must be undertaken to reach consensus on standardized content and definition.

- Because they recognize the significance of this project, respondents also recommended a number of additional items that they would like evaluated and possibly included in a core set of standardized data elements.

6. Recommendations to the Department

1. The Committee supports the HHS Data Council in its formation of the Health Data Standards Committee to focus attention on the needs for standardized data both within the Department and in the health care community at large and to foster collaboration and consensus with the major standards-setting organizations. To this end, the Committee recommends that the Data Council:

- Circulate the report within the Department for review and constructive criticism.

- Investigate the formation of leadership sites within the Department for each of the standards-setting organizations.

- Refer the core health data elements recommendations to the National Uniform Claim Committee for their consideration as they study the issue of uniform data elements for paper and electronic collection in Fall 1996.

- Provide stable resources to the project to establish an interdepartmental work group, with DHHS taking the lead, to work with the key standards-setting organizations in the area of core health data elements.

2. The Committee recommends the following actions specifically related to the core data elements:

- For those elements that the Committee recommends as being ready to standardize, request each of the data collection entities within the Department to review the set of data elements and to match data contents and definitions with similar items that they are currently collecting or plan to collect. Report to the HHS Data Council on the viability of these elements and definitions being adopted in their program. If a reporting entity is using a different element or definition, explain why their current usage is preferable.

- Support implementation and testing activities for those data elements for which agreement on definitions has been reached and those for which minimal additional work is needed on definitional agreement. Public and private participants have indicated a willingness to work together to disseminate information, test data elements, and utilize electronic means to ensure the widest dissemination of these activities.

- For those data elements which have been recognized as significant core elements, but for which there is not consensus on definition, support the formation of a public-private working group to conduct or coordinate additional study or research and to further refine definitions. This group, or a separate group, could also be the focus for evaluating additions to the list of core data elements and for setting up methods for testing and promulgating the final products.

- Place the Committee's report, elements and definitions on an appropriate departmental Home Page as guidance to the field and as a means of encouraging use and soliciting further comments and suggestions while the report is under review within the Department.

3. Because agreement on a unique personal identifier is recognized as a key element to the successful establishment of core data elements, and their use, support the formation of a public-private working group to study and provide recommendations in this area.

4. Support the NCVHS continuing its work in this area, especially using its expertise to discuss research issues, to assist in consensus building, and to participate with the Data Council in the implementation of the core data element project recommendations.

7. Future Activities

As highlighted earlier, the Committee has identified a number of areas that should be considered for implementation by the HHS Data Council. These include the review and implementation of core data elements and definitions within departmental data collection activities; formation of public-private work groups to assist in promulgating data elements for which consensus has been reached or for undertaking additional study on critical elements for which there are no standardized definitions. Additionally, a consensus must be reached on the unique personal identifier.

Participants in the various meetings had discussed ways to disseminate new data items, seek input, and inform data collectors of recommended elements and definitions. It was felt that the Committee should consider designing a WEB page on the Internet that could be used for these activities. The Committee could recommend such an activity, but it would require departmental staff to actually design, input data, and monitor and update the site.

Several organizations have volunteered to facilitate dissemination and feedback of the core data elements project. These activities could take several forms. One would be through the use of a state-level or regional-level organization that already has a line of communication with other organizations. An example of this could be NAHDO which could undertake to work with its members. Another form would be through an organization that already has a WEB page; several organizations indicated that they would be willing to test the sharing of this information through their Internet sites.

It is of vital importance to participate in and/or be members of the numerous data standards groups. Currently there is little or no input from the public health field for several reasons. One major reason is the staff and dollar resources required to travel to and participate in several meetings per group per year. Another problem is that, although the HHS Data Council has recently established a Health Data Standards Committee, until the past few months, there has been no central location within the Department for monitoring the activities of the data standards groups. Throughout the meetings it became apparent that many standards-setting groups are moving ahead without broader input, for example, from those in the public health and epidemiology fields. Place holders will be set, and, in some cases data items and definitions decided on, before national and local public health agencies and organizations will be able to act.

It became obvious early in the meetings that the identification of core data elements, their definitions, and the consensus-building needed to encourage use of these items would be an ongoing and full-time activity for several years. Although the Committee serves a very useful purpose in bringing together the experts to discuss and consider these elements, it takes dedicated departmental staff to keep the process underway on a day-to-day basis. The Committee recommends that the Department fund these activities on an ongoing basis.

D

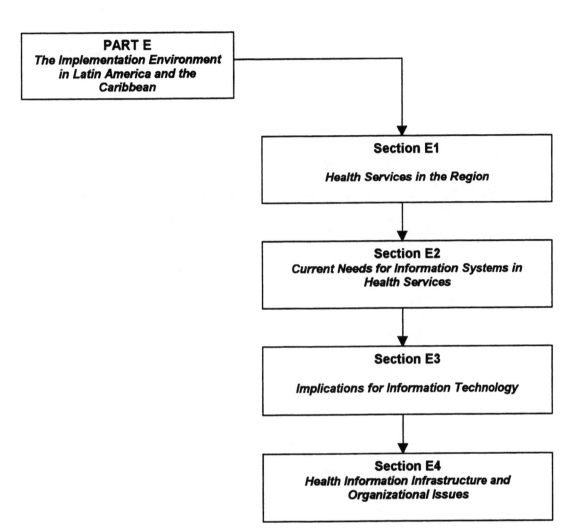

PART E
The Implementation Environment in Latin America and the Caribbean

Section E1

Health Services in the Region

Section E2
Current Needs for Information Systems in Health Services

Section E3

Implications for Information Technology

Section E4
Health Information Infrastructure and Organizational Issues

E

Part E. The Implementation Environment in Latin America and the Caribbean

E

Part E.   The Implementation Environment in Latin America and the Caribbean

He that will not apply new remedies, must expect new evils.

Francis Bacon (1561–1626)

Healthcare delivery systems (health services) in the Region of Latin America and the Caribbean have different kinds of organizations aimed to provide curative and preventive-oriented services to their respective target populations. As a whole, these organizations involve the utilization of a large amount of resources — organized at different levels of technological complexity — that have been developed and allocated to deal with even greater needs for provision of healthcare.

E.1.   Health Services in the Region

Health services have a high degree of heterogeneity in their size, organization, resources, production, and population coverage, both between and within countries. The specific characteristics of health services are determined by multiple macrocontext and health sector factors such as:

- National overall socioeconomic development

- In-country distribution pattern of socioeconomic development

- Prevailing characteristics of the political and economic system

- Legal and normative framework of the healthcare system

- Structure of service provision by type and mix of ownership of facilities and type of payer (public, private, or a mixture)

- Financing framework and the mode of reimbursement for services provided

- Administrative and clinical organization of health services

- Geographical distribution of healthcare

- Geographical and financial coverage of public and private services, at different care levels

- Historical trends in healthcare utilization

E

• Strategies adopted for the development, adequacy and reform of health services

The simultaneous influence of these factors — some of them rapidly changing throughout time and geographical area — leads to a remarkable diversity in the features and form of operation of health services. The added variability, even in the same geographical area, of the health condition of populations makes it nearly impossible to define a single "model" of healthcare service even for an individual country. The level of economic development and degree of industrialization has a significant influence on health systems, which are also influenced by other macro-environmental factors of political and social nature; by the historical development of the health sector; and by the way each country organized its health system. Within countries, wide differences are commonly found among different geographical areas and different socioeconomic groups of the population.

Figure 1. Expenditure in Health per Capita and GDP/Per Capita in Selected Countries of Latin America and the Caribbean, 1994

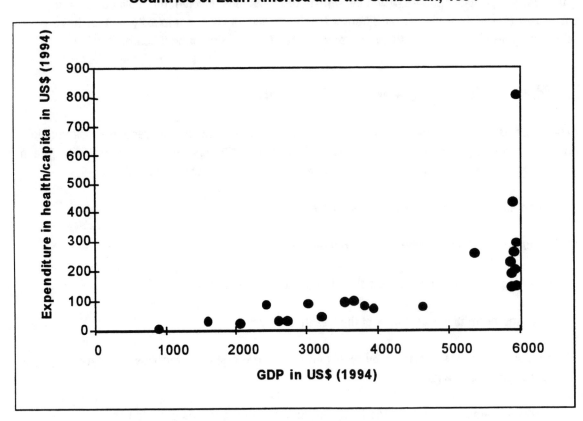

Note: Eighteen countries with less than 0.5 million population are excluded.
Source : PNUD, 1997 (based on 1994 data)

According to the World Bank (1993), no country of the Latin America and Caribbean Region is categorized as industrialized. According to the United Nations Development Program, the gross domestic product (GDP) per capita for 1994, used as a proxy for national socioeconomic development in countries of the Region, ranged from US$896 to US$11,051 for Haiti and Barbados, respectively. The proportion of national expenditure in health per capita, taken as a proportion of GDP, ranged from 1.5% (Haiti) to 13% (Argentina).

Some countries have very small or mid-sized populations (e.g., Anguila and Turks and Caicos Islands with 8 and 15 thousand inhabitants, respectively; in the Eastern Caribbean country population range from 250,000 to 40,000) and, therefore, small-sized health services. When countries with less than half million population are excluded, the expenditure in health per capita ranges between a few dollars to about US$100 per year. Only when the GDP approaches US$6,000 there is an abrupt increase in the per capita health expenditure (Figure 1), and even then the variation is very broad (from US$200 to US$800). These data suggest that, in practice, health services are highly dependent upon the available resources allocated to health, which in turn is related to the overall level of socioeconomic development.

Health systems involve different stakeholders, such as the State, financial agencies, insurers, and providers of healthcare. Specific institutions may comprise one or more of these types of stakeholders (e.g., a social security system institution insuring and providing healthcare). The population participates not only as the target of the services produced but also as direct or indirect payer and user of healthcare. Most countries in the Region have a public-private mix in their health system, with different degrees of predominance of each sector; the proportion of the public-private mix varies with individual countries.

There are large segments of populations without or with limited access to healthcare, mainly the poor and rural groups. The public sector segment can involve different aspects: ownership, funding, contracting, or just the utilization of healthcare by public beneficiaries. The role assumed by the public sector may change in relation to the process of health sector reform and privatization, in practically all countries of the Region.

The characteristics of the private sector and private healthcare networks are difficult to determine, due to the great variety in the specific types of services provided, the capital and investments involved, the population or market coverage, and the technological complexity of different organizations. This results in a great diversity of private health services, with great internal heterogeneity of care levels – ambulatory, diagnostic, and therapeutic services, and hospitals of different sizes, coverage and technical complexity. This diversity is greater still in ambulatory centers, which range from community centers with low technological complexity to centers of high level of specialization and technology.

Available health service statistics, originated from the countries, are mainly focused on the public sector or social security subsectors. At the ambulatory level, the private sector covers highly diverse dimensions; from outpatient care provided at the individual level, sometimes by the same personnel contracted in the public sector, to large and complex healthcare facilities.

E.1.1. Hospitals

Most of the healthcare delivery resources are allocated to hospitals at the secondary and tertiary care levels. According to size and level of specialization, hospitals are complex institutions, where information is needed in several internal centers of intermediate and final production of health services, including managerial and general services supporting the clinical provision of healthcare. The number of hospitals and hospital beds in each country of the region is shown in Figure 2, which plots data from 16,566 institutions surveyed during 1996-1997. There is probably minor under-registration of hospitals and beds in some countries and sectors, especially Argentina, which did not report the number of beds in 885 of its hospitals.

Figure 2.   Hospitals and Hospital Beds in Countries of the LAC Region and GDP Per Capita

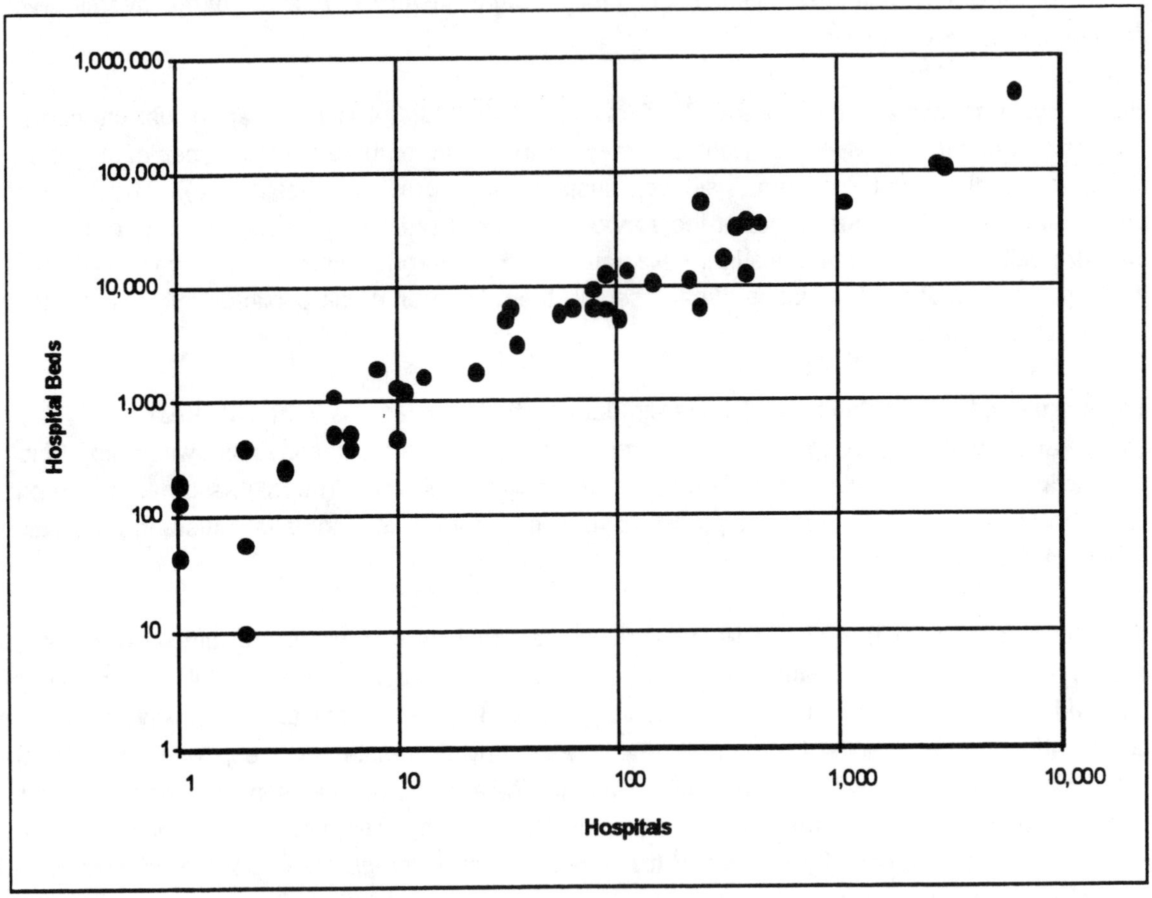

Source: HSP/HSO Directory of Hospitals of Latin America and the Caribbean (1996)
Note: Data represented in log scales

Two-thirds of the hospitals have 50 beds or fewer, and 16% between 51 and 100 beds. In total, 73% of the hospitals have 100 beds or fewer. These hospitals represent 37.3% of the total number of beds. Hospitals with more than 500 beds represent only 1.3% of the total number of hospitals, but have 13% of all beds. A higher proportion of hospitals belong to the private sector (46.9%) as opposed to the public (44.4%). The latter group is composed of a greater number (39.2%) of general public hospitals, and only 5.2% are run by the social security system. The philanthropic sector has 7.8% of the hospitals, while military hospitals represent 0.7% of the total.

The proportion of beds in the public sector is greater than in any other sector (45.1%), while only a third of the beds are in the private sector. At secondary and tertiary level, public hospitals tend to have a greater number of beds, including teaching institutions and those with beds devoted to chronic and psychiatric in-patient care. The beds of the social security system correspond to 7.6%, 11.4% are in philanthropic hospitals, and 1% are in military centers.

In ten countries, all hospitals belong to the public sector, while in the remaining there exists a mixture of ownership. Private ownership varies — it represents 69% of hospitals in Mexico and 62% in Honduras. In Brazil, nearly a fifth (19.5%) of the hospitals are of philanthropic nature, while in the other countries, except for Honduras (23.4%) there is only a small proportion of institutions in the philanthropic subsector. In a survey of hospitals of the Region, conducted by the Pan American Health Organization in 1996-1997, a total of 16,566 hospitals responded, representing a total of 1.1 million beds. The countries with greater availability of beds per population are smaller than half million inhabitants (U.S. Virgin Islands, Turks and Caicos Islands, the Eastern Caribbean island states, and the Netherlands Antilles). In the countries with more than half million inhabitants, the availability of beds per 1,000 population ranges between 5.1 per 1,000 in Cuba to 0.7 in Haiti. Figure 3 depicts the relationship between hospitals beds per 1,000 population and socioeconomic development represented by GDP, for countries over half million population.

**Figure 3. Beds per 1,000 Population in
Latin America and the Caribbean, 1996**

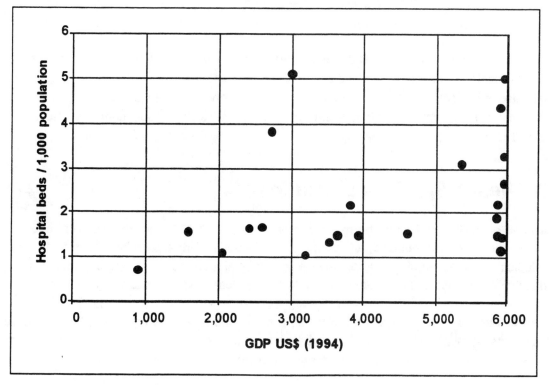

Source: Directory of Hospitals of Latin America and the Caribbean (1996)
Note: Countries with less than 0.5 million inhabitants were excluded

Most countries have between one and two beds per thousand, irrespective of GDP level; on the other hand, availability of beds ranges from 1 to 5 per thousand in the countries with higher GDP (close to US$6,000). The availability of beds according to affiliation sectors per country has a distribution similar to the one observed with regard to hospitals, but is mostly concentrated in the public sector, because public hospitals are usually larger — for example, although almost 70% of hospitals in Mexico are private, they have only 30% of the beds.

E.1.2. Primary Healthcare

Although each healthcare system may have specific operational definitions of its levels of care, there is more agreement on what is primary healthcare (PHC) than what constitute the more complex levels of care. The definition of PHC is mainly based on the roles and responsibilities assumed at primary level, which is preventive-oriented and based on relatively simple curative-oriented services.

No clear patterns are found in PHC centers when comparing different countries. However, some characteristics are common: the basic clinical personnel team is based on professionals (such as doctors, nurses, visiting community health officers, midwives, dentists) and auxiliary personnel, working in ambulatory centers. Maternal and child programs may be performed (including activities such as checkups, vaccination, family planning), and simple curative services, including general medical consultation, are usually provided. Less complex centers exist (rural posts, dispensary centers), as centers complementary to those PHC centers, usually staffed by auxiliary professionals. The simple rural centers are important where there is no availability of direct healthcare personnel, physicians, or when easy access to more complex centers is not possible.

As the highest level of complexity, PHC depends on general practitioners supported by specialists in pediatrics, gynecology, obstetrics, and others, and by equipment that can be used in relatively unsophisticated environments, providing basic laboratory, X-rays, sterilization, dentistry, and cold chain for vaccine maintenance services. Vehicles and communication equipment are also highly relevant in PHC.

E.1.3. Health Services Utilization

The utilization of health services is the result of multiple factors influencing the biological need for health interventions, access, demand, and actual service usage. Information related to demographic, epidemiological, socioeconomic, cultural, and environmental conditions of target populations is required in order to assess and monitor the use of health services, and as a basis for planning.

Health services are productive organizations within a social and market environment, but they have special characteristics and cannot be fully equated to other open market organizations that sell services. Some of those differentiating characteristics include:

- *Asymmetry of demand* - Whilst access to health services is linked to ability to pay, if no equitable measures to ensure access are applied, a great proportion of unfulfilled demand is concentrated in the poorer groups of population, which carry a higher burden of health problems. Not only marketing but also epidemiological approaches are required to analyze access and utilization of health services.

- *Induced demand* - Demand is influenced by the opinion of epidemiologists and clinical professionals, by the existence of specialists that tend to induce demand, as well as by previous experience in using health services. Besides, physicians have great influence in the selection of the form and content of healthcare interventions needed by each patient. They control both the supply and demand and very little "choice" is left to the patient.

- *Market perspective* - Two approaches are complementary in the assessment of health services: health services as provider organizations — a supply-side view — and the population seen both as the user (a very special kind of customer) and as a target group of people with differential needs for healthcare — a demand-side view.

- *Measurement difficulties* - The use of health services means actual access of people to health services, so the most direct approach to its estimation comes from household surveys. However, an indirect approach is the estimate of the rate of services provided per unit of target population.

E.1.4. Health Services and Health Sector Reform

Following different goals and demands, many countries of the Region have embarked on political and economic reform processes involving the State, the market, the public sector, and the health sector. According to the Report of the Interagency Special Meeting on Health Sector Reform organized by PAHO and held in Washington D.C. in December 1995:

Health Sector Reform is a process aimed at introducing substantive changes into the different agencies of the health sector, their relationships, and the roles they perform, with a view to increasing equity in benefits, efficiency in management, and effectiveness in satisfying the health needs of the population. This process is dynamic, complex, and deliberate; it takes place within a given time frame and is based on conditions that make it necessary and workable.

From the above statement, the following main objectives of health sector reform are identified:

- To improve health and living conditions of the peoples of the Americas

- To become part of the social reform in the Region, one of the pillars of development, along with justice, well-being, and equity

- To reduce health status inequities, improve access to good quality health services, and foster shared responsibility among institutions, individuals, and communities

E

- To modernize the organizations and operation of public institutions providing health services

- To balance the public and private health subsectors in order to achieve complementarity in their efforts

- To ensure that reasonable financial resources are available in the sector at a sustainable level to allow its objectives to be met.

According to the main goals and objectives pursued by the reform processes, some key aspects of healthcare are subject to information and evaluation:

- The role of the State and organizational modernization

- Equity in health and access to healthcare

- Administrative, technical, economic, allocative, and social efficiency

- Productivity and cost containment.

- Cost-effectiveness of healthcare interventions

- Priority-setting and definition of a basic package of benefits

- Quality of care and user satisfaction.

E.2. Current Needs for Information Systems in Health Services

A variety of implications for health information depend on the characteristics adopted by specific health services, at different levels and geographical areas and by the practical issue raised by health sector reform. The complexity of health services and the healthcare network imply a great challenge to the design, development, and running of health service information systems. In general, there are specific systems of information systems at the local level, including the coexistence of several particular information systems within more complex centers, such as specialty hospitals.

Information systems are essential tools to address the need to know at the delivery level and to understand and guide health reform processes. They contribute to the discernment of the determinants, the socioeconomic and epidemiological context around the changing sector, and the attributable impact of the reform processes, both in the sector itself and in the health conditions of the population. Information systems are, therefore, tools to support the adequate development of health services. New implications have been raised from the health sector reforms occurring in countries of the Region:

- The pursuit for quality of care and the quest for efficiency — both in terms of technical productivity, resource allocation, and economic efficiency, and

- The search for more effective outcomes, through economic and epidemiological analysis supported by information.

The decentralization process has occurred in both local management and adaptation of information systems to local realities and needs, where information supports local decision-making.

E

E.3. Implications for Information Technology

Information technology must be adapted to the volume and complexity of the information that is required and used at different levels of healthcare organizations. While at large specialty hospitals there is a need for multiple functional operational units, implying therefore the need for a complete set of information system (e.g., pharmacy, laboratory, personnel management, accountability), in small general hospitals there is a more basic requirement for information technology. In PHC centers the information technology may be as simple as the level of complexity in healthcare.

All this has implications in the selection and deployment of appropriate technology, through the combination of technology of different complexities, depending on the level of action and decision in which data will be processed and information will be provided. Supporting appropriate technology, the application of suitable and user-friendly software to be used primarily by healthcare personnel — not trained in information technology — at the PHC level for service operation, individual patient care, and epidemiological analysis is to be the major goal of systems developers.

In order to preserve the functional integration of healthcare networks, the use of information network should involve different institutions, in both the public and private sectors. Common standards and criteria are needed for those concepts, measures, and reports to be shared and integrated. Major organizational challenges regarding the deployment of health and healthcare informatics applications faced by managers, political decision-makers, and developers in the Region, especially in the public sector, are mostly related to:

- Inadequate health information infrastructure

- Organizational deficiencies

- Great diversity of user needs

- Access to and appropriate deployment and utilization of technology.

E.4. Health Information Infrastructure and Organizational Issues

These components are poorly developed in the Region. They require clear responsibility and accountability structures, setting of objectives and targets for individuals and departments, and mechanisms for motivating people and for providing feedback about their achievements.

Lack of organizational rationality, limited organizational skills, and inability to manage and use information for decision-making constitute significant issues. Illiteracy is a barrier to the growing area of consumer-oriented health applications or "consumer informatics", the basis for individual access to health information and self-help. Adequate institutional infrastructure requires the presence of a framework that allows information to be used in a way that encourages individuals to take advantage of existing data according to their particular needs and the objectives of the organization.

A recent survey of the health information infrastructure in the Region revealed major problems and constraints related to data collection, information utilization and dissemination, and the capacitation of human resources. The survey (PAHO/WHO Health Services Information Systems Resources Survey), conducted in 1996, had the objective of determining the status of development of the information function in the Region, including organizational development and infrastructure. Key informants in twenty-four countries responded to the survey.

E.4.1. Data Collection, Processing, and Information Utilization

Data capture and its accuracy represent the most serious problem in the operation of information systems, and major stumbling blocks confronted by systems operators relate to the quality of data sources and timely data collection and recording. An analysis of the degree of development of nine core information systems functions studied by the PAHO/WHO Health Services Information Systems Resources Survey showed that nearly all countries conduct systematic health data collection, recording, and archiving, based on norms and standards defined at the national level (Table 1).

Most of the information collected refers to services provided and epidemiological surveillance. In two-thirds of the countries it was considered to be of intermediate level of detail and data organization, in about one-sixth to be of low level of detail and data organization, and in only 12 to 16% of cases considered to be advanced. Significantly, data related to users and their families, the environment, health risk factors, user satisfaction with health services and violence to women and children were not collected or sporadically collected in about two-thirds of the countries surveyed. When data are processed and information is available, its utilization by health professionals is another important problem. Of the seven areas of application studied, the level of information use was reported consistently as absent or low. In the area of service evaluation and support to service operation, the level of utilization was considered to be intermediate to advanced in one-third of the countries. Significantly, very little use is made of data in the areas of clinical decision-making, cost of service, and clinical and administrative research (Table 2).

E

Table 1. Degree of Development of Nine Core Information Function Activities in Twenty-four Latin American and Caribbean Countries in 1996 Categorized by Level of Detail and Data Organization and Expressed as Percentage of Respondents

CORE INFORMATION FUNCTION	ABSENT	LOW	INTERMEDIATE	ADVANCED
Systematic data collection following national standards	4.2	20.6	62.5	12.5
Recording and archiving	4.2	12.5	66.7	16.7
Information about services provided	0.0	20.8	62.5	16.7
Information about users and their families	29.2	50.0	20.8	0.0
Information related to epidemiological surveillance	0.0	12.5	75.0	12.5
Information about the environment	12.5	41.7	37.5	8.3
Information about health risk factors	20.8	50.0	25.0	4.2
Information about violence (women and children)	20.8	70.8	8.3	0.0
Information about user satisfaction with health services	25.0	54.2	20.8	0.0

Table 2. Utilization of Data and Information by Areas of Application in Twenty-four Latin American and Caribbean Countries in 1996 Categorized by Level of Utilization Expressed as Percentage of Respondents

AREA OF APPLICATION	ABSENT	LOW	INTERMEDIATE	ADVANCED
Type of service provided	16.7	62.5	16.7	4.2
Support to service operation	4.2	58.3	33.3	4.2
Clinical decision-making	25.0	50.0	25.0	0.0
Evaluation of service processes	12.5	54.2	29.2	4.2
Evaluation of staff performance	33.3	41.7	25.0	0.0
Cost of services	45.8	29.2	16.7	8.3
Clinical and administrative research	37.5	50.0	12.5	0.0

Countries are confronted with continuing constraints in their infrastructure for the generation, analysis, summarization, reporting, communication, and especially in using health data and information for the better management of their health programs and services. In summary, the following problems and constraints characterize most of the information systems in the Region:

- Requirements for data recording and reporting by service staff are excessive in that much of the required data are not used in the tasks they perform in case and facility management, with the result that there is an unnecessary recording and reporting burden on service staff.

Such extensive reporting also leads to great amounts of data accumulating at all levels of the system, little of which are analyzed and used;

- Lack of awareness by health policy-makers and program managers of the strategic importance and practical usefulness of health information for planning and management results in low demand for information;

- Data routinely reported by health services are considered of dubious quality in terms of validity and completeness, and therefore are frequently not relied upon;

- Data on the health of those without access to services, or who use private sector services are missing from government-run health information systems;

- There is increasing use of general and special-purpose surveys, often supported by international agencies, to capture data, some of which should be available within routine reporting systems. Such surveys further lessen reliance on the routine data;

- In many countries, disease surveillance systems do not function adequately;

- Data capture at the point of care, and data entry or recording in manual or automated databases represent two significant problem areas in health data management;

- Despite considerable investment in computers and data processing, inadequate use is being made of available technological options for the better management and communications of health data;

- Various departments, programs, and institutions within the health sector tend to develop their own data collection systems. Effective coordination of health information is often lacking, which results in duplication and gaps in data collection, reporting, use, and management;

- Analysis, reporting, and feedback of health data and information from the central level to the services are rare and not well prepared, and reports to international agencies are inconsistent and dominate the indicators promoted by the agencies, which may not be relevant for national use;

- The greatest need remains the establishment of information systems that enable the recovery of patient-oriented, problem-oriented, and procedure-oriented data to assist in the assessment of the impact of health services on the health status of individuals and populations.

E

E.4.2. Education and Training in Health Informatics

Nearly one-third of the countries do not have training programs in health information systems for mid-level and higher management. When programs do exist, in half of the countries they are considered inadequate (Table 3). In about two-thirds of the countries training is conducted at the local, regional, and national levels. Very few countries participate in international training schemes.

Table 3. Degree of Development of User Training in the Generation and Utilization of Information in Twenty-four Latin American and Caribbean Countries in 1996 Categorized by Level of Management Expressed as Percentage of Respondents

MANAGEMENT LEVEL	ABSENT	LOW	INTERMEDIATE	ADVANCED
Operative Level	13.0	52.2	30.4	4.3
Mid-Level Administration	26.1	43.5	26.1	4.3
Higher Management	26.1	43.5	21.7	8.7

E.4.3. Hospital Information Systems

The hospital subsector is the area better served by information systems. Of the 16,566 hospitals registered in PAHO's Directory of Latin American and Caribbean Hospitals database, 6,267 (37.83%) indicated that they had formal information systems in place. Of these, a total of 5,230 hospitals (83.45%) reported using computers (or 31.57% of the 16,566 hospitals). Table 4 presents details of the legal ownership of hospital institutions.

Table 4. Legal Ownership of 16,566 Hospitals and of 6,267 Hospitals with Formal Information Systems in Latin America and the Caribbean, period 1995-1997 (Percent Values Refer to the Total Number of Facilities in each Group)

GROUP OWNERSHIP	NO INFO SYST		WITH INFO SYST		WITH COMPUTERS		ALL FACILITIES	
	No.	%	No.	%	Total	%	No.	%
Public Non-Social Security	4,952	48.08	1,546	24.67	1,399	26.74	6,498	39.22
Public Social Security	409	3.97	467	7.45	438	8.37	876	5.29
Private	4,073	39.55	3,710	59.20	2,859	54.66	7,783	46.98
Philanthropic	770	7.47	514	8.20	505	9.65	1,284	7.75
Military	95	0.92	30	0.47	29	0.55	125	0.75
Total	10,229	100.0	6,267	100.0	5,230	100.0	16,566	100.0

Considering all facilities, public hospitals, including those of the social security, account for 44.51%; private 46.98%; philanthropic 7.75% and military the remaining 0.75%. There are, however, significant differences in the existence of information systems among institutions according to ownership. Of hospitals reporting having information systems, in terms of absolute numbers, nearly 60% are private and slightly less than one-third are public (32.1%).

The relative distribution of information systems and computer utilization provides a different picture. Although the social security hospital facilities constitute only 5.29% of all establishments, they proportionally (Table 5) have the higher number of information systems, 467 out of 876 (53.31%), followed by private (47.67%), philanthropic (40.03%), military (24%), and public non-social security (23.79%).

Table 5. Proportion of Hospitals with Information Systems by Ownership Category

OWNERSHIP	HOSPITALS	INFO SYST	PROPORTION	COMPUTERS	% COMPUTERS
Public Non-Social Security	6,498	1,546	23.79	1,399	90.49
Public Social Security	876	467	53.31	438	93.79
Private	7,783	3,710	47.67	2,859	77.06
Philanthropic	1,284	514	40.03	505	98.24
Military	125	30	24.0	29	96.66

It is noteworthy that above 93% of the social security hospitals with information systems are computerized. The disparity between the existence of information systems in the two types of public hospitals, public social security and public non-social security, is evident, even though the relative percentage of computer utilization is not that great.

Only about 40% of philanthropic hospitals have information systems. However, considered as a group, computer utilization is highest (98.24%) in this category, followed by military (96.66%) and public hospitals (91.25%). Private hospitals reported having information systems, on the other hand, have the lowest utilization of computers (77.06%).

Figure 4 shows the distribution, as percentage, of Latin American and Caribbean hospitals regarding their number of beds. In Table 6 the absolute and percent values of hospitals and beds are presented according to categories of hospital size in the 15,479 hospitals that reported bed number.

Of all hospitals, 10,027 (60.53%), representing 20% of all beds, have 50 or fewer beds. Of those, 5,621 (56%) are private, 3,806 (37.95%) are public, 529 (5.27%) are philanthropic, and 71 (0.7%) are military. It is important to note that 60% of all beds are in hospitals with 200 or fewer beds. Smaller hospitals have fewer information systems in place but it is noteworthy that again, social security and private small hospitals (50 or fewer beds) have a high proportion of institutions with systems that parallels that of larger hospitals (Table 7).

E

Figure 4. Distribution of Hospital Size (Number of Beds) in 16,566 Hospitals of Latin America and the Caribbean

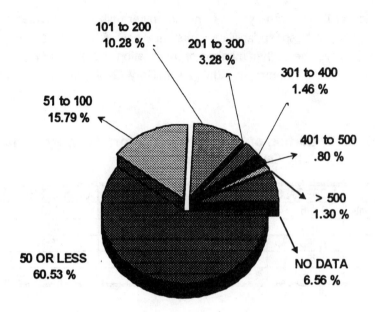

Table 6. Proportion of Hospitals and Beds According to Hospital Size

Hospital Size (Beds)	Hospitals		Beds	
	No.	%	No.	%
1-50	10,027	60.5	219,383	20.0
51-100	2,615	15.8	189,559	17.3
101-200	1,703	10.3	242,770	22.1
201-300	544	3.3	133,225	12.1
301-400	242	1.5	84,811	7.7
401-500	133	0.8	58,951	5.4
501-1000	186	1.1	126,169	11.5
>1000	29	0.2	43,097	3.9
Total	15,479	93.4	1,097,965	100.0
No Data	1,087	6.5		
Grand Total	16,566	100.0		

Source: HSP/HSO Directory of Latin America and Caribbean Hospitals, 1996-1997. Data not available for 1,087 hospitals (of which 885 or 81.4% are in Argentina)

Table 7. Hospitals with 1-50 Beds and Information Systems
by Ownership Category

OWNWERSHIP	HOSPITALS	1-50 BEDS	PROPORTION	INFO SYST	% INFO SYST
Public Non-Social Security	6,498	3,382	52.04	603	17.82
Public Social Security	876	424	48.40	199	46.93
Private	7,783	5,621	72.22	2,325	41.36
Philanthropic	1,284	529	41.19	120	22.68
Military	125	71	56.80	5	7.04

Table 8 shows the distribution of hospitals with and without information systems categorized by grouping countries considering the percentage of institutions with information systems. Group 3, which includes countries with information systems in 31% to 50% of their hospitals, comprises the largest number of instances, 5,447 institutions, which represent 39.96% of 13,630 hospitals (82.27% of the total number of hospitals in the database).

The representative countries in this group, ordered by number of implemented institutions, include: Brazil, Mexico, Argentina, Colombia, Chile, and Paraguay. Only 439 institutions (7% of the hospitals with information systems) comprise Groups 1 and 2 (countries with information systems in more than 51% of their facilities). Most information systems are automated, of the 6,267 institutions with information systems, and 5,230 (83.45%) have computers. There are, however, no details available regarding type and level of implemented applications.

It is interesting to note that there is no association of clinical residency programs and the existence of information systems — of the total universe of 16,566 hospitals, 5,764 (34.79%) have clinical residency while of the 6,267 hospitals with information systems, only 1,735 (27.68%) indicated having residency programs.

E.4.4. Implementation Issues

A review of the experience shows that there is a broad spectrum of possible applications that can take advantage of current technology and there are many options for each application area. The selection of one or other technological option will depend on existing infrastructure and local requirements.

Chief concerns regarding the development and implementation of health information systems applications, is the search for solutions to infrastructure problems, user interfaces, and health-specific developments. Another significant issue in most developing countries, besides access to technology, relates to the availability, level, quality and cost of technical staff support and technical services.

E

Table 8. Information Systems in 16,566 Hospitals of Latin America and the Caribbean Grouped by Percentage of Hospitals with Systems

GROUP	COUNTRY	TOTAL NUMBER HOSPITALS	% TOTAL No. HOSP	WITHOUT INFO SYS	WITH INFO SYSTEM NUMBER HOSPITALS	% WITH IS	WITH COMPUTER NUMBER HOSPITALS	% WITH COMPUTER
Group 1 – Above 71%	TURKS & CAICOS	1	0.006	0	1	100.00	1	100.00
	BAHAMAS	5	0.030	1	4	80.00	4	80.00
	PUERTO RICO	90	0.543	20	70	77.78	64	71.11
	Subtotal Group 1	96	0.580	21	75	78.13	69	71.88
Group 2 – Between 51-70%	GUADELOUPE	10	0.060	4	6	60.00	6	60.00
	URUGUAY	111	0.670	45	66	59.46	66	59.46
	PERU	443	2.674	180	263	59.37	262	59.14
	COSTA RICA	33	0.199	14	19	57.58	19	57.58
	NETH ANTILLES	11	0.066	5	6	54.55	6	54.55
	BERMUDA	2	0.012	1	1	50.00	1	50.00
	MARTINIQUE	6	0.036	3	3	50.00	3	50.00
	Subtotal Group 2	616	3.718	252	364	59.09	363	58.93
Group 3 – Between 31-50%	PARAGUAY	236	1.425	121	115	48.73	57	24.15
	MEXICO	3033	18.309	1603	1430	47.15	693	22.85
	COLOMBIA	1053	6.356	618	435	41.31	417	39.60
	BRAZIL	6124	36.967	3786	2338	38.18	2313	37.77
	CHILE	385	2.324	241	144	37.40	144	37.40
	ARGENTINA	2780	16.781	1801	979	35.22	812	29.21
	ST LUCIA	6	0.036	4	2	33.33	2	33.33
	SURINAME	13	0.078	9	4	30.77	4	30.77
	Subtotal Group 3	13630	82.277	8183	5447	39.96	4442	32.59
Group 4 – Between 11-30%	EL SALVADOR	77	0.465	54	23	29.87	23	29.87
	HONDURAS	89	0.537	66	23	25.84	23	25.84
	PANAMA	55	0.332	41	14	25.45	13	23.64
	GUATEMALA	145	0.875	109	36	24.83	36	24.83
	VENEZUELA	348	2.101	271	77	22.13	54	15.52
	US VIRGIN ISLANDS	23	0.139	18	5	21.74	5	21.74
	ECUADOR	299	1.805	240	59	19.73	59	19.73
	NICARAGUA	78	0.471	66	12	15.38	12	15.38
	CUBA	243	1.467	206	37	15.23	37	15.23
	BOLIVIA	385	2.324	327	58	15.06	58	15.06
	DOMINICAN REPUBLIC	213	1.286	183	30	14.08	30	14.08
	BARBADOS	8	0.048	7	1	12.50	1	12.50
	Subtotal Group 4	1963	11.850	1588	375	19.10	351	17.88
Group 5 – Less 10%	BELIZE	10	0.060	9	1	10.00	1	10.00
	HAITI	103	0.622	99	4	3.88	3	2.91
	TRINIDAD & TOBAGO	64	0.386	63	1	1.56	1	1.56
	Subtotal Group 5	177	1.068	171	6	3.39	5	2.82
Group 6 – None	ANGUILLA	2	0.012	2	0	0.00	0	0.00
	ANTIGUA & BARBUDA	3	0.018	3	0	0.00	0	0.00
	BRITISH VIRGIN ISLANDS	2	0.012	2	0	0.00	0	0.00
	DOMINICA	1	0.006	1	0	0.00	0	0.00
	GRENADA	5	0.030	5	0	0.00	0	0.00
	GUYANA	35	0.211	35	0	0.00	0	0.00
	JAMAICA	31	0.187	31	0	0.00	0	0.00
	MONTSERRAT	1	0.006	1	0	0.00	0	0.00
	ST KITTS & NEVIS	3	0.018	3	0	0.00	0	0.00
	ST VINCENT & GRENADINES	1	0.006	1	0	0.00	0	0.00
	Subtotal Group 6	84	0.507	84	0	0	0	0.00
	TOTAL	16566		10299	6267	37.83	5230	31.57

Source: Directory of Latin American and Caribbean Hospitals, 1996-1997 (PAHO/WHO Div. Health Systems and Services Development)

Technology assessment is too important to be left to technologists, medical specialists, and service providers alone, as they have a tendency to focus exclusively on innovations with narrow applications. Appropriateness of the technology, cultural and language issues, models of healthcare institutional organization and delivery, and acceptance and cost-benefit of systems are major concerns of developers and users. They all play a fundamental part in the selection, form of implementation, and operation of informatics and telecommunications applications. The fact is that although the lack of information systems has been shown to be one reason for inequalities of access and care quality among individuals and society groups, the inappropriate implementation of applications may indeed widen the gulf between the haves and the have-nots.

E.4.5. *Sustainability of Initiatives*

A retrospective of project experiences shows that continuity and sustainability of information systems projects continue to be a major problem in the Region. A common observation is that externally funded projects frequently collapse upon funding termination, and this fact demonstrates that all projects need justification in terms of cost-benefit and long-term financial sustainability besides organizational capacity to develop and implement information systems. This further indicates that spreading the financial risk across several stakeholders may be appropriate, as cost-sharing increases overall awareness, utilization, and long-term potential for success.

E.4.5.1. Technological Infrastructure

Investment in information systems and technology must be linked to the right strategy to achieve long-term benefits. Greater value and longer life cycles of application products can be achieved in information systems projects when effort is directed to technology-independent development of common information functions, data standards, and data manipulation methods established across all applications.

E.4.5.2. Systems Specification Issues

A major problem in systems specification refers to persistent ambiguity in objectives and functions wanted — health sector applications may reflect the chronic problems of the sector: lack of agreement on priorities, lack of a coordinated approach to problem solving, poor definition of contents of care, and lack of definition of minimum data sets to support decision-making. Failing to resolve ambiguity in application development represents a serious risk and may surface as organizational conflicts, low usability, and inappropriateness.

A shared mission statement, robust requirements process, peer reviews of critical specifications, and user involvement in the design process will go a long way to prevent future problems. Given today's rapid and often unpredictable changes in the economics of health, in the organization and strategies of health services, the growing competitiveness among healthcare providers, and the changing of

E

information requirements, health organizations must realistically expect that their information systems will be changing accordingly.

An appropriate systems specification process addresses the logical requirements of systems and avoids the temptation of technology-driven or imposed development solutions. The objective is to detach issues related to the physical implementation of an informatics solution, with its questions of software and hardware platform options, functional access, and actual application development, from the more permanent logical "knowledge" assets, represented by information structures standardized at a higher level of the systems architecture.

The aim of the model is to separate long-term knowledge assets from the implementation environment-associated short-term technological assets, particular procedures, hardware, and code-related issues. This will leave room for autonomy regarding physical systems development, implementation, and adaptation to user needs. The idea, therefore, is to be able to carry the knowledge-sharing assets of systems specification across different generations of systems without suffering from losses due to technology-induced innovations, for instance, the introduction of a new database management platform or operating system, and to avoid being caught in a short-term reactive behavior dictated by the "*du jour*" technological option.

E.4.5.3. Promoting the Use of Common Specification Standards

When designing health applications the aim should be to promote the utilization of an agreed common set of functional and data content specifications standards defined for the whole health sector at a national or even international level, as has been the case in the European Union. It involves the definition of the characteristics of systems application modules, functionalities desired, and the selection of core data elements in the context of an integrated, scalable, and platform-independent logical solution.

Appropriateness of the technology, cultural and language issues, models of healthcare institutional organization and delivery, acceptance, and systems cost-benefit are major concerns of developers and users. They all play a fundamental part in the selection, form of implementation, and operation of informatics applications.

Use of common specification standards will enable health application developers to draw on a pool of common knowledge and avoid redundant or repetitive developments. Such specifications will help the exchange of data across different providers, financing agents, and governmental agencies. They will further assist systems professionals to focus on any particular area of application using a general framework that will ensure consistency across different applications — this is especially valuable for the drive toward corporate approaches to management and integration of information systems and longer application life cycles.

By providing consistent specifications for all application areas, common systems standards also will leave developers and users free to concentrate on the issues that are particular to each implementation environment, such as local priorities and organizational structures.

E.4.5.4. Access to Technology

A significant issue in Latin America and the Caribbean continues to be access to technology and the availability, level, quality, and cost of telecommunication services. The technology infrastructure is generally poor compared to other regions. The human and organizational resources and capabilities and the level of technological development of providers and consumers vary widely among different countries. In most places only few computers or old generation equipment are available to direct patient care users, and generally most health professionals lack basic computer knowledge.

Frequently, there is an obsolete telecommunications infrastructure with low coverage as well as poor quality of communication lines. Although monopolies are gradually disappearing, or being significantly reduced, many countries still have a monopolistic telecommunications market with regulations and tariff structures that inhibit the utilization of the type of services that are required by health and healthcare telecommunications applications.

Only in a small number of countries and, even in those, in only limited geographical areas is the telecommunications infrastructure capable of supporting cost-effective broad-band applications. In most healthcare sites only few computers or old generation equipment is available to direct patient care professionals and, throughout the health sector, there is poor knowledge of the potentialities of computers. Most health information implementations found in the health sector in Latin America and the Caribbean correspond to applications directed towards the automation of the "back-office" and a limited number of "front-office" functions.

The information infrastructure of Latin America and the Caribbean is poorly developed and ranks just above that of Africa and some Eastern European countries but, although information technology expenditures in Latin America and the Caribbean represent only about 5% of the world total (Figure 5), the growth of information technology in the region has been consistently the world's highest since 1985 (Figure 6).

Figure 7 shows the ranking of five regions (North America, Latin America and the Caribbean, Western Europe, Eastern Europe/Middle East/Africa, and Asia/Pacific) regarding the Information Society Index (ISI), which considers the information infrastructure as developed by World Times, Inc. and the International Data Corporation, and the Expenditures in Information Technology as percentage of the Gross Domestic Product (IT$/GDP).

Major problems to be dealt with relate to the disparity among Latin America and Caribbean countries regarding technological infrastructure, investment capability, and consistency of political support to ensure continuity of projects and adequate flow of resources to purchase and maintain relatively expensive capital equipment, products, and services. The design and deployment of information systems is complicated by the complexity and variety of objectives, functions, and technical contents of the health systems as they necessarily must be aligned to the institutional goals.

E

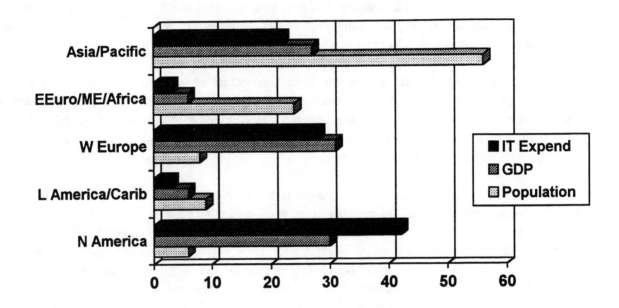

Figure 5. Information Technology Expenditures, Gross Domestic Product and Population as Percentage for Five World Regions (source: International Data Corporation, 1996)

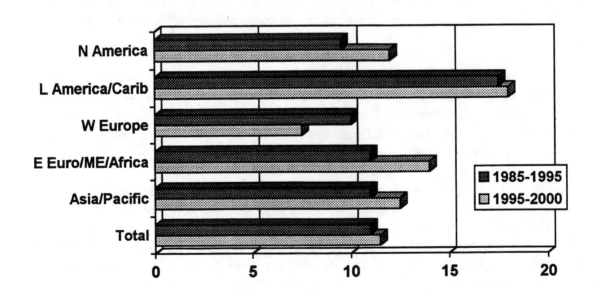

Figure 6. Information Technology Growth 1985-1995 and 1995-2000 (source: International Data Corporation, 1996)

Figure 7. Information Society Index and IT Expenditure/GDP Ranking for World Regions and for Selected Latin American Countries

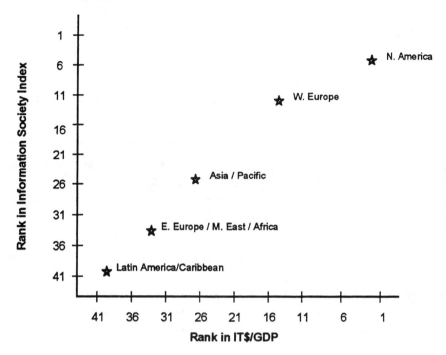

SOURCE: International Data Corporation, 1996

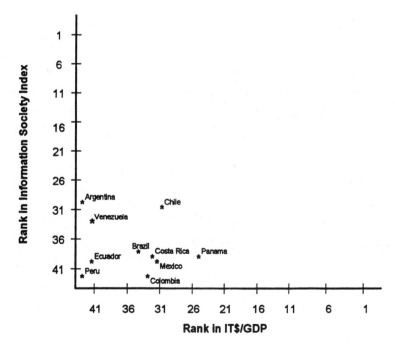

SOURCE: International Data Corporation, 1996

Many Ministries have embarked on the computerization of their services, aiming at providing better information for management and service delivery. Most of the initiatives have been centralized in health information units, but there is a growing tendency towards decentralization. However, systems rarely have been implemented at the level of primary or community care centers. These systems have positively impacted on the timeliness and accuracy in retrieving data and information about service utilization, patient flow, resource utilization, disease surveillance, morbidity and mortality patterns, and in the operation of healthcare and ancillary services. In the Eastern Caribbean a major project funded by the Inter American Development Bank was initiated in 1995 with the objective of deploying community health services information systems, but its impact is still to be evaluated.

Countries with on-going information systems projects of significance which consider a broader scope of information utilization include: Argentina, Chile, Uruguay, Brazil, Bolivia, Venezuela, Colombia, Barbados, Belize, Grenada, St. Vincent and the Grenadines, St. Lucia, Dominica, Jamaica, Cuba, Panama, Guatemala, Costa Rica, and Mexico. In Costa Rica, Chile, Brazil, and Mexico important telecommunications-based projects have been recently initiated.

In the past three years there has been a brisk growth of the Internet connectivity in the Latin America and the Caribbean, as measured by the number of hosts (164,051 by January 1997) registered under the corresponding geographic domain. Although the numbers do not reflect the real total number of hosts in each country, because organizational domain hosts were not included in the above figure, they demonstrate the growing number of hosts in every country.

An analysis of the distribution of Internet hosts exhibits wide variation, which becomes more evident when one considers the corresponding country population — the number of inhabitants per host being a good indicator of the penetration of Internet-related technologies in Latin American and Caribbean Region (Table 9). The number of telephone lines per 100 inhabitants is still low (average 11.69 lines per 100 persons) when, for example, compared to the U.S. (57.4 per 100 persons) or Canada (59.2 per 100 persons). The same is valid for television and radio receivers for 1,000 inhabitants. Increased connectivity and access to the Internet will require major expansion of the telecommunications infrastructure in nearly all countries.

Table 9. Geographic Internet Domain Hosts, Telephone Lines, and Television and Radio Receivers in Selected Latin American and Caribbean Countries Ranked by Population/Host Index

COUNTRIES	POPULATION x 1,000	REGISTERED HOSTS	% TOTAL	POPULATION PER HOST	TELEPHONES PER 100 PERS	TV RECEIVERS PER 1,000 PERS	RADIO RECEIVERS PER 1,000 PERS
ANTIGUA	66	169	0.103	47	28.9	356	417
CHILE	14,641	15,885	9.683	922	11.0	210	344
COSTA RICA	3,575	3,491	2.128	1,024	11.1	141	258
DOMINICA	71	55	0.034	1,291	19.1	72	587
BAHAMAS	284	195	0.119	1,456	30.3	225	592
URUGUAY	3,221	1,823	1.111	1,767	16.8	166	232
BRAZIL	167,046	77,148	47.027	2,165	7.5	208	386
ARGENTINA	35,405	12,688	7.734	2,790	12.3	221	683
MEXICO	97,245	29,840	18.189	3,259	8.8	149	255
DOMINICAN REPUBLIC	8,098	2,301	1.403	3,519	7.4	87	171
PANAMA	2,722	751	0.458	3,625	10.2	167	224
COLOMBIA	36,200	9,054	5.519	3,998	11.3	117	177
PERU	24,691	5,192	3.165	4,756	2.9	98	254
ST LUCIA	146	21	0.013	6,952	15.4	190	759
NICARAGUA	4,731	531	0.324	8,910	1.7	66	262
VENEZUELA	22,777	2,417	1.473	9,424	9.9	163	448
TRINIDAD & TOBAGO	1,335	141	0.086	9,468	15.0	316	494
JAMAICA	2,483	249	0.152	9,972	10.6	134	421
BARBADOS	264	21	0.013	12,571	31.8	280	876
HONDURAS	5,981	408	0.249	14,659	2.1	73	387
GUYANA	854	52	0.032	16,423	5.1	40	493
BOLIVIA	7,774	430	0.262	18,079	3.0	103	613
ECUADOR	11,937	590	0.360	20,232	5.3	85	318
ST KITTS & NEVIS	41	2	0.001	20,500	29.6	206	648
PARAGUAY	5,220	187	0.114	27,914	3.1	52	66
GUATEMALA	11,241	274	0.167	41,026	2.3	82	171
EL SALVADOR	6,027	132	0.080	45,659	3.2	93	413
SURINAME	432	4	0.002	108,000	11.6	132	639
	474,508	164,051	100	2,892 (a)	11.69 (a)	151.14 (a)	413.86 (a)

- Internet Hosts represents the number of hosts registered under geographic domains and does not include hosts registered in organizational domains (.com, .org, .net, etc.). Data for January 1997.
- Data for telephone lines are for 1993
- Data for television and radio receivers are for 1992

(a) Average values

Sources: Organization of American States RedHUCyT Project United Nations 1995 Statistical Yearbook (40th Edition)

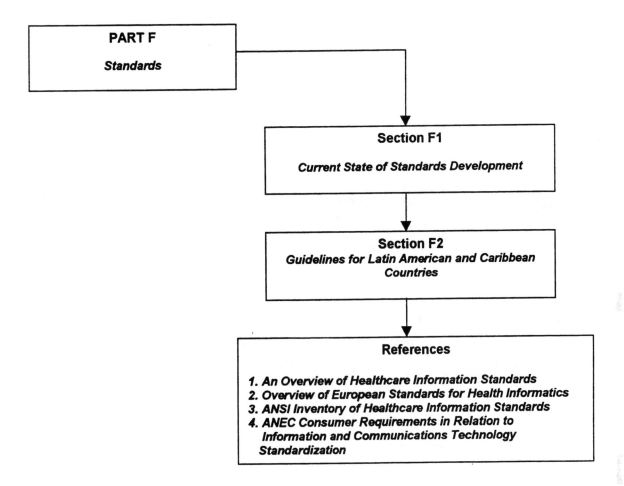

PART F

Standards

Section F1

Current State of Standards Development

Section F2
Guidelines for Latin American and Caribbean Countries

References

1. An Overview of Healthcare Information Standards
2. Overview of European Standards for Health Informatics
3. ANSI Inventory of Healthcare Information Standards
4. ANEC Consumer Requirements in Relation to Information and Communications Technology Standardization

F

Part F. Standards

F

Part F. Standards

*Ideals are like stars; you will not succeed in touching them with your hands.
But like the seafaring man on the desert of waters, you choose them
as your guides, and following them you will reach your destiny.*

Carl Schurz (1829–1906)

The dramatic changes in the healthcare industry discussed thus far have led to an increased sense of urgency in the development of new healthcare delivery models, broad organizational restructuring, and the redesign of healthcare administrative and clinical processes. These changes are also creating new demands for healthcare information technology. In particular, the drive to open systems architectures is gaining speed throughout the world. In health as in other data transmission application fields, users generally demand open, distributed, interconnected, highly reliable, and inter-operable systems, with increasingly stringent security requirements. The integrated management of health services and the continuity of medical care require the adoption of commonly accepted messages, formats, codification, and medical record structure.

F.1. Current State of Standards Development

One of the characteristics of health data transmission applications is the integration of technologies, information, and communication systems. The role of standards in traditional sectors is well known. Well-founded arguments exist for considering similar effects for the application to health, an area characterized by market fragmentation, the proliferation of incompatible applications, the high costs of developing individual solutions, a short life cycle, maintenance problems, and the barriers to achieving the operative integration of different and isolated systems. Logically, the coordination of this sector and the adoption of common standards for users, manufacturers, and service providers would seem likely to foster the production of more cost-effective and stable solutions.

The central element of open systems, therefore, is the use of standards. Without easy, reliable, approved ways to connect the necessary components, open systems cannot work. Within the healthcare industry there are a number of categories of information that each have separate standards. They are listed here, along with a brief description of the category, and applicable examples of well-known standards:

- *Identifier Standards* - These are themselves subdivided into patient, provider, site-of-care, and product. Not surprisingly, there is no universal acceptance and/or satisfaction with these systems.

F

- *Communications (Message Format) Standards* - Although the standards in this area are still in various stages of development, they are generally more mature than those of the other groups.

- *Content and Structure Standards* - Work in this area is primarily directed at developing standards for the design of the Computer-based Patient Record, and on dental records.

- *Clinical Data Representations (Codes)* - These are widely used to document diagnoses and procedures. There are over 150 known coding systems, such as the International Classification of Diseases (ICD) system, promoted by the World Health Organization. The Current Procedural Terminology (CPT) coding system is promoted in the United States by the American Medical Association (AMA). Another common standard for medical terms is the Systematized Nomenclature of Human and Veterinary Medicine (SNOMED). It has eleven separate axes for categorizing semantic relationships among medical terms. Laboratory Observation Identifier Names and Codes (LOINC) has been developed to create universal test codes for laboratory results and observation messages.

- *Confidentiality, Data Security, and Authentication* - The development of both the Computer-based Patient Record and Healthcare Networks has spurred the need for more definitive confidentiality, data security, and authentication guidelines and standards. Numerous activities are underway to address these issues.

- *Quality Indicators, Data Sets, and Guidelines* - Although there is not an accredited standard to measure healthcare quality, there are several quality indicators, data sets, and guidelines that are gaining acceptance. In the United States the Health Plan Employer Data and Information Set (HEDIS) has been developed with the support of the National Committee for Quality Assurance (NCQA). It identifies data to support performance measurement in the areas of quality, access and patient satisfaction, membership and utilization, and finance.

- *International Standards* - The International Organization for Standardization (ISO) is a worldwide federation of national standards organizations. It has 90 member countries. The purpose of ISO is to promote the development of standardization and related activities in the world. To this end there are many organizations, committees, and subgroups which promote the evolution of healthcare standards worldwide.

From a healthcare standards perspective, the area of standards is in constant flux and one must be attentive to the evolution of the recommendations of the international and national technical agencies and professional organizations that work on standards research. The knowledgeable healthcare executive will do well to stay current on healthcare standards development. In addition, vendors demonstrating present and future commitment to standards are those most likely to survive in the very competitive healthcare IS&T marketplace, and should be given top consideration by healthcare enterprises in the process of systems selection.

F.2. Guidelines for Latin American and Caribbean Countries

In light of the inexorable move towards standards development and convergence, Latin American and Caribbean countries should take steps, individually and collectively, to foster the development and acceptance of internationally agreed IS&T standards, in order to facilitate the advantages of standards-based systems.

It is evident that the harmonious operation of disparate modules provided by different manufacturers is possible only if specific standards are adhered to, in the technical context of information systems and communications as well as in that of medicine. The definition of the clinical record, including aspects of its structure, semantics, codification, etc., are also important questions that cry out for standardization, without which the desired degree of interoperability would be impossible.

Finally, the issue is germane to specific security issues that address medical ethics, not to mention legislative implications, especially in the case of Latin America. In the Region the policies and elements related to health information infrastructure show an evident delay in comparison with developed countries, which results in a formal limitation not only to provide more economic and steadier solutions but for the performance of coordinated health policies and plans. The area of standards offers the opportunity to consider the elements which primary care information systems should contain. Very soon multimedia facilities will be integrated in the design of these systems with the objective of facilitating patient care and reducing costs.

The evolution of standards will depend on the attitude developed by all stakeholders. This is a particularly important time, given the revolution occurring in the information world in which we are immersed. In the commercial sector, companies that remain indifferent to the standardization process and allow others to decide its key aspects run the serious risk of being excluded from any possibility for competitiveness. Moreover, health institution administrators that are indifferent to the standardization processes may see their investments endangered and themselves burdened by technological solutions inappropriate for their real needs.

F

REFERENCE 1

AN OVERVIEW OF HEALTHCARE INFORMATION STANDARDS

Jeffrey S. Blair, Program Manager, IBM Healthcare Solutions, Atlanta, Georgia

INTRODUCTION

The rising cost of health care throughout the world has created an urgency to improve healthcare productivity and quality. This sense of urgency has led to the development of new healthcare delivery models, broad organizational restructuring, and the redesign of healthcare business and clinical processes. Not only are these changes redefining the healthcare environment, they are also creating a demand for a new healthcare information infrastructure.

The creation of this healthcare information infrastructure requires the integration of existing and new architectures, application systems, and services. Core elements of this infrastructure include patient-centered care facilitated by Computer-based Patient Record (CPR) systems, continuity of care enabled by the sharing of patient information across information networks, and outcomes measurement aided by the greater availability and specificity of healthcare information.

To make these diverse components work together, healthcare information standards (classifications, guides, practices, and terminology) are required. This article gives you an overview of the major existing and emerging healthcare information standards, as well as the efforts to coordinate, harmonize, and accelerate these standards activities. It is organized into the following topics:

- Identifier standards
- Communications (message format) standards
- Content and structure standards
- Clinical data representations (codes)
- Confidentiality, data security, and authentication
- Quality indicators, data sets, and guidelines
- International standards
- Standards coordination and promotion activities

IDENTIFIER STANDARDS

There is a universal need for healthcare identifiers to uniquely specify each patient, provider, site-of-care, and product; however, there is not universal acceptance and/or satisfaction with these systems.

Patient Identifiers

The Social Security Number (SSN) is being considered for use as a patient identifier in the United States today. However, critics point out that it is not an ideal identifier. They say that not everyone has an SSN; several individuals may use the same SSN; and the SSN is so widely used for other 1 purposes that it presents an exposure to violations of confidentiality. On the other hand, it may be some time before funding is available to develop, disseminate, and maintain a more ideal patient identifier.

Two work efforts have emerged to address these issues: ASTM's (formerly known as the American Society for Testing and Materials) E31.12 Subcommittee developed the "Guide for the Properties of a Universal Health Care Identifier (UHID) E1714.95." It presents a set of requirements outlining the properties of a national system creating a UHID, includes critiques of the SSN, and creates a sample UHID (ASTM, 1995). The Computer-based Patient Record Institute's (CPRI's) Codes and Structures Work Group has a Patient Identifier Project Team. This project team has also investigated these issues and is preparing a comprehensive position paper (CPRI, 1995).

Provider Identifiers

The Health Care Financing Administration (HCFA) has created a widely used provider identifier known as the Universal Physician Identifier Number (UPIN) (Terrell et al., 1991). The UPIN is only assigned to physicians who handle Medicare patients. To address this limitation, HCFA is developing the National Provider File (NPF). It will create a new provider identifier for Medicare, which will include all caregivers and sites-of-care. It will also be available for use by Medicaid programs and other government agencies if they decide to adopt it. This new provider identifier is targeted to be available April, 1996. However, there are no plans at this time to extend HCFA's new provider identifier to the private sector (HCFA, 1995).

F

Site-of-Care Identifiers

Two site-of-care identifier systems are widely used. One is the Health Industry Number (HIN), issued by the Health Industry Business Communications Council (HIBCC). The HIN is an identifier for healthcare facilities, practitioners, and retail pharmacies. HCFA has also defined provider of service identifers for Medicare usage. Both HCFA's provider of service identifer and the UPIN identifier will be replaced by HCFA's National Provider File for Medicare usage (HIBCC, 1994).

Product and Supply Labeling Identifiers

Three identifiers are widely accepted. The Labeler Identification Code (LIC) identifies the manufacturer or distributor and is issued by HIBCC (HIBCC, 1994). The LIC is used both with and without bar codes for products and supplies distributed within a healthcare facility. The Universal Product Code (UPC) is maintained by the Uniform Code Council and is typically used to label products that are sold in retail settings. The National Drug Code (NDC) also serves as an identifier and is described later in the Clinical Data Representations section.

COMMUNICATIONS (MESSAGE FORMAT) STANDARDS

Although the standards in this topic area are still in various stages of development, they are generally more mature than those in most of the other topic areas. They are typically developed by committees within standards development organizations (SDOs) and have generally been accepted by users and vendors. The profiles of these standards below were derived from many sources, but considerable content came from the CPRI's "Position Paper on Computer-based Patient Record Standards" (CPRI, 1994), and the Agency for Health Care Policy and Research's (AHCPR's) "Current Activities of Selected Health Care Informatics Standards Organizations" (Moshman Associates, 1995).

- Accredited Standards Committee (ASC) X12N: This committee is developing message format standards for transactions between payors and providers. They are being accepted by both users and vendors. They define the message formats for the following transaction types (DISA, 1995):

  - 148 - Report of Injury, Illness, or Incident
  - 270 - Eligibility, Coverage, or Benefit Inquiry
  - 271 - Eligibility, Coverage, or Benefit Information
  - 276 - Healthcare Claim Status Request
  - 277 - Healthcare Claim Status Notification
  - 278 - Healthcare Service Review Information
  - 834 - Benefit Enrollment and Maintenance
  - 835 - Healthcare Claim Payment/Advice
  - 837 - Healthcare Claim (Submission).

  ASC X12N has also developed the following interactive UN/EDIFACT message standards:

  - X12.345 Interactive Healthcare Eligibility/Benefit Information Message (IHCEBR) - X12.346 Interactive Healthcare Eligibility/Benefit Inquiry Message (IHCEBI).

  ASC X12N is also working on the following standards to be published in the near future:

  - 274 - Healthcare Provider Information
  - 275 - Patient Information.

The above transactions (274 and 275) will be used to request and send patient data (tests, procedures, surgeries, allergies, etc.) between a requesting party and the party maintaining the database. This patient data message format has the ability to encapsulate Health Level 7, ASTM, or American College of Radiology - National Electrical Manufacturers' Association (ACR-NEMA) clinical data (McDonald, 1995).

The secretariat for ASC X12 and the Pan American EDIFACT Board is the Data Interchange Standards Association (DISA). ASC X12N is recognized as an Accredited Standards Committee (ASC) by the American National Standards Institute (ANSI).

- **ASTM Message Format Standards.** The following standards were developed within ASTM Committee E31. This committee is recognized as an accredited organization by ANSI:

  - ASTM E1238 Standard Specification for Transferring Clinical Observations Between Independent Systems: E1238 was developed by ASTM Subcommittee E31.11. This standard is being used by most of the largest commercial laboratory vendors in the United States to transmit laboratory results. It has been incorporated into the Japanese Image Store and Carry (ISAC) standard. Health Level Seven (HL7) has incorporated E1238 as a subset within its laboratory results message format (CPRI, 1994; McDonald, 1995).

  - ASTM E1394 Standard Specification for Transferring Information Between Clinical Instruments: E1394 was developed by ASTM Subcommittee E31.14. This standard is being used for communication of information from laboratory instruments to computer systems. This standard has been developed by a consortium consisting of most U.S. manufacturers of clinical laboratory instruments (CPRI, 1994).

  - ASTM E1460 Specification for Defining and Sharing Modular Health Knowledge Bases (Arden Syntax): E1460 was developed by ASTM Subcommittee E31.15. The Arden Syntax provides a standard format and syntax for representing medical logic and for writing rules and guidelines that can be automatically executed by computer systems. Medical logic modules produced in one site-of-care system can be sent to a different system within another site-of-care and then customized to reflect local usage (CPRI, 1994).

  - ASTM E1467 Specification for Transferring Digital Neurophysical Data Between Independent Computer Systems: E1467 was developed by ASTM Subcommittee E31.16. This standard defines codes and structures needed to transmit electrophysiologic signals and results produced by electroencephalograms (EEG) and electromyograms. The standard is similar in structure to ASTM E1238 and HL7, and it is being adopted by all of the EEG systems manufacturers (CPRI, 1994).

- Digital Imaging and Communications (DICOM): This standard is developed by the American College of Radiology - National Electrical Manufacturers' Association (ACR-NEMA). It defines the message formats and communications standards for diagnostic and therapeutic images. DICOM is supported by most radiology Picture Archiving and Communications Systems (PACS) vendors. It has also been incorporated into the European MEDICOM (Medical Image Communication) standard and the Japanese "second common" standard for medical communications over

F

networks. DICOM medical content is supported by the Japanese Image Store and Carry (ISAC) optical disk system and is being planned for incorporation by Kodak's PhotoCD. ACR-NEMA is considering applying for recognition as an accredited standards committee by ANSI. (CPRI, 1994)

- Health Level Seven (HL7): HL7 defines transactions for transmitting data about patient registration, admission, discharge and transfers, insurance, charges and payors, orders and results for laboratory tests, image studies, nursing and physician observations, diet orders, pharmacy orders, supply orders, and master files. The HL7 standard is supported by most system vendors and used in most large U.S. hospitals today. It also is used in Australia, Austria, Canada, Germany, Israel, Japan, New Zealand, The Netherlands, and the United Kingdom.

  HL7 is also developing transactions to exchange information about appointment scheduling, problem lists, clinical trial enrollments, patient permissions, voice dictation, advanced directives, and physiological signals. Furthermore, task forces in HL7 are developing prototype transactions with new object oriented technologies such as CORBA and Microsoft's OLE objects. HL7 is recognized as an accredited organization by ANSI (CPRI, 1994; McDougall, 1995).

- Institute of Electrical and Electronic Engineers, Inc. (IEEE) P1157 Medical Data Interchange Standard (MEDIX): IEEE Engineering in Medicine and Biology Society (EMB) is developing the MEDIX standards for the exchange of data between hospital computer systems. (Harrington, 1993; CPRI, 1994) Based on the International Standards Organization (ISO) standards for all seven layers of the OSI reference model, MEDIX is working on a framework model to guide the development and evolution of a compatible set of standards. This activity has been carried forward as a joint working group under ANSI HISPP's Message Standards Developers Subcommittee (MSDS), described later in this article. IEEE is recognized as an accredited organization by ANSI.

- IEEE P1073 Medical Information Bus (MIB): This standard defines the linkages of medical instrumentation (e.g., critical care instruments) to point-of-care information systems. (CPRI, 1994)

- National Council for Prescription Drug Programs (NCPDP): This council has developed standards for communication of billing and eligibility information between community pharmacies and third party payors. They have been in use since 1985 and now serve almost 90 percent of the nation's community pharmacies. They are working on standards for adverse drug reactions and utilization review. NCPDP has applied for recognition as an accredited organization by ANSI. (CPRI, 1994; McDonald, 1995).

CONTENT AND STRUCTURE STANDARDS

Guidelines and standards for the content and structure of computer-based patient record systems are being developed within ASTM Subcommittees E31.12 and E31.19. They have been acknowledged by other standards organizations, and they are now beginning to gain some user acceptance.

A major revision to E1384, now called a "Standard Description for Content and Structure of the Computer-based Patient Record," has been made within Subcommittee E31.19. (ASTM, 1994) This revision includes work from HISPP on data modeling and an expanded framework that includes master tables and data views by user. It has been selected as the foundation CPR content requirement in the I/S plans for Group Health Cooperative of Puget Sound, as well as a component in the CPR plans of the Veterans' Administration (VA) (Goverman, 1994).

Companion standards to E1384 have been developed within Subcommittee E31.19. They are:

- E1633, "A Standard Specification for the Coded Values Used in the Automated Primary Record of Care"

- E1239-94, "A Standard Guide for Description of Reservation/Registration-A/D/T Systems for Automated Patient Care Information Systems" (ASTM, 1994).

- E1715-95, "Practice For An Object-Oriented Model for Registration, Admitting, Discharge, and Transfer (RADT) Functions in Computer-based Patient Record Systems."

Within the E31.12 Subcommittee, domain-specific guidelines for emergency room data within the CPR (E1744) are available and domain-specific guidelines for nursing and anesthesiology within the CPR are being developed (Moshman Associates, 1995; Waegemann, 1995)

The newly formed E31.22 Subcommittee on Health Information Transcription and Documentation is developing standards for the processes, systems, and management of medical transcription and its integration with other modalities of report generation.

A Computer-based Oral Health Record (COHR) Concept Model has been developed by the COHR Working Group of the Council on Dental Practice (CDP) of the American Dental Association (ADA). The ADA has released this document for comment. (ADA, 1995).

CLINICAL DATA REPRESENTATIONS (CODES)

Clinical data representations have been widely used to document diagnoses and procedures. There are over 150 known code systems. The codes with the widest acceptance in the United States include:

- International Classification of Diseases (ICD) codes, now in the ninth edition (ICD-9): These codes are maintained by the World Health Organization (WHO) and are accepted worldwide. In the United States, HCFA and the National Center for Health Statistics (NCHS) have supported the development of a clinical modification of the ICD codes (ICD-9-CM). WHO has been developing ICD-10 and HCFA has formed a voluntary technical panel to assist with the development of the ICD-10 Procedure Coding System (ICD-10-PCS). However, HCFA projects that ICD-10 will not be available for use within the United States for a few years. Payors require the use of ICD-9-CM codes for reimbursement purposes, but they have limited value for clinical and research purposes due to their lack of clinical specificity (Chute, 1995).

F

- Current Procedural Terminology (CPT) codes: These codes are maintained by the American Medical Association (AMA) and are widely used in the United States for reimbursement and utilization review purposes. The codes are derived from medical specialty nomenclatures and are updated annually (Chute, 1995).

- The Systematized Nomenclature of Human and Veterinary Medicine (SNOMED) International: This code structure is maintained by the College of American Pathologists (CAP) and is widely accepted for describing pathological test results. It has a multi-axial (eleven fields) coding structure that gives it greater clinical specificity than the ICD and CPT codes, and it has considerable value for clinical purposes. The CAP has begun to coordinate SNOMED development with the message standards organizations HL7 and ACR-NEMA. SNOMED is a leading candidate to become the standardized nomenclature for computer-based patient record systems (Chute, 1995).

- Laboratory Observation Identifier Names and Codes (LOINC): These codes were developed by an ad hoc group of clinical pathologists, chemists, and laboratory service vendors with support from the Hartford Foundation, the NLM, and the AHCPR. The goal of this project is to create universal test codes to be used in the context of existing ASTM E1238 and HL7 Version 2.2 laboratory results and observation messages. The LOINC database contains records representing more than 6300 laboratory observations including chemistry, toxicology, serology, microbiology, and some clinical variables. It is being incorporated into the Unified Medical Language System (UMLS) and is being adopted by at least two medical information system vendors. It is now available for downloading and free public use on the Internet (McDonald, 1995).

- Diagnostic and Statistical Manual of Mental Disorders (DSM), now in its fourth edition (DSM-IV): This code structure is maintained by the American Psychiatric Association (APA). It sets forth a standard set of codes and descriptions for use in diagnoses, prescriptions, research, education, and administration (Chute, 1995).

- Diagnostic Related Groups (DRGs): These codes are maintained by HCFA. They are derivatives of ICD-9-CM codes and are used to facilitate reimbursement and case-mix analysis. They lack the clinical specificity to be of value in direct patient care or clinical research (Chute, 1995).

- The National Drug Code (NDC): This code is maintained by the Food and Drug Administration (FDA) and is required for reimbursement by Medicare, Medicaid, and insurance companies. It is sometimes included within the UPC format.

- Gabrieli Medical Nomenclature (GMN): This nomenclature was developed and is maintained by Computer-based Medicine, Inc. It is designed to represent every medical word or phrase in a canonical or vernacular form that may occur in clinical records. It is a computer-based nomenclature that self-updates with new words. The nomenclature partitions the entire field of medicine into six main branches or axes. It includes 189,000 primary terms and 300,000 synonyms. The Australian Medical Society is testing the GMN (Gabrieli, 1995).

- Unified Medical Language System (UMLS): This system is maintained by the National Library of Medicine (NLM). It contains a metathesaurus that links biomedical terminology, semantics, and formats of the major clinical coding and reference systems. It links medical terms (e.g., ICD, CPT, SNOMED, DSM, CO-STAR, and D-XPLAIN) to the NLM's medical index subject headings (MeSH codes) and to each other. The UMLS also contains a specialist lexicon, a semantic network, and an information sources map. Together, these elements should eventually represent all of the codes, vocabularies, terms, and concepts that will become the foundation for an emerging medical informatics infrastructure. The 1995 UMLS metathesaurus contains 223,000 concepts and 442,000 terms (Cimino et al., 1993; EHRR, 1995).

The Large Scale Testing of Health Vocabularies is a project co-sponsored by the NLM and the AHCPR. It will determine the completeness of the metathesaurus of the UMLS and of the vocabularies that soon will be added to it. At least eight medical institutions are contributing domain-specific medical vocabularies for this project. The test, which is targeted to begin in November of 1995, will probably involve many of these same medical institutions plus several federal and state healthcare departments/agencies. The importance of this test is its potential to define both the framework and much of the content of a common medical vocabulary which would be available for use by developers and vendors of computer-based patient record systems (CPRI, 1995; EHRR, 1995).

An evaluation of clinical code systems has been made by participants of the Codes and Structures Work Group of the CPRI. This work effort was supported in part by NIH grants. It evaluated eight major clinical classifications for their content coverage. This research was based on clinical text from four major medical centers. Although no classification system captured all concepts, SNOMED International demonstrated the highest score in every category. This paper has been reviewed by the CPRI Board of Directors and has been submitted for publication (CPRI, 1995).

CONFIDENTIALITY, DATA SECURITY, AND AUTHENTICATION

The development of computer-based patient record systems and healthcare information networks have created the need for more definitive confidentiality, data security, and authentication guidelines and standards. The following activities address this need:

- The Fair Health Information Practices Act (HR 435), sponsored by Rep. Gary Condit (D-CA), was re-introduced in the House of Representatives in January, 1995. A companion bill, The Healthcare Privacy Protection Act, sponsored by Sen. Robert Bennett (R-UT), is being drafted for introduction in the Senate. These bills address the need for uniform, comprehensive, federal rules governing the use and disclosure of identifiable health information of individuals. They specify the responsibilities of those who collect, use, and maintain health information about patients. They also define the rights of patients and provide a variety of mechanisms that will allow patients to enforce their rights (Frawley, 1995).

F

- ASTM Subcommittee E31.12 on Computer-based Patient Records is developing "Guidelines for Minimal Data Security Measures for the Protection of Computer-based Patient Records" (Moshman Associates, 1995).

- ASTM Subcommittee E31.17 on Access, Privacy, and Confidentiality of Medical Records is working on standards to address these issues. They are expected to be approved by ASTM before the end of 1995 (Moshman Associates, 1995).

- ASTM Subcommittee E31.20 is developing standard specifications for electronic authentication of health information. They are expected to be approved by ASTM before the end of 1995 (Moshman Associates, 1995).

- The Committee on Regional Health Data Networks convened by the Institute of Medicine (IOM) has completed a definitive study and published its findings in a book titled, "Health Data in the Information Age: Use, Disclosure, and Privacy" (Donaldson & Lohr, 1994).

- The Computer-based Patient Record Institute's (CPRI) Work Group on Confidentiality, Privacy, and Security has completed a white paper that addresses access to patient data and another that addresses authentication. (CPRI, 1995) They are also developing a series of guidelines on information security and, as of this date, have published, "Guidelines for Establishing Information Security: Policies at Organizations Using Computer-based Patient Records" (CPRI, 1994), and "Guidelines for Information Security Education Programs at Organizations Using Computer-based Patient Record Systems" (CPRI, 1995).

- The American Association for Medical Transcription (AAMT) is preparing guidelines on confidentiality, privacy, and security of patient care documentation through the process of medical dictation and transcription (Tessier, 1995).

QUALITY INDICATORS, DATA SETS, AND GUIDELINES

Although there is not an accredited standard to measure healthcare quality, there are several quality indicators, data sets, and guidelines which have been developed and are gaining acceptance. They include:

- The Joint Commission on Accreditation of Health Care Organizations (JCAHO) has been developing and testing the Indicator Measurement System (IMSystem). The IMSystem includes 25 indicators addressing obstetrics, perioperative, oncology, trauma, and cardiovascular care. These indicators are intended to facilitate measurements of provider performance. Several vendors are planning to include JCAHO clinical indicators in their performance measurement systems (JCAHO, 1994; JCAHO, 1995).

- The Health Plan Employer Data and Information Set (HEDIS) version 2.0 and 2.5 has been developed with the support of the National Committee for Quality Assurance (NCQA). It identifies data to support performance measurement in the areas of quality (e.g., preventive medicine, prenatal care, acute and chronic disease, and mental health), access and patient satisfaction, membership and utilization, and finance. The development of HEDIS has been supported by several large employers and managed care organizations (NCQA, 1993; NCQA, 1995).

- There are many organizations that have developed practice guidelines/parameters during the last several years. These guidelines have been developed by national, regional, and local organizations, such as professional associations, government agencies, providers, consulting firms, and vendors. The AMA publishes the Directory of Practice Parameters, which includes about 1600 listings (including 100 developed by the AMA) (Business and Health, 1994).

- Within the federal government, the AHCPR has developed 16 practice guidelines written by interdisciplinary panels of practitioners. The AHCPR is within the Public Health Service, which is part of the Department of Health and Human Services.

- Additionally, there are some private organizations which have developed and marketed practice guidelines (Business and Health, 1994). The organizations include:

    - Health Risk Management's Institute for Healthcare Quality: It has developed over 480 diagnosis-based guidelines for more than 2000 treatment options for its self-insured clients nationwide.

    - Value Health Sciences: It has developed the Medical Review System, which uses practice guidelines to evaluate the appropriateness of a proposed procedure. The Medical Review system is being used to pre-certify 34 major medical and surgical procedures for more than 10 million individuals in the United States.

    - Milliman & Robertson, Inc.: It has developed healthcare management guidelines for inpatient and surgical care, return to work planning, ambulatory care, and home health care.

INTERNATIONAL STANDARDS

- The International Organization for Standardization (ISO) is a worldwide federation of national standards organizations. It has 90 member countries. The purpose of ISO is to promote the development of standardization and related activities in the world. ANSI was one of the founding members of ISO and is the representative for the United States (Waegemann, 1995).

    ISO has established a communications model for Open Systems Interconnection (OSI). IEEE/MEDIX and HL7 have recognized and built upon the ISO/OSI framework. Further, ANSI HISPP has stated as one of its objectives the encouragement of U.S. healthcare standards compatibility with ISO/OSI. The ISO activities related to information technology take place within the Joint Technical Committee (JTC) 1.

    A proposal to form an ISO Technical Committee (TC) on Healthcare Informatics, with ANSI as the Secretariat, was presented to ANSI HISPP in August 1995. The ISO TC's scope includes: healthcare models; healthcare records and care functions; privacy, confidentiality,

F

and security; content and structure; concept representations; communications; and application functions. ANSI HISPP declared its intent to support this initiative and plans to review and vote on the actual proposal document by November 1995.

- The Comité Europeen de Normalisation (CEN) is a European standards organization with 16 TCs. Two TCs are specifically involved in health care: TC 251 (Medical Informatics) and TC 224 WG12 (Patient Data Cards) (Waegemann, 1995).

  The CEN TC 251 on Medical Informatics includes work groups on: Modeling of Medical Records; Terminology, Coding, Semantics, and Knowledge Bases; Communications and Messages; Imaging and Multimedia; Medical Devices; and Security, Privacy, Quality, and Safety. The CEN TC 251 has established coordination with healthcare standards development in the United States through ANSI HISPP.

- United Nations (UN) Electronic Data Interchange For Administration, Commerce, and Transport (EDIFACT) is a generic messaging-based communications standard with health-specific subsets. UN/EDIFACT is often parallel to X12 and HL7 in terms of message content, although X12 and HL7 have a different syntax (transaction-based). Recently, X12.345 and X12.346 were developed and are recognized as UN/EDIFACT message format standards. They support interactive healthcare eligibility/information and inquiry. UN/EDIFACT is widely used in Europe and in several Latin American countries. As indicated earlier, the Data Interchange Standards Association, Inc. (DISA) is the Secretariat and administrative arm for the Pan American EDIFACT Board (PAEB) and for ASC X12 (DISA, 1995; UNECE, 1994).

- The READ Classification System (RCS) is a multi-axial medical nomenclature used in the United Kingdom. It is sponsored by the National Health Service and has been integrated into computer-based ambulatory patient record systems in the United Kingdom (CAMS, 1994).

- A Japanese consortium that includes Sony, Toshiba, and Canon has implemented a video disk-based patient record system called Image Store and Carry (ISAC). This standard provides structures for storing patients' demographic data, all kinds of medical images, electrocardiograms, laboratory data, and clinical information. (McDonald, 1995) ISAC includes both the ASTM E1238 and DICOM standards.

- The Japanese Association of Healthcare Information Systems Industry (JAHIS) was established in April 1994 for the purpose of: contributing to the development of the healthcare information systems industry; the improvement in the health, medical treatment, and welfare of the nation; technological improvement; the ensuring of quality and safety; and the promotion of the standardization of healthcare information systems. It also plans to promote international cooperation in the fields of health, medical treatment, and welfare (CPRI, 1995).

STANDARDS COORDINATION AND PROMOTION ACTIVITIES

In the United States, there are several organizations and/or initiatives to help coordinate, promote, or accelerate the development of healthcare information standards. For the last several years, the primary organization working to coordinate healthcare information standards was the ANSI Healthcare Informatics Standards Planning Panel (HISPP). A transition plan has been developed to evolve ANSI HISPP into the ANSI Healthcare Informatics Standards Board (HISB), which would give it greater authority to achieve its missions.

- The major missions of ANSI HISSP have been:

  1. To facilitate the coordination of SDOs for healthcare data interchange (e.g., ACR/NEMA, ASTM, HL7, IEEE/MEDIX, X12) and other relevant standards groups (e.g., X3, ASC MD156) toward achieving the evolution of a unified set of non-redundant, non-conflicting standards. This activity has occurred within the ANSI HISPP Message Standards Developers Subcommittee (MSDS).

  2. To interact with and provide input to CEN TC 251 (Medical Informatics) in a coordinated fashion and explore avenues of international standards development.

- While some have been frustrated with the rate of progress of the ANSI HISPP MSDS, many of the SDO collaborations fostered by this subcommittee are likely to continue on their own. These include:

  - NCPDP continues to meet with HL7 and X12 to ensure compatibility with the drug prescription messages of HL7 and the billing messages of X12 (McDonald, 1995).

  - ACR-NEMA has prepared a draft proposal to create a joint working relationship with HL7 to develop message formats for the Information System - Imaging System interface (Bidgood, 1995; ACR-NEMA, 1995).

  - The Joint Working Group to Create a Common Data Model, formed by IEEE/MEDIX and MSDS, continues as an open standards effort to support the development of a common data model that can be shared by developers of healthcare informatics standards (IEEE, 1994).

  - HL7's working groups continue to work with other SDOs: The HL7 Automated Data and Waveforms Working Group is coordinating with ASTM E31.16, IEEE P1073 MIB, and LOINC; the Control/Query Working Group is coordinating with CEN and the CDC; the Inter-Enterprise Working Group is coordinating with ASC X12N; and, the Order Entry/Ancillary Working Group is coordinating with the CDC (Health Level Seven, 1995).

Several Joint Standards Developers' Meetings on Healthcare Information Process Modeling have recently been held. These meetings have included representatives from ASTM, ACR-NEMA, ASC X12N, ADA, IEEE\MEDIX and MIB, HL7 and NCPDP. It plans to define healthcare scenarios, the

F

roles of significant individuals involved in these scenarios, the resulting healthcare information system processes, as well as include specific examples of these processes.

The Computer-based Patient Record Institute (CPRI) is not an SDO, but its mission includes the promotion of standards related to computer-based patient record systems. Activities within several CPRI working groups reflect this mission of standards promotion:

- The CPR Description Work Group has work efforts to promote common definitions and concepts for the computer-based patient record system; o The Codes and Structures Work Group has a work effort to evaluate clinical code systems which was described in the Clinical Data Representations (Codes) section earlier

;

- The Confidentiality, Privacy, and Security Work Group has created several white papers and guidelines which were mentioned in the Confidentiality, Data Security, and Authentication section earlier (CPRI, 1995).

CPRI is partnering with the Center for Healthcare Information Management (CHIM) on the Health Information Interchange Standards Implementation Project (HIISIP). CHIM is an association of healthcare software vendors. The HIISIP project would help identify standard vocabularies which could be used in vendor-developed CPR products. It also plans to demonstrate the use of these standard healthcare vocabularies among vendor systems by 1997 (CHIM/CPRI HIISIP, 1995).

The Workgroup on Electronic Data Interchange (WEDI) was a voluntary, public/private task force formed in 1991 as a result of the call for healthcare administrative simplification by the director of the Department of Health and Human Services. WEDI incorporated as a formal organization in 1995. They have developed an action plan to promote healthcare EDI which includes promotion of EDI standards, architectures, confidentiality, identifiers, health cards, legislation, and publicity (CPRI, 1995).

SUMMARY

This article has presented an overview of major existing and emerging healthcare information standards. It describes the efforts to coordinate, harmonize, and accelerate these standards activities. Healthcare informatics is a dynamic area characterized by changing business and clinical processes, functions, and technologies. The effort to create healthcare informatics standards is therefore also dynamic. For the most current information on standards, refer to the "For More Information" section at the end of this article.

AKNOWLEDGEMENTS

This article is a significant update of the subject matter included in "Overview of Standards Related to the Emerging Health Care Information Infrastructure" published by CRC Press as a chapter in The Biomedical Engineering Handbook in May 1995.

While many contributed information to this article, the following individuals deserve special acknowledgement:

- Margret Amatayakul, M.B.A.
- W. Dean Bidgood, Jr., M.D.
- Christopher G. Chute, M.D., Ph.D.
- Paul Clayton, Ph.D.
- Kathleen Frawley, J.D., R.R.A.
- W. Edward Hammond, Ph.D.
- Terri L. Luthy
- Clement J. McDonald, M.D.
- Claudia Tessier
- C. Peter Waegemann

REFERENCES

- ACR-NEMA, 1995. "Proposal to HL7 from ACR-NEMA," July 95, Washington, D.C.
- American Dental Association (ADA), 1995. "American Dental Association Computer-based Oral Health Record Concept Model," Version 0.9, July, 1995, Chicago, IL.
- American National Standards Institute's Health Care Informatics Standards Planning Panel, 1994. "Charter Statement," New York, NY.
- American National Standards Institute's Health Care Informatics Standards Planning Panel, 1994. "Task Group on Provider Identifiers, February 4, 1994," New York, NY.
- ASTM, 1995. "Guide for the Properties of a Universal Health Care Identifier, E1714.95," ASTM Subcommittee E31.12, Philadelphia, PA.
- ASTM, 1994. "Membership Information Packet: ASTM Committee E31 on Computerized Systems," Philadelphia, PA.
- ASTM, 1995. "A Standard Description for Content and Structure of the Computer-based Patient Record, E1384-91/95 Revision," ASTM Subcommittee E31.19, Philadelphia, PA.
- ASTM, 1994. "Standard Guide for Description of Reservation/ Registration-Admission, Discharge, Transfer (R-ADT) Systems for Automated Patient Care Information Systems, E1239-94," ASTM Subcommittee E31.19, Philadelphia, PA.
- ASTM 1995. "A Standard Specification for the Coded Values Used in the Automated Primary Record of Care, E1633-95," ASTM Subcommittee E31.19, Philadelphia, PA.
- Bidgood, W.D., 1995. Personal communication, August 95.
- Business and Health, 1994. "Special Report on Guidelines," Montvale, NJ.
- Cannavo, M.J., 1993. "The Last Word Regarding DEFF & DICOM," Healthcare Informatics, October 93: 32-34.
- CHIM/CPRI Health Information Interchange Standards Implementation Project, 1995. "Minutes of Meeting, May 16, 1995," Atlanta, GA.
- Chute, C.G., November, 1991. "Tutorial 19: Clinical Data Representations," Symposium on Computer Applications in Medical Care, Washington, D.C.
- Chute, C.G., 1995. Personal communication, August 95.
- Cimino, J.J., Johnson, S.B., Peng, P., Aguirre, A., 1993. "From ICD9-CM to MeSH Using the UMLS: A How-to-Guide," SCAMC, Washington, D.C.

F

- Computer Aided Medical Systems Limited, 1994. "CAMS News," Vol. 4/1, January, 94, Leicestershire, U.K.
- Computer-based Patient Record Institute, 1994. "CPRI-Mail," Vol. 3/1, February 94, Chicago, IL.
- Computer-based Patient Record Institute, 1994. "Position Paper on Computer-based Patient Record Standards," Chicago, IL.
- Computer-based Patient Record Institute, 1995. "CPRI-Mail," Vol. 4/ 2, April 95, Chicago, IL.
- Computer-based Patient Record Institute, 1995. "Codes and Structures Patient Identifier Work Group Working Paper, June 1995" Version 2.1, Chicago, IL.
- Computer-based Patient Record Institute, 1995. "CPRI Major Codes Evaluation, Phase II," CPRI Codes and Structures Work Group, July 95, Chicago, IL.
- Data Interchange Standards Association, 1995. "ASC X12 Status Report, June 1995," Alexandria, VA.
- Donaldson, M.S. & Lohr, K.N. (Eds.), 1994. "Health Data in the Information Age: Use, Disclosure, and Privacy," Institute of Medicine, National Academy Press, Washington, D.C.
- Electronic Health Records Report, 1995. "Move Aside, Roget, Make Room for Metathesaurus. But Is It Ready For Records Prime Time?" August 1, 1995.
- Evans, D.A., Cimino, J.J., Hersh, W.R., Huff, S.M., Bell, D.S. 1994. "Toward a Medical-concept Representation Language," Journal of the American Medical Informatics Association, 1(3):207-217.
- Frawley, K., 1995. Personal communication, August 95.
- Gabrieli, E.R., 1995. Personal communication, August 95.
- Goverman, I.L., 1994. "Orienting Health Care Information Systems Toward Quality: How Group Health Cooperative of Puget Sound Did It," Journal on Quality Improvement, 20(11):595.
- Hammond, W.E., 1993. "Overview of Health Care Standards and Understanding What They All Accomplish," HIMSS Proceedings, American Hospital Association, Chicago, IL.
- Hammond, W.E., McDonald, C., Beeler, G., Carlson, D., Barrett, L., Bidgood, D., McDougall, M. 1994. "Computer Standards: Their Future Within Health Care Reform," HIMSS Proceedings, Health Care Information and Management Systems Society, Chicago, IL.
- Harrington, J.J. 1993. "IEEE P1157 MEDIX: A Standard for Open Systems Medical Data Interchange," Institute of Electrical and Electronic Engineers, New York City, NY.
- Health Care Financing Administration, 1995. "National Provider Identifier/National Provider File," Baltimore, MD.
- Health Industry Business Communications Council, 1994. "Description of Present Program of Standards Activity," Phoenix, AZ.
- Health Level Seven, 1995. "HL7 News," Summer 1995, Ann Arbor, MI.
- Humphreys, B., November, 1991. "Tutorial 20: Using and Assessing the UMLS Knowledge Sources," Symposium on Computer Applications in Medical Care, Washington, D.C.
- Institute of Electrical and Electronics Engineers, 1994. "Trial-Use Standard for Health Care Data Interchange - Information Model Methods: Data Model Framework," IEEE Standards Department, New York, NY.
- Joint Commission on Accreditation of Healthcare Organizations, 1994. "The Joint Commission Journal on Quality Improvement," Oakbrook Terrace, IL.
- Joint Commission on Accreditation of Healthcare Organizations, 1995. "The 1995 Guide to Hospital Accreditation Resources," Oakbrook Terrace, IL.
- McDonald, C., 1995. "Laboratory Observation Identifier Names and Codes (LOINC) Users Guide vs. 1.0," Regenstrief Institute, Indianapolis, IN.

- McDonald, C., 1995. "News on U.S. Health Informatics Standards," M.D. Computing, New York, NY.
- McDougall, M., 1995. "Standard Gains Healthcare Industry Acceptance & Support," Healthcare Informatics, July 1995.
- Medical Records Institute, 1995. "International Directory of Organizations, Standards, and Developments in the Creation of Electronic Health Records, Second Edition," August, 1995, Newton, MA.
- Moshman Associates, Inc., 1995. "Current Activities of Selected Health Care Informatics Standards Organizations," Office of Science and Data Development, Agency for Health Care Policy and Research, Bethesda, MD.
- National Committee for Quality Assurance, 1993. "Hedis 2.0: Executive Summary," Washington, D.C.
- National Committee for Quality Asurance, 1995. "HEDIS 2.5: Updated Specifications for HEDIS 2.0," Washington, D.C.
- Rothwell, D.J., Cote, R.A., Cordeau, J.P., Boisvert, M.A., 1993. "Developing a Standard Data Structure for Medical Language - The SNOMED Proposal," SCAMC, Washington, D.C.
- Terrell, S.A., Dutton, B.L., Porter, L., Cowles, C.M., American Health Care Association, 1991. "In Search of the Denominator: Medicare Physicians - How many are there?" Health Care Financing Administration, Baltimore, MD.
- Tessier, C., 1995. Personal communication, August 95.
- United Nations Economic Commission for Europe, 1994. "UN/EDIFACT: A Short Introduction," Geneva, Switzerland.
- Waegemann, C.P., 1995. Personal communication, August 95.
- Workgroup for Electronic Data Interchange, 1993. "WEDI Report: October 1993," Convened by the Department of Health and Human Services, Washington, D.C.

FOR FURTHER INFORMATION

- For copies of AAMT's guidelines on confidentiality, privacy, and security of patient care documentation through the process of medical dictation and transcription, contact the American Association for Medical Transcription, P.O. Box 576187, Modesto, CA 95357-6187, (209) 551-0883.
- For copies of standards accredited by ANSI, contact the American National Standards Institute, 11 West 42nd St., NYC, NC 10036, (212) 642-4900. For information on ANSI Health Care Informatics Standards Planning Panel (HISPP), contact Steven Cornish, (212) 642-4900.
- For copies of individual ASTM standards, contact ASTM Customer Service, 1916 Race Street, Philadelphia, PA 19103-1187, (215) 299-5585, fax: (215) 977-9679, email: service@local.astm.org.
- For more information on CEN TC 251, contact Georges De Moor, at Comite Europeen de Normalisation (CEN), Central Secretariat, Rue de Stassart 36, B-1050, Brussels, Belgium, telephone: 011-32-9-240-3436.
- For more information on CPRI publications and services, contact the Computer-based Patient Record Institute, Margret Amatayakul, 1000 E. Woodfield Road, Suite 102, Schaumburg, IL 60173, (847) 706-6746.

F

- For more information on electronic data interchange standards by ASC X12 and EDIFACT, contact the Data Interchange Standards Association (DISA), 1800 Diagonal Road, Suite 200, Alexandria, VA 22314, (703) 548-7005 ext. 155, fax: (703) 548-5738.
- For information on the Gabrieli Medical Nomenclature, contact Computer Based Medicine, Inc., 4 Cambridge Center, Cambridge MA, 02042, (617) 494-0909, fax: (617) 621-6982.
- For information on provider identifier standards and proposals, contact the Health Care Financing Administration (HCFA), Bureau Program Operations, 6325 Security Blvd., Baltimore, MD 21207, (410) 966-5798.
- For information on ICD-9-CM codes, contact HCFA, Medical Coding, 401 East Highrise Bldg., 6325 Security Blvd., Baltimore, MD 21207, (410) 966-5318.
- For information on site-of-care and supplier labeling identifiers, contact the Health Industry Business Communications Council (HIBCC), 5110 N. 40th Street, Suite 250, Phoenix, AZ 85018, (602) 381-1091.
- For copies of standards developed by Health Level 7, contact HL7, 3300 Washtenaw Avenue, Suite 227, Ann Arbor, MI 48104, (313) 677-7777. For draft proposals, meeting minutes, and proceedings, contact HL7 electronically, e-mail: dumccss.mc.duke.edu.
- For copies of standards developed by the Institute of Electrical and Electronic Engineers/Engineering in Medicine and Biology Society, in New York City, call (212) 705-7900. For information on IEEE/MEDIX meetings, contact Jack Harrington, Hewlett-Packard, 3000 Minuteman Rd., Andover, MA 01810, (508) 681-3517.
- For more information on the Japanese Association of Healthcare Information Systems Industry (JAHIS), please contact JAHIS, Toranomon TBL Building, 1-19-9, Toranomon, Minto-Ku, Tokyo 105. Phone: 011-81-3-3506-8010, fax: 011-81-3-3506-8070.
- For more information on clinical indicators, contact the Joint Commission on Accreditation of Health Care Organizations (JCAHO), Department of Indicator Measurement, One Renaissance Blvd., Oakbrook Terrace, IL 60181, (708) 916-5600.
- For more information on ISAC, contact the ISAC Committee, 2-3-4-10F Akasaka, Minato Ku, Tokyo 107, Japan, fax: 011-81-3-3505-1996.
- For more information on LOINC, contact Kathy Hutchins at the Regenstrief Institute, 1001 W. 10th Street, RG-5, Indianapolis, IN 46202, (317)630-7400, fax: (317)630-6962, and Internet address: loinc@regenstrief.iupui.edu.
- For information on pharmaceutical billing transactions, contact the National Council for Prescription Drug Programs (NCPDP), 2401 N. 24th Street, Suite 365, Phoenix, AZ 85016, (602) 957-9105.
- For information on HEDIS, contact the National Committee for Quality Assurance (NCQA), Planning and Development, 1350 New York Avenue, Suite 700, Washington, D.C. 20005, (202) 628-5788.
- For copies of ACR/NEMA DICOM standards, contact David Snavely, National Electrical Manufacturers Association (NEMA), 2101 L. Street N.W., Suite 300, Washington, D.C. 20037, (202) 457-8400.
- For information on standards development in the areas of computer-based patient record concept models, confidentiality, data security, authentication, and patient cards, and for information on standards activities in Europe, contact Peter Waegemann, Medical Records Institute (MRI), 567 Walnut Street, P.O. Box 289, Newton, MA 02160. (617) 964-3923.

- For information on the UMLS and the Large Scale Testing of Health Vocabularies project, contact the National Library of Medicine, Betsy Humphries, 8600 Rockville Pike, Bethesda, MD 20894 Bldg, 38, Room 2W06,(301) 496-6921, fax: (301) 496-6923.

F

REFERENCE 2

OVERVIEW OF EUROPEAN STANDARDS FOR HEALTH INFORMATICS

In Europe, the activities of normalization of the Information and Communication Technologies for Health began in April 1990 with the creation of the Technical Committee CEN/TC251 (Medical Informatics), within the European Committee of Normalization (CEN).

EUROPEAN POLICY DOCUMENTS AND OBLIGATIONS WITH RESPECT TO THEM

EN (European Standard) -   EUROPEAN STANDARDS. To be adopted as Standards of the European Union, revoking divergent national standards.

HD (Harmonization Document) -   HARMONIZATION DOCUMENTS. They are necessary to revoke divergent national standards.

ENV (European Pre-standard) -   EXPERIMENTAL EUROPEAN STANDARD. Announced as they are defined.

European Standards in Health Informatics

Revised July 9, 1998

Published standards can be obtained from the National Standards Bodies of the CEN countries. From non-European countries, the standards may be ordered from any National Standards Body of the CEN member countries.

Identification	Year of availability	Subject
ENV 1064	1993	Medical informatics – Standard communication protocol - Computer-assisted electrocardiography
ENV 1068	1993	Medical Informatics – Healthcare information interchange - Registration of coding schemes (Replaced by ISO/IEC 7826-1 and 7826-2)
CR 1350	1993	CEN Report: Investigation of syntaxes for existing interchange formats to be used in healthcare
ENV 1613	1995	Medical informatics - Messages for exchange of laboratory information
ENV 1614	1995	Healthcare informatics - Structure for nomenclature, classification and coding of properties in clinical laboratory sciences
ENV 1828	1995	Medical informatics - Structure for classification and coding of surgical procedures
ENV 12017	1997	Medical Informatics - Vocabulary
ENV 12018	1997	Identification, administrative, and common clinical data structure for intermittently connected devices used in healthcare (including machine readable cards)
ENV 12052	1997	Medical Informatics - Medical imaging communication
ENV 12264	1997	Medical informatics - Categorical structures of systems of concepts - Model for semantical representation
prENV 12265	1997	Medical informatics - Electronic healthcare record architecture
ENV 12381	1996	Medical informatics - Time standards for healthcare specific problems
ENV 12388	1996	Medical Informatics - Algorithm for digital signature services in Healthcare
prENV 12435		Medical informatics - Expression of the results of measurements in health sciences
prENV 12443		Medical informatics - Medical informatics healthcare information framework
ENV 12537-1	1997	Medical informatics - Registration of information objects used for electronic data interchange (EDI) in healthcare – Part 1: The Register

F

ENV 12537-2	1997	Medical informatics - Registration of information objects used for EDI in healthcare – Part 2: Procedures for the registration of information objects used for EDI in healthcare
ENV 12538	1997	Medical informatics - Messages for patient referral and discharge
ENV 12539	1997	Medical Informatics - Request and report messages for diagnostic service departments
CR 12587	1996	CEN Report: Medical Informatics – Methodology for the development of healthcare messages
ENV 12610	1997	Medical informatics - Medicinal product identification
ENV 12611	1997	Medical informatics – Categorical structure of systems of concepts – Medical devices
ENV 12612	1997	Medical Informatics – Messages for the exchange of healthcare administrative information
ENV 12623	1997	Medical Informatics - Media Interchange in medical imaging communications
CR 12700	1997	CEN Report: Supporting document to ENV 1613:1994 – Messages for exchange of laboratory information
ENV 12922-1	1997	Medical image management - Part 1: Storage commitment service class
ENV 12924	1997	Medical Informatics - Security categorization and protection for healthcare information systems
ENV 12967-1	1998	Medical Informatics – Healthcare information systems Architecture – Part 1: Healthcare middleware layer

REFERENCE 3

American National Standards Institute
Healthcare Informatics Standards Board

Inventory of Health Care Information Standards

Pertaining to

The Health Insurance Portability and Accountability Act (HIPAA) of 1996 (P.L. 104-191)

January 1997

Table of Contents

F

Supporting Standards   115

F

Security, Safeguards and Electronic Signatures 153

Executive Summary

Introduction

The Health Insurance Portability and Accountability Act of 1996 (HIPAA) was signed into law on August 21, 1996. The administrative simplification portion of HIPAA requires the Secretary of Health and Human Services (HHS) to adopt standards for the electronic transmission of specific administrative health transactions. These standards will apply to health plans, health care clearinghouses, and health care providers who transmit any health information in electronic form in connection with the following transaction:

- Health Claims or equivalent encounter information
- Health Claims Attachments
- Enrollment and Disenrollment in a Health Plan
- Eligibility For a Health Plan
- Health Care Payment and Remittance Advice
- Health Plan Premium Payments
- First Report of Injury
- Health Claim Status
- Referral Certification and Authorization
- Coordination of Benefits

Unless there is no existing standard, or a different standard will substantially reduce administrative costs to health care providers and health plans, the Secretary must adopt "a standard that has been developed, adopted, or modified by a standard setting organization."

The American National Standards Institute's Healthcare Informatics Standards Board (ANSI HISB) provides an open, public forum for the voluntary coordination of healthcare informatics standards among all United States' standard developing organizations. Every major developer of healthcare informatics standards in the United States participates in ANSI HISB. The ANSI HISB has 34 voting members and more than 100 participants, including ANSI-accredited and other standards developing organizations, professional societies, trade associations, private companies, federal agencies, and others. In response to the passage of HIPAA, ANSI HISB offered its services to the Secretary of HHS to prepare an inventory of existing healthcare information standards that pertained to the transactions specified by P.L.104-191. It also offered to assign them into appropriate HIPAA transaction categories and supporting standards sections. The Secretary accepted the offer and this report is the result.

The purpose of this report is to supply the Secretary of HHS with an inventory of existing healthcare informatics standards appropriate for the administrative simplification requirements of HIPAA and to map them into the relevant categories. To obtain the information for this report, HISB developed a set of templates asking for the following characteristics for each standard or set of standards:

- Category/classification of standard
- Standards Development Organization
- ANSI accreditation status
- Name of standard
- Contact for more information

F

- Description of standard
- Readiness of standard
- Indicators of market acceptance
- Level of specificity
- Relationships with other standards
- Identifiable costs

These templates were distributed to HISB participants with a request for a quick turnaround. Responses were received from ANSI-accredited standards developers, other organizations, and government agencies. The responses were coordinated into the administrative simplification standards categories, reviewed by HISB for appropriate classification and accuracy, and returned to the submitting standards organizations following the review for revision and resubmission. The final judgment for the placement of the existing standards in these categories and the accuracy of the information rests with the standard developing organization submitting the information, such as level of specificity and market acceptance. This report does not recommend specific standards but provides relevant comparative information to support the Secretary's analyses and decisions.

The vision for improved efficiency and effectiveness of the U.S. health care system through applications of information technology to health care is shared by Congress, the Secretary of HHS, and ANSI HISB. Administrative and clinical data standards are nationally important to improve the uniformity, accuracy, and automation of patient care data. Such data will support the development and dissemination of timely information needed to make good health care and payment decisions. By providing this report on existing administrative data standards and making it widely available, ANSI HISB hopes to contribute to a foundation that will improve the cost and medical effectiveness of health care in the public and private sectors, nationally and internationally.

Acknowledgments

ANSI HISB acknowledges the contributions provided by the following individuals:
Jeff Blair - Overall coordination and template design
Jean Narcisi - Response coordination and creation of the report
Alison Turner - Secretarial Coordination within ANSI

The following individuals provided input into the report:

Solomon Appavu
Christopher G. Chute, MD
J. Michael Fitzmaurice, PhD
Debbie Jenkins
Robert Owens
Rick Peters, MD
Daniel Staniec
C. Peter Waegemann

Transaction Standards

Health Claims or Equivalent Encounter Information

Accredited Standards Committee (ASC) X12, Health Care Task Group

The main objective of ASC X12 is to develop standards to facilitate electronic interchange relating to such business transactions as order placement and processing, shipping and receiving, invoicing, payment, cash application data, insurance transactions, and other data associated with the provision of products and services. The aim of ASC X12 is to structure standards so that computer programs can translate data to and from internal formats without extensive reprogramming. In this way, by using internally developed or commercially available software and private or public-access communication networks, ASC X12 believes that all sizes of firms and institutions using intelligent computational devices can benefit from the use of the standard. The efficiencies of standard interchange format can minimize the difficulties and expenses that could be incurred if each institution were to impose its own formats on every institution with which it does business. In ASC X12, the various subcommittees develop new standards that become recommendations for the full ASC X12 membership. The full ASC X12 membership must go through a consensus process before a proposed standard (or any change to a standard) is published as a Draft Standard for Trial Use. After a reasonable trial period, these standards are submitted to ANSI to start the process of consensus approval and registration.

ASC X12 has eleven Subcommittees including ASC X12N - Insurance. The ASC X12 subcommittees have maintained liaison with and obtained membership from a broad spectrum of businesses, government agencies, and institutions throughout the world. Communication is maintained with many organizations having experience in similar activities. A list of those participating in the development of the standards may be secured by contacting the Data Interchange Standards Association (DISA), Secretariat to ASC X12.

ANSI Accreditation:

X12 was accredited as an ANSI accredited standards committee in 1979. Subsequent X12 procedure changes have required ANSI re-accreditation which was last granted in 1987.

The main objective of ASC X12 is to develop Electronic Data Interchange (EDI) standards to facilitate electronic business transactions (i.e. order placement and processing, shipping and receiving, invoicing, payment, cash application data, insurance transactions). ASC X12 endeavors to structure standards in a manner that computer programs can translate data to and from internal formats without extensive reprogramming.

This strategy allows companies to maximize their resources required for internally developed or commercial software (recommended) and private or public-access communication networks. ASC X12 believes that all sizes of companies using intelligent computational devices can benefit from the use of the standard. The efficiencies of standard interchange format can minimize the difficulties incurred from each organization using its own formats to transact business. Within ASC X12, the various subcommittees are responsible for developing standards in their area of expertise. Once a subcommittee has developed a draft standard the full ASC X12 membership reviews and approves it

F

according to the operating policies and procedures. All standards (new or changed) require the consensus approval of the full ASC X12 membership. The approved standard becomes a draft standard for trial use for a reasonable trial period. After the trial period the draft standards are submitted to ANSI to become an American National Standard (ANS).

ASC X12N Health Care Claim (837)

Contact For More Information: Data Interchange Standards Association (DISA) 703-548-7005.

Description of Standard:

A) The objective of the Health Care Claim (837) is to support the administrative reimbursement processing as it relates to the submission of health care claims for both health care products and services.

B) This transaction set can be used to submit health care claim billing information, encounter information, or both, from providers of health care services to payers, either directly or via intermediary billers and claims clearinghouses. It can also be used to transmit health care claims and billing payment information between payers with different payment responsibilities where coordination of benefits is required or between payers and regulatory agencies to monitor the rendering, billing, and/or payment of health care services within a specific health care/insurance industry segment.

C) This transaction is used for administrative reimbursement for health care products and services for medical, hospital, dental, pharmaceutical, durable medical equipment claims as well as for workers compensation jurisdictional reporting.

D) This standard may be used from any operating system, network, or hardware platform.

E) The standard has been developed with widespread input from the health care industry incorporating all business needs into its functionality.

F) The ANSI ASC X12 is the only nationally recognized EDI standards development organization in the United States for all types of electronic commerce. ASC X12 is the organization assigned by ANSI to represent the United States in the development of International EDI standards.

G) Standards. These standards are developed using a consensus process by the users in the health care industry.

H) The standards developed by ASC X12 may be translated to/from application systems using off the shelf translation software products which are used by all industries utilizing the ASC X12 standards.

Readiness of Standard:

A) The Health Care Claim (837) is not a guideline.

B) The Health Care Claim (837) standard is fully implementable. The transaction set was approved as a Draft Standard for Trial Use (DSTU) in October of 1992 as Version 003030.

C) The standard can be obtained by contacting the Data Interchange Standards Association (DISA) at 703-548-7005.

D) This standard does not require an implementation guide. ASC X12 has published four Type II Tutorial reports or tutorials for version 003041 in October of 1994, version 003050 in October

1995, version 003051 in February 1996, and version 003060 in April of 1996. To facilitate consistent implementation across the health care industry, the X12 Insurance Subcommittee is currently in the process of completing five implementation guides for version 003070 encompassing medical, hospital, dental, pharmaceutical claims, and workers compensation jurisdictional reporting with an anticipated publication date of June 1997.

E) There will be only one implementation guide per claim type for each version of the standards the X12 Health Care Task Group selects in accordance with the industry.

F) The implementation guides will specify the conformance to the standards.

G) Conformance tools are commercially available.

H) The same tools used for conformance may also be used as testing tools.

I) The standard is complete. The current version of the standard is 003070. As business needs dictate, enhancements may be made to the standard three times per year, one major release along with two subsequent sub-releases. The X12 Health Care Task Group has developed procedures to determine when to move to the next version of the standard as well as when to retire past versions. The Health Care Task Group will also determine the need for new versions of the implementation guides (not more frequently than once per year).

J) Currently no enhancements are under development.

AA)This standard has been completed.

BB) This standard has been completed and undergoing industry implementation.

Indicator of Market Acceptance:

A) The X12 standards are made available via many sources including from the Data Interchange Standards Association, Washington Publishing (ASC X12 Insurance Subcommittee's publisher), industry user groups and associations, and the Internet. Due to the multiplicity and diversity of these distribution methods, it is not possible to determine how many copies have been distributed and to whom.

B) All Medicare carriers and intermediaries have implemented ASC X12 standards for claims. Many other payers have followed HCFA's lead and implemented the standard as well.

C) ASC X12 represents international standards development. North American and other countries have implemented ASC X12 standards for purchasing and financial transactions. It would be to their benefit to further leverage their investment in EDI translation software, hardware and communication infrastructure to utilize the health care transactions.

Over 300 payer, provider, vendor, and plan sponsor organizations currently participate in the development of the ASC X12 standards and implementation guides to meet the business needs of the entire health care industry. These organizations have experienced the benefits of mature standards because costs associated with developing and maintaining proprietary formats far exceed the investment necessary to implement a single set of health care EDI transactions.

Level of Specificity:

A) The ASC X12 EDI transactions have been developed to meet the specific business needs identified by the standards developers and the health care industry.

B) See attached table of contents from the ASC X12 Insurance Committee's implementation guides.

F

C) ASC X12 standards incorporate the business requirements for exchanging information contained within other standards. The ASC X12 standards provides a vehicle for communicating other standards within the standards.

D) ASC X12 maintains over one thousand internal code sets to support the standards. Along with the internal code sets the ASC X12 standards reference over 350 external code sources such as:
- Current Procedural Terminology (CPT) Codes from American Medical Association
- Current Dental Terminology (CDT) Codes from American Dental Association
- International Classification of Diseases Clinical Modification - (ICD-9-CM) Diagnosis from U.S. National Center for Health Statistics.

E) There are too many code sets to describe here. Refer to the ASC X12 standards publication.

F) Internal code sets are included within the ASC X12 standards publications and implementation guides. When external code sets are referenced within these documents, the source where the code sets can be obtained is listed.

G) When possible, the implementation guides will either include the external code sets or provide further information on how to obtain the external code sets. Internal code sets are included within the implementation guides.

H) Internal code sets are available to all users of the ASC X12 standards. Usage of the external code sets will vary by source and their ability to promote the usage of their code sets.

I) ASC X12 internal code sets follow the same processes defined for the development and maintenance of the EDI transactions. External code lists are maintained by the external code source's internal development procedures.

Relationships with Other Standards:

A) ASC X12 strives to coordinate and incorporate the needs of the other standards development organizations such as Health Level 7 (HL7), National Council for Prescription Drug Programs (NCPDP), and the American Society for Testing and Materials into the ASC X12 standards.

B) See A).

C) See A).

D) Open communication in the development of the standards amongst the standards development organizations.

E) ASC X12 is the ANSI appointed standards development organization responsible for international EDI standards within the United States.

F) None

G) Given the scope and responsibility for the development and maintenance of the EDI standards for the United States and the international community with respect to United States international standards, ASC X12 is only privy to the business needs which are brought forward and coordinated with other health care organizations. At this time, we are unaware of any gaps in the current standards for insurance.

Identifiable Costs:

A) None applicable. ASC X12 does not license it standards.

B) B)The cost of acquiring the ASC X12 standards publication varies depending upon the source of the publications. Currently they are available from:
- Data Interchange Standards Association (DISA) 703-548-7005.
- Washington Publishing Corporation 800-972-4334
- Industry user groups and associations
- The Internet (http://www.disa.org, http://www.wpc-edi.com)

C) The typical cost ranges from free to $415.00 for the full ASC X12 standards publication in either paper form or CD-ROM.

D) The cost/timeframe for education and training will depend upon the individuals and skill levels of the individuals within an organization. Some organizations have completed education and training within one week while others have taken longer.

E) The cost/timeframe for implementation depends upon the internal systems capabilities, systems development philosophy, hardware platform selected, EDI translator software, communication methodology and individual resources within an organization. Costs can range anywhere from free for a personal computer solution to well over $150,000 for midsize and mainframe systems. Some organizations have implemented the standards within a matter of days while other have taken months to achieve the same end result.

F) The current use of proprietary formats such as the National Standard Format (NSF) and the costs of maintaining these formats far outweigh the costs associated with implementing a single set of the health care industry standards from ASC X12.

ASC X12N Interactive Healthcare Claim/Encounter (IHCLME)

Contact For More Information: Data Interchange Standards Association (DISA) 703-548-7005.

Description of Standard:

A) The objective of the Interactive Healthcare Claim/Encounter (IHCLME) is to support the administrative reimbursement processing as it relates to the submission of health care claims for both health care products and services in an interactive environment.

B) This message can be used to submit health care claim billing information, encounter information, or both, from providers of health care services to payers, either directly or via intermediary billers and claims clearinghouses interactively with the possibility for automatic adjudication and an immediate response.

C) This message can be used for the administrative reimbursement of health care products and services for medical, hospital, dental, pharmaceutical and durable medical equipment claims.

D) This standard may be used from any operating system, network, or hardware platform.

E) The standard has been developed with widespread input from the health care industry incorporating all business needs into its functionality.

F) The ANSI ASC X12 is the only nationally recognized EDI standards development organization in the United States for all type of electronic commerce. ASC X12 is the organization assigned by ANSI to represent the United States in the development of International EDI standards.

G) This standard is developed using a consensus process by the users in the health care industry.

H) The standards developed by ASC X12 may be translated to/from application systems using off the shelf translation software products which are used by all industries utilizing the ASC X12 standards.

F

Readiness of Standard:

A) The Interactive Healthcare Claim/Encounter (IHCLME) is not a guideline.

B) The message is expected to be approved as a Draft Standard for Trial Use (DSTU) in October 1997.

C) The standard can be obtained by contacting the Data Interchange Standards Association (DISA) at 703-548-7005 once approved.

D) This standard does not require an implementation guide. ASC X12 has published four Type II Tutorial reports or tutorials for version 003041 in October of 1994, version 003050 in October 1995, version 003051 in February 1996, and version 003060 in April of 1996. To facilitate consistent implementation across the health care industry, the X12 Insurance Subcommittee is currently in the process of completing five implementation guides for version 003070 encompassing medical, hospital, dental, pharmaceutical claims, and workers compensation jurisdictional reporting with an anticipated publication date of April 1997.

E) There will be only one implementation guide for the Interactive Healthcare Claim/Encounter (IHCLME).

F) The implementation guides will specify the conformance to the standards.

G) Yes, conformance tools are commercially available.

H) The same tools used for conformance may also be used as testing tools.

I) The standard has been defined and currently is undergoing review by the members of the X12 Health Care Task Group. As business needs dictate, enhancements may be made to the standard three times per year, one major release along with two subsequent subreleases. The X12 Health Care Task Group has developed procedures to determine when to move to the next version of the standard, as well as, when to retire past versions. The Health Care Task Group will also determine the need for new versions of the implementation guides (not more frequently than once per year).

J) Currently no enhancements are under development.

AA) This standard must be balloted by ANSI X12 followed by a ballot within UN/EDIFACT.

BB) This message is expected to be approved as a Draft Standards for Trail Use (DSTU) in October 1997.

Indicator of Market Acceptance:

A) The X12 standards are made available via many sources including from the Data Interchange Standards Association, Washington Publishing (ASC X12 Insurance Subcommittee's publisher), industry user groups and associations, and the Internet. Due to the multiplicity and diversity of these distribution methods, it is not possible to determine how many copies have been distributed and to whom.

B) Every government contractor has been funded by the Health Care Financing Administration (HCFA) to implement the ASC X12 standards. Many other payers have followed HCFA's lead and implemented the standards as well.

C) Yes. ASC X12 represents international standards development. North American and other countries have implemented ASC X12 standards for purchasing and financial transactions. It would be to their benefit to further leverage their investment in EDI translation software, hardware and communication infrastructure to utilize the health care transactions.

Over 300 payer, provider, vendor, and plan sponsor organizations currently participate in the development of the ASC X12 standards and implementation guides to meet the business needs of the entire health care industry. These organizations have experienced the benefits of mature standards because costs associated with developing and maintaining proprietary formats far exceed the investment necessary to implement a single set of health care EDI transactions.

Level of Specificity:

A) The ASC X12 EDI transactions have been developed to meet the specific business needs identified by the standards developers and the health care industry.

B) See attached table of contents from the ASC X12 Insurance Committee's implementation guides.

C) ASC X12 standards incorporate the business requirements for exchanging information contained within other standards. The ASC X12 standards provides a vehicle for communicating other standards within the standards.

D) ASC X12 maintains over one thousand internal code sets to support the standards. Along with the internal code sets the ASC X12 standards reference over 350 external code sources such as:
- Current Procedural Terminology (CPT) Codes from American Medical Association
- Current Dental Terminology (CDT) Codes from American Dental Association
- International Classification of Diseases Clinical Modification - (ICD-9-CM) Diagnosis from U.S. National Center for Health Statistics.

E) There are too many code sets to describe here. Refer to the ASC X12 standards publication.

F) Internal code sets are included within the ASC X12 standards publications and implementation guides. When external code sets are referenced within these documents, the source where the code sets can be obtained is listed.

G) When possible, the implementation guides will either include the external code sets or provide further information on how to obtain the external code sets. Internal code sets are included within the implementation guides.

H) Internal code sets are available to all users of the ASC X12 standards. Usage of the external code sets will vary by source and their ability to promote the usage of their code sets.

I) ASC X12 internal code sets follow the same processes defined for the development and maintenance of the EDI transactions. External code lists are maintained by the external code source's internal development procedures.

Relationships with Other Standards:

A) ASC X12 strives to coordinate and incorporate the needs of the other standards development organizations such as Health Level 7 (HL7), National Council for Prescription Drug Programs (NCPDP), and the American Society for Testing and Materials into the ASC X12 standards.

B) See A).

C) See A).

D) Open communication in the development of the standards amongst the standards development organizations.

E) ASC X12 is the ANSI appointed standards development organization responsible for international EDI standards within the United States

F) None

G) Given the scope and responsibility for the development and maintenance of the EDI standards for the United States and the international community with respect to United States international standards, ASC X12 is only privy to the business needs which are brought forward and coordinated with other health care organizations. At this time, we are unaware of any gaps in the current standards for insurance.

Identifiable Costs:

A) None applicable. ASC X12 does not license it standards.

B) The cost of acquiring the ASC X12 standards publication varies depending upon the source of the publications. Currently they are available from:
- Data Interchange Standards Association (DISA) 703-548-7005.
- Washington Publishing Corporation 800-972-4334
- Industry user groups and associations
- The Internet (http://www.disa.org, http://www.wpc-edi.com)

C) The typical cost ranges from free to $415.00 for the full ASC X12 standards publication in either paper form or CD-ROM.

F

D) The cost/timeframe for education and training will depend upon the individuals and skill levels of the individuals within an organization. Some organizations have completed education and training within one week while others have taken longer.

E) The cost/timeframe for implementation depends upon the internal systems capabilities, systems development philosophy, hardware platform selected, EDI translator software, communication methodology and individual resources within an organization. Costs can range anywhere from free for a personal computer solution to well over $150,000 for midsize and mainframe systems. Some organizations have implemented the standards within a matter of days while other have taken months to achieve the same end result.

F) ASC X12 Interactive Healthcare Claims Encounter (IHCLME) is used to transmit claims/encounters interactively, coordinating with the possibility for automatic adjudication and an immediate response. Identifying data requirements, determining business scenarios, grouping data needs into segments and defining the structure of the messages. Claims being considered for interactive transactions include pharmacy, institutional, professional and dental. One message will cover all four claim types. The response message covers the claim status and adjudication information. These will be EDIFACT messages utilizing ASC X12 data dictionaries. This message is currently under development.

National Council for Prescription Drug Programs (NCPDP)

The scope of the standards that NCPDP develops are those for information processing for the pharmacy services sector of the health care industry.

ANSI Accredited:

NCPDP was accredited by ANSI on August 6, 1996. The type of accreditation was the Accredited Organization Method.

NCPDP Standard Claims Billing Version 2.0

This batch format is compatible to and consistent with the standard Universal Claim Form to enable logical progression from a manual paper claims submission system to an automated billing process. The Standard Claims Billing format utilizes both data elements and program logic that include the following items or understandings:

- Use of industry accepted data elements (National Drug Code Number (NDC), National Association of Boards of Pharmacy Number (NABP) Processor number, etc.).
- Contingency allowance for future enhancements.
- Compatibility of the format to most existing processing systems.

NCPDP Telecommunications Standard Format Version 3.2

NCPDP recommends the use of a standardized format for electronic communication of claims between pharmacy providers, insurance carriers, third-party administrators, and other responsible parties. This standard addresses the data format and content, the transmission protocol, and other appropriate telecommunication requirements and was developed to accommodate the eligibility verification process at the point-of-sale and to provide a consistent format for electronic claims processing. The standard supports the submission and adjudication of third party prescription drug claims in an on-line, real-time environment.

NCPDP Version 3 Release 2 was a standard created by the NCPDP Telecommunication Work Group (Work Group One). The objective of the standard is to provide a standard format for on-line real time adjudication for pharmacy claims. Functions include billing of pharmaceutical products including compound medications; billing of professional drug utilization review situations. Users of the standard include administrative/reimbursement and clinical environment. Pharmacies submit claims for drugs and professional services and when applicable receive clinical DUR information derived from payer/prescription benefit manager databases. The standard is used in all operating system environments and claims are submitted and then adjudicated directly from pharmacy to payer and via network. The standard satisfies the needs of public and private prescription benefit plans for well over 100,000,000 health plan members. In addition, this standard facilitates a specific type of business communication between a large number of diverse parties within the third party environment. To do this successfully, it must accomplish the following tasks:

- Support the needs of as wide a base of potential users as possible.
- Maximize use of existing relevant standards wherever possible (e.g. Version 1.0 of this standard).
- Be flexible enough to change as needs and technology change.
- Be unambiguous.
- Be easy to implement by payers and pharmacy management software developers.

User Environment.

A given organization might serve multiple roles (for example, Administrator and Processor). Certain roles might be split between multiple organizations, the administrator and processor could be different.

This standard addresses the submission of a claim and/or professional service by a dispenser to an administrator/processor, and identifies the response of the administrator/processor to the dispenser. For the purpose of this document, the term "processor" will be used to identify the identity actually performing the authorization/adjudication function.

Types of Messages:

This standard addresses two types of communication between the dispenser (sender) and the processor (receiver). These communication types **are claim submission/response** and **claim reversal/response**. These are described in detail below:

Claim Submission/Response:

This transaction is used by the dispenser to request the administrator verify the eligibility of a specific claimant according to the appropriate plan parameters. The message sent by the dispenser contains four types of data:
1) Control Data: This identifies the message type, destination, etc.
2) Dispenser Data: This identifies the provider of the service.
3) Claimant Data: This identifies the person for whom the service is being provided.
4) Prescription Data: This describes the specific service being provided by the Dispenser.

F

Each claim submission message contains control, dispenser, and claimant data, and up to four occurrences of prescription data. A special case message is where there are zero occurrences of the prescription data. This identifies a request to only verify the eligibility of the claimant.

Depending upon the particular claim submission message, the processor can provide one of the following general types of responses:

- Eligibility verification only- This occurs when the processor is verifying the eligibility of the claimant. The claim must be submitted for processing at another time.
- Claim capture only- This occurs when the processor acknowledges receipt of the claim, but is not making any judgment regarding eligibility of the claimant.
- Claim capture, eligibility verification, and adjudication- This occurs when the processor captures and processes the claim, and returns to the originator the dollar amounts allowed under the terms of the plan.

Claim Reversal/Response:

This transaction is used by the dispenser to request the administrator to reverse a previously submitted claim. The results of a successfully submitted reversal are as if the claim was not submitted in the first place. The message sent by the dispenser contains four types of data:

1) Control Data: This identifies the message type, destination, etc.
2) Dispenser Data: This identifies the provider of the service.
3) Prescription Data: This describes the specific service being provided by the Dispenser.

Each claim reversal message contains control, dispenser, and one occurance of prescription data.
The claim reversal response tells the dispenser if the administrator was able to reverse the claim or not.

Business Flow:

The prescription information is transmitted electronically either through a value-added network switch or directly to a payer or pharmacy benefit management company, where the various transaction functions described above are completed. A paid or rejected response is sent back either through a value-added network switch or directly to the pharmacy in a matter of seconds. This is completed in an on-line real-time environment.

Application Function/Domain Completeness:

Version 3.2 was completed in February 1992 and ongoing maintenance continues. A Drug Utilization Review (DUR) component and a Professional Pharmacy Services (PPS) component have been added to enhance the standard to fit the business needs of the pharmacy community. Drug Utilization Review provides information to the pharmacist regarding potential drug interactions of the prescription drug being billed with the claimant's drug history. In addition, a compound standard has also been developed.

TABLE OF NCPDP TELECOMMUNICATION

STANDARD VERSION/RELEASE

Standard/ Version/ Release	Standard Approved by NCPDP	Dictionary Complete	Implementation Guide Complete	Widely Used & Implemented	Highlights
3.2	Feb. 1992	Yes	Yes	Yes	1 billion transactions in 1996
3.3	Feb. 1996	March 1997	No	Somewhat	Compound Drugs
3.4	June 1996	March 1997	No	Somewhat	Prior Authorization
3.5	Oct. 1996	March 1997	No	No	New Data Elements
4.0	Feb. 1997	March 1997	No	No	New/Revised Data Elements

This standard has no competing standard to date. The membership of NCPDP has established this widely accepted and implemented standard for on-line real-time prescription claims processing. Implementing this standard required the coordinated efforts and timely response of software developers, payers/claims processors, managed care organizations, pharmacy providers, and numerous other organizations. This standard is being used to process over 1 billion prescription drug claims per year.

Readiness of Standard:

A) NCPDP Version 3.2 is not a guideline, but a completed standard. This standard was submitted recently to ANSI to become an American National Standard.
B) This standard has been implemented by the vast majority of the pharmacy benefits industry since 1992. It was developed to be a natural progression from the previously implemented version.
C) The standard can be obtained by contacting NCPDP's office at (602) 957-9105.
D) NCPDP Version 3.2 has a separate implementation guide. Work is under way for 3.3 and 3.4 implementation guides.
E) There is only one implementation guide. There are no major options that impact compatibility.
F) Yes, a conformance standard is specified (certification procedures). It is important to note that trading partners accomplish this, not NCPDP
G) Yes, conformance test tools are available.
H) The test tools are developed by trading partners based on business agreements.
I) The standard is complete and undergoes periodic enhancements.
J) A compound drug enhancement was recently completed, as well as different data elements for new versions and releases.
AA) A data element request form (DERF) process (data maintenance) has been developed at NCPDP to enable the standard to be modified by the NCPDP membership to fit the business needs of the industry.
BB) This standard is modified periodically upon review of DERFs.

Indicator of Market Acceptance:

A) The standard is virtually used by every pharmacy processor, PBM (Pharmacy Benefit Management Company) submitting on-line real-time pharmacy claims. Every Pharmacy Practice Management Software Vendor in the United States supports the standard. Over 1,000,000,000

F

claims from 100,000,000 health plan members were submitted in 1996 using the standard. The standard will be used in South Africa in early 1997. In addition, 43 State Medicaid Agencies utilize our standard for their business needs.

B) The language will be English only.

Level of Specificity:

A) Version 3.2 allows for both fixed length transactions or variable length transactions. Implementation of variable length transactions gives the sender and receiver the option of compressing or eliminating optional data elements to reduce message length where these data elements are not required by the processor. As of Version 3.3, fixed length transactions are no longer supported.

B) There is no implementation guideline for the Compound standard for V3.2. There is one for Compounds (V3.3) and Prior Authorization (V3.4).

C) Data sets referenced include :
   1. FDA's National Drug Code (NDC)
   2. NABP #s - National Association for Boards of Pharmacy Number, an universal identifier for pharmacies in the United States
   3. DAW codes - Dispense as written codes

D) The code sets are updated as new data elements are approved by the membership.

E) The data dictionary can be acquired by contacting NCPDP's office at 602-957-9105.

F) There is an instruction sheet.

G) It is used by virtually all users of the standard. (in the hundreds).

H) It is not under development.

Relationships with Other Standards:

A) PPS and DUR are used as part of the NCPDP standard.

B) The X12 835 is used to report on the remittances for claims submitted.

C) Not applicable.

D) Not applicable.

E) No, this standard is not consistent with international standards.

F) There are no gaps.

G) Not applicable.

Identifiable Costs:

The costs for licenser, cost of acquisition, cost time frames for education, training, and implementation are contingent upon the usage and trading partner agreements.

Contact For More Information:

NCPDP, Inc. 4201 North 24th Street, Suite 365, Phoenix, AZ 850160-6268,
Phone (602) 957-9105,
Lee Ann C. Stember - President,
Daniel J. Staniec, R.Ph., MBA Executive Vice President of External Affairs

Health Care Financing Administration (HCFA)

ANSI Accredited:

Not ANSI accredited. Have not applied for accreditation.

HCFA National Standard Format (NSF), Version 002.00

Contact for more information: Joy Glass - Email Jglass@hcfa.gov, 410-786-6125, FAX 410-786-4047

Description of Standard:

The NSF consists of fixed-length (320 bytes) records. Each record has a unique identifier and logically related data elements.
A) Objective - The NSF was designed to standardize and increase the submission of electronic claims and coordination of benefits exchange.
B) Function - The NSF is used to electronically submit health care claims and encounter information from providers of health care services to payers. It is also used to exchange health are claims and payment information between payers with different payment responsibility.
C) User Environment - NSF users consist of a variety of health care providers, such as, professional, dental, chiropractic, Indian health service providers, and suppliers of medical equipment and supplies. A variety of payers also use the format to exchange claim and payment information.
D) Systems Environment - The NSF is a file format and is platform/operating system independent.
E) Application Function/Domain Completeness - All codes used in the NSF are complete.
F) The NSF is "user friendly" and easily implemented. It contains detailed record and data descriptions as well as unambiguous data definitions. It is widely used by providers of health care and payers. In FY96, 668,650,936 Medicare claims were submitted electronically. Ninety eight (98) percent of those claims were in the NSF. The NSF does not have to be translated prior to application processing. The use of compression techniques eliminates at least 50% overhead when transmitting the NSF. With compression, the NSF is more economical than an ANSI X12 837 to transport.

Readiness of Standard:

A) The NSF is a guideline for building electronic claims. The NSF supports policy requirements for users. The NSF defines processes using validation statements. The NSF provides a structured design for building claims.
B) The NSF was fully implemented for Medicare in 1991 and continues to be supported. The NSF has been implemented by about 200 other payers.
C) The NSF is available on the HCFA BPO bulletin board 410-786-0215. The file name is NSF.EXE and is located in area 3. There are no restrictions and it is free of charge.
D) The NSF implementation guide is built into the specifications and people may build standard claims from it.
E) Some payers provide a guide to identify payer specific requirements.
F) The NSF specifies conformity. Because it is in the public domain some people choose not to conform. This would easily be fixed if it was recognized by Federal statute. The specifications are clear and conformity is easy to achieve.

F

G) HCFA's Office of Analysis and Systems has developed a software conformance/enforcement tool for the NSF.

H) Other Indicators of Readiness: The NSF has been available since 1991.

Indicator of Market Acceptance:

A) Medicare implemented the standard in 1991. Copies of the NSF are requested almost daily. The NSF is available on a bulletin board. Diskettes were previously distributed. Since the NSF is free of charge, the number of copies distributed is not maintained.

B) The following government agencies have implemented the NSF:
   1) Medicare
   2) Medicaid
   3) Indian Health Services
   4) Champus
   5) Numerous Blue Shield plans and some 200 organizations use the NSF.

C) We are not aware of other countries that implemented the NSF.

D) We constantly receive praise from software vendors, clearinghouses and health care providers

E) regarding the usefulness of the NSF and ease of implementation.

Level of Specificity:

A) The NSF is very detailed. Record descriptions exist, as well as, unambiguous data element definitions and format descriptions.

B) The NSF framework is detailed down to the smallest named unit of information.

C) The NSF does not reference or assume other standards to achieve more specificity.

D) thru H) The NSF includes a code set for the place of service, podiatry codes, and type of service. The NSF assumes the following codes sets:

CODE SET	AVAILABLE FORM
Health Care Procedure Codes (HCPCS)	HCFA
Provide Specialty Codes	HCFA
ICD-9 CM Procedure Codes	National Center For Health Statistics
CPT Codes	
Physicians Current Procedure Terminology Manual	
National Drug Code	
Blue Book, Price Alert, National	Drug Data File
Claim Adjustment Reason Code	BCBS Association
Health Care Professional Shortage Area	HCFA
National Association of Insurance Committee Code	NAIC Code List Manual
Medicare Inpatient/Outpatient Message	HCFA
Investigational Device Exemption Number	FDA

Relationship with Other Standards:

The ANSI X12 837 health care claim is not suitable for use in an application program and must be translated into the NSF prior to claims processing. The NSF does not have to be translated and, in turn, reduces administrative costs.

Identifiable Costs:

The NSF is distributed free of charge. The NSF can be implemented within 3 to 6 months of receipt of the standard specifications. Implementation costs vary depending on how a payer implements the standard. Health care provider costs are minimal. The average cost for software is less than $200, and sometimes as little as $25.00. Implementation costs can range from $100,00 to $500,000. If a complete system rewrite is performed, the cost could be $500,000. If the change is at the interface, the cost could be less than $100,000. These costs include comprehensive systems testing.

HCFA Uniform Bill-92 (UB-92), Version 4.1

Contact for more information: Jean M. Harris – E-mail: JHarris2@hcfa.gov, 410-786-6168,
Fax: 410-786-4047

Description of Standard:

The UB92 consists of fixed-length (192 bytes) records. Each record has an unique identifier and logically related data elements.
Objective - The UB92 was designed to standardize and increase the submission of electronic claims and coordination of benefits exchange.

Function - The UB92 is used to electronically submit claims for health care received in an institutional setting to payers. It is also used to exchange health Care claims and payment information between payers with different payment responsibility.

User Environment - UB92 users are institutional providers. A variety of payers also use the format to exchange claim and payment information.

Systems Environment - The UB92 is a file format and is platform/operating system independent.

Application Function/Domain Completeness - All codes used in the UB92 are complete.
The UB92 is "user friendly" and easily implemented. It contains detailed record and data descriptions as well as unambiguous data definitions. It is widely used by providers of health care and payers. It is conservatively estimated that 60,000 providers use the UB92. In FY96, 141,872,119 Medicare institutional claims were submitted electronically. Ninety six point eight (96.8) percent of those claims were in the UB92. The UB92 does not have to be translated prior to application processing. The use of compression techniques eliminates at least 50% overhead when transmitting the UB92. With compression, the UB92 is more economical than an ANSI X12 837 to transport.

Readiness of Standard:

A) The UB92 is a guideline for building electronic claims. The UB92 supports policy requirements for users. The UB92 defines processes using procedure statements.
B) The UB92 was fully implemented for Medicare in 1993 (the UB83 was implemented in 1983) and continues to be supported. The UB92 has been implemented by about 73 other major payers.
C) The UB92 is available on the HCFA BPO bulletin board 410-786-0215. The file name is UB92BBS.EXE and is located in area 3. There are no restrictions and it is free of charge.

F

D) The UB92 implementation guide is built into the specifications, and people may build standard claims from it.

E) Some payers provide a guide to identify payer specific requirements.

F) The UB92 specifies conformity. Because it is in the public domain some people choose not to conform. This would easily be fixed if it was recognized by Federal statute. The specifications are clear and conformity is easy to achieve.

G) & H) HCFA's Office of Analysis and Systems has developed a software conformance/enforcement tool for the UB92.

I) thru, M) The UB92 has been available since 1993.

Indicator of Market Acceptance:

A) Medicare implemented the standard (UB83) in 1983. Copies of the UB92 are requested frequently. The UB92 is available on a bulletin board. Diskettes were previously distributed. Since the UB92 is free of charge, the number of copies distributed is not maintained.

B) The following government agencies have implemented the UB92:
   - Medicare
   - Medicaid

   Numerous Blue Cross plans use the UB92. Approximately, 73 other payers have implemented the standard.

C) We are not aware of other countries that implemented the UB92.

D) We constantly receive praise from software vendors, clearinghouses and health care providers regarding the usefulness of the UB92 and ease of implementation.

Level of Specificity:

A) The UB92 is very detailed. Record descriptions exist, as well as unambiguous data element definitions and format descriptions.

B) The UB92 framework is detailed down to the smallest named unit of information.

C) The UB92 does not reference or assume other standards to achieve more specificity.

D) thru H) The UB92 includes a code set for the patient status, accommodation revenue codes, ancillary revenue codes, and condition codes. The UB92 assumes the following code sets:

CODE SETS	AVAILABLE FROM
Health Care Procedure Codes (HCPCS)	HCFA
ICD-9 CM Procedure Codes	National Center for Health Statistics
CPT Codes	
Physicians Current Procedure Terminology Manual	
Claim Adjustment Reason Code	BCBS Association
Medicare Inpatient/Outpatient Message	HCFA
Investigation Device Exemption Number	FDA
Revenue, Value and Occurrence Codes	National Uniform Billing Committee

Relationship with Other Standards:

The ANSI X12 837 health care claim is not suitable for use in an application program and must be translated into the UB92 prior to claims processing. The UB92 does not have to be translated and, in turn, reduces administrative costs.

Identifiable Costs:

The UB92 is distributed free of charge. Typically, it takes one year from statement of intent for the UB92 to be in full production. Implementation costs vary depending on how a payer implements the standard. If a complete system rewrite is performed, the cost could be $1,000,000. If the change is at the interface, the cost could be as little as $100,000. These costs include comprehensive systems testing.

American Dental Association (ADA) Accredited Standards Committee MD 156

The American Dental Association (ADA) is sponsor and secretariat of the Accredited Standards Committee (ASC) MD156 for Dental Materials, Instruments and Equipment. In 1992 there was interest in the standardization of clinical information systems. After evaluating current informatics activities, the ADA initiated several projects relating to clinical technology. A task group of the ASC MD156 was created by the Association to initiate the development of technical reports, guidelines, and standards on electronic technologies used in dental practice.

Components of the task group include five working groups for clinical information systems. The working groups were established to promote the concept of a dental computerized clinical work station and allow the integration of different software and hardware components into one system in order to provide for all of a clinician's information needs. Clinical information systems include all areas of computer-based information technologies such as digital radiography, digital intraoral video cameras, digital voice-text-image transfer, periodontal probing devices, CAD/CAMs, etc. By establishing standards for these modules, the need for several stand-alone systems in the dental office will be eliminated.

Each working group encompasses a broad spectrum of projects under a central theme. Within each working group, subcommittees are responsible for the specific projects. Each subcommittee has been researching standards already in existence to determine if they could be applicable to dentistry. Participants are also interfacing with standards groups active in medical informatics.

The ADA also sponsors participation in ANSI activities of the International Organization for Standardization (ISO) Technical Committee 106 on dentistry and acts as secretariat for ANSI for Working Group 2 of ISO/TC 106. Thus, the ADA works both nationally and internationally in the formation of standards for dentistry.

ANSI Accredited:

The American Dental Association has been sponsoring a standards program for dental materials, instruments and equipment since 1928. From 1928 to 1953, all specifications for dental materials, instruments and equipment were developed at the National Bureau of Standards by the federal government in cooperation with the ADA. Between 1953 and 1970, the Dental Materials Group of the International Association for Dental Research (IADR) acted as advisor to the ADA in developing specifications. In 1970, American National Standards Committee MD156 (ANSC MD156) was established by the American National Standards Institute, replacing the Dental Materials Group.

In 1983, the ANSC MD156 became an accredited committee by ANSI making the committee the Accredited Standards Committee MD156 (ASC MD156).

F

To date, 56 specifications for dental materials, instruments and equipment have been adopted by ANSI as American National Standards. In addition, the ADA acts as proprietary sponsor on a project to handle standards for dental radiographic film. This activity is conducted under the Accredited Canvas Method of ANSI.

ADA Implementation Guide for ASC X12 837

The standards which are being developed for electronic insurance transactions focus on the "envelope" used to transmit data electronically. The ADA has been working with the ASC X12 in order to define the data content placed in that envelope. The ADA has been responsible for the data content as it pertains to dental claims while the National Uniform Claim Committee (NUCC) and the National Uniform Billing Committee (NUBC) focus on the non-institutional and institutional data sets.

The ADA released an Implementation Guide for dental claims submission based upon the ANSI ASC X12 837 transaction set. The Association provided the data content for a dental claim based upon the ADA Dental Claim Format for the Implementation Guide. The Guide will assist practice management vendors, third-party payers and clearinghouses in the execution of the ASC X12 standards. Future versions of the 837 Dental Implementation Guide will be developed by ASC X12. However, the ADA will continue to provide the data content for the development of an Implementation Guide for dental applications.

The ADA developed two versions of the Implementation Guide (Versions 3041 and 3051) which were adopted by the ASC MD156 and recommended for use by practice management vendors for electronic dental claims transactions. Future versions of the Guide will be developed within the ASC X12. However, the ASC MD156 will continue to work with the ASC X12 Insurance Subcommittee. ANSI/ADA 1000 A Standard Clinical Data Architecture for the Structure and Content of a Computer-based Patient Record. Detailed information pertaining to the ANSI 1000 standard is entitled Activities to Promote Interoperability of Standards - Frameworks, Architectures, and Models.

Description of Standard:

The ADA Dental Implementation Guide is based upon the ASC X12 837 claims submission transaction. It was developed to assist users such as practice management vendors, third-party payers, and clearinghouses, in the execution of the 837 for dental claims transactions.

Readiness of Standard:

The ASC X12 claims submission 837 is being used for submitting some dental claims. However, utilization of the standard is very low at this time. Currently, most dental claims are submitted using proprietary formats. The 837 is the first standard to be developed for claims transactions. Therefore, the Association encourages that electronic dental claims transactions continue to be submitted in the current electronic formats, whether the transactions are proprietary formats or the 837, and a migration should occur to require ASC X12 formats only. The 837 transaction is the only approved ANSI draft standard for trial use. However, the ASC X12 Interactive Claim standard will soon be finalized and when approved it will be the preferred standard to be used for dental claims transactions.

Identifiable Costs:

The ADA's Implementation Guide version 3051 is free of charge from the ADA. Future versions of the Dental Implementation Guide will be available through DISA.

Contact for more information:

Ms. Sharon Stanford
Asst. Director,
Guidelines and Standards Development
American Dental Association
211 East Chicago Avenue
Chicago, Illinois 60611
Phone: (312) 440-2509
Fax: (312) 440-7494
email: stanfors@ada.org

Health Level Seven, Inc. (HL7)

Category/Classification of Standard

- Health Claims or Equivalent Encounter Information - Health Level Seven provides healthcare organizations such as hospitals and clinics the ability to consolidate patient billing information between computer systems. HL7 also provides the ability to transmit appropriate healthcare claims to the Health Care Financing Administration using their proprietary formats: UB82 for HL7 Versions 1.0 through 2.1 and the UB92 for HL7 Versions 2.2 and 2.3. In particular the UB82 part of the HL7 Standard predates the X12 835 transaction set by five years. If "equivalent encounter information" is to mean the clinical data associated with an encounter, then HL7 is currently uniquely positioned to have an existing standard to send this data. It is reasonable to expect that this type of clinical data would be included in the NCQA and HEDIS reporting requirements.
- Health Claims Attachments - In all versions, HL7 provides data interchange formats for consolidating patient-specific clinical information to support most healthcare claims, including physician's orders, prescriptions, laboratory and clinical tests, diagnostic procedures (excluding imaging) and resulting outcomes. HL7 version 2.2 is the only ANSI approved clinical data interchange standard in these areas. HL7 has also defined segments to transmit data (including clinical data) associated with an injury or accident.
- First Report Of Injury - In collaboration with the Centers for Disease Control (CDC), Health Level Seven is developing an Emergency Room data interchange format to report specific first encounter disease information.
- Referral Certification And Authorization - Health Level Seven has specific segments and trigger events to perform the data interchange necessary for referral and authorization. This request most frequently requires detailed clinical data over several encounters. Health Level Seven is uniquely positioned to meet these requirements.

Health Level Seven became an ANSI accredited SDO, Accredited Organization Method, on June 12, 1994.

F

Health Level Seven Versions 1.0 through 3.0

1) Health Level Seven Version 1.0 (published in 1987)
2) Health Level Seven Version 2.0 (published in 1989)
3) Health Level Seven Version 2.1 (published in 1990)
4) Health Level Seven Version 2.2 Application Protocol for Electronic Data Exchange in Healthcare (published in 1994, ANSI approved on February 8, 1996)
5) Health Level Seven Version 2.3 Application Protocol for Electronic Data Exchange in Healthcare is currently in the final stages of revision (expected publish date is March, 1997; currently in process for ANSI approval)
6) Health Level Seven Version 3.0 Application Protocol for Electronic Data Exchange in Healthcare is in the development stage (anticipated publish date is December 1998)

Contact For More Information:

Mark McDougall
Executive Director
Health Level Seven
3300 Washtenaw Avenue, Suite 227
Ann Arbor, MI 48104-4250
Phone: (313) 677-7777
Fax: (313) 677-6622
E-mail: hq@hl7.org

Description of Standard:

Objectives

To facilitate the interchange of health informatics and administrative and financial data needed to support clinical practice. By creating messages with sufficient granularity of data to support clinical practices, HL7 also creates support for the interchange of health informatics data needed for research (e.g., clinical trials messages; the use of the results messages to build clinical research databases), public health (e.g., the use of immunization query/reporting to track immunization needs of populations, the use of product experience messages to support drug and equipment adverse effects), and epidemiology (detailed clinical data can be collected on specific diseases).
Functions.

HL7 supports the following functions. (Please refer to Attachments 1 and 2 for a complete listing of HL7 event type codes and HL7 order control codes, respectively; to Attachment 3 for a listing of UB2 segments; and to Attachment 4 for product experience segments.) Those specific to Version 2.3 are denoted by an asterisk (*):
- Administrative functions, including messages for:
  - administrative support for clinical practice
  - ADT (admitting, discharge, and transfer within an institution)
  - registration (inpatient, outpatient, group and private practice)
- Financial support for clinical practice including:
  - notifying a billing/financial system of work performed
  - adding / updating patient accounts
  - purging patient accounts
  - generating bills and accounts receivable statements (a display query)

- generating and transmitting UB92 data (including charges, payments and adjustments)
  - updating account*
  - ending account*
- Scheduling*, including resources for:
  - inpatient
  - outpatient
  - clinic
  - private practice
- Orders, including but not limited to:
  - clinical laboratory
  - radiology
  - pharmacy (various types and levels including inpatient and outpatient)
  - EKG
  - EEG
  - dietary
  - requisitions
- Results, including, but not limited to:
  - clinical laboratory
  - radiology
  - pharmacy
  - images (by reference in HL7 Version 2.2, and directly in HL7 Version 2.3)
  - discharge summaries
  - op-notes
  - clinic notes
  - pharmacy administrations
  - Support for reporting results containing waveform data* (e.g. EEG, ICU 'strip' data, etc.)
- Immunization queries and reporting*, including:
  - patient identification
  - next of kin
  - patient visit
  - insurance information
  - common order
  - pharmacy administration
  - pharmacy route
  - observation/result
  - notes (regarding immunization)
- Clinical trials definition and reporting*
- Product experience reporting* (e.g. adverse drug/equipment reporting messages), including:
  - sender
  - observation
  - causal relationship
  - product summary
  - product detail
  - facility
  - Clinical master files support
  - Clinical referrals*
  - Problems, goals, and pathways*
  - Clinical transcription*
  - General query support for all of the above areas in both display and record-oriented formats

User Environment

The user environment for HL7 includes administrative, financial, and clinical information in support of clinical practice, research, adverse product experience, and epidemiology. The specific user 'environments' include any settings where this type of information needs to be transmitted between healthcare applications, such as:

- hospitals
- groups of hospitals (with associated clinics, and associated private or small practice groups)
- clinics
- private practices
- small group practices

Specific applications environments/settings where HL7 is currently being used include: workstation/desktop applications; message routing applications (e.g. 'gateways,' communications components such as the Andover Working Group's "Enterprise Communicator"), clinical data repositories (important components of the 'electronic medical record'), and systems comprised of these three software 'tiers.' Some of these already operate over the Internet.

Systems Environment

HL7 is a specification for healthcare informatics messages to be sent between applications, and thus, has no specific requirements for any of the above (i.e. no specific requirements for operating systems, network, hardware or other requirements). However, the HL7 Versions 2.2 and 2.1 do require an ASCII-based message encoding syntax, which is defined in Chapter 2 of the standard. HL7 Version 2.3 allows non-ASCII encoding schemes as defined in Chapter 2 of the standard, but does not directly support binary data. (Binary data objects may be referenced in HL7 Version 2.2 messages via the use of the 'Reference Pointer' data type.) HL7 Version 2.3 does contain a specific data type (ED, for encapsulated data) which allows for a MIME-encoding of binary data. By using this method, binary data may be transmitted in HL7 Version 2.3 messages.

It is important to note that even within HL7 Versions 2.1-2.3, the messages are defined abstractly, without reference to a specific encoding syntax. This allows implementors to use non-HL7 encoding syntaxes as needed (e.g., there is an HL7 Version 2.2 implementation using ASN.1 BER encoding syntax). This same paradigm will be followed in Version 3.0: the messages will be defined without regard to the encoding syntax used to send them between applications.

Although its messages will be defined abstractly, HL7 Version 3.0 plans to support 4 different 'encoding' layers: character based (an improved version of the current Version 2 encoding syntax), CORBA, OLE, and EDIFACT.

Application Function/Domain Completeness

With HL7 Version 2.3, HL7 has doubled the scope of messages supporting clinical practice, and the administrative and financial data needed to support clinical practice. HL7 believes that the core areas of clinical data are covered at this point. However, there is additional work to be completed. The members of HL7 have created the following special interest groups (SIGs) to define and research additions to the specification. The SIGs will determine if the area of interest can be addressed within one of the current HL7 technical committees, or whether a new technical committee needs to be formed. The list of current HL7 SIGs gives an indication of future areas that HL7 will address:

- Object brokering technologies (OBT) SIG (CORBA, OLE). Their goal is to demonstrate "proof of concept" for new technologies. A second demonstration was held at HIMSS '96. Full HL7 support requires completion of the HL7 object data model. The Andover Working Group is using a version of this approach that supports both CORBA and OLE versions of HL7 Version 2.2 messages.
- Automated Data (enhanced coverage of waveforms, ICU-systems, etc.)
- Home Health
- Image Management (with DICOM and related input)
- Professional Certification

- Security
- Codes and Vocabularies
- Clinical Decision Support (e.g. Arden Syntax)
- SGML

In addition, the Quality Assurance/Data Modeling technical committee, which is doing the bulk of the work on the methodology for HL7 Version 3.0, will split into two separate technical committees, one concerned with the Version 3.0 methodology (including object data modeling), and the other concerned with quality assurance.

HL7 Version 3.0 will be based on an object modeling framework, including the message development framework created by the IEEE Joint Working Group on the Common Data Model, and also using work developed by CEN TC-251, WG-3, Project Team 25, for developing messages from object models. This work has been expanded and adapted to HL7's needs by HL7's Quality Assurance/Data Modeling technical committee. Many of the relevant documents are available on the Duke University Healthcare Informatics Standards Web Site (use http://www.mcis.duke.edu/standards/guide.htm for all standards, and use http://www.mcis.duke.edu/standards/HL7/hl7.htm for just HL7). In addition to the Message Development Framework and detailed instructional materials, HL7 has created a Reference Information Model that will be used to define and harmonize sub-models for each technical committee. Over the next year to 18 months, HL7 will use this work to develop Version 3.0.

The Version 3.0 approach has been demonstrated at two HIMSS's conferences and validated by the work of the Andover Working Group in their Enterprise Communicator specification and implementation. (Supported already by over 100 vendors and institutions.)

Ways In Which This Standard Is Superior To Other Standards In This Category/Classification

The HL7 standard is superior in its completeness of coverage of scope of messages supporting clinical practice, and the administrative and financial data needed to support clinical practice. It has gained market acceptance and very widespread use, not only within the U.S., but internationally in such countries as Canada, The Netherlands, Germany, Australia, New Zealand, Finland and Japan. It provides ease of implementation, flexibility, and has gained acceptance by major vendors and academic sites.

Other Relevant Characteristics

HL7 is actively working to harmonize its work with other SDO's and with other relevant areas. For example, HL7 recently formed a codes and vocabularies SIG which will work to standardize the code sets in use for clinical data fields and transactions. HL7 is participating in the IEEE JWG/Common Data Model and convenes meetings jointly with X12N. HL7 has an MOU with NCPDP and is working to harmonize the NCPDP's SCRIPT specification with the HL7 Pharmacy messages.

Readiness of Standard:

Is It A Guideline?

HL7 is not a guideline, but an actual standard for healthcare informatics messages supporting clinical practice, and the administrative and financial data needed to support clinical practice. Insofar as HL7 Version 2 messages are based on 'trigger events,' they address actual processes within the healthcare environment. HL7 Version 3.0 will be based on objects derived from analysis of scenarios and business cases in the healthcare environment: in that sense Version 3.0 will address actual

F

processes of information flows within the healthcare environment. The exchange of such information can be used to support clinical practice, but does not per se, define practice. In the same sense, HL7 messages do not imply the design of applications, but can be used to create or request data which is needed by healthcare clinical applications.

Is It Implementable?

HL7 Versions 2.1 and 2.2 are fully implementable, since they have been balloted standards since 1990 and 1994 respectively. In addition to the standards themselves, HL7 has published Implementation Guides for Version 2.1 and 2.2. HL7 Version 2.3 will be finalized during the first quarter of 1997, at which time it will be fully implementable. As with Versions 2.1 and 2.2, HL7 will publish an Implementation Guides for Version 2.3. There are thousands of installations using HL7 Version 2.1 and 2.2, and many sites using 2.3 draft versions. In addition, an Access database will be available with Version 2.3 to help users create their own interface specifications. This database consists of tables for HL7 components, tables, fields, messages and segments and includes several predefined queries (e.g., alpha sort of tables, numeric sort of tables, fields and components, etc.).
Version 3.0 is planned for release during the fourth quarter of 1998 and will provide both a standard and an Implementation Guide. In addition, formal conformance profiles will be available for Version 3.0.

How Can The Standard Be Obtained?

Copies of the HL7 standard V2.1, 2.2, and 2.3 are available for $125 each from HL7 Headquarters at:
3300 Washtenaw Avenue, Suite 227
Ann Arbor, MI 48104-4250
Phone: (313) 677-7777
Fax: (313) 677-6622
E-mail: hq@hl7.org

Does This Require A Separate Implementation Guide?

HL7 has published Implementation Guides for Version 2.1 and 2.2. HL7 Version 2.3 will be published during the first quarter of 1997, at which time it will be fully implementable. As with Version 2.1 and 2.2, HL7 will publish an Implementation Guide for Version 2.3.

Is There Only One Implementation Guideline?

For the 2.x versions of HL7 there is a single Implementation Guide. Version 3.0 will provide four Implementation Guide sections, one for each of the four implementable message specifications: character-based; OLE, CORBA, and OLE.

Is A Conformance Standard Specified?

The Conformance SIG is working on this part of the standard. A conformance standard will definitely be provided for Version 3.0, and the Conformance SIG may also develop conformance standards for HL7 Versions 2.x.

Are Conformance Test Tools Available?

Conformance test tools will be part of Version 3.0, and the Conformance SIG may also develop them for Version 2.3.

Source Of Test Tools?

The source of HL7 V3.0 test tools has not yet been selected. Additionally, the Conformance SIG may develop or contract them for Version 2.3.

If The Standard Is Under Development, What Parts Of It Are Ready Now?

Version 2.1 and 2.2 are available now; Version 2.3 is currently available in draft form and will be available in its final, published form during the first quarter of 1997.

What Extensions Are Now Under Development?

As indicated earlier, these include:
- Object brokering technologies
- Automated Data (enhanced coverage of waveforms, ICU-systems, etc.)
- Home Health
- Image Management (with DICOM and related input)
- Professional Certification
- Security
- Codes and Vocabularies
- Clinical Decision Support (e.g. Arden Syntax)
- SGML
- Andover Working Group's "Enterprise Communicator"

Major Milestones Toward Standards Completion?

Version 2.3:
- Final balloting

Version 3.0
- Completion of the "Strawman" Reference Information Model
- Completion of the Hierarchical Message Descriptions
- Completion of Implementable Message Specifications for OLE/CORBA and printable character streams

Projected Dates For Final Balloting And/Or Implementation.
- V2.3 - Final balloting will be completed by mid January, 1997. Anticipated publish date is March, 1997.
- V3.0 - Work will begin in January, 1997 with the objective of having the first ballots completed by the end of 1998.

Other Indicators Of Readiness That May Be Appropriate.

One company has been using the proposed Referral chapter specification (new with Version 2.3) in two state-wide and three regional healthcare information networks for the past two years. Much of the information in this chapter was derived from prototyping the work being accomplished in these information networks. They have utilized inter-enterprise transactions for 80% of the events in the Referral chapter. In addition, one hospital vendor has implemented the Scheduling transactions (also new with Version 2.3) and has been using them successfully since January, 1996.

F

Indicators of Market Acceptance:

Based on our membership records of over 1,600 total members in HL7, approximately 739 vendors, 652 healthcare providers, 104 consultants, and 111 general interest/payor agencies are utilizing the HL7 standard. HL7 standards have been installed thousands of times. For example, one vendor alone has installed 856 interfaces per HL7 standards as of mid 1996. In addition the HL7 standard is being used and implemented in Canada, Australia, Finland, Germany, The Netherlands, New Zealand, and Japan.

Another relevant indicator of market acceptance in the public sector is the Andover Working Group's implementation of the Enterprise Communicator (and the accompanying tightly coupled, zero optionality conformance specification for sections of HL7 Version 2.2): the Andover Working Group is a 'test implementation' of the Version 3.0 functionality (it has CORBA, OLE, and character-based encoding structures, and is scheduled for production during the fourth quarter of 1996 or the first quarter of 1997.

Level of Specificity:

Description Of Framework Detail And Level Of Granularity.

The granularity of the HL7 standard is sufficient to support clinical practice (i.e., it is much more granular that the reimbursement standards). It's framework, in terms of scope, is also sufficient to support clinical practices.

Does The Standard Reference Or Assume Other Standards To Achieve More Specificity?

The HL7 standard does not reference or assume other standards to achieve more specificity. HL7 is, in general, more granular than other standards. It allows the use of standard code sets as needed by implementors via the HL7 CE data type.

Assumed Code Sets.

Current HL7 assumes code sets for a small number of single 'data elements.' These are termed 'HL7 tables,' and are so marked and so defined within the current specification.
For other data elements, HL7 allows the use of either 'site-defined' (e.g., HL7 IS data type) or 'standard (external) code sets' (e.g., using the CE coded element data type).
HL7 has hundreds of users who are using the HL7 tables.

Sources Of Code Sets.

HL7 tables are defined within the HL7 standard. User defined tables are defined at implementation time. Standard (external) tables (e.g. SNOMED, ICD9, CPT) are defined externally by their source-creating institutions, and may be obtained from their usual suppliers.

Available Assistance On The Use Of Code Sets.

It is expected that the new HL7 Codes and Vocabularies SIG will make recommendations for code sets, including means for obtaining the various standard external code sets. It is also expected that Version 3.0 will specify more completely all three types of code sets (HL7, user-defined, and external standards). Chapter 7 contains an extensive list of external standard code sets (including where to obtain them).

Projected Dates Of Completion And Implementation For Code Sets Currently Under Development.

The vocabulary SIG is expected to publish these dates sometime after the January 1997 HL7 meeting.

Relationships with Other Standards:

Other Standards
- HL7 and X12N. No overlap.
- HL7 and NCPDP Script. Conceptual overlap in the area of prescription messages (including authorization and refills).
- HL7 and ASTM Lab information and Waveform messages. Conceptual overlap.
  Standards Reconciliation Or Coordination Activities
- HL7 and X12N are convening simultaneously so that members may attend and learn what each group is doing. Harmonization at the object model level is being addressed in that both groups are members of the IEEE-JWG/Common Data Model. Both groups have agreed not to create overlapping, redundant messages. HL7 and NCPDP have created an MOU and are working to harmonize the NCPDP script messages and the HL7 Pharmacy messages in terms of content and vocabulary so that a one-pass, unambiguous, translator can translate from one form to another. (The market dictates this approach.)
- HL7 and ASTM lab messages have been harmonized by having members of both groups work on both standards, thus guaranteeing interoperability.
- HL7 and ASTM waveform messages have been harmonized by having members of both groups work on both standards, thus guaranteeing interoperability.
- HL7 and IEEE Medix have been co-meeting and working with the IEEE JWG/CDM to harmonize their data models.
- HL7 has been harmonizing with DICOM via the HL7 IMSIG (Image Management SIG).
- HL7 is working with various groups to harmonize code sets/vocabularies for clinical data.
- HL7 has also been engaged in unofficial coordination with CEN TC 251 WG3 by sharing members working on various projects (including US 'experts' attending WG3 meetings). HL7 would also like to do some formal reconciliation of the object data models used by WG3.

What Portion Of The Specification And Functionality Is Affected By This Coordination?
(See above).

What Conditions Are Assumed In Order For This Coordination To Be Effective?
Cooperation and openness from the other SDO's.

Is This Standard Consistent With International Standards? If So, Which Standards?

In terms of the scope of HL7, to our knowledge there are no ISO standards that cover the HL7 scope (see definition above). Version 3.0 will be compatible with EDIFACT, CORBA and OLE as encoding syntaxes. Additionally, the Andover Working Group has demonstrated a means to use CORBA or OLE with Version 2.3 messages.

What Gaps Remain Among Related Standards That Should Be Addressed?

Agreement on standard code sets/terminologies for various clinical items need to be addressed. In addition, the listing of HL7 SIGs above identifies gaps in the clinical support coverage.

F

Describe What Is Being Done To Address These Gaps?
See above.

Attachment 1

HL7 Event Type Codes

Value	Description
A01	ADT/ACK - Admit / visit notification
A02	ADT/ACK - Transfer a patient
A03	ADT/ACK - Discharge/end visit
A04	ADT/ACK - Register a patient
A05	ADT/ACK - Pre-admit a patient
A06	ADT/ACK - Change an outpatient to an inpatient
A07	ADT/ACK - Change an inpatient to an outpatient
A08	ADT/ACK - Update patient information
A09	ADT/ACK - Patient departing - tracking
A10	ADT/ACK - Patient arriving - tracking
A11	ADT/ACK - Cancel admit/visit notification
A12	ADT/ACK - Cancel transfer
A13	ADT/ACK - Cancel discharge/end visit
A14	ADT/ACK - Pending admit
A15	ADT/ACK - Pending transfer
A16	ADT/ACK - Pending discharge
A17	ADT/ACK - Swap patients
A18	ADT/ACK - Merge patient information
A19	QRY/ACK - Patient query
A20	ADT/ACK - Bed status update
A21	ADT/ACK - Patient goes on a "leave of absence"
A22	ADT/ACK - Patient returns from a "leave of absence"
A23	ADT/ACK - Delete a patient record
A24	ADT/ACK - Link patient information
A25	ADT/ACK - Cancel pending discharge
A26	ADT/ACK - Cancel pending transfer
A27	ADT/ACK - Cancel pending admit
A28	ADT/ACK - Add person information
A29	ADT/ACK - Delete person information
A30	ADT/ACK - Merge person information
A31	ADT/ACK - Update person information
A32	ADT/ACK - Cancel patient arriving - tracking
A33	ADT/ACK - Cancel patient departing - tracking
A34	ADT/ACK - Merge patient information - patient ID only
A35	ADT/ACK - Merge patient information - account number only
A36	ADT/ACK - Merge patient information - patient ID and account number
A37	ADT/ACK - Unlink patient information
A38	ADT/ACK - Cancel pre-admit
A39	ADT/ACK - Merge person - external ID
A40	ADT/ACK - Merge patient - internal ID
A41	ADT/ACK - Merge account - patient account number
A42	ADT/ACK - Merge visit - visit number

A43	ADT/ACK - Move patient information - internal ID
A44	ADT/ACK - Move account information - patient account number
A45	ADT/ACK - Move visit information - visit number
A46	ADT/ACK - Change external ID
A47	ADT/ACK - Change internal ID
A48	ADT/ACK - Change alternate patient ID
A49	ADT/ACK - Change patient account number
A50	ADT/ACK - Change visit number
A51	ADT/ACK - Change alternate visit ID
B01	PPR/ACK - Patient problem
C01	CRM - Register a patient on a clinical trial
C02	CRM - Cancel a patient registration on clinical trial (for clerical mistakes only)
C03	CRM - Correct/update registration information
C04	CRM - Patient has gone off a clinical trial
C05	CRM - Patient enters phase of clinical trial
C06	CRM - Cancel patient entering a phase (clerical mistake)
C07	CRM - Correct/update phase information
C08	CRM - Patient has gone off phase of clinical trial
C09	CSU - Automated time intervals for reporting, like monthly
C10	CSU - Patient completes the clinical trial
C11	CSU - Patient completes a phase of the clinical trial
C12	CSU - Update/correction of patient order/result information
G01	PGL/ACK - Patient goal
I01	RQI/RPI - Request for insurance information
I02	RQI/RPL - Request/receipt of patient selection display list
I03	RQI/RPR - Request/receipt of patient selection list
I04	RQD/RPI - Request for patient demographic data
I05	RQC/RCI - Request for patient clinical information
I06	RQC/RCL - Request/receipt of clinical data listing
I07	PIN/ACK - Unsolicited insurance information
I08	RQA/RPA - Request for treatment authorization information
I09	RQA/RPA - Request for modification to an authorization
I10	RQA/RPA - Request for resubmission of an authorization
I11	RQA/RPA - Request for cancellation of an authorization
I12	REF/RRI – Patient referral
I13	REF/RRI – Modify patient referral
I14	REF/RRI – Cancel patient referral
I15	REF/RRI – Request patient referral status
M01	MFN/MFK - Master file not otherwise specified (for backward compatibility only)
M02	MFN/MFK - Master file - Staff Practitioner
M03	MFN/MFK - Master file - Test/Observation
varies	MFQ/MFR - Master files query (use event same as asking for e.g., M05 - location)
M04	MFD/ACK - Master files delayed application acknowledgement
M05	MFN/MFK - Patient location master file
M06	MFN/MFK - Charge description master file
M07	MFN/MFK - Clinical study with phases and schedules master file
M08	MFN/MFK - Clinical study without phases but with schedules master file
O01	ORM – Order message (also RDE, RDS, RGV, RAS)
O02	ORR – Order response (also RRE, RRD, RRG, RRA)
Q06	OSQ/OSR - Query for order status
P01	BAR/ACK - Add and update patient account
P02	BAR/ACK - Purge patient account
P03	DFT/ACK - Post detail financial transaction
P04	QRY/DSP - Generate bill and A/R statements

F

P05	BAR/ACK - Update account
P06	BAR/ACK - End account
P07	PEX - Unsolicited initial individual product experience report
P08	PEX - Unsolicited update individual product experience report
P09	SUR - Summary product experience report
PC1	PPR - PC/ Problem Add
PC2	PPR - PC/ Problem Update
PC3	PPR - PC/ Problem Delete
PC4	PRQ - PC/ Problem Query
PC5	PRR - PC/ Problem Response
PC6	PGL - PC/ Goal Add
PC7	PGL - PC/ Goal Update
PC8	PGL - PC/ Goal Delete
PC9	PGQ - PC/ Goal Query
PCA	PGR - PC/ Goal Response
PCB	PPP - PC/ Pathway (Problem-Oriented) Add
PCC	PPP - PC/ Pathway (Problem-Oriented) Update
PCD	PPP - PC/ Pathway (Problem-Oriented) Delete
PCE	PTQ - PC/ Pathway (Problem-Oriented) Query
PCF	PTR - PC/ Pathway (Problem-Oriented) Query Response
PCG	PPG - PC/ Pathway (Goal-Oriented) Add
PCH	PPG - PC/ Pathway (Goal-Oriented) Update
PCJ	PPG - PC/ Pathway (Goal-Oriented) Delete
PCK	PTU - PC/ Pathway (Goal-Oriented) Query
PCL	PTV - PC/ Pathway (Goal-Oriented) Query Response
Q01	QRY/DSR - Query sent for immediate response
Q02	QRY/ACK - Query sent for deferred response
Q03	DSR/ACK - Deferred response to a query
Q05	UDM/ACK - Unsolicited display update
R01	ORU/ACK - Unsolicited transmission of an observation
R02	QRY – Query for results of observation
R03	Display-oriented results, query/unsol. Update (for backward compatibility only)
R04	ORF – Response to query; transmission of requested observation
RAR	RAR – Pharmacy administration information query response
RDR	RDR – Pharmacy dispense information query response
RER	RER – Pharmacy encoded order information query response
RGR	RGR – Pharmacy dose information query response
ROR	ROR – Pharmacy prescription order query response
S01	SRM/SRR - Request new appointment booking
S02	SRM/SRR - Request appointment rescheduling
S03	SRM/SRR - Request appointment modification
S04	SRM/SRR - Request appointment cancellation
S05	SRM/SRR - Request appointment discontinuation
S06	SRM/SRR - Request appointment deletion
S07	SRM/SRR - Request addition of service/resource on appointment
S08	SRM/SRR - Request modification of service/resource on appointment
S09	SRM/SRR - Request cancellation of service/resource on appointment
S10	SRM/SRR - Request discontinuation of service/resource on appointment
S11	SRM/SRR - Request deletion of service/resource on appointment
S12	SIU/ACK – Notification of new appointment booking
S13	SIU/ACK – Notification of appointment rescheduling
S14	SIU/ACK - Notification of appointment modification
S15	SIU/ACK - Notification of appointment cancellation
S16	SIU/ACK - Notification of appointment discontinuation

S17	SIU/ACK - Notification of appointment deletion
S18	SIU/ACK - Notification of addition of service/resource on appointment
S19	SIU/ACK - Notification of modification of service/resource on appointment
S20	SIU/ACK - Notification of cancellation of service/resource on appointment
S21	SIU/ACK - Notification of discontinuation of service/resource on appointment
S22	SIU/ACK - Notification of deletion of service/resource on appointment
S23	SIU/ACK - Notification of blocked schedule time slot(s)
S24	SIU/ACK - Notification of open ("unblocked") schedule time slot(s)
S25	SQM/SQR - Query schedule information
T01	MDM/ACK - Original document notification
T02	MDM/ACK - Original document notification and content
T03	MDM/ACK - Document status change notification
T04	MDM/ACK - Document status change notification and content
T05	MDM/ACK - Document addendum notification
T06	MDM/ACK - Document addendum notification and content
T07	MDM/ACK - Document edit notification
T08	MDM/ACK - Document edit notification and content
T09	MDM/ACK - Document replacement notification
T10	MDM/ACK - Document replacement notification and content
T11	MDM/ACK - Document cancel notification
T12	QRY/DOC - Document query
V01	VXQ - Query for vaccination record
V02	VXX – Response to vaccination query returning multiple PID matches
V03	VXR – Vaccination record response
V04	VXU – Unsolicited vaccination record update
W01	ORU – Waveform result, unsolicited transmission of requested information
W02	QRF – Waveform result, response to query
X01	PEX – Product experience

Attachment 2

HL7 Order Control Codes and Their Meaning

Value	Description	Originator	Field Note
NW	New order	P	I
OK	Order accepted & OK	F	I
UA	Unable to Accept Order	F	n
CA	Cancel order request	P	a
OC	Order canceled	F	
CR	Canceled as requested	F	
UC	Unable to cancel	F	b
DC	Discontinue order request	P	c
OD	Order discontinued	F	
DR	Discontinued as requested	F	
UD	Unable to discontinue	F	
HD	Hold order request	P	
OH	Order held	F	
UH	Unable to put on hold	F	
HR	On hold as requested	F	

RL	Release previous hold	P	
OE	Order released	F	
OR	Released as requested	F	
UR	Unable to release	F	
RP	Order replace request	P	e,d,h
RU	Replaced unsolicited	F	f,d,h
RO	Replacement order	P,F	g,d,h,l
RQ	Replaced as requested	F	d,e,g,h
UM	Unable to replace	F	
PA	Parent order	F	l
CH	Child order	F,P	i
XO	Change order request	P	
XX	Order changed, unsol.	F	
UX	Unable to change	F	
XR	Changed as requested	F	
DE	Data errors	P,F	
RE	Observations to follow	P,F	j
RR	Request received	P,F	k
SR	Response to send order status request	F	
SS	Send order status request	P	
SC	Status changed	F,P	
SN	Send order number	F	l
NA	Number assigned	P	l
CN	Combined result	F	m
RF	Refill order request	F, P	o
AF	Order refill request approval	P	p
DF	Order refill request denied	P	q
FU	Order refilled, unsolicited	F	r
OF	Order refilled as requested	F	s
UF	Unable to refill	F	t
LI	Link order to patient care message	u	
UN	Unlink order from patient care message	u	

Attachment 3

UB92 Segments

The UB2 segment contains data necessary to complete UB92 bills. Only UB92 fields that do not exist in other HL7 defined segments appear in this segment. Patient Name and Date of Birth are required; they are included in the PID segment and therefore do not appear here. When the field locators are different on the UB92, as compared to the UB82, the element is listed with its new location in parentheses ( ).

UB2 attributes

SEQ	LEN	DT	OPT	RP/#	TBL#	ITEM#	ELEMENT NAME
1	4	SI	O			00553	Set ID - UB2
2	3	ST	O			00554	Co-Insurance Days (9)
3	2	IS	O	Y/7	0043	00555	Condition Code (24-30)
4	3	ST	O			00556	Covered Days (7)
5	4	ST	O			00557	Non-Covered Days (8)
6	11	CM	O	Y/12	0153	00558	Value Amount & Code
7	11	CM	O	Y/8		00559	Occurrence Code & Date (32-35)
8	28	CM	O	Y/2		00560	Occurrence Span Code/Dates (36)
9	29	ST	O	Y/2		00561	UB92 Locator 2 (State)
10	12	ST	O	Y/2		00562	UB92 Locator 11 (State)
11	5	ST	O			00563	UB92 Locator 31 (National)
12	23	ST	O	Y/3		00564	Document Control Number
13	4	ST	O	Y/23		00565	UB92 Locator 49 (National)
14	14	ST	O	Y/5		00566	UB92 Locator 56 (State)
15	27	ST	O			00567	UB92 Locator 57 (National)
16	2	ST	O	Y/2		00568	UB92 Locator 78 (State)
17	3	NM	O			00815	Special Visit Count

PID attributes

SEQ	LEN	DT	OPT	RP/#	TBL#	ITEM#	ELEMENT NAME
1	4	SI	O			00104	Set ID - Patient ID
2	20	CX	O			00105	Patient ID (External ID)
3	20	CX	R	Y		00106	Patient ID (Internal ID)
4	20	CX	O	Y		00107	Alternate Patient ID - PID
5	48	XPN	R			00108	Patient Name
6	48	XPN	O			00109	Mother's Maiden Name
7	26	TS	O			00110	Date/Time of Birth
8	1	IS	O		0001	00111	Sex
9	48	XPN	O	Y		00112	Patient Alias
10	1	IS	O		0005	00113	Race
11	106	XAD	O	Y		00114	Patient Address
12	4	IS	B			00115	County Code
13	40	XTN	O	Y		00116	Phone Number - Home
14	40	XTN	O	Y		00117	Phone Number - Business
15	60	CE	O		0296	00118	Primary Language
16	1	IS	O		0002	00119	Marital Status
17	3	IS	O		0006	00120	Religion
18	20	CX	O			00121	Patient Account Number
19	16	ST	O			00122	SSN Number - Patient
20	25	CM	O			00123	Driver's License Number - Patient
21	20	CX	O	Y		00124	Mother's Identifier
22	3	IS	O		0189	00125	Ethnic Group
23	60	ST	O			00126	Birth Place
24	2	ID	O		0136	00127	Multiple Birth Indicator
25	2	NM	O			00128	Birth Order
26	4	IS	O	Y	0171	00129	Citizenship
27	60	CE	O		0172	00130	Veterans Military Status
28	80	CE	O			00739	Nationality
29	26	TS	O			00740	Patient Death Date and Time

F

30	1	ID	O		0136	00741	Patient Death Indicator

Attachment 4

Product Experience Segments

PES - product experience sender segment

PES attributes

SEQ	LEN	DT	OPT	RP/ #	TBL #	ITEM #	ELEMENT NAME
1	80	XON	O			01059	Sender Organization Name
2	60	XCN	O	Y		01060	Sender Individual Name
3	200	XAD	O	Y		01062	Sender Address
4	44	XTN	O	Y		01063	Sender Telephone
5	75	EI	O			01064	Sender Event Identifier
6	2	NM	O			01065	Sender Sequence Number
7	600	FT	O	Y		01066	Sender Event Description
8	600	FT	O			01067	Sender Comment
9	26	TS	O			01068	Sender Aware Date/Time
10	26	TS	R			01069	Event Report Date
11	3	ID	O	Y/2	0234	01070	Event Report Timing/Type
12	1	ID	O		0235	01071	Event Report Source
13	1	ID	O	Y	0236	01072	Event Reported To

PEO - product experience observation segment

Details related to a particular clinical experience or event are embodied in the PEO segment. This segment can be used to characterize an event which might be attributed to a product to which the patient was exposed. Products with a possible causal relationship to the observed experience are described in the following PCR (possible causal relationship) segments. The message format was designed to be robust and includes many optional elements which may not be required for a particular regulatory purpose but allow a complete representation of the drug experience if needed.
A PEX message can contain multiple PEO segments if the patient experienced more than one event but must contain at least one PEO segment.

PEO attributes

SEQ	LEN	DT	OPTC	RP/ #	TBL #	ITEM #	ELEMENT NAME
1	60	CE	O	Y		01073	Event Identifiers Used
2	60	CE	O	Y		01074	Event Symptom/Diagnosis Code
3	26	TS	R			01075	Event Onset Date/Time
4	26	TS	O			01076	Event Exacerbation Date/Time
5	26	TS	O			01077	Event Improved Date/Time
6	26	TS	O			01078	Event Ended Data/Time
7	106	XAD	O			01079	Event Location Occurred Address
8	1	ID	O	Y	0237	01080	Event Qualification
9	1	ID	O		0238	01081	Event Serious
10	1	ID	O		0239	01082	Event Expected
11	1	ID	O	Y	0240	01083	Event Outcome
12	1	ID	O		0241	01084	Patient Outcome

13	600	FT	O	Y		01085	Event Description From Others
14	600	FT	O	Y		01086	Event From Original Reporter
15	600	FT	O	Y		01087	Event Description From Patient
16	600	FT	O	Y		01088	Event Description From Practitioner
17	600	FT	O	Y		01089	Event Description From Autopsy
18	60	CE	O	Y		01090	Cause Of Death
19	46	XPN	O			01091	Primary Observer Name
20	106	XAD	O	Y		01092	Primary Observer Address
21	40	XTN	O	Y		01093	Primary Observer Telephone
22	1	ID	O		0242	01094	Primary Observer's Qualification
23	1	ID	O		0242	01095	Confirmation Provided By
24	26	TS	O			01096	Primary Observer Aware Date/Time
25	1	ID	O		0243	01097	Primary Observer's identity May Be Divulged

PCR - possible causal relationship segment

The PCR segment is used to communicate a potential or suspected relationship between a product (drug or device) or test and an event with detrimental effect on a patient. This segment identifies a potential causal relationship between the product identified in this segment and the event identified in the PEO segment.

More than one PCR segment can be included in the message if more than one product is possibly causally related to the event.

PCR attributes

SEQ	LEN	DT	OPT	RP/ #	TBL #	ITEM #	ELEMENT NAME
1	60	CE	R			01098	Implicated Product
2	1	IS	O		0239	01099	Generic Product
3	60	CE	O			01100	Product Class
4	8	CQ	O			01101	Total Duration Of Therapy
5	26	TS	O			01102	Product Manufacture Date
6	26	TS	O			01103	Product Expiration Date
7	26	TS	O			01104	Product Implantation Date
8	26	TS	O			01105	Product Explanation Date
9	8	IS	O		0239	01106	Single Use Device
10	60	CE	O			01107	Indication For Product Use
11	8	IS	O		0239	01108	Product Problem
12	30	ST	O	Y/3		01109	Product Serial/Lot Number
13	1	IS	O		0239	01110	Product Available For Inspection
14	60	CE	O			01111	Product Evaluation Performed
15	60	CE	O		0247	01112	Product Evaluation Status
16	60	CE	O			01113	Product Evaluation Results
17	8	ID	O		0248	01114	Evaluated Product Source
18	26	TS	O			01115	Date Product Returned To Manufacturer
19	1	ID	O		0242	01116	Device Operator Qualifications
20	1	ID	O		0250	01117	Relatedness Assessment
21	2	ID	O	Y/6	0251	01118	Action Taken In Response To The Event
22	2	ID	O	Y/6	0232	01119	Event Causality Observations
23	1	ID	O	Y/3	0253	01120	Indirect Exposure Mechanism

F

PSH - product summary header segment

PSH attributes

SEQ	LEN	DT	OPT	RP/#	TBL #	ITEM #	ELEMENT NAME
1	60	ST	R			01233	Report Type
2	60	ST	O			01234	Report Form Identifier
3	26	TS	R			01235	Report Date
4	26	TS	O			01236	Report Interval Start Date
5	26	TS	O			01237	Report Interval End Date
6	12	CQ	O			01238	Quantity Manufactured
7	12	CQ	O			01239	Quantity Distributed
8	1	ID	O		0329	01240	Quantity Distributed Method
9	600	FT	O			01241	Quantity Distributed Comment
10	12	CQ	O			01242	Quantity in Use
11	1	ID	O		0329	01243	Quantity in Use Method
12	600	FT	O			01244	Quantity in Use Comment
13	2	NM	O	Y/8		01245	Number of Product Experience Reports Filed by Facility
14	2	NM	O	Y/8		01246	Number of Product Experience Reports Filed by Distributor

PDC - product detail country segment

PDC attributes

SEQ	LEN	DT	OPT	RP/#	TBL #	ITEM #	ELEMENT NAME
1	80	XON	R			01247	Manufacturer/Distributor
2	60	CE	R			01248	Country
3	60	ST	R			01249	Brand Name
4	60	ST	O			01250	Device Family Name
5	60	CE	O			01251	Generic Name
6	60	ST	O	Y		01252	Model Identifier
7	60	ST	O			01253	Catalogue Identifier
8	60	ST	O	Y		01254	Other Identifier
9	60	CE	O			01255	Product Code
10	4	ID	O		0330	01256	Marketing Basis
11	60	ST	O			01257	Marketing Approval ID
12	12	CQ	O			01258	Labeled Shelf Life
13	12	CQ	O			01259	Expected Shelf Life
14	26	TS	O			01260	Date First Marked
15	26	TS	O			01261	Date Last Marked

FAC - facility segment

FAC attributes

SEQ	LEN	DT	OPT	RP/#####	TBL #	ITEM #	ELEMENT NAME
1	20	EI	R			01262	Facility ID
2	1	ID	O		0331	01263	Facility Type
3	200	XAD	R			01264	Facility Address
4	44	XTN	R			01265	Facility Telecommunication
5	60	XCN	O	Y		01266	Contact Person

66

6	60	ST	O	Y	01267	Contact Title
7	200	XAD	O	Y	01268	Contact Address
8	44	XTN	O	Y	01269	Contact Telecommunication
9	60	XCN	R		01270	Signature Authority
10	60	ST	O		01271	Signature Authority Title
11	200	XAD	O		01272	Signature Authority Address
12	44	XTN	O		01273	Signature Authority Telecommunication

National Uniform Claim Committee (NUCC)

The National Uniform Claim Committee was organized in May 1995 to develop, promote, and maintain a standard data set for use by the non-institutional health care community to transmit claim and encounter information to and from all third-party payers. The data set includes data elements, definitions, and code sets. Providers and suppliers may submit the NUCC data set using either a paper or electronic envelope.

The NUCC has received a formal consultative role regarding standards for health care transactions selected by the Secretary of Health and Human Services (HHS) as specified in the administrative simplification section of the Health Insurance Portability and Accountability Act of 1996 (P.L. 104-191). As specified in Act, American National Standards Institute (ANSI) accredited organizations must consult with the NUCC, the National Uniform Billing Committee (NUBC), the Workgroup for Electronic Data Interchange (EDI), and the American Dental Association (ADA). If the Secretary selects a standard different from one developed by an ANSI-accredited organization, she also must consult with the NUCC, NUBC, WEDI, and ADA.

The NUCC is chaired by the American Medical Association (AMA) with the Health Care Financing Administration (HCFA) as a critical partner. The Committee includes representation from key provider and payer organizations, as well as standards setting organizations, state and federal regulators, and the NUBC. As such, the NUCC is intended to have an authoritative voice regarding national standard data content and data definitions for non-institutional health care claims and encounters. The following organizations serve on the Committee as voting members:
- American Medical Association
- Health Care Financing Administration
- Alliance for Managed Care
- American Association of Health Plans
- ANSI ASC X12 Insurance Subcommittee
- Blue Cross and Blue Shield Association
- Health Insurance Association of America
- Medical Group Management Association
- National Association for Medical Equipment Services
- National Association of Insurance Commissioners
- National Association of State Medicaid Directors
- National Uniform Billing Committee

The NUCC will finalize its recommended data set in the first quarter of 1997 and make it available to the public. The NUCC also will provide formal comments into the ANSI ASC X12 Professional Implementation Guide for the Claim (837). Subsequently, the NUCC will address all other transactions specified in P.L 104-191.

F

ANSI Accredited:

The NUCC is not ANSI accredited; however, ANSI ASC X12 Insurance Subcommittee is a voting member of the NUCC, and several NUCC members are active in X12 and the HISB and are members of ANSI.

National Uniform Claim Committee Recommended Data Set for a Non-Institutional Claim or Encounter

Description of Standard:

The NUCC data set is intended for the transmission of claim and encounter information to and from all third-party payers, regardless of whether the envelope is paper or electronic.

Readiness of Standard:

The NUCC will make its recommendation available to the public in the first quarter of 1997.

Identifiable Costs:

No or minimal costs.

Contact For More Information:

Mark J. Segal, Ph.D.
Chair, National Uniform Claim Committee
Director, American Medical Association
515 N. State Street
Chicago, IL 60610
Phone: 312/464/4726
Fax: 312/464/5836
E-mail: Mark_Segal@ama-assn.org

Indicator of Market Acceptance:

Voting members of the NUCC represent key provider and public and private payer organizations. Constituencies of these organizations were surveyed twice during the development of NUCC recommendations.

Health Claim Attachments

There are several standards developing organizations working on clinical data models, technical reports, guidelines and standards for clinical data. Some of these SDOs include HL7, ADA, X12, IEEE, ACR/NEMA/DICOM, and ASTM. Information regarding some of the standards being developed by HL7 and ADA appeared in the previous claims and encounter section and detailed information regarding their other projects appears in the Appendix explaining the activities to promote interoperability of standards - frameworks, architectures and models. Additional information regarding ASTM appears in the Security section. Claim attachment information pertaining to X12, IEEE, DICOM, and ASTM standards is listed below.

Accredited Standards Committee (ASC) X12 Insurance Subcommittee, Health Care Task Group.

ANSI Accreditation

X12 was accredited as an ANSI accredited standards committee in 1979. Subsequent X12 procedure changes have required ANSI re-accreditation which was last granted in 1987.

The main objective of ASC X12 is to develop Electronic Data Interchange (EDI) standards to facilitate electronic business transactions (i.e. order placement and processing, shipping and receiving, invoicing, payment, cash application data, insurance transactions). ASC X12 endeavors to structure standards in a manner that computer programs can translate data to and from internal formats without extensive reprogramming.

This strategy allows companies to maximize their resources required for internally developed or commercial software (recommended) and private or public-access communication networks. ASC X12 believes that all sizes of companies using intelligent computational devices can benefit from the use of the standard. The efficiencies of standard interchange format can minimize the difficulties incurred from each organization using its own formats to transact business. Within ASC X12, the various subcommittees are responsible for developing standards in their area of expertise. Once a subcommittee has developed a draft standard the full ASC X12 membership reviews and approves it according to the operating policies and procedures. All standards (new or changed) require the consensus approval of the full ASC X12 membership. The approved standard becomes a draft standard for trial use for a reasonable trial period. After the trial period the draft standards are submitted to ANSI to become an American National Standard (ANS).

ASC X12 Patient Information (275)

Contact for more information: Data Interchange Standards Association (DISA) 703-548-7005.

Description of Standard:

A) The objective of the Patient Information (275) is to support the exchange of demographic, clinical and other supporting patient information to support administrative reimbursement processing as it relates to the submission of health care claims for both health care products and services.

B) This transaction set can be used to communicate individual patient information requests and patient information (either solicited or unsolicited) between separate health care entities in a variety of settings to be consistent with confidentiality and use requirements.

C) This transaction is used to provide additional patient information to support administrative reimbursement for health care products and services.

D) This standard may be used from any operating system, network, or hardware platform.

E) The standard has be developed with widespread input from the health care industry incorporating all business needs into its functionality.

F

F) The ANSI ASC X12 is the only nationally recognized EDI standards development organization in the United States for all type of electronic commerce. ASC X12 is the organization assigned by ANSI to represent the United States in the development of International EDI standards.

G) Standards. These standards are developed using a consensus process by the users in the health care industry.

H) The standards developed by ASC X12 may be translated to/from application systems using off the shelf translation software products which are used by all industries utilizing the ASC X12 standards.

Readiness of Standard:

A) The Patient Information (275) is not a guideline. However the X12 Insurance Subcommittee is currently developing implementation guides.

B) The Patient Information (275) standard is fully implementable. The transaction set was approved as a Draft Standard for Trial Use (DSTU) in June of 1995 as Version 0030?2.

C) The standard can be obtained by contacting the Data Interchange Standards Association (DISA) at 703-548-7005.

D) This standard does not require an implementation guide. ASC X12 has published four Type II Tutorial reports or tutorials for version 003041 in October of 1994, version 003050 in October 1995, version 003051 in February 1996, and version 003060 in April of 1996. To facilitate consistent implementation across the health care industry, the X12 Insurance Subcommittee is currently in the process of completing five implementation guides for version 003070 encompassing medical, hospital, dental, pharmaceutical claims, and workers compensation jurisdictional reporting with an anticipating publication date of April 1997.

E) There currently is only one implementation guide for the Patient Information (275) transaction.

F) The implementation guides will specify the conformance to the standards.

G) Yes, conformance tools are commercially available.

H) The same tools used for conformance may also be used as testing tools.

I) The standard is complete. The current version of the standard is 003070. As business needs dictate, enhancements may be made to the standard three times per year, one major release along with two subsequent sub-releases. The X12 Health Care Task Group has developed procedures to determine when to move to the next version of the standard as well as when to retire past versions. The Health Care Task Group will also determine the need for new versions of the implementation guides (not more frequently than once per year).

J) Currently no enhancements are under development.

AA) This standard has been completed.

BB) This standard has been completed and undergoing industry implementation.

Indicator of Market Acceptance:

A) The X12 standards are made available via many sources including from the Data Interchange Standards Association, Washington Publishing (ASC X12 Insurance Subcommittee's publisher), industry user groups and associations, and the Internet. Due to the multiplicity and diversity of these distribution methods, it is not possible to determine how many copies have been distributed and to whom.

B) Yes. ASC X12 represents international standards development. North American and other countries have implemented ASC X12 standards for purchasing and financial transactions. It would be to their benefit to further leverage their investment in EDI translation software, hardware and communication infrastructure to utilize the health care transactions.

C) Over 300 payer, provider, vendor, and plan sponsor organizations currently participate in the development of the ASC X12 standards and implementation guides to meet the business needs of the entire health care industry. These organizations have experienced the benefits of mature standards as costs associated with developing and maintaining proprietary formats far exceed the investment necessary to implement a single set of health care EDI transactions.

Level of Specificity:

A) The ASC X12 EDI transactions have been developed to meet the specific business needs identified by the standards developers and the health care industry.

B) See attached table of contents from the ASC X12 Insurance Committee's implementation guides.

C) ASC X12 standards incorporate the business requirements for exchanging information contained within other standards. The ASC X12 standards provides a vehicle for communicating other standards within the standards.

D) ASC X12 maintains over one thousand internal code sets to support the standards. Along with the internal code sets the ASC X12 standards reference over 350 external code sources such as:
   - Current Procedural Terminology (CPT) Codes from American Medical Association
   - International Classification of Diseases Clinical Modification - (ICD-9-CM) Diagnosis from U.S. National Center for Health Statistics.

E) There are too many code sets to describe here. Refer to the ASC X12 standards publication.

F) Internal code sets are included within the ASC X12 standards publications and implementation guides. When external code sets are referenced within these documents, the source where the code sets can be obtained is listed.

G) When possible, the implementation guides will either include the external code sets or provide further information on how to obtain the external code sets. Internal code sets are included within the implementation guides.

H) Internal code sets are available to all users of the ASC X12 standards. Usage of the external code sets will vary by source and their ability to promote the usage of their code sets.

I) ASC X12 internal code sets follow the same processes defined for the development and maintenance of the EDI transactions. External code lists are maintained by the external code source's internal development procedures.

Relationships with other standards:

A) ASC X12 strives to coordinate and incorporate the needs of the other standards development organizations such as Health Level 7 (HL7), National Council for Prescription Drug Programs (NCPDP), and the American Society for Testing and Materials into the ASC X12 standards.

B) See A).

C) See A).

D) Open communication in the development of the standards amongst the standards development organizations.

E) ASC X12 is the ANSI appointed standards development organization responsible for international EDI standards within the United States

F) None

G) Given the scope and responsibility for the development and maintenance of the EDI standards for the United States and the international community with respect to United States international standards, ASC X12 is only privy to the business needs which are brought forward and coordinated with other health care organizations. At this time, we are unaware of any gaps in the current standards for insurance.

F

Identifiable Costs:

A) None applicable. ASC X12 does not license it standards.
B) The cost of acquiring the ASC X12 standards publication varies depending upon the source of the publications. Currently they are available from:
   - Data Interchange Standards Association (DISA) 703-548-7005.
   - Washington Publishing Corporation 800-972-4334
   - Industry user groups and associations
   - The Internet (http://www.disa.org, http://www.wpc-edi.com)
C) The typical cost ranges from free to $415.00 for the full ASC X12 standards publication in either paper form or CD-ROM.
D) The cost/timeframe for education and training will depend upon the individuals and skill levels of the individuals within an organization. Some organizations have completed education and training within one week while others have taken longer.
E) The cost/timeframe for implementation depends upon the internal systems capabilities, systems development philosophy, hardware platform selected, EDI translator software, communication methodology and individual resources within an organization. Costs can range anywhere from free for a personal computer solution to well over $150,000 for midsize and mainframe systems. Some organizations have implemented the standards within a matter of days while other have taken months to achieve the same end result.

IEEE 1157 MEDIX Project

Institute of Electrical and Electronics Engineers, Medical Information Bus (MIB) General Committee.

ANSI Accreditation:

IEEE is a charter member of ANSI and is an Accredited Standards Developing Organization.

IEEE 1073, Standard for Medical Device Communications

A family of documents that defines the entire seven layer communications requirements for the "Medical Information Bus" (MIB). This is a robust, reliable communication service designed for Intensive Care Unit, Operating Room, and Emergency Room bedside devices.

Approved Standards:

1) IEEE 1073.3.1 - Standard for Medical Device Communications, Transport Profile - Connection Mode: This document defines the services and requirements for a bedside subnetwork. It defines services similar to those defined in Ethernet and TCP/IP. Combined with 1073.4.1, it defines the hardware required to offer hospitals to ensure ease of use for clinician initiated automatic data capture from bedside devices. An approved ANSI Standard since August, 1995.
2) IEEE 1073.4.1 - Standard for Medical Device Communications, Physical Layer, Cable Connected: This document defines the cables, connectors, data rates, and bit level encoding for the MIB. It is coupled with IEEE 1073.3.1 to complete the "lower layers" for 1073. An approved ANSI Standard since August, 1995.
3) IEEE 1073 - Standard for Medical Device Communications, Overview and Framework: This document serves as an overview of the 1073 family of standards and a roadmap of which

documents, present and planned, contain information on different facets of communication. It defines the underlying philosophy in the 1073 family of standards. Approved by the IEEE Standards Board in March, 1996.

On-going Standards Work:

- IEEE 1073.1 - Standard for Medical Device Communications, Medical Device Data Language (MDDL) Overview and Framework: This document defines the ISO Standards and conventions for using Object-Oriented Technology to define communications services for bedside medical devices. This is expected to go to ballot in late 1996.
- IEEE 1073.1.1 - Standard for Medical Device Communications, MDDL Common Definitions: This document defines the common definitions for the object oriented communications services for medical devices.
- IEEE 1073.1.2 - Standard for Medical Device Communications, MDDL Virtual Medical Device, Generalized: This document defines the general features of all virtual medical devices, in an object oriented environment. This is highly harmonized with CEN TC251, PT021 First Working Draft "Vital Signs Representations".
- IEEE 1073.1.3 - Standard for Medical Device Communications, MDDL Virtual Medical Device, Specialized: This document defines the general features of specialized virtual medical devices for specific device categories. This is highly harmonized with CEN TC251, PT021 First Working Draft "Vital Signs Representation".
- IEEE 1073.1.3.1 - Standard for Medical Device Communications, MDDL Virtual Medical Device, Specialized, Infusion Device: Defines the specific object oriented communications services for infusion devices. This project should have a first draft by the end of 1996.
- IEEE 1073.1.3.2 - Standard for Medical Device Communications, MDDL Virtual Medical Device, Specialized, Vital Signs Monitor: Defines the specific object oriented communications services for vital signs monitors.
- IEEE 1073.1.3.1 - Standard for Medical Device Communications, MDDL Virtual Medical Device, Specialized, Ventilator: Defines the specific object oriented communications services for ventilators. This project was started in April, 1996.
- IEEE 1073.2 - Standard for Medical Device Communications, Application Profile, Overview and Framework: Describes the common theory and rules for all application profiles to be defined for the 1073 family. This was approved by the ballot group in late 1995, but is in editing stage. Should be approved by IEEE Standards Board in September, 1996.
- IEEE 1073.2.0 - Standard for Medical Device Communications, Application Profile, Medical Device Encoding Rules: An optimization of ISO Basic Encoding Rules made for bedside medical devices. This should go to ballot in late 1996.
- IEEE 1073.2.1 - Standard for Medical Device Communications, Application Profile, Minimum Set: Defines the minimum application profile for bedside medical devices. The service provided allows for one way capture of device data. This should go to ballot in late 1996.
- IEEE 1073.2.2 - Standard for Medical Device Communications, Application Profile, Basic Capabilities: Defines the basic set of communications services for an application profile for bedside medical devices. The services provided allow for two way getting and setting of attribute values, and for creating and deleting of objects.

F

Contact For More Information:

Bob Kennelly
Chair, IEEE 1073 General Committee
LinkTech
30 Orville Drive
Bohemia, NY 11716
(P) 516-567-5656, ext. 7482
(F) 516-563-2819
(E) bobk@linktech.ilcddc.com

Description of Standard:

The IEEE 1073 Family of Standards serves to achieve the following: Objectives: To standardize data communications for patient connected bedside devices, optimized for the acute care setting, to allow clinicians to set up device communications in a "plug and play" fashion.

Functions:

The function of this family of standards is to permit real time, continuous, and comprehensive capture of device data from patient connected bedside devices. This data includes physiological parameter measurements and device settings.

User Environment:

This family of standards is used in any setting containing patient connected bedside devices, but was optimized in its design for acute care settings such as intensive care, operating rooms, and emergency rooms.

Systems Environment:

IEEE 1073 defines a bedside sub-network where devices communicate with a bedside communications controller. The standard is strongly based on ISO Open Systems Interconnect, and as such is able to be compatible with most computer industry standard implementations. Prototype implementations have been done with DOS, Windows, Windows NT, TCP/IP and Ethernet.

Application Function/Domain Completeness:

The lower layers, or hardware, for this standard is completed as an IEEE and ANSI Standard. Drafts exist for many of the upper layer pieces required to do prototyping. Several documents are going to ballot in 1997.

In what way(s) is this standard superior to other standards in this category/classification?

The IEEE 1073 is the first attempt to standardize device interfaces. The previous data interfaces provided by device manufacturers were based on RS-232, in which only the very basic voltage levels and data rates are defined. Each device manufacturer needed to invent heir own language for device communications. Device manufacturers frequently changed this language in large and small ways across product lines and product revisions. The result was an entirely impossible quagmire of differing device interfaces for devices that tend to be portable and able to plug into multiple ports, each requiring a specific device driver to talk. It is similar to needed a different phone plug for each area code you want to call.

Readiness of Standard:

A) The IEEE 1073 family of standards are design standards that must be implemented during device design, or in after market converters. The implementation of 1073 allows for comprehensive, automatic collection of device data, which will affect clinician practice.

B) IEEE 1073 is presently implementable, and is in the process of being done at McKay-Dee Hospital in Ogden, Utah. The lower layers standards are supported by commercially available silicon and boards. The upper layers exist as drafts, using available object oriented models. To implement 1073 in 1996, a hospital must know its device type population, and design tables in their HIS to interpret the specific message structure, format, and content from their medical devices. The delivery of this message is standardized today.

C) The IEEE 1073 Standards are available from IEEE by calling 908-562-3800.

D) There is presently no implementation guide for the IEEE 1073 Standards.

E) There is presently no implementation guide for the IEEE 1073 Standards.

F) A conformance test plan and method is intended future work of the IEEE 1073 General Committee.

G) There are no conformance test tools available for IEEE 1073.

H) There are no conformance test tools available for IEEE 1073.

I) The lower layers of the standard are completed and implementable today. The lower layers are analogous to using ethernet and TCP/IP. The upper layers are still being developed, with several documents expected to be approved in 1997.

J) There are no extensions being developed, since the scope for this standard includes all communication layers for bedside medical devices.

AA) Ballot groups for 5 upper layer documents are being formed and will be closed by the end of 1996. Balloting for these documents will occur in the second quarter of 1997, with approval by the IEEE Standards Board in September or December 1997.

BB) Upon approval of the documents in 1997, a full implementation of IEEE 1073 will be achievable. Prototype implementations will be done in the first half of 1997.

Indicator of Market Acceptance:

A) As of January 1996, approximately 400 copies of the approved standards had been sold by IEEE.

B) IEEE 1073 is in the early adopter stage in the market. There are people at LDS Hospital, Univ. of West Virginia, Univ. Texas Houston Medical School, Texas Children's Hospital, and Naval Hospital San Diego doing prototyping work. One medical device vendor, Siemens, is shipping product in Europe with IEEE 1073 embedded.

C) There is prototype and evaluation work on IEEE 1073 being done in UK, Germany, Spain, Norway, and Japan.

D) There is growing demand for 1073 from US Hospitals, which is being recognized by US device vendors, and being considered for their new product designs. Also, the Hewlet-Packard led Andover Working Group has stated their intent to do prototype implementations of 1073 in 1997.

F

Level of Specificity:

Notes:

A) IEEE 1073 is a family of standards that describe in specific detail what needs to be implemented to be compliant.
B) The lower layers of 1073 are very specifically defined and are supported by a commercially available integrated circuit product. The upper layer drafts define very specific message contents and structure for specific types of bedside medical devices.
C) IEEE 1073 references many ISO communications standards to define the communications protocol. These include ISO Standards for RS-485, HDLC, Basic Encoding Rules, ASN.1, and the Guide to Developing Managed Objects.
D) There is a defined nomenclature within IEEE 1073 that defines the parameter name and a code structure for physiologic parameters and device settings.
E) The code set is a subset of the Medical Device Data Language (MDDL), and is listed as the MDDL Nomenclature, IEEE 1073.1.1
F) IEEE 1073.1.1 is a draft available from IEEE. It has also been submitted to LOINC for inclusion in that work.
G) There is presently no users' guide for the code set. However, one of the vendor members of the general committee has developed a tool in-house that may be released for public use in 1997.
H) The IEEE 1073 nomenclature is not presently being used in any commercial application.
I) IEEE 1073.1.1 should be balloted in 1997.

Relationships with Other Standards:

A) IEEE 1073 is a bedside subnetwork that collects device data. In any application that requires this data, 1073 has a relationship with that standard. The relationship will most likely be expressed through application gateways. Such examples may include: conversion of device data to HL7 format for inclusion of device parameters in an HL7 based clinical data depository; conversion of device data into an X12 message for inclusion in billing applications; use of device data by an electronic medical record standardized any other SDO.
B) IEEE 1073 has been having its meeting in conjunction with the HL7 working group meetings to ensure rapid convergence of ideas.
C) The most important aspect of our coordination efforts is elimination of workscope overlap. For example, at the last HL7 meeting we received a presentation on LOINC that resulted in formal submittal of our work to LOINC.
D) The only assumed condition we have is that our work will be viewed as valuable and taken as a contribution.
E) IEEE 1073 is entirely based on the ISO Open System Interconnect model and multiple ISO communications standards such as HDLC, BER, ASN.1, MOSI, GDMO.
F) The remaining gaps are mainly in areas of implementations to ensure that the goals of standardization are achievable in actual practice.
G) The nearest term efforts on implementations will be done in the Andover Working Group.

Identifiable Costs:

- Please indicate the cost or your best estimate for the following:
- Cost of licensure: There is no licensure cost for IEEE 1073.
- Cost of acquisition : Medical device with embedded IEEE 1073 interfaces should have minimal cost difference from present purchase prices. The hospital infrastructure to support bedside data capture will likely be similar to the costs of putting PC's at bedsides.

- Cost/timeframes for education and training: Unknown
- Cost/timeframes for implementation: Unknown

Please note any other cost considerations: The probable investment in IEEE 1073 infrastructure for hospitals will be small compared to the benefits from being able to have comprehensive data on the conditions of the most gravely ill, and costly, patients.

Digital Imaging Communication in Medicine (DICOM) Standards Committee

Membership: Professional specialty societies, industry (National Electrical Manufacturers Association and other industry), and government, industry, and trade association liaison members.

ANSI Accreditation:

NEMA is an ANSI-Accredited standards developing organization. The DICOM Standards Committee, through NEMA, can develop American National Standards via the ANSI Canvass Procedure. The DICOM Standards Committee is considering applying for ANSI Accredited Standards Committee status in 1997.

DICOM Standard. NEMA PS3.x - 1992, 1993, 1995

Contact For More Information

DICOM Secretariat: NEMA
Mr. David Snavely, 1300 North 17th Street, Suite 1847, Rosslyn, VA 22209
e-mail: dav_snavely@nema.org

DICOM Liaison Working Group Secretariat: American College of Radiology
Mr. James Potter, 1891 Preston White Drive, Reston, VA 22091
e-mail: jamesp@acr.org

DICOM Structured Reporting Secretariat: College of American Pathologists
Ms. Karen Kudla, 325 Waukegan Road, Northfield, IL 60093-2750
e-mail: kkudla@cap.org

DICOM Visible Light Working Group Secretariat: Am. Soc. of Gastro. Endoscopy
Dr. Louis Korman, Washington VA Medical Center
e-mail: lkorman@erols.com

DICOM ANSI HISB Liaison: W. Dean Bidgood, Jr., M.D., M.S.
Box 3321, Duke University Medical Center, Durham, NC 27710
e-mail: bidgood@nlm.nih.gov

Description of Standard

DICOM specifies a generic digital format and a transfer protocol for biomedical images and image-related information. The specification is usable on any type of computer and is useable to transfer

F

images over the Internet. DICOM interfaces are available for nearly all types of imaging devices sold by all of the leading vendors of radiology imaging equipment. DICOM is now being adopted for use outside of radiology (for example, in pathology, internal medicine, veterinary medicine, and dentistry). The most commonly used diagnostic and therapeutic biomedical image types are fully covered by DICOM. DICOM has been adopted by the U.S. Veterans Affairs Administration and the U.S. Armed Forces.

DICOM enables interchange of text information, coded information, measurements, images, and other binary data. The systems domain focus is on all aspects of image management. Interfacing with other text-based information systems is also specified. Trial implementation of a new structured report interface will begin in January, 1997.

Readiness of Standard

All radiology image specifications of DICOM are fully implementable. The visible light (color) image types and the structured reporting interfaces will be available for trial implementation in January, 1997. Additional draft specifications for radiation oncology, PostScript™ Print management, Positron Emission Tomography, image data compression, security, image presentation (standardized display) parameters are under development at the time of this writing.

DICOM is an implementable standard. There is no official implementation guide. Public domain software implementations are available on the Internet. Several companies offer implementation software "tool kits" for sale. Further information about DICOM resources may be obtained on the NEMA WWW site: (http://www.nema.org).

Indicator of Market Acceptance

DICOM is the dominant non-prominent data interchange message standard in biomedical imaging. All major radiology equipment vendors have implemented the standard. Acceptance is growing rapidly outside of radiology. Interconnectivity among many vendors has been demonstrated to the public in many international meetings since 1992.

Level of Specificity

DICOM is a highly specific and explicit specification. The standard specifies all data interchange parameters from hardware factors (industry standards adopted) up through the bit/byte stream, services, protocols, to the domain knowledge layer. A very practical and useful level of interoperability can be achieved with the standard. The need for local configuration agreements is minimized. The SNOMED DICOM Microglossary™ is the preferred *coding system -to- message data element* Mapping Resource. SNOMED (Systematized Nomenclature of Human and Veterinary Medicine, © College of American Pathologists) and LOINC (Logical Observation Identifiers, Names, and Codes) database are the preferred coding systems. DICOM also supports locally-defined (or private) coding systems.

Relationships with Other Standards

DICOM has a close relationship to the HL7 Standard in the area of Imaging System - Information System interfacing. DICOM has entered into standards developing partnership with the SNOMED Authority of the College of American Pathologists. Ultrasound, cardiovascular, and other DICOM measurement codes are being developed in close cooperation with the LOINC Committee. Internationally, DICOM is compatible with the CEN/TC 251 WG4 MEDICOM Standard and the Japanese JIRA and MEDIS-DC Standards for network interchange of images and image-related information.

Enhancement of the Information System - Imaging System interface specifications of DICOM and related standards is underway at the time of this writing. DICOM offers advanced capabilities for management of binary data objects (such as images) that are not available in the current versions text-based data interchange standards (HL7 and X-12).

Identifiable Costs

The printed specification of the DICOM Standard is available from NEMA for approximately $300. Implementation training is available from private consulting and training companies. Due to the complexity of imaging technology, the DICOM specification is complex. Significant training is required in order to write compatible software. However, the availability of software implementation "tool kits" from several commercial sources has greatly simplified the implementation of DICOM for most vendors.

ASTM Committee E31 on Healthcare Informatics

The category/classification of this standard is: **Data Content Vocabulary** for Computer-Based Patient Records

The standards development organization is ASTM. ASTM is an ANSI accredited standards development organization.

Organized in 1898, ASTM (the American Society for Testing and Materials) has grown into one of the largest voluntary standards development systems in the world. ASTM is a not-for profit organization that provides a forum for producers, users, ultimate consumers, and those having a general interest (representatives of government and academia) to meet on common ground and write standards for materials, products, systems, and services. From the work of 132 standards-writing committees, ASTM publishes more that 9000 standards. ASTM headquarters has no technical research or testing facilities; such work is done voluntarily by 35,000 technically qualified ASTM members located throughout the world. ASTM provides continuing education and training in the use and application of ASTM standards through Technical and Professional Training courses. In 1987, ASTM formed the Institute for Standards and Research (ISR). The purpose of the Institute is to provide a mechanism for conducting research to improve the quality and timeliness of ASTM standards. It does no research, but serves as the intermediary between the standards-writing community and the public or private agencies that could provide appropriate research and technical services, or supply funding for such research.

F

Accreditation

ASTM is an ANSI Accredited by the Organization Method. All ASTM Committee E31 standards are approved as American National Standards

ASTM E1384-96 Standard Guide for Content and Structure of the Computer-Based Patient Record

Contact for more information:

Manager - Committee E31, ASTM
100 Barr Harbor Drive
West Conshohocken, PA 19373
Ph: 610-832-9500
Fax: 610-832-9666

Standard Description

This standard guide is intended to provide the framework vocabulary for the computer-based patient record content. It proposes a minimum essential content drawn from a developing annex of dictionary elements.

Elements are populated using master tables which range from standard code systems to reference tables harmonized with HL-7 Version 2.2. It calls for unique data views specified for clinical settings. The standard contains an annex of dictionary items intended as a reference standard for designers and developers.

Functions: Implementation Independent Content Organization
Master Tables
Data Views
User Environment: Administrative And Clinical Users
Software Developers - Data Base Design
Educators - Health Informatics
Systems Environment: Does Not Specify System Environment
Evolving Standard - Ongoing Development
Most Complete CPR Content Standard

Value

There are no other standards that address the overall content vocabulary for computer-based patient records. This standard offers an initial data model intended for application in all healthcare settings. It currently serves as a reference model for vendors and institutions working to build data base content for CPRs.

Readiness of the Standard

A) This standard is a guideline that addresses policy and design. Since it offers an overall data model, users would incorporate the elements of the standard that apply to their situation. For example, requests for this standard come from designers working on the data content of the CPR. The proposed content is being used as a base data model and for data definitions.

B) This standard does not require a separate implementation guide. It should be used in conjunction with the Standard Specification for Coded Values for the Computer-Based Patient Record E1633 to achieve more specificity. Vocabulary data elements are defined in E1384, which include limited code values and pointers to E1633 for the specific master tables and code systems and values needed for the data elements. Code sets are assumed, referenced in E1633 for data elements; and harmonized with code sets in HL-7 where feasible.

C) How can the standard be obtained? ASTM standards are available through the ASTM Customer Service Department by calling 610-832-9585. Standards can also be ordered through the ASTM Web Site at www. astm.org

The standard is fully usable now as a reference guide for designers/developers of Computer-Based Patient Records.

Milestones

Milestones identified are additional content, harmonization with companion standards and joint development work on new vocabulary. The most recent ballot was in 1996. Proposed revisions are already in development and updates will be balloted in 1997.

Indicator of Market Acceptance

A) If the standard is a guideline, how many copies have been requested and distributed? Approximately 2300 copies of the E31 standards have been distributed.

B) If the standard is an implementable standard, how many vendors, healthcare organizations, and/or government agencies are using it?

This type of information is difficult to obtain for the E31 standards. It is indicated where available under the document specific information to follow.

This standard is included in the ASTM 1996 Book of standards made available to people who join ASTM. Currently, the membership of E31 Committee on Healthcare Informatics is over 300. Actual numbers of interested individuals who have requested this standard far exceeds the membership.

The Veterans Administration reports using this as a reference standard.

Other indicators of market acceptance include users who are currently involved in developing CPR applications within individual hospitals and hospital consortiums; vendors who are working on CPR data repository models; and CPR project planners who are in the process of defining content standards for their enterprise.

This standard is also included in a 1996 publication that has been adopted by all Health Information Administration programs in the United States.

Level of Specificity

This standard is a guide. It calls for standard content expressed in a uniform manner. It does not provide data dictionary specificity. It identifies the common information framework that is part of patient records in multiple settings.

Relationship with Other Standards

As indicated, this standard depends on ASTM E1633 for specified coded values; uses some HL-7 data elements and a limited number of master tables. Ongoing analysis is performed to continue work on harmonizing elements with collaborative work, e.g. the Minimum Data Set from the National Committee on Vital and Health Statistics. Harmonization with message standards are proposed for revisions where possible. Functionality will be strengthened by coordination. Conditions assumed for coordination to be effective include joint work initiatives among standards developers and representatives from the user community who currently use this standard.

E1384 can be obtained from ASTM at:

F

100 Barr Harbor Drive, West Conshohocken, PA 19428
(610) 832-9500 Web Site: http://www.astm.org

Category/Classification of the Standard

Health Claim Attachments

ASTM E1769-95 Standard Guide for Properties of Electronic Health Records and Record Systems

Contact for more information:

Manager - Committee E31, ASTM
100 Barr Harbor Drive
West Conshohocken, PA 19373
Ph: 610-832-9500
Fax: 610-832-9666

Description of Standard

This standard defines the requirements, properties, and attributes of a computer-based patient record. It serves as an agreement among all the parties about the goals and constraints of the computer-based patient record, and provides criteria for making tradeoffs and decisions about how the record will be configured. The guide defines a computer-based record as the structured set of demographic, environmental, social, financial, and clinical data elements in electronic form needed to document the healthcare given to a single patient. It discusses how information is entered, dealing with such questions as who can enter, how is information identified, how is it validated, and who is accountable. It describes data attributes, such as permanence, accessibility, reliability, internal consistency, and security. System response time and the ability to process data are considered. Output criteria are addressed, including who can access information, the level of fact detail available, customization of display, multimedia outputs, and export to other systems. The system must protect the rights of the patient to confidentiality and the rights of the care provider to privacy. The concept of connecting together various encounter records of a patient to produce a longitudinal patient record is described. Systems to implement computer-based medical records must support local clinical functions. In addition, they should also be considered nodes of a national clinical network. The data content of the records must meet the needs of all legitimate users, such as payers, regulatory agencies, public health workers, researchers, and quality of care/outcome studies personnel. The records must be mobile and accessible to all authorized users. This ensures easy transport of records when patients move or change care providers. It also permits the extraction of billing, monitoring, and research data into other computer systems. Full logical compatibility among data banks is essential for these purposes.

Readiness of Standard

The standard is published and is an American National Standard. How can the standard be obtained? ASTM standards are available through the ASTM Customer Service Department by calling 610-832-9585. Standards can also be ordered through the ASTM Web Site at www. astm.org

Indicators of Market Acceptance

Approximately 2300 copies of the E31 standards have been distributed.
A wide variety of vendors are implementing EHR systems. The standard describes many of the features which are being incorporated into these systems and includes many features which have yet to be implemented by vendors. There has been no feedback to the standards committee from vendors indicating any objection to the features described in the standard other than the technical difficulty of achieving some of the functions described therein.

Level of Specificity

The standard describes EHR functions at a functional level. It makes no attempt to recommend a specific implementation strategy but rather attempts to outline how the various functions described can interact to provide a functional EHR.

Relationship with Other Standards

Related ASTM standards, notably E 1384, provide information on topics such as the data elements which should be included in an EHR system. Numerous additional standards such as HL7 for data exchange and various coding schemes to determine data content are also relevant.

Identifiable Costs

The cost to implement this standard depends heavily on the technology and methodologies chosen by a specific vendor.

Category/Classification of the Standard

Health Claim Attachments

ASTM E1633-95 Standard Specification for Coded Values Used in the Computer-Based Patient Record

Contact for more information:
Manager - Committee E31, ASTM
100 Barr Harbor Drive
West Conshohocken, PA 19373
Ph: 610-832-9500
Fax: 610-832-9666

F

Description of Standard

This specification identifies the lexicons to be used for the data elements identified in the Annex portion of Standard E1384, Guide for the Content and Structure of the Computer-Based Patient Record. It is intended to unify the representations for (1) the identified data elements for the computer-based patient record, (2) data elements contained in other standard statistical data standards, (3) data elements used in other healthcare data message exchange format standards, or (4) in data gathering forms for this purpose, and (5) in data derived from these elements so that data recorded in the course of patient care can be exchangeable and provide consistent devel0pment of CPR content vocabulary that can. also provide an accurate source for statistical and resource management data. Code values are specified using master tables which range from standard code value sets identified directly for the data element to standard code systems such as ICD9 to reference tables harmonized with HL7 Version 2.2. It promotes consistent data views specified for clinical settings. The standard is intended as a reference standard for designers and developers.

Functions: Implementation independent content organization
Identifies data representation for vocabulary elements
Includes an initial catalog of coded value sets
References known mater tables
User Environment: Administrative and clinical users
Software developers - data base design
Educators - health informatics
Systems Environment: Does not specify system environment
Evolving standard - ongoing development is focused on alignment with value sets used in companion standards

Value: Provides the 2nd edition of detailed representation for the listed data elements contained in the vocabulary content in Standard ASTM E1384. It currently serves as a reference model for vendors and institutions working to build data base content for CPRs.

Readiness of Standard

This standard is a specification that addresses data structure and data dictionary design. Since it combines with E1384 to offer an overall data model, users would incorporate the elements of the standard that apply to their situation. Requests for this standard come from designers working on the data content of the CPR. The proposed content is being used as a base data model and for data definitions.

This standard does not require a separate implementation guide. It should be used in conjunction with the Standard E1384. Vocabulary data elements are defined in E1384, which include limited code values and point to this specification for the specific delineations for the data form, coded values to be used in representing the element and where appropriate, and more formally identified master tables and code systems needed for the data elements. Code sets are assumed, referenced in E1633 for data elements and harmonized with code sets is ASTM Standards E 1238, E1239 and HL7 where feasible.

The standard is fully usable now as a reference guide for designers/developers of computer-based patient records.

Milestones identified are continued code value expansions, harmonization with companion standards and joint development work on new vocabulary. The most recent ballot was 1996. Proposed revisions and updates will be balloted in early 1997.

The standard is published and is an American National Standard. How can the standard be obtained? ASTM standards are available through the ASTM Customer Service Department by calling 610-832-9585. Standards can also be ordered through the ASTM Web Site at www. astm.org

Indicators of Market Acceptance

Approximately 2300 copies of the E31 standards have been distributed.

The Veterans Administration reports using this as a reference standard. Other indicators include users who are currently involved in developing CPR applications within individual hospitals and hospital consortiums; vendors who are working on CPR data repository models; and CPR project planners who are in the process of defining content standards for their enterprise.

This standard is also included in a 1996 publication that has been adopted by all Health Information Administration programs in the United States. Another text due out in 1997 on data dictionaries for healthcare recommends usage of this specification in conjunction with E1384 for constructing data dictionaries in healthcare organizations.

Level of Specificity

This standard calls for content to be expressed in a uniform manner. It does provide some data dictionary specificity. It identifies the common representation for data to be part of computer-based patient records in multiple settings.

Relationship with Other Standards

As indicated, this standard is written to provide the detailed specificity to ASTM E1384 for specified code values. Major work on this standard continues to be comparison and reconciliation with other standards and evolving data sets such as the Minimum Data Set from the National Committee on Vital and Health Statistics; and the National Provider Identification efforts underway in the Health Care Financing Administration. Harmonization with message standards and data element values included in X12 are proposed for revisions where possible. Functionality will be strengthened by coordination. Conditions assumed for coordination to be effective include joint work initiatives among standard developers and representatives from the user community who currently use this standard.

Enrollment and Disenrollment in a Health Plan

Accredited Standards Committee (ASC) X12, Health Care Task Group

ASC X12 Benefit Enrollment and Maintenance (834)

Contact for more information - Data Interchange Standards Association (DISA) 703-548-7005.

F

Description of Standard

A) The objective of the - Benefit Enrollment and Maintenance (834) is to support the administration of enrollment and disenrollment of covered individuals within various insurance products.

B) This transaction set can be used to enroll and disenroll covered individuals for insurance products such as health, life, flexible spending accounts, and retirement products.

C) This transaction is used for administration of insurance benefit plans.

D) This standard may be used from any operating system, network, or hardware platform.

E) The standard has be developed with widespread input from the health care industry incorporating all business needs into its functionality.

F) The ANSI ASC X12 is the only nationally recognized EDI standards development organization in the United States for all type of electronic commerce. ASC X12 is the organization assigned by ANSI to represent the United States in the development of International EDI standards.

G) Standards. These standards are developed using a consensus process by the users in the health care industry.

H) The standards developed by ASC X12 may be translated to/from application systems using off the shelf translation software products which are used by all industries utilizing the ASC X12 standards.

Readiness of Standard

A) The Benefit Enrollment and Maintenance (834) is not a guideline. However X12 has published implementation guides.

B) The Benefit Enrollment and Maintenance (834) standard is fully implementable. The transaction set was approved as a Draft Standard for Trial Use (DSTU) in February of 1992 as Version 003021.

C) The standard can be obtained by contacting the Data Interchange Standards Association (DISA) at 703-548-7005.

D) Each X12 transaction must have an implementation guide and a complete and unambiguous data dictionary if identical implementations are to be obtained. The X12 began writing implementations guides during calendar year 1996 for version 3070. None have yet been tested between operating trading partners. No draft data dictionary is yet available.

E) There is only one implementation guide for the Benefit Enrollment and Maintenance (834).

F) The implementation guides will specify the conformance to the standards.

G) Yes, conformance tools are commercially available.

H) The same tools used for conformance may also be used as testing tools.

I) The standard is complete. The current version of the standard is 003070. As business needs dictate, enhancements may be made to the standard three times per year, one major release along with two subsequent sub-releases. The X12 Health Care Task Group has developed procedures to determine when to move to the next version of the standard as well as when to retire past versions. The Health Care Task Group will also determine the need for new versions of the implementation guides (not more frequently than once per year).

J) Currently no enhancements are under development.

AA) This standard has been completed.

BB) This standard has been completed and undergoing industry implementation.

Indicator of Market Acceptance

A) The X12 standards are made available via many sources including from the Data Interchange Standards Association, Washington Publishing (ASC X12 Insurance Subcommittee's publisher), industry user groups and associations, and the Internet. Due to the multiplicity and diversity of these distribution methods, it is not possible to determine how many copies have been distributed and to whom.

B) Yes. ASC X12 represents international standards development. North American and other countries have implemented ASC X12 standards for purchasing and financial transactions. It would be to their benefit to further leverage their investment in EDI translation software, hardware and communication infrastructure to utilize the health care transactions.

C) Over 300 payer, provider, vendor, and plan sponsor organizations currently participate in the development of the ASC X12 standards and implementation guides to meet the business needs of the entire health care industry. These organizations have experienced the benefits of mature standards as costs associated with developing and maintaining proprietary formats far exceed the investment necessary to implement a single set of health care EDI transactions.

Level of Specificity

A) The ASC X12 EDI transactions have been developed to meet the specific business needs identified by the standards developers and the health care industry.

B) See attached table of contents from the ASC X12 Insurance Committee's implementation guides.

C) ASC X12 standards incorporate the business requirements for exchanging information contained within other standards. The ASC X12 standards provides a vehicle for communicating other standards within the standards.

D) ASC X12 maintains over one thousand internal code sets to support the standards. Along with the internal code sets the ASC X12 standards reference over 350 external code sources such as:
   - Current Procedural Terminology (CPT) Codes from American Medical Association
   - Current Dental Terminology (CDT) Codes from American Dental Association
   - International Classification of Diseases Clinical Modification - (ICD-9-CM) Diagnosis from U.S. National Center for Health Statistics.

E) There are too many code sets to describe here. Refer to the ASC X12 standards publication.

F) Internal code sets are included within the ASC X12 standards publications and implementation guides. When external code sets are referenced within these documents, the source where the code sets can be obtained is listed.

G) When possible, the implementation guides will either include the external code sets or provide further information on how to obtain the external code sets. Internal code sets are included within the implementation guides.

H) Internal code sets are available to all users of the ASC X12 standards. Usage of the external code sets will vary by source and their ability to promote the usage of their code sets.

I) ASC X12 internal code sets follow the same processes defined for the development and maintenance of the EDI transactions. External code lists are maintained by the external code source's internal development procedures.

Relationships with Other Standards

A) ASC X12 strives to coordinate and incorporate the needs of the other standards development organizations such as Health Level 7 (HL7), National Council for Prescription Drug Programs (NCPDP), and the American Society for Testing and Materials into the ASC X12 standards.

F

B) See A).
C) See A).
D) Open communication in the development of the standards amongst the standards development organizations.
E) ASC X12 is the ANSI appointed standards development organization responsible for international EDI standards within the United States
F) None
G) Given the scope and responsibility for the development and maintenance of the EDI standards for the United States and the international community with respect to United States international standards, ASC X12 is only privy to the business needs which are brought forward and coordinated with other health care organizations. At this time, we are unaware of any gaps in the current standards for insurance.

Identifiable Costs:

A) None applicable. ASC X12 does not license it standards.
B) The cost of acquiring the ASC X12 standards publication varies depending upon the source of the publications. Currently they are available from:
   - Data Interchange Standards Association (DISA) 703-548-7005.
   - Washington Publishing Corporation 800-972-4334
   - Industry user groups and associations
   - The Internet (http://www.disa.org, http://www.wpc-edi.com)
C) The typical cost ranges from free to $415.00 for the full ASC X12 standards publication in either paper form or CD-ROM.
D) The cost/timeframe for education and training will depend upon the individuals and skill levels of the individuals within an organization. Some organizations have completed education and training within one week while others have taken longer.
E) The cost/timeframe for implementation depends upon the internal systems capabilities, systems development philosophy, hardware platform selected, EDI translator software, communication methodology and individual resources within an organization. Costs can range anywhere from free for a personal computer solution to well over $150,000 for midsize and mainframe systems. Some organizations have implemented the standards within a matter of days while other have taken months to achieve the same end result.

National Council for Prescription Drug Programs (NCPDP)

NCPDP Member Enrollment Standard

NCPDP recommends the use of a standardized format for member enrollment among insurance carriers, third-party administrators, and other providers. The Member Enrollment Standard was developed to enhance the enrollment verification process and provide a consistent format for enrollment verification processing.

Eligibility for a Health Plan

Accredited Standards Committee X12 Insurance Subcommittee, Health Care Task Group

ANSI Accreditation:

X12 was accredited as an ANSI accredited standards committee in 1979. Subsequent X12 procedure changes have required ANSI re-accreditation which was last granted in 1987.

The main objective of ASC X12 is to develop Electronic Data Interchange (EDI) standards to facilitate electronic business transactions (i.e. order placement and processing, shipping and receiving, invoicing, payment, cash application data, insurance transactions). ASC X12 endeavors to structure standards in a manner that computer programs can translate data to and from internal formats without extensive reprogramming.

This strategy allows companies to maximize their resources required for internally developed or commercial software (recommended) and private or public-access communication networks. ASC X12 believes that all sizes of companies using intelligent computational devices can benefit from the use of the standard. The efficiencies of standard interchange format can minimize the difficulties incurred from each organization using its own formats to transact business. Within ASC X12, the various subcommittees are responsible for developing standards in their area of expertise. Once a subcommittee has developed a draft standard the full ASC X12 membership reviews and approves it according to the operating policies and procedures. All standards (new or changed) require the consensus approval of the full ASC X12 membership. The approved standard becomes a draft standard for trial use for a reasonable trial period. After the trial period the draft standards are submitted to ANSI to become an American National Standard (ANS).

ASC X12, Health Care Eligibility/Benefit Inquiry (270)

ASC X12, Health Care Eligibility/Benefit Information (271)

Contact For More Information: Data Interchange Standards Association (DISA) 703-548-7005.

Description of Standard:

A) The objective of the Health Care Eligibility/Benefit Inquiry (270) - Health Care Eligibility/Benefit Information (271) is to provide for the exchange of eligibility inquiry and response to individuals within a health plan.

B) This transaction set can be used by health care providers to request and receive coverage and payment information on the member/insured in a batch environment where real time processing is not required.

C) This transaction is used to provide additional patient eligibility information to support administrative reimbursement for health care products and services.

D) This standard may be used from any operating system, network, or hardware platform.

E) The standard has be developed with widespread input from the health care industry incorporating all business needs into its functionality.

F) The ANSI ASC X12 is the only nationally recognized EDI standards development organization in the United States for all type of electronic commerce. ASC X12 is the organization assigned by ANSI to represent the United States in the development of International EDI standards.

G) Standards. These standards are developed using a consensus process by the users in the health care industry.

H) The standards developed by ASC X12 may be translated to/from application systems using off the shelf translation software products which are used by all industries utilizing the ASC X12 standards.

F

Readiness of Standard:

A) The Health Care Eligibility/Benefit Inquiry (270) - Health Care Eligibility/Benefit Information (271) is not a guideline. However the X12 Insurance Subcommittee is currently developing implementation guides.

B) The Health Care Eligibility/Benefit Inquiry (270) - Health Care Eligibility/Benefit Information (271) standard is fully implementable. The transaction set was approved as a Draft Standard for Trial Use (DSTU) in February of 1993 as Version 003031.

C) The standard can be obtained by contacting the Data Interchange Standards Association (DISA) at 703-548-7005.

D) This standard does not require an implementation guide. ASC X12 has published four Type II Tutorial reports or tutorials for version 003041 in October of 1994, version 003050 in October 1995, version 003051 in February 1996, and version 003060 in April of 1996. To facilitate consistent implementation across the health care industry, the X12 Insurance Subcommittee is currently in the process of completing five implementation guides for version 003070 encompassing medical, hospital, dental, pharmaceutical claims, and workers compensation jurisdictional reporting with an anticipating publication date of April 1997.

E) There currently is only one implementation guide for the Health Care Eligibility/Benefit Inquiry (270) - Health Care Eligibility/Benefit Information (271) transaction.

F) The implementation guides will specify the conformance to the standards.

G) Yes, conformance tools are commercially available.

H) The same tools used for conformance may also be used as testing tools.

I) The standard is complete. The current version of the standard is 003070. As business needs dictate, enhancements may be made to the standard three times per year, one major release along with two subsequent sub-releases. The X12 Health Care Task Group has developed procedures to determine when to move to the next version of the standard as well as when to retire past versions. The Health Care Task Group will also determine the need for new versions of the implementation guides (not more frequently than once per year).

J) Currently no enhancements are under development.

AA) This standard has been completed.

BB) This standard has been completed and undergoing industry implementation.

Indicator of Market Acceptance:

A) The X12 standards are made available via many sources including from the Data Interchange Standards Association, Washington Publishing (ASC X12 Insurance Subcommittee's publisher), industry user groups and associations, and the Internet. Due to the multiplicity and diversity of these distribution methods, it is not possible to determine how many copies have been distributed and to whom.

B) Every Medicare carrier and intermediary has implemented ASC X12 standards for healthcare eligibility. All carriers have implemented the 270/271 for eligibility. Many other payers have followed HCFA's lead and implemented the standard as well.

C) Yes. ASC X12 represents international standards development. North American and other countries have implemented ASC X12 standards for purchasing and financial transactions. It would be to their benefit to further leverage their investment in EDI translation software, hardware and communication infrastructure to utilize the health care transactions.

D) Over 300 payer, provider, vendor, and plan sponsor organizations currently participate in the development of the ASC X12 standards and implementation guides to meet the business needs of the entire health care industry. These organizations have experienced the benefits of mature standards as costs associated with developing and maintaining proprietary formats far exceed the investment necessary to implement a single set of health care EDI transactions.

Level of Specificity:

A) The ASC X12 EDI transactions have been developed to meet the specific business needs identified by the standards developers and the health care industry.

B) See attached table of contents from the ASC X12 Insurance Committee's implementation guides.

C) ASC X12 standards incorporate the business requirements for exchanging information contained within other standards. The ASC X12 standards provides a vehicle for communicating other standards within the standards.

D) ASC X12 maintains over one thousand internal code sets to support the standards. Along with the internal code sets the ASC X12 standards reference over 350 external code sources such as:
- Current Procedural Terminology (CPT) Codes from American Medical Association
- Current Dental Terminology (CDT) Codes from American Dental Association
- International Classification of Diseases Clinical Modification - (ICD-9-CM) Diagnosis from U.S. National Center for Health Statistics.

E) There are too many code sets to describe here. Refer to the ASC X12 standards publication.

F) Internal code sets are included within the ASC X12 standards publications and implementation guides. When external code sets are referenced within these documents, the source where the code sets can be obtained is listed.

G) When possible, the implementation guides will either include the external code sets or provide further information on how to obtain the external code sets. Internal code sets are included within the implementation guides.

H) Internal code sets are available to all users of the ASC X12 standards. Usage of the external code sets will vary by source and their ability to promote the usage of their code sets.

I) ASC X12 internal code sets follow the same processes defined for the development and maintenance of the EDI transactions. External code lists are maintained by the external code source's internal development procedures.

Relationships with Other Standards:

A) ASC X12 strives to coordinate and incorporate the needs of the other standards development organizations such as Health Level 7 (HL7), National Council for Prescription Drug Programs (NCPDP), and the American Society for Testing and Materials into the ASC X12 standards.

B) See A).

C) See A).

D) Open communication in the development of the standards amongst the standards development organizations.

E) ASC X12 is the ANSI appointed standards development organization responsible for international EDI standards within the United States

F) None

G) Given the scope and responsibility for the development and maintenance of the EDI standards for the United States and the international community with respect to United States international standards, ASC X12 is only privy to the business needs which are brought forward and coordinated with other health care organizations. At this time, we are unaware of any gaps in the current standards for insurance.

F

Identifiable Costs

A) None applicable. ASC X12 does not license it standards.
B) The cost of acquiring the ASC X12 standards publication varies depending upon the source of the publications. Currently they are available from:
   - Data Interchange Standards Association (DISA) 703-548-7005.
   - Washington Publishing Corporation 800-972-4334
   - Industry user groups and associations
   - The Internet (http://www.disa.org, http://www.wpc-edi.com)
C) The typical cost ranges from free to $415.00 for the full ASC X12 standards publication in either paper form or CD-ROM.
D) The cost/timeframe for education and training will depend upon the individuals and skill levels of the individuals within an organization. Some organizations have completed education and training within one week while others have taken longer.
E) The cost/timeframe for implementation depends upon the internal systems capabilities, systems development philosophy, hardware platform selected, EDI translator software, communication methodology and individual resources within an organization. Costs can range anywhere from free for a personal computer solution to well over $150,000 for midsize and mainframe systems. Some organizations have implemented the standards within a matter of days while other have taken months to achieve the same end result.

ASC X12, Health Care Task Group

Interactive Health Care Eligibility/Benefit Inquiry (IHCEBI)

Interactive Health Care Eligibility/Benefit Response (IHCEBR)

Contact For More Information:

Data Interchange Standards Association (DISA) 703-548-7005.

Description of Standard:

A) The objective of the Interactive Health Care Eligibility/Benefit Inquiry (IHCEBI) - Interactive Health Care Eligibility/Benefit Response (IHCEBR) is to provide for the exchange of eligibility inquiry and response to individuals within a health plan.
B) This interactive message can be used by health care providers to request and receive coverage and payment information on the member/insured in an online real time environment.
C) This message is used to provide additional patient eligibility information to support administrative reimbursement for health care products and services.
D) This standard may be used from any operating system, network, or hardware platform.
E) The standard has be developed with widespread input from the health care industry incorporating all business needs into its functionality.
F) The ANSI ASC X12 is the only nationally recognized EDI standards development organization in the United States for all type of electronic commerce. ASC X12 is the organization assigned by ANSI to represent the United States in the development of International EDI standards.
G) Standards. These standards are developed using a consensus process by the users in the health care industry.

H) The standards developed by ASC X12 may be translated to/from application systems using off the shelf translation software products which are used by all industries utilizing the ASC X12 standards.

Readiness of Standard

A) The Interactive Health Care Eligibility/Benefit Inquiry (IHCEBI) - Interactive Health Care Eligibility/Benefit Response (IHCEBR) is not a guideline. However the X12 Insurance Subcommittee is currently developing implementation guides.

B) The Interactive Health Care Eligibility/Benefit Inquiry (IHCEBI) - Interactive Health Care Eligibility/Benefit Response (IHCEBR) standard is fully implementable. The message was approved as a Draft Standard for Trial Use (DSTU) in October of 1994 as Version 003050.

C) The standard can be obtained by contacting the Data Interchange Standards Association (DISA) at 703-548-7005.

D) Each X12 transaction must have an implementation guide and a complete and unambiguous data dictionary if identical implementations are to be obtained. The X12 began writing implementations guides during calendar year 1996 for version 3070. None have yet been tested between operating trading partners. No draft data dictionary is yet available.

E) There currently is only one implementation guide for the Interactive Health Care Eligibility/Benefit Inquiry (IHCEBI) - Interactive Health Care Eligibility/Benefit Response (IHCEBR).

F) The implementation guides will specify the conformance to the standards.

G) Yes, conformance tools are commercially available.

H) The same tools used for conformance may also be used as testing tools.

I) The standard is complete. The current version of the standard is 003070. As business needs dictate, enhancements may be made to the standard three times per year, one major release along with two subsequent sub-releases. The X12 Health Care Task Group has developed procedures to determine when to move to the next version of the standard as well as when to retire past versions. The Health Care Task Group will also determine the need for new versions of the implementation guides (not more frequently than once per year).

J) Currently no enhancements are under development.

AA) This standard has been completed.

BB) This standard has been completed and undergoing industry implementation.

Indicator of Market Acceptance

A) The X12 standards are made available via many sources including from the Data Interchange Standards Association, Washington Publishing (ASC X12 Insurance Subcommittee's publisher), industry user groups and associations, and the Internet. Due to the multiplicity and diversity of these distribution methods, it is not possible to determine how many copies have been distributed and to whom.

B) Every Medicare carrier and intermediary has implemented ASC X12 standards for payment and remittance advice. Many other payers have followed HCFA's lead and implemented the standard as well.

C) Yes. ASC X12 represents international standards development. North American and other countries have implemented ASC X12 standards for purchasing and financial transactions. It would be to their benefit to further leverage their investment in EDI translation software, hardware and communication infrastructure to utilize the health care transactions.

D) Over 300 payer, provider, vendor, and plan sponsor organizations currently participate in the development of the ASC X12 standards and implementation guides to meet the business needs of the entire health care industry. These organizations have experienced the benefits of mature

F

standards as costs associated with developing and maintaining proprietary formats far exceed the investment necessary to implement a single set of health care EDI transactions.

Level of Specificity

A) The ASC X12 EDI transactions have been developed to meet the specific business needs identified by the standards developers and the health care industry.

B) See attached table of contents from the ASC X12 Insurance Committee's implementation guides.

C) ASC X12 standards incorporate the business requirements for exchanging information contained within other standards. The ASC X12 standards provides a vehicle for communicating other standards within the standards.

D) ASC X12 maintains over one thousand internal code sets to support the standards. Along with the internal code sets the ASC X12 standards reference over 350 external code sources such as:
   - Current Procedural Terminology (CPT) Codes from American Medical Association
   - Current Dental Terminology (CDT) Codes from American Dental Association
   - International Classification of Diseases Clinical Modification - (ICD-9-CM) Diagnosis from U.S. National Center for Health Statistics.

E) There are too many code sets to describe here. Refer to the ASC X12 standards publication.

F) Internal code sets are included within the ASC X12 standards publications and implementation guides. When external code sets are referenced within these documents, the source where the code sets can be obtained is listed.

G) When possible, the implementation guides will either include the external code sets or provide further information on how to obtain the external code sets. Internal code sets are included within the implementation guides.

H) Internal code sets are available to all users of the ASC X12 standards. Usage of the external code sets will vary by source and their ability to promote the usage of their code sets.

I) ASC X12 internal code sets follow the same processes defined for the development and maintenance of the EDI transactions. External code lists are maintained by the external code source's internal development procedures.

Relationships with Other Standards

A) ASC X12 strives to coordinate and incorporate the needs of the other standards development organizations such as Health Level 7 (HL7), National Council for Prescription Drug Programs (NCPDP), and the American Society for Testing and Materials into the ASC X12 standards.

B) See A).

C) See A).

D) Open communication in the development of the standards amongst the standards development organizations.

E) ASC X12 is the ANSI appointed standards development organization responsible for international EDI standards within the United States

F) None

G) Given the scope and responsibility for the development and maintenance of the EDI standards for the United States and the international community with respect to United States international standards, ASC X12 is only privy to the business needs which are brought forward and coordinated with other health care organizations. At this time, we are unaware of any gaps in the current standards for insurance.

Identifiable Costs

A) None applicable. ASC X12 does not license it standards.
B) The cost of acquiring the ASC X12 standards publication varies depending upon the source of the publications. Currently they are available from:
   - Data Interchange Standards Association (DISA) 703-548-7005.
   - Washington Publishing Corporation 800-972-4334
   - Industry user groups and associations
   - The Internet (http://www.disa.org, http://www.wpc-edi.com)
C) The typical cost ranges from free to $415.00 for the full ASC X12 standards publication in either paper form or CD-ROM.
D) The cost/timeframe for education and training will depend upon the individuals and skill levels of the individuals within an organization. Some organizations have completed education and training within one week while others have taken longer.

The cost/timeframe for implementation depends upon the internal systems capabilities, systems development philosophy, hardware platform selected, EDI translator software, communication methodology and individual resources within an organization. Costs can range anywhere from free for a personal computer solution to well over $150,000 for midsize and mainframe systems. Some organizations have implemented the standards within a matter of days while other have taken months to achieve the same end result.

Health Care Payment and Remittance Advice

Accredited Standards Committee X12 Insurance Subcommittee, Health Care Task Group

ANSI Accreditation:

X12 was accredited as an ANSI accredited standards committee in 1979. Subsequent X12 procedure changes have required ANSI re-accreditation which was last granted in 1987.

The main objective of ASC X12 is to develop Electronic Data Interchange (EDI) standards to facilitate electronic business transactions (i.e. order placement and processing, shipping and receiving, invoicing, payment, cash application data, insurance transactions). ASC X12 endeavors to structure standards in a manner that computer programs can translate data to and from internal formats without extensive reprogramming.

This strategy allows companies to maximize their resources required for internally developed or commercial software (recommended) and private or public-access communication networks. ASC X12 believes that all sizes of companies using intelligent computational devices can benefit from the use of the standard. The efficiencies of standard interchange format can minimize the difficulties incurred from each organization using its own formats to transact business. Within ASC X12, the various subcommittees are responsible for developing standards in their area of expertise. Once a subcommittee has developed a draft standard the full ASC X12 membership reviews and approves it according to the operating policies and procedures. All standards (new or changed) require the consensus approval of the full ASC X12 membership. The approved standard becomes a draft standard for trial use for a reasonable trial period. After the trial period the draft standards are submitted to ANSI to become an American National Standard (ANS).

F

ASC X12N Health Care Claim Payment/Advice (835).

Contact For More Information:

Data Interchange Standards Association (DISA) 703-548-7005.

Description of Standard:

A) The objective of the Health Care Claim Payment/Advice (835) is to support reimbursement processing for health care products and services.

B) This transaction set can be used to make a payment, send an Explanation of Benefits (EOB) remittance advice, or make a payment and send an EOB remittance advice only from a health insurer to a health care provider either directly or via a financial institution.

C) This transaction is used for administrative reimbursement for health care products and services.

D) This standard may be used from any operating system, network, or hardware platform.

E) The standard has be developed with widespread input from the health care industry incorporating all business needs into its functionality.

F) The ANSI ASC X12 is the only nationally recognized EDI standards development organization in the United States for all type of electronic commerce. ASC X12 is the organization assigned by ANSI to represent the United States in the development of International EDI standards.

G) Standards. These standards are developed using a consensus process by the users in the health care industry.

H) The standards developed by ASC X12 may be translated to/from application systems using off the shelf translation software products which are used by all industries utilizing the ASC X12 standards.

Readiness of Standard

A) The Health Care Claim Payment/Advice (835) is not a guideline. However X12 has published implementation guides.

B) The Health Care Claim Payment/Advice (835) standard is fully implementable.

C) The standard can be obtained by contacting the Data Interchange Standards Association (DISA) at 703-548-7005.

D) This standard does not require an implementation guide. ASC X12 has published four Type II Tutorial reports or tutorials for version 003041 in October of 1994, version 003050 in October 1995, version 003051 in February 1996, and version 003060 in April of 1996. To facilitate consistent implementation across the health care industry, the X12 Insurance Subcommittee is currently in the process of completing five implementation guides for version 003070 encompassing medical, hospital, dental, pharmaceutical claims, and workers compensation jurisdictional reporting with an anticipating publication date of April 1997.

E) There are currently two versions of the implementation guide for the Health Care Claim Payment/Advice (835) one for version 003051 and one for version 003070.

F) The implementation guides will specify the conformance to the standards.

G) Yes, conformance tools are commercially available.

H) The same tools used for conformance may also be used as testing tools.

I) The standard is complete. The current version of the standard is 003070. As business needs dictate, enhancements may be made to the standard three times per year, one major release along with two subsequent sub-releases. The X12 Health Care Task Group has developed procedures to determine when to move to the next version of the standard as well as when to retire past versions. The Health Care Task Group will also determine the need for new versions of the implementation guides (not more frequently than once per year).

J) Currently no enhancements are under development.

AA) This standard has been completed.

BB) This standard has been completed and undergoing industry implementation.

Indicator of Market Acceptance

A) The X12 standards are made available via many sources including from the Data Interchange Standards Association, Washington Publishing (ASC X12 Insurance Subcommittee's publisher), industry user groups and associations, and the Internet. Due to the multiplicity and diversity of these distribution methods, it is not possible to determine how many copies have been distributed and to whom.

B) Every Medicare carrier and intermediary has implemented ASC X12 standards for claim and remittance advice. All carriers have implemented the 270/271 for eligibility. Many other payers have followed HCFA's lead and implemented the standard as well.

C) Yes. ASC X12 represents international standards development. North American and other countries have implemented ASC X12 standards for purchasing and financial transactions. It would be to their benefit to further leverage their investment in EDI translation software, hardware and communication infrastructure to utilize the health care transactions.

D) Over 300 payer, provider, vendor, and plan sponsor organizations currently participate in the development of the ASC X12 standards and implementation guides to meet the business needs of the entire health care industry. These organizations have experienced the benefits of mature standards as costs associated with developing and maintaining proprietary formats far exceed the investment necessary to implement a single set of health care EDI transactions.

Level of Specificity

A) The ASC X12 EDI transactions have been developed to meet the specific business needs identified by the standards developers and the health care industry.

B) See attached table of contents from the ASC X12 Insurance Committee's implementation guides.

C) ASC X12 standards incorporate the business requirements for exchanging information contained within other standards. The ASC X12 standards provides a vehicle for communicating other standards within the standards.

D) ASC X12 maintains over one thousand internal code sets to support the standards. Along with the internal code sets the ASC X12 standards reference over 350 external code sources such as:
    - Current Procedural Terminology (CPT) Codes from American Medical Association
    - Current Dental Terminology (CDT) Codes from American Dental Association
    - International Classification of Diseases Clinical Modification - (ICD-9-CM) Diagnosis from U.S. National Center for Health Statistics.

E) There are too many code sets to describe here. Refer to the ASC X12 standards publication.

F) Internal code sets are included within the ASC X12 standards publications and implementation guides. When external code sets are referenced within these documents, the source where the code sets can be obtained is listed.

G) When possible, the implementation guides will either include the external code sets or provide further information on how to obtain the external code sets. Internal code sets are included within the implementation guides.

H) Internal code sets are available to all users of the ASC X12 standards. Usage of the external code sets will vary by source and their ability to promote the usage of their code sets.

F

I) ASC X12 internal code sets follow the same processes defined for the development and maintenance of the EDI transactions. External code lists are maintained by the external code source's internal development procedures.

Relationships with Other Standards

A) ASC X12 strives to coordinate and incorporate the needs of the other standards development organizations such as Health Level 7 (HL7), National Council for Prescription Drug Programs (NCPDP), and the American Society for Testing and Materials into the ASC X12 standards.

B) See A).

C) See A).

D) Open communication in the development of the standards amongst the standards development organizations.

E) ASC X12 is the ANSI appointed standards development organization responsible for international EDI standards within the United States

F) None

G) Given the scope and responsibility for the development and maintenance of the EDI standards for the United States and the international community with respect to United States international standards, ASC X12 is only privy to the business needs which are brought forward and coordinated with other health care organizations. At this time, we are unaware of any gaps in the current standards for insurance.

Identifiable Costs:

A) None applicable. ASC X12 does not license it standards.

B) The cost of acquiring the ASC X12 standards publication varies depending upon the source of the publications. Currently they are available from:
- Data Interchange Standards Association (DISA) 703-548-7005.
- Washington Publishing Corporation 800-972-4334
- Industry user groups and associations
- The Internet (http://www.disa.org, http://www.wpc-edi.com)

C) The typical cost ranges from free to $415.00 for the full ASC X12 standards publication in either paper form or CD-ROM.

D) The cost/timeframe for education and training will depend upon the individuals and skill levels of the individuals within an organization. Some organizations have completed education and training within one week while others have taken longer.

E) The cost/timeframe for implementation depends upon the internal systems capabilities, systems development philosophy, hardware platform selected, EDI translator software, communication methodology and individual resources within an organization. Costs can range anywhere from free for a personal computer solution to well over $150,000 for midsize and mainframe systems. Some organizations have implemented the standards within a matter of days while other have taken months to achieve the same end result.

Health Care Premium Payments

Accredited Standards Committee X12 Insurance Subcommittee, Health Care Task Group

Consolidated Service Invoice/Statement (811)

Payment Order/Remittance Advice (820)

Contact For More Information:

Data Interchange Standards Association (DISA) 703-548-7005.

Description of Standard:

A) The objective of the Consolidated Service Invoice/Statement (811) - Payment Order/Remittance Advice (820) is to facilitate health plan premium billing and payment.

B) These transaction sets can be used by health care prayers and plan sponsors for the purpose of premium billing (Consolidated Service Invoice/Statement 811) and collection (Order/Remittance Advice 820).

C) These transactions are used for the administrative reimbursement for health plans between health care payers and plan sponsors.

D) This standard may be used from any operating system, network, or hardware platform.

E) The standard has be developed with widespread input from the health care industry incorporating all business needs into its functionality.

F) The ANSI ASC X12 is the only nationally recognized EDI standards development organization in the United States for all type of electronic commerce. ASC X12 is the organization assigned by ANSI to represent the United States in the development of International EDI standards.

G) Standards. These standards are developed using a consensus process by the users in the health care industry.

H) The standards developed by ASC X12 may be translated to/from application systems using off the shelf translation software products which are used by all industries utilizing the ASC X12 standards.

Readiness of Standard:

A) The Consolidated Service Invoice/Statement (811) - Payment Order/Remittance Advice (820) is not a guideline. However the X12 Insurance Subcommittee is currently developing implementation guides.

B) The Consolidated Service Invoice/Statement (811) - Payment Order/Remittance Advice (820) standard is fully implementable. The transaction has been approved as a Draft Standard for Trial Use (DSTU).

C) The standard can be obtained by contacting the Data Interchange Standards Association (DISA) at 703-548-7005.

D) Each X12 transaction must have an implementation guide and a complete and unambiguous data dictionary if identical implementations are to be obtained. The X12 began writing implementations guides during calendar year 1996 for version 3070. None have yet been tested between operating trading partners. No draft data dictionary is yet available.

F

E) There currently is only one implementation guide for the Consolidated Service Invoice/Statement (811) - Payment Order/Remittance Advice (820) for the purposes of health plan premium payments.

F) The implementation guides will specify the conformance to the standards.

G) Yes, conformance tools are commercially available.

H) The same tools used for conformance may also be used as testing tools.

I) The standard is complete. The current version of the standard is 003070. As business needs dictate, enhancements may be made to the standard three times per year, one major release along with two subsequent sub-releases. The X12 Health Care Task Group has developed procedures to determine when to move to the next version of the standard as well as when to retire past versions. The Health Care Task Group will also determine the need for new versions of the implementation guides (not more frequently than once per year).

J) Currently no enhancements are under development.

AA) This standard has been completed.

BB) This standard has been completed and undergoing industry implementation.

Indicator of Market Acceptance:

A) The X12 standards are made available via many sources including from the Data Interchange Standards Association, Washington Publishing (ASC X12 Insurance Subcommittee's publisher), industry user groups and associations, and the Internet. Due to the multiplicity and diversity of these distribution methods, it is not possible to determine how many copies have been distributed and to whom.

B) Yes. ASC X12 represents international standards development. North American and other countries have implemented ASC X12 standards for purchasing and financial transactions. It would be to their benefit to further leverage their investment in EDI translation software, hardware and communication infrastructure to utilize the health care transactions.

C) Over 300 payer, provider, vendor, and plan sponsor organizations currently participate in the development of the ASC X12 standards and implementation guides to meet the business needs of the entire health care industry. These organizations have experienced the benefits of mature standards as costs associated with developing and maintaining proprietary formats far exceed the investment necessary to implement a single set of health care EDI transactions.

Level of Specificity:

A) The ASC X12 EDI transactions have been developed to meet the specific business needs identified by the standards developers and the health care industry.

B) See attached table of contents from the ASC X12 Insurance Committee's implementation guides.

C) ASC X12 standards incorporate the business requirements for exchanging information contained within other standards. The ASC X12 standards provides a vehicle for communicating other standards within the standards.

D) ASC X12 maintains over one thousand internal code sets to support the standards. Along with the internal code sets the ASC X12 standards reference over 350 external code sources such as:
   - Current Procedural Terminology (CPT) Codes from American Medical Association
   - Current Dental Terminology (CDT) Codes from American Dental Association
   - International Classification of Diseases Clinical Modification - (ICD-9-CM) Diagnosis from U.S. National Center for Health Statistics.

E) There are too many code sets to describe here. Refer to the ASC X12 standards publication.

F) Internal code sets are included within the ASC X12 standards publications and implementation guides. When external code sets are referenced within these documents, the source where the code sets can be obtained is listed.

G) When possible, the implementation guides will either include the external code sets or provide further information on how to obtain the external code sets. Internal code sets are included within the implementation guides.

H) Internal code sets are available to all users of the ASC X12 standards. Usage of the external code sets will vary by source and their ability to promote the usage of their code sets.

I) ASC X12 internal code sets follow the same processes defined for the development and maintenance of the EDI transactions. External code lists are maintained by the external code source's internal development procedures.

Relationships with Other Standards:

A) ASC X12 strives to coordinate and incorporate the needs of the other standards development organizations such as Health Level 7 (HL7), National Council for Prescription Drug Programs (NCPDP), and the American Society for Testing and Materials into the ASC X12 standards.

B) See A).

C) See A).

D) Open communication in the development of the standards amongst the standards development organizations.

E) ASC X12 is the ANSI appointed standards development organization responsible for international EDI standards within the United States

F) None

G) Given the scope and responsibility for the development and maintenance of the EDI standards for the United States and the international community with respect to United States international standards, ASC X12 is only privy to the business needs which are brought forward and coordinated with other health care organizations. At this time, we are unaware of any gaps in the current standards for insurance.

Identifiable Costs:

A) None applicable. ASC X12 does not license it standards.

B) The cost of acquiring the ASC X12 standards publication varies depending upon the source of the publications. Currently they are available from:
   - Data Interchange Standards Association (DISA) 703-548-7005.
   - Washington Publishing Corporation 800-972-4334
   - Industry user groups and associations
   - The Internet (http://www.disa.org, http://www.wpc-edi.com)

C) The typical cost ranges from free to $415.00 for the full ASC X12 standards publication in either paper form or CD-ROM.

D) The cost/timeframe for education and training will depend upon the individuals and skill levels of the individuals within an organization. Some organizations have completed education and training within one week while others have taken longer.

E) The cost/timeframe for implementation depends upon the internal systems capabilities, systems development philosophy, hardware platform selected, EDI translator software, communication methodology and individual resources within an organization. Costs can range anywhere from free for a personal computer solution to well over $150,000 for midsize and mainframe systems. Some organizations have implemented the standards within a matter of days while other have taken months to achieve the same end result.

F

First Report of Injury
Accredited Standards Committee X12 Insurance Subcommittee,

Property And Casualty Task Group

ANSI Accreditation:

X12 was accredited as an ANSI accredited standards committee in 1979. Subsequent X12 procedure changes have required ANSI re-accreditation which was last granted in 1987.

The main objective of ASC X12 is to develop Electronic Data Interchange (EDI) standards to facilitate electronic business transactions (i.e. order placement and processing, shipping and receiving, invoicing, payment, cash application data, insurance transactions). ASC X12 endeavors to structure standards in a manner that computer programs can translate data to and from internal formats without extensive reprogramming.

This strategy allows companies to maximize their resources required for internally developed or commercial software (recommended) and private or public-access communication networks. ASC X12 believes that all sizes of companies using intelligent computational devices can benefit from the use of the standard. The efficiencies of standard interchange format can minimize the difficulties incurred from each organization using its own formats to transact business. Within ASC X12, the various subcommittees are responsible for developing standards in their area of expertise. Once a subcommittee has developed a draft standard the full ASC X12 membership reviews and approves it according to the operating policies and procedures. All standards (new or changed) require the consensus approval of the full ASC X12 membership. The approved standard becomes a draft standard for trial use for a reasonable trial period. After the trial period the draft standards are submitted to ANSI to become an American National Standard (ANS).

Report of Injury, Illness or Incident (148)

Contact For More Information:

Data Interchange Standards Association (DISA) 703-548-7005.

Description of Standard:

A) The objective of the Report of Injury, Illness or Incident (148) is to facilitate the first report of an injury, incident or illness.
B) This transaction set can be used to report information pertaining to an injury, illness or incident to entities interested in the information for statistical, legal, and claims and risk management processing requirements.
C) This transaction is used for administrative reporting requirements.
D) This standard may be used from any operating system, network, or hardware platform.
E) The standard has been developed with widespread input from the health care industry incorporating all business needs into its functionality.

F) The ANSI ASC X12 is the only nationally recognized EDI standards development organization in the United States for all type of electronic commerce. ASC X12 is the organization assigned by ANSI to represent the United States in the development of International EDI standards.

G) Standards. These standards are developed using a consensus process by the users in the health care industry.

H) The standards developed by ASC X12 may be translated to/from application systems using off the shelf translation software products which are used by all industries utilizing the ASC X12 standards.

Readiness of Standard:

A) The Report of Injury, Illness or Incident (148) is not a guideline. However the X12 Insurance Subcommittee is currently developing an implementation guide.

B) The Report of Injury, Illness or Incident (148) standard is fully implementable. The transaction set was approved as a Draft Standard for Trial Use (DSTU).

C) The standard can be obtained by contacting the Data Interchange Standards Association (DISA) at 703-548-7005.

D) This standard does not require an implementation guide. ASC X12 has published four Type II Tutorial reports or tutorials for version 003041 in October of 1994, version 003050 in October 1995, version 003051 in February 1996, and version 003060 in April of 1996. To facilitate consistent implementation across the health care industry, the X12 Insurance Subcommittee is currently in the process of completing five implementation guides for version 003070 encompassing medical, hospital, dental, pharmaceutical claims, and workers compensation jurisdictional reporting with an anticipating publication date of April 1997.

E) There currently is only one implementation guide for the Report of Injury, Illness or Incident (148).

F) The implementation guides will specify the conformance to the standards.

G) Yes, conformance tools are commercially available.

H) The same tools used for conformance may also be used as testing tools.

I) The standard is complete. The current version of the standard is 003070. As business needs dictate, enhancements may be made to the standard three times per year, one major release along with two subsequent sub-releases. The X12 Health Care Task Group has developed procedures to determine when to move to the next version of the standard as well as when to retire past versions. The Health Care Task Group will also determine the need for new versions of the implementation guides (not more frequently than once per year).

J) Currently no enhancements are under development.

AA) This standard has been completed.

BB) This standard has been completed and undergoing industry implementation.

Indicator of Market Acceptance:

A) The X12 standards are made available via many sources including the Data Interchange Standards Association, Washington Publishing (ASC X12 Insurance Subcommittee's publisher), industry user groups and associations, and the Internet. Due to the multiplicity and diversity of these distribution methods, it is not possible to determine how many copies have been distributed and to whom.

B) Every government contractor has been funded by the Health Care Financing Administration (HCFA) to implement the ASC X12 standards. Many other payers have followed HCFA's lead and implemented the standards as well. Many other payers have followed HCFA's lead and implemented the standard as well.

C) Yes. ASC X12 represents international standards development. North American and other countries have implemented ASC X12 standards for purchasing and financial transactions. It

F

would be to their benefit to further leverage their investment in EDI translation software, hardware and communication infrastructure to utilize the health care transactions.

D) Over 300 payer, provider, vendor, and plan sponsor organizations currently participate in the development of the ASC X12 standards and implementation guides to meet the business needs of the entire health care industry. These organizations have experienced the benefits of mature standards as costs associated with developing and maintaining proprietary formats far exceed the investment necessary to implement a single set of health care EDI transactions.

Level of Specificity:

A) The ASC X12 EDI transactions have been developed to meet the specific business needs identified by the standards developers and the health care industry.

B) See attached table of contents from the ASC X12 Insurance Committee's implementation guides.

C) ASC X12 standards incorporate the business requirements for exchanging information contained within other standards. The ASC X12 standards provides a vehicle for communicating other standards within the standards.

D) ASC X12 maintains over one thousand internal code sets to support the standards. Along with the internal code sets the ASC X12 standards reference over 350 external code sources such as:
- Current Procedural Terminology (CPT) Codes from American Medical Association
- Current Dental Terminology (CDT) Codes from American Dental Association
- International Classification of Diseases Clinical Modification - (ICD-9-CM) Diagnosis from U.S. National Center for Health Statistics.

E) There are too many code sets to describe here. Refer to the ASC X12 standards publication.

F) Internal code sets are included within the ASC X12 standards publications and implementation guides. When external code sets are referenced within these documents, the source where the code sets can be obtained is listed.

G) When possible, the implementation guides will either include the external code sets or provide further information on how to obtain the external code sets. Internal code sets are included within the implementation guides.

H) Internal code sets are available to all users of the ASC X12 standards. Usage of the external code sets will vary by source and their ability to promote the usage of their code sets.

I) ASC X12 internal code sets follow the same processes defined for the development and maintenance of the EDI transactions. External code lists are maintained by the external code source's internal development procedures.

Relationships with Other Standards:

A) ASC X12 strives to coordinate and incorporate the needs of the other standards development organizations such as Health Level 7 (HL7), National Council for Prescription Drug Programs (NCPDP), and the American Society for Testing and Materials into the ASC X12 standards.

B) See A).

C) See A).

D) Open communication in the development of the standards amongst the standards development organizations.

E) ASC X12 is the ANSI appointed standards development organization responsible for international EDI standards within the United States

F) None

G) Given the scope and responsibility for the development and maintenance of the EDI standards for the United States and the international community with respect to United States international standards, ASC X12 is only privy to the business needs which are brought forward and coordinated with other health care organizations. At this time, we are unaware of any gaps in the current standards for insurance.

Identifiable Costs:

A) None applicable. ASC X12 does not license it standards.
B) The cost of acquiring the ASC X12 standards publication varies depending upon the source of the publications. Currently they are available from:
   - Data Interchange Standards Association (DISA) 703-548-7005.
   - Washington Publishing Corporation 800-972-4334
   - Industry user groups and associations
   - The Internet (http://www.disa.org, http://www.wpc-edi.com)
C) The typical cost ranges from free to $415.00 for the full ASC X12 standards publication in either paper form or CD-ROM.
D) The cost/timeframe for education and training will depend upon the individuals and skill levels of the individuals within an organization. Some organizations have completed education and training within one week while others have taken longer.
E) The cost/timeframe for implementation depends upon the internal systems capabilities, systems development philosophy, hardware platform selected, EDI translator software, communication methodology and individual resources within an organization. Costs can range anywhere from free for a personal computer solution to well over $150,000 for midsize and mainframe systems. Some organizations have implemented the standards within a matter of days while other have taken months to achieve the same end result.

Health Level Seven (HL7)

Emergency room message being developed with Centers for Disease Control (CDC). See detailed information regarding HL7 in the Claims section.

ASTM Committee E31 on Healthcare Informatics

Organized in 1898, ASTM (the American Society for Testing and Materials) has grown into one of the largest voluntary standards development systems in the world. ASTM is a not-for profit organization that provides a forum for producers, users, ultimate consumers, and those having a general interest (representatives of government and academia) to meet on common ground and write standards for materials, products, systems, and services. From the work of 132 standards-writing committees, ASTM publishes more that 9000 standards. ASTM headquarters has no technical research or testing facilities; such work is done voluntarily by 35,000 technically qualified ASTM members located throughout the world. ASTM provides continuing education and training in the use and application of ASTM standards through Technical and Professional Training courses. In 1987, ASTM formed the Institute for Standards and Research (ISR). The purpose of the Institute is to provide a mechanism for conducting research to improve the quality and timeliness of ASTM standards. It does no research, but serves as the intermediary between the standards-writing community and the public or private agencies that could provide appropriate research and technical services, or supply funding for such research.

F

ANSI Accreditation:

ASTM is an ANSI Accredited by the Organization Method. All ASTM Committee E31 standards are approved as American National Standards.

E1744-95, Standard Guide for a View of Emergency Medical Care in the Computerized Patient Record

Contact For More Information

Manager - Committee E31, ASTM
Barr Harbor Drive
West Conshohocken, PA 19373
Ph: 610-832-9500
Fax: 610-832-9666

Description of Standard

This guide covers the identification of the information that is necessary to document emergency medical care in a computerized patient record that is part of a paperless patient record system designed to improve efficiency and cost-effectiveness. It details the use of data elements already established for emergency care in the field or in a treatment facility and places them in the context of the object models for health care that will be the vehicle for communication standards for health care data. The codes for the data elements referred to in the document will be developed in consideration of national or professional guidelines whenever available. The EMS definitions are based on those generated from the national consensus conference sponsored by NHTSA and from ASTM F30.03.03 on EMS management information systems. The Emergency Department (ED) definitions will consider those recommended by the Data Elements for Emergency Department Systems workshop sponsored by CDC, NHTSA, and other public and private organizations. The hospital discharge definitions will be developed in consideration of existing requirements for Medicare and Medicaid payment. The ASTM process allows for the definitions to be updated as the national consensus changes. When national or professional definitions do not exist, or whenever there is a conflict in the definitions, the committee will recommend a process for resolving the conflict or present the various definitions within the document along with an explanation for the purpose of each definition.

This view reinforces the concepts set forth in E-1239 and E-1384 that documentation of care in all settings must be seamless and be conducted under a common set of precepts using a common logical record structure and common terminology. The computerized patient record focuses on the patient and includes information about the occurrence of the emergency, symptoms requiring emergency medical treatment, medical/mental assessment/diagnoses established, treatment rendered, outcome and disposition of the patient after emergency treatment. It consists of subsets of the data computerized by multiple care providers at the time of onset/scene and enroute, in the emergency department, in the hospital or other emergency health care settings. The computerized patient record focuses on the documentation of information that is necessary to support patient care but does not define appropriate care.

Readiness of Standard

This guide is a "view" of the data elements to document the types of emergency medical information that would be valuable if available in the computerized patient record. As a view of the computerized patient record, the information presented will conform to the structure defined in other ASTM standards for the computerized patient record. This guide is intended to amplify Guides E 1239, E 1384, and F 1629 and the formalisms described in Practice E 1715. It is implementable in that it consists of a list of data elements important to emergency medical care that vendors can include in their data systems. The guide does not include attribute values for each of the data elements. However, most of these data elements are already defined in the other documents as indicated in Section VI. (The EMS definitions are based on those generated from the national consensus conference sponsored by NHTSA and from ASTM F30.03.03 on EMS management information systems. The Emergency Department (ED) definitions will consider those recommended by the Data Elements for Emergency Departments Workshop sponsored by CDC, NHTSA, and other public and private organizations. The hospital discharge definitions will be developed in consideration of existing requirements for Medicare and Medicaid payment.) The guide is currently being revised to include the attribute values. The guide may be obtained for a fee from ASTM.

The standard is published and is an American National Standard. How can the standard be obtained? ASTM standards are available through the ASTM Customer Service Department by calling 610-832-9585. Standards can also be ordered through the ASTM Web Site at www.astm.org

Indicators of Market Acceptance

Approximately 2300 copies of the E31 standards have been distributed.
The Guide will be incorporated into the overall standards for the computerized patient record and is not designed to stand alone.

Level of Specificity

Same as information under VII.

Relationships with other Standards

There are no other similar Standards related to emergency medical care that have been developed by an authorized SDO. Defacto standards developed by the organizations listed in VI include data sets that have been developed during a formal consensus process (EMS), through broad participation by all stakeholders (ED) or through the payment of public funds (hospital). The definitions developed during these efforts will be incorporated into the next revision of E-1744.

F

Health Claim Status

Accredited Standards Committee X12 Insurance Subcommittee, Property and Casualty Task Group

ANSI Accreditation:

X12 was accredited as an ANSI accredited standards committee in 1979. Subsequent X12 procedure changes have required ANSI re-accreditation which was last granted in 1987. The main objective of ASC X12 is to develop Electronic Data Interchange (EDI) standards to facilitate electronic business transactions (i.e. order placement and processing, shipping and receiving, invoicing, payment, cash application data, insurance transactions). ASC X12 endeavors to structure standards in a manner that computer programs can translate data to and from internal formats without extensive reprogramming.

This strategy allows companies to maximize their resources required for internally developed or commercial software (recommended) and private or public-access communication networks. ASC X12 believes that all sizes of companies using intelligent computational devices can benefit from the use of the standard. The efficiencies of standard interchange format can minimize the difficulties incurred from each organization using its own formats to transact business. Within ASC X12, the various subcommittees are responsible for developing standards in their area of expertise. Once a subcommittee has developed a draft standard the full ASC X12 membership reviews and approves it according to the operating policies and procedures. All standards (new or changed) require the consensus approval of the full ASC X12 membership. The approved standard becomes a draft standard for trial use for a reasonable trial period. After the trial period the draft standards are submitted to ANSI to become an American National Standard (ANS).

Health Care Claim Status Request (276)

Health Care Claim Status Notification (277)

Contact For More Information:

Data Interchange Standards Association (DISA) 703-548-7005.

Description of Standards

A) The objective of the Health Care Claim Status Request (276) - Health Care Claim Status Notification (277) is to determine the status of a submitted claim.
B) This transaction set pair can be used to request the status of a submitted claim by the health care provider using the Health Care Claim Status Request (276) and the payer to respond to these inquiries using the Health Care Claim Status Notification (277). The Health Care Claim Status Notification (277) can be used independently of the Health Care Claim Status Request (276) for the purposes of an unsolicited claim status from the payer to the health care provider as well as payer requests for additional information from the health care provider.
C) This transaction is used to support administrative reimbursement for health care products and services.
D) This standard may be used from any operating system, network, or hardware platform.
E) The standard has been developed with widespread input from the health care industry incorporating all business needs into its functionality.
F) The ANSI ASC X12 is the only nationally recognized EDI standards development organization in the United States for all type of electronic commerce. ASC X12 is the organization assigned by ANSI to represent the United States in the development of International EDI standards.

G) Standards. These standards are developed using a consensus process by the users in the health care industry.

H) The standards developed by ASC X12 may be translated to/from application systems using off the shelf translation software products which are used by all industries utilizing the ASC X12 standards.

Readiness of Standard

A) The Health Care Claim Status Request (276) - Health Care Claim Status Notification (277) is not a guideline. However the X12 Insurance Subcommittee is currently developing an implementation guide.

B) The Health Care Claim Status Request (276) - Health Care Claim Status Notification (277) standard is fully implementable. The transaction set was approved as a Draft Standard for Trial Use (DSTU) in October of 1993 as Version 003040.

C) The standard can be obtained by contacting the Data Interchange Standards Association (DISA) at 703-548-7005.

D) This standard does not require an implementation guide. ASC X12 has published four Type II Tutorial reports or tutorials for version 003041 in October of 1994, version 003050 in October 1995, version 003051 in February 1996, and version 003060 in April of 1996. To facilitate consistent implementation across the health care industry, the X12 Insurance Subcommittee is currently in the process of completing five implementation guides for version 003070 encompassing medical, hospital, dental, pharmaceutical claims, and workers compensation jurisdictional reporting with an anticipating publication date of April 1997.

E) There currently is only one implementation guide for the Health Care Claim Status Request (276) - Health Care Claim Status Notification (277).

F) The implementation guides will specify the conformance to the standards.

G) Yes, conformance tools are commercially available.

H) The same tools used for conformance may also be used as testing tools.

I) The standard is complete. The current version of the standard is 003070. As business needs dictate, enhancements may be made to the standard three times per year, one major release along with two subsequent sub-releases. The X12 Health Care Task Group has developed procedures to determine when to move to the next version of the standard as well as when to retire past versions. The Health Care Task Group will also determine the need for new versions of the implementation guides (not more frequently than once per year).

J) Currently no enhancements are under development.

AA) This standard has been completed.

BB) This standard has been completed and undergoing industry implementation.

Indicator of Market Acceptance

A) The X12 standards are made available via many sources including from the Data Interchange Standards Association, Washington Publishing (ASC X12 Insurance Subcommittee's publisher), industry user groups and associations, and the Internet. Due to the multiplicity and diversity of these distribution methods, it is not possible to determine how many copies have been distributed and to whom.

B) Yes. ASC X12 represents international standards development. North American and other countries have implemented ASC X12 standards for purchasing and financial transactions. It would be to their benefit to further leverage their investment in EDI translation software, hardware and communication infrastructure to utilize the health care transactions.

C) Over 300 payer, provider, vendor, and plan sponsor organizations currently participate in the development of the ASC X12 standards and implementation guides to meet the business needs

F

of the entire health care industry. These organizations have experienced the benefits of mature standards as costs associated with developing and maintaining proprietary formats far exceed the investment necessary to implement a single set of health care EDI transactions.

Level of Specificity:

A) The ASC X12 EDI transactions have been developed to meet the specific business needs identified by the standards developers and the health care industry.
B) See attached table of contents from the ASC X12 Insurance Committee's implementation guides.
C) ASC X12 standards incorporate the business requirements for exchanging information contained within other standards. The ASC X12 standards provides a vehicle for communicating other standards within the standards.
D) ASC X12 maintains over one thousand internal code sets to support the standards. Along with the internal code sets the ASC X12 standards reference over 350 external code sources such as:
    - Current Procedural Terminology (CPT) Codes from American Medical Association
    - Current Dental Terminology (CDT) Codes from American Dental Association
    - International Classification of Diseases Clinical Modification - (ICD-9-CM) Diagnosis from U.S. National Center for Health Statistics.
E) There are too many code sets to describe here. Refer to the ASC X12 standards publication.
F) Internal code sets are included within the ASC X12 standards publications and implementation guides. When external code sets are referenced within these documents, the source where the code sets can be obtained is listed.
G) When possible, the implementation guides will either include the external code sets or provide further information on how to obtain the external code sets. Internal code sets are included within the implementation guides.
H) Internal code sets are available to all users of the ASC X12 standards. Usage of the external code sets will vary by source and their ability to promote the usage of their code sets.
I) ASC X12 internal code sets follow the same processes defined for the development and maintenance of the EDI transactions. External code lists are maintained by the external code source's internal development procedures.

Relationships with Other Standards

A) ASC X12 strives to coordinate and incorporate the needs of the other standards development organizations such as Health Level 7 (HL7), National Council for Prescription Drug Programs (NCPDP), and the American Society for Testing and Materials into the ASC X12 standards.
B) See A).
C) See A).
D) Open communication in the development of the standards amongst the standards development organizations.
E) ASC X12 is the ANSI appointed standards development organization responsible for international EDI standards within the United States
F) None
G) Given the scope and responsibility for the development and maintenance of the EDI standards for the United States and the international community with respect to United States international standards, ASC X12 is only privy to the business needs which are brought forward and coordinated with other health care organizations. At this time, we are unaware of any gaps in the current standards for insurance.

Identifiable Costs:

A) None applicable. ASC X12 does not license it standards.

B) The cost of acquiring the ASC X12 standards publication varies depending upon the source of the publications. Currently they are available from:
   - Data Interchange Standards Association (DISA) 703-548-7005.
   - Washington Publishing Corporation 800-972-4334
   - Industry user groups and associations
   - The Internet (http://www.disa.org, http://www.wpc-edi.com)

C) The typical cost ranges from free to $415.00 for the full ASC X12 standards publication in either paper form or CD-ROM.

D) The cost/timeframe for education and training will depend upon the individuals and skill levels of the individuals within an organization. Some organizations have completed education and training within one week while others have taken longer.

E) The cost/timeframe for implementation depends upon the internal systems capabilities, systems development philosophy, hardware platform selected, EDI translator software, communication methodology and individual resources within an organization. Costs can range anywhere from free for a personal computer solution to well over $150,000 for midsize and mainframe systems. Some organizations have implemented the standards within a matter of days while other have taken months to achieve the same end result.

F) The current use of proprietary formats such as the National Standard Format (NSF) and the costs of maintaining these formats far outweigh the costs associated with implementing a single set of the health care industry standards from ASC X12.

ASC X12 Claim Status (276/277) was approved October 1993. This transaction is used to determine the status of a submitted claim. The Implementation Guide is in development and is expected to be approved June 1997.

Referral Certification and Authorization

Accredited Standards Committee X12 Insurance Subcommittee, Property and Casualty Task Group

ANSI Accreditation:

X12 was accredited as an ANSI accredited standards committee in 1979. Subsequent X12 procedure changes have required ANSI re-accreditation which was last granted in 1987.

The main objective of ASC X12 is to develop Electronic Data Interchange (EDI) standards to facilitate electronic business transactions (i.e. order placement and processing, shipping and receiving, invoicing, payment, cash application data, insurance transactions). ASC X12 endeavors to structure standards in a manner that computer programs can translate data to and from internal formats without extensive reprogramming.

This strategy allows companies to maximize their resources required for internally developed or commercial software (recommended) and private or public-access communication networks. ASC X12 believes that all sizes of companies using intelligent computational devices can benefit from the use of the standard. The efficiencies of standard interchange format can minimize the difficulties incurred from each organization using its own formats to transact business. Within ASC X12, the various subcommittees are responsible for developing standards in their area of expertise. Once a

F

subcommittee has developed a draft standard the full ASC X12 membership reviews and approves it according to the operating policies and procedures. All standards (new or changed) require the consensus approval of the full ASC X12 membership. The approved standard becomes a draft standard for trial use for a reasonable trial period. After the trial period the draft standards are submitted to ANSI to become an American National Standard (ANS).

Health Care Service Review Information (278)

Contact For More Information:

Data Interchange Standards Association (DISA) 703-548-7005.

Description of Standard:

A) The objective of the Health Care Service Review Information (278) is used for referral certification and authorization.
B) This transaction set can be used to request and transmit demographic, utilization, certification and referral information. Includes no Utilization Management treatment information.
C) This transaction is used to support administration of health care services review between payers, providers, plan sponsors, and utilization review organizations..
D) This standard may be used from any operating system, network, or hardware platform.
E) The standard has be developed with widespread input from the health care industry incorporating all business needs into its functionality.
F) The ANSI ASC X12 is the only nationally recognized EDI standards development organization in the United States for all type of electronic commerce. ASC X12 is the organization assigned by ANSI to represent the United States in the development of International EDI standards.
G) Standards. These standards are developed using a consensus process by the users in the health care industry.
H) The standards developed by ASC X12 may be translated to/from application systems using off the shelf translation software products which are used by all industries utilizing the ASC X12 standards.

Readiness of Standard:

A) The Health Care Service Review Information (278) is not a guideline. However the X12 Insurance Subcommittee is currently developing implementation guides for this transaction.
B) The Health Care Service Review Information (278) standard is fully implementable. The transaction set was approved as a Draft Standard for Trial Use (DSTU) in October of 1994 as Version 003050.
C) The standard can be obtained by contacting the Data Interchange Standards Association (DISA) at 703-548-7005.
D) This standard does not require an implementation guide. ASC X12 has published four Type II Tutorial reports or tutorials for version 003041 in October of 1994, version 003050 in October 1995, version 003051 in February 1996, and version 003060 in April of 1996. To facilitate consistent implementation across the health care industry, the X12 Insurance Subcommittee is currently in the process of completing five implementation guides for version 003070 encompassing medical, hospital, dental, pharmaceutical claims, and workers compensation jurisdictional reporting with an anticipating publication date of April 1997.

E) There currently is only one implementation guide for the Health Care Service Review Information (278).

F) The implementation guides will specify the conformance to the standards.

G) Yes, conformance tools are commercially available.

H) The same tools used for conformance may also be used as testing tools.

I) The standard is complete. The current version of the standard is 003070. As business needs dictate, enhancements may be made to the standard three times per year, one major release along with two subsequent sub-releases. The X12 Health Care Task Group has developed procedures to determine when to move to the next version of the standard as well as when to retire past versions. The Health Care Task Group will also determine the need for new versions of the implementation guides (not more frequently than once per year).

J) Currently no enhancements are under development.

AA) This standard has been completed.

BB) This standard has been completed and undergoing industry implementation.

Indicator of Market Acceptance:

A) The X12 standards are made available via many sources including from the Data Interchange Standards Association, Washington Publishing (ASC X12 Insurance Subcommittee's publisher), industry user groups and associations, and the Internet. Due to the multiplicity and diversity of these distribution methods, it is not possible to determine how many copies have been distributed and to whom.

B) Yes. ASC X12 represents international standards development. North American and other countries have implemented ASC X12 standards for purchasing and financial transactions. It would be to their benefit to further leverage their investment in EDI translation software, hardware and communication infrastructure to utilize the health care transactions.

C) Over 300 payer, provider, vendor, and plan sponsor organizations currently participate in the development of the ASC X12 standards and implementation guides to meet the business needs of the entire health care industry. These organizations have experienced the benefits of mature standards as costs associated with developing and maintaining proprietary formats far exceed the investment necessary to implement a single set of health care EDI transactions.

Level of Specificity:

A) The ASC X12 EDI transactions have been developed to meet the specific business needs identified by the standards developers and the health care industry.

B) See attached table of contents from the ASC X12 Insurance Committee's implementation guides.

C) ASC X12 standards incorporate the business requirements for exchanging information contained within other standards. The ASC X12 standards provides a vehicle for communicating other standards within the standards.

D) ASC X12 maintains over one thousand internal code sets to support the standards. Along with the internal code sets the ASC X12 standards reference over 350 external code sources such as:
- Current Procedural Terminology (CPT) Codes from American Medical Association
- Current Dental Terminology (CDT) Codes from American Dental Association
- International Classification of Diseases Clinical Modification - (ICD-9-CM) Diagnosis from U.S. National Center for Health Statistics.

E) There are too many code sets to describe here. Refer to the ASC X12 standards publication.

F) Internal code sets are included within the ASC X12 standards publications and implementation guides. When external code sets are referenced within these documents, the source where the code sets can be obtained is listed.

F

G) When possible, the implementation guides will either include the external code sets or provide further information on how to obtain the external code sets. Internal code sets are included within the implementation guides.

AA) Internal code sets are available to all users of the ASC X12 standards. Usage of the external code sets will vary by source and their ability to promote the usage of their code sets.

BB) ASC X12 internal code sets follow the same processes defined for the development and maintenance of the EDI transactions. External code lists are maintained by the external code source's internal development procedures.

Relationships with Other Standards:

A) ASC X12 strives to coordinate and incorporate the needs of the other standards development organizations such as Health Level 7 (HL7), National Council for Prescription Drug Programs (NCPDP), and the American Society for Testing and Materials into the ASC X12 standards.

B) See A).

C) See A).

D) Open communication in the development of the standards amongst the standards development organizations.

E) ASC X12 is the ANSI appointed standards development organization responsible for international EDI standards within the United States

F) None

G) Given the scope and responsibility for the development and maintenance of the EDI standards for the United States and the international community with respect to United States international standards, ASC X12 is only privy to the business needs which are brought forward and coordinated with other health care organizations. At this time, we are unaware of any gaps in the current standards for insurance.

Identifiable Costs:

A) None applicable. ASC X12 does not license it standards.

B) The cost of acquiring the ASC X12 standards publication varies depending upon the source of the publications. Currently they are available from:
- Data Interchange Standards Association (DISA) 703-548-7005.
- Washington Publishing Corporation 800-972-4334
- Industry user groups and associations
- The Internet (http://www.disa.org, http://www.wpc-edi.com)

C) The typical cost ranges from free to $415.00 for the full ASC X12 standards publication in either paper form or CD-ROM.

D) The cost/timeframe for education and training will depend upon the individuals and skill levels of the individuals within an organization. Some organizations have completed education and training within one week while others have taken longer.

E) The cost/timeframe for implementation depends upon the internal systems capabilities, systems development philosophy, hardware platform selected, EDI translator software, communication methodology and individual resources within an organization. Costs can range anywhere from free for a personal computer solution to well over $150,000 for midsize and mainframe systems. Some organizations have implemented the standards within a matter of days while other have taken months to achieve the same end result.

F) The current use of proprietary formats such as the National Standard Format (NSF) and the costs of maintaining these formats far outweigh the costs associated with implementing a single set of the health care industry standards from ASC X12.

ASC X12 Healthcare Service Review (278) was approved February 1996. This transaction is used to request and transmit demographic, utilization, certification and referral information. The Implementation Guide is in development and is expected to be approved June 1997.

Supporting Standards

Codes and Code Sets (including issues of maintenance)

World Health Organization (WHO)

The WHO Collaborating Center for the Classification of Diseases for North America, located at the National Center for Health Statistics, is responsible for the coordination of all official disease classification activities in the United States relating to the ICD and its use, interpretation and periodic revision.

ANSI Accreditation:

The WHO Collaborating Center for North America is not an ANSI accredited body. The Collaborating Center is part of an international network of Collaborating Centers coordinated by the World Health Organization (WHO).

International Classification of Diseases, Ninth Revision (ICD-9)

International Classification of Diseases, Tenth Revision (ICD-10)

There are no separate templates for ICD-9 and ICD-10. On the following page, however, is a template developed by the National Center for Health Statistics (NCHS) for ICD-9 CM and ICD-10 CM.

National Center for Health Statistics (NCHS)

International Classification of Diseases, Ninth Revision, Clinical Modification (ICD-9-CM)
International Classification of Diseases, Tenth Revision, Clinical Modification (ICD-10-CM)
International Classification of Diseases Procedure Coding System (ICD-10-PCS)

Name of Standard: (1) International Classification of Diseases (ICD); Ninth Revision, Clinical Modification (ICD-9-CM) currently in use for morbidity reporting.

Contact For More Information

Marjorie S. Greenberg
Ph: 301-436-4253 Ext. 107
Fax: 301-436-4233)
E-mail: MSG1@NCH11A.EM.CDC.GOV; or

F

Donna Pickett
Ph: 301-436-7050 Ext.142
Fax: 301-436 4233)
E-mail: DFP4@NCH11A.EM.CDC.GOV

Description of Standard

The ICD-9-CM is the latest version of a classification that originated as the International List of Causes of Deaths, adopted in 1893 by the International Statistical Institute. The classification was revised at ten-yearly intervals and at the Sixth Revision Conference in 1948, the first undertaken by the WHO, its scope was extended to include non-fatal conditions and its use was recommended for morbidity statistics as well as for mortality. Subsequent revisions have enhanced its usefulness for morbidity applications by increasing the specificity of rubrics and by emphasizing manifestations of disease. Effective January 1979, the ICD-9-CM became the sole classification system used for morbidity reporting in the United States.

The ICD-9-CM, widely accepted and used in the health care industry, has been adopted by the federal government and the private sector for a number of purposes: data collection, quality of care analyses, resource utilization, research and reimbursement, and statistical reporting.

ICD-10-CM is currently under development, with a planned implementation date of October 1, 2000.

Readiness of Standard:

There are official coding guidelines used to instruct users on the classification. The ICD-9-CM classification and the guidelines are in the public domain and are available on CDROM from the Government Printing Office.

Is it implementable? (If so, is it fully or partially implementable?, explain)

The guidelines and classification are both in current use.

How can the standard be obtained?

The ICD-9-CM classification and the official national coding guidelines are in the public domain and are widely available. Both can be obtained through the Government Printing Office or through various publishers.

Does it require a separate implementation guide? (If so is the guide approved by the SDO?

Not applicable

Is there only one implementation guideline (or are there major options that impact compatibility)?

Not applicable

Is a conformance standard identified?

Not applicable

Are conformance test tools available?

Not applicable

Source of test tools?

Not applicable

If the standard is under development, what parts of it are ready now?

Work on the clinical modification (CM) of the International Classification of Diseases and Related Health Problems (ICD-10) is currently underway; it will undergo review in the Department of Health and Human Services in 1997. The final version is scheduled to be available by October 1, 1998.

What extensions are now under development?
What are the major milestones toward standards completion?
What are the projected dates for final balloting and/or implementation?

The planned implementation of ICD-10-CM, in conjunction with the Health Care Financing Administration's Procedure Coding System (ICD-10-PCS), is tentatively scheduled for October 1, 2000.

Please note any other indicators of readiness that may be appropriate.

Indicator of Market Acceptance

Both the classification and guidelines for it are in wide use with thousands of copies being used nationally for the submission of health insurance claims and for statistical data collection, performance measures, research, etc.

If the standard is an implementable standard, how many vendors, healthcare organizations and/or government agencies are using it?

N/A

Is this standard being used in other countries (which are they)?

The ICD-9 is used internationally for cause of death tabulation. The ICD-9-CM, the morbidity version of the ICD-9, is used in the United States primarily, but Australia and Israel use the ICD-9-CM for morbidity. These countries will be implementing the ICD-10 for both morbidity and mortality prior to the United States.

Please note any other relevant indicator of market acceptance within the public or private sector.

Many private vendors produce a variety of software and book products based on the ICD-9-CM.

F

Level of Specificity

If your standard is a guideline, how detailed is it?

The guidelines for the ICD-9-CM are broad guidelines for coding. They are not teaching manuals.

If it is an implementable standard, describe how detailed its framework is and its level of granularity.

N/A

Does the standard(s) reference or assume other standards to achieve more specificity?

N/A

If it includes or assumes code sets, which ones are they?

The ICD-9-CM is code set.

What is the description of the code set?

A medical statistical classification

How is the code set acquired?

The ICD-9-CM classification and the official national coding guidelines are in the public domain and are widely available. Both can be obtained through the Government Printing Office or through various publishers.

Is there a users' guide or some other assistance available on the code set?

WHO published an official rule book for mortality rules. The U.S. publishes official guidelines for the use of the ICD-9-CM for morbidity applications.

If the code set is currently in use, what is the extent of its use (e.g., approximate number of users)?

All health care claims must list the ICD-9-CM diagnosis code.

If the code set is under development, what are the projected dates of completion and implementation?

N/A

Relationships with other standards

Volume 3 of ICD-9-CM is the classification of procedures used in the inpatient setting. CPT is used by physicians and hospital-based outpatient departments for the coding of procedures. The Health Care Financing Administration is developing ICD-10-PCS to replace Volume 3.

Identify specific standards reconciliation or coordination activities.

NCHS serves as the North American Collaborating Center for the Classification of Diseases (ICD) and for the International Classification of Impairments, Disabilities, and Handicaps (ICIDH). NCHS is responsible for the coordination of all official disease classification activities in the United States relating to the ICD and its use, interpretation and periodic revision. [See also III (A)].

The ICD-9-CM Coordination and Maintenance Committee is the process by which the classification (Volumes 1, 2, and 3) is maintained and updated each year. The Coordination and Maintenance process ensures stability of the classification system and it s comparability with its parent system, ICD-9. Established in 1985, this Committee was formed to provide a public forum to discuss possible updates and revisions to the ICD-9-CM.

What portion of the specification and functionality is affected by this coordination?

N/A

What conditions are assumed in order for this coordination to be effective?

All requests for modification are handled through the ICD-9-CM Coordination and Maintenance Committee. The Committee discusses such topics as the need to update the ICD-9-CM due to changes in medical technology, the need to provide greater specificity in classifying diagnoses (adding clinical detail and accuracy), and the need to correct inaccuracies in the classification. No official changes are made without being brought before this committee.

Although the Committee is a federal committee, suggestions for modifications come from both the public and private sectors, and interested parties are asked to submit recommendations for modification prior to a scheduled meeting.

Modifications are not considered without the expert advice of clinicians, epidemiologists, and nosologists (both public and private sectors).

Is this standard consistent with international standards? If so, which standards?

Yes. The ICD-9-CM is consistent with ICD-9, and ICD-10-CM similarly will be consistent with ICD-10.

What gaps remain among related standards that should be addressed?

Describe what is being done to address these gaps.

Identifiable Costs

Notes: ICD-10-CM
- Please indicate the cost or your best estimate for the following:
  - Cost of licensure: None, the classification is in the public domain
  - Cost of acquisition (if different from licensure)
  - Cost/timeframes for education and training/implementation
A two-year timeframe is planned to allow for training and system modifications and software development for the transition to ICD-10-CM.
- Please note any other cost considerations.

F

American Medical Association (AMA)

Physicians' Current Procedural Terminology (CPT)

Physicians' Current Procedural Terminology , Fourth Edition (CPT) is a listing of descriptive terms and identifying codes for reporting medical services and procedures. The purpose of the terminology is to provide a uniform languages that will accurately describe medical, surgical and diagnostic services, and will thereby provide an effective means for reliable nationwide communication among health professionals, patients and third-parties. The first edition of CPT appeared in 1966.

Developing Organization

CPT was created and is authored by the American Medical Association (AMA).

ANSI Accreditation:

The AMA is a member of ANSI. CPT is copyrighted by the AMA.

Names

Physicians' Current Procedural Terminology, Fourth Edition (CPT)

Description

CPT contains the American Medical Association's listing of descriptive terms and identifying codes. It also contains numeric modifiers, notes, guidelines and an index designed to provide explanatory information and facilitate the correct usage of the coding system.

Contact For More Information:

Celeste G. Kirschner
Director, Coding and Nomenclature
American Medical Association
515 N. State Street
Chicago, IL 60610
Phone: 312-464-5932
Fax: 312-464-5849

Indicator of Market Acceptance

CPT is used as the reporting mechanism by physicians and many other health professionals in the United States. It is the coding system used by Medicare and virtually all third party payors, including workers compensation and Medicaid. Hospitals use CPT codes to report outpatient service to Medicare. Its usage internationally is growing, particularly by United States companies that have international components. CPT was recently selected as the coding system of choice by the Medical Association of South Africa. CPT is Level I of HCPCS (HCFA Common Procedure Coding System).

Level of Specificity

CPT contains over 7300 codes to describe medical and surgical procedures. CPT is divided into 6 major sections, including Evaluation and Management Services, Anesthesia, Surgery, Radiology,

Pathology and Medicine. The section heads, subheads, and titles provide an implicit hierarchy. The Surgery section is subdivided anatomically. The Medicine Section is divided by medical subspecialties. A series of two digit modifiers are also included to make the coding system more specific, to allow the reporting of a procedure under specific circumstances. For example, modifiers may be used to describe the use of assistant surgeons, a bilateral procedure, or a return to the operating room during the postoperative period.

Maintenance of CPT

CPT is authored by the American Medical Association. The CPT Editorial Panel is made up of 15 physicians, 10 nominated by the AMA and one each nominated by the Blue Cross and Blue Shield Association, the Health Insurance Association of America, the Health Care Financing Administration and the American Hospital Association. A non-physician representative of the Health Care Professionals Advisory Committee (HCPAC) also serves as a member of the Panel.

The Panel's Executive Committee includes the chairman, the vice chairman and three other members of the Panel, as elected by the entire Panel. One of the three members-at-large of the executive committee must be a third-party payer representative. The AMA provides staff support for the CPT Editorial Panel and appoints a staff secretary. Supporting the Editorial Panel in its work is the CPT Advisory Committee. Committee members are primarily physicians nominated by the national medical specialty societies represented in the AMA House of Delegates. The Health Care Professional Advisory Committee allows for participation of organizations representing limited license practitioners and allied health professionals. Most members of the Advisory Committee serve as Chair of a specialty society committee and thus form a network of approximately 1000 physicians and other health professionals actively working to maintain the clinical integrity of the system.

Readiness

Current Procedural Terminology (CPT) is available in the following print and electronic formats:

1 volume spiral-bound edition;
1 volume soft bound edition;
1 volume spiral-bound Professional edition;
1 volume three-ring bound Professional edition

Electronic versions in EBCDIC or ASCII for full and short description magnetic tape formats; also available in diskette format, short or long description which can be used with any software that allows import of an ASCII file. A CD-ROM version, that includes CPT, is available for 1997.

In addition, CPT is currently licensed to many software system vendors and publishing companies.

Identifiable Costs

CPT is available at low cost through the AMA or through the AMA's licensing activities. CPT can be purchased from the AMA in print formats for as low as $38. CPT can be licensed from the AMA in electronic formats for as low as $149. Licenses are granted to those that distribute CPT in print and electronic formats. Licenses for CPT in print products are granted for as low as $10 per product. Licenses for CPT in electronic products are granted for $50 per product license with a minimal additional user fee for multi-user versions. The codes are revised yearly.

F

College of American Pathologists

Systematized Nomenclature of Human and Veterinary Medicine (SNOMED) International

SNOMED® International is recognized throughout the world as a comprehensive, multiaxial nomenclature classification system created for the indexing of the entire medical vocabulary, including symptoms, diagnoses, and procedures. Its design provides the framework for representing the activities, observations, and diagnoses found in the medical record and coding them into a computer-processable form. The structure of SNOMED® International, together with its ability to index and retrieve comprehensive patient information, makes this system a strong candidate for the standard vocabulary and data model that is essential for the computer-based patient record.

Developing Organization

SNOMED® International is owned and managed by the College of American Pathologists (CAP). The CAP is a national medical specialty society serving more than 15,000 physician members and the laboratory community in the United States and internationally. College fellows elect a 12-member Board of Governors and three officers who serve as the governing body. Supporting the Board of Governors are a hierarchy of Councils, Commissions and Committees. These groups develop and oversee College and projects and programs. Administrative support and overall coordination and implementation of College programs is provided by staff located at the CAP Headquarters office in Northfield, Illinois.

The Council on Practice and Education is responsible for the operation of several CAP committees including the SNOMED® Editorial Board (SEB). Through the work of the SNOMED® Editorial Board chaired by College member, Roger A. Cote, MD, new terms and codes are continuously added to the SNOMED® vocabulary, with at least two updates provided annually. Via relationships with other medical specialty societies, the SEB is responsible for the design, development and maintenance of the SNOMED® vocabulary.

ANSI Accreditation:

SNOMED® International is not a standard. It is a registered trademark owned and copyrighted by the College of American Pathologists. As an organization, the CAP is not directly involved in standards development.

Name:

SNOMED® International

Contact For More Information:
Karen Kudla
SNOMED Program Manager
College of American Pathologists
325 Waukegan Road
Northfield, IL 60093
Phone: 847-832-7446
Fax: 847-832-8170
E-Mail: kkudla@cap.org

Description

SNOMED® International is a comprehensive, multiaxial nomenclature classification system created for the indexing of the entire medical vocabulary, including signs and symptoms, diagnoses, and procedures. Introduced in September 1993 and traceable to its roots in the early 1960s as the Systematized Nomenclature of Pathology (SNOP), SNOMED® is being rapidly accepted worldwide as the standard for indexing medical record information. It has been translated from English into 12 other languages. The American Veterinary Medical Association and the American Dental Association have recognized SNOMED®'s strength as a comprehensive nomenclature and have endorsed its use. In addition, the American College of Radiology/National Equipment Manufacturers Association will be using a subset of SNOMED® in their Digital Imaging and Communications in Medicine standard (DICOM).

Of the major factors required for successful computer-based patient record development, a common medical vocabulary for use in records and standards for integrating multiple and disparate sources of information are critical elements. The eleven modules of the current version of SNOMED® contain more than 144,000 terms and term codes, with new updates provided to SNOMED® users at least twice per year. Many electronic records proponents are concluding that SNOMED® International offers the best prospects for a standardized vocabulary.

Readiness

SNOMED® International is available in the following print and electronic formats: four-volume hard-bound printed set electronic version on CD-ROM in a tab-delimited ASCII format
In addition, the following information systems vendors are licensed to distribute SNOMED® International:
ACT Medisys
ANATROL
Antrim Corporation
Cerner Corporation
Citation Computer Systems
Collaborative Medical Systems
Computer Trust Corp.
Dentente Corporation
Dynacor Inc.
Dynamic Healthcare Tech, Inc.
Galen Group, Ltd.
Health Data Science Corp.
Healthpoint GP
Kaiser Permanente
Laboratory Consulting, Inc.
MedicaLogic
Orbis Systems
Psyche Systems
Science Applications Int'l Corp.
Sunquest Information Systems
Univ. Of Alabama at Birmingham

F

Indicator of Market Acceptance

SNOMED® International is widely used and distributed throughout the United States and worldwide. SNOMED® International was ranked on top in a study conducted by the Computer-based Patient Record Institute (CPRI) which evaluated all available coding systems for their ability to be used as a common medical terminology.

SNOMED® International has been translated into Greek, Chinese, Czech, French, German, Hungarian, Italian, Japanese, Norwegian, Portuguese, Russian, Slovakian, and Spanish.
The American Veterinary Medical Association and the American Dental Association have recognized SNOMED®'s strength as a comprehensive nomenclature and have endorsed its use. In addition, the American College of Radiology/National Equipment Manufacturers Association will be using a subset of SNOMED® in their Digital Imaging and Communications in Medicine standard (DICOM).

Level of Specificity

SNOMED® International is a detailed coded nomenclature and classification of preferred medical terms and concepts, consisting of more than 144,000 terms and term codes divided into eleven linked hierarchical modules: Topography; Morphology; Function; Living Organisms; Chemicals, Drugs, and Biological Products; Physical Agents, Activities and Forces; Social Context; Diseases/Diagnoses; Procedures; and general Linkage Modifiers

Identifiable Costs

SNOMED® International is available to individuals for a single fee.
In addition, licenses are granted to distribute SNOMED® International for commercial or institutional use. Licensing fees are determined by the number of users per site, and are renewed annually

American Dental Association (ADA)

Current Dental Terminology (CDT)

The ADA's Current Dental Terminology (CDT) is a manual that is intended to be of practical use to those in dental offices who deal with patients' dental plans, by providing assistance in accurately reporting dental treatment and procedures to third-party payers. The document used for reporting treatment is the American Dental Association's Code on Dental Procedures and Nomenclature which is contained in the CDT. The Code is structured so that it can be used by dentists and/or their staff to report care provided to patients. Within CDT, many code numbers are accompanied by additional information or explanations to help clarify how the codes should be applied.

Developing Organization

CDT is maintained by the American Dental Association through its Council on Dental Benefit Programs.

ANSI Accreditation:

CDT is not a standard. It is a copyrighted document of the American Dental Association. However, as an organization, the ADA is directly involved in standards development as sponsor and secretariat of the ASC MD156.

Name

Current Dental Terminology (CDT)

Contact For More Information:

Thomas Conway
American Dental Association
211 East Chicago Avenue
Chicago, Illinois 60611
Phone: 312/440-2752
Fax: 312/440-2520
E-mail: conwayt@ada.org

Description

The CDT contains the American Dental Association's codes for dental procedures and nomenclature and is the nationally accepted set of numeric codes and descriptive terms for reporting dental treatments. CDT also contains a description of the ADA Dental Claim Form; clinical and dental benefit terminology; and a description of the tooth numbering system.

Readiness

CDT is available in the following print and electronic formats:
1 volume spiral bound manual;

Electronic version in MS DOS diskette, an ASCII file, and a database program. Must have IBM compatible computer with at least 512K RAM.
In addition, CDT is currently licensed to many practice management software systems vendors.

Indicator of Market Acceptance

CDT is used as a reporting tool by all practicing dentists in the United States. It is also used by third-party payers for claims processing. The ADA's procedure codes are also included in the HCFA Procedural Coding System (HCPCS) as the dental (D) codes.

Level of Specificity

CDT includes the ADA's Code on Dental Procedures and Nomenclature consisting of over 400 distinct dental procedures. The codes and nomenclature have been divided into 12 categories of service: Diagnostic, Preventive, Restorative, Endodontics, Periodontics, Prosthodontics; removable,

F

Maxillofacial Prosthetics, Implant Services, Prosthodontics;fixed, Oral Surgery, Orthodontics, and Adjunctive General Services.

Identifiable Costs

CDT is available to individuals for $29.95. Licenses are granted for $500 for a five year period to those that distribute CDT in software systems, continuing education programs and other products. The codes are revised on a five-year cycle.

Advisory Committee on Dental Electronic Nomenclature Indexing and Classification (ACODENIC)

Microglossary of SNOMED for Dentistry

The American Dental Association established this advisory committee to develop standardized clinical terminology for the dental profession in an electronic environment. All segments of the health care process must be addressed, such as patient history, presenting conditions, physical findings, services, risk factors, outcomes, or other important details. In addition, all facets of health care, independent of profession, discipline or specialty must be included in standardized terminology. Therefore, the Advisory Committee has engaged in the difficult task of creating a clinical terminology and coding system which will provide the dental profession with varying degrees of utility.

In order to accomplish this charge, the American Dental Association recognized the strength of the SNOMED International system and began working with the College of American Pathologists on the development of a microglossary of SNOMED for dentistry. The ADA's Microglossary is currently in development and is expected to be completed in 1997. The ADA is participating with a sample of terms from the Microglossary in the Large Scale Vocabulary Test conducted by the National Library of Medicine (NLM). The proposed dental terms are being tested against the NLM's Unified Medical Language System (UMLS). The goal of the NLM Large Scale Vocabulary Test is to contribute to an understanding of the controlled terminology that will be needed for electronic health care systems, whether these are for direct patient care, clinical or health services research, or public health surveillance. The Test seeks to determine the extent to which a combination of existing health-related terminologies cover vocabulary needed in health information systems. The terminology that the participants submit to should provide the basis for realistic resouce estimates for developing and maintaining a comprehensive "standard" health vocabulary that is based on existing terminologies. In addition, the ADA's dental terms were recently used to update the dental terminology for the NLM's 1997 Medical Subject Headings (MeSH). MeSH is the vocabulary used to index articles in the National Library of Medicine's MEDLINE database and its derivative publications, including *Index Medicus* and the American Dental Association's *Index to Dental Literature*.

The ADA's procedure codes will also be mapped to the SNOMED terms in the Dental Microglossary.
Comprehensive Glossary of Dental Terms - Standardized terminology must have explicit definitions. A collective guide is important for consistent interpretation of terms by the profession and aggregate data analysts. Therefore, the American Dental Association's ACODENIC is also developing a comprehensive glossary of dental terms. In addition to defining the terms in the Microglossary, the definitions will be useful for the NLM's MeSH and UMLS knowledge sources.

Center for Nursing Classification, University of Iowa College of Nursing

Nursing Interventions Classification (NIC)

The **Nursing Interventions Classification** (NIC) is a comprehensive, standardized language describing treatments that nurses perform in all settings and in all specialties. NIC interventions include both the physiological (e.g. Acid-Base Management) and the psychosocial (e.g. Anxiety Reduction). There are interventions for illness treatment (e.g. Hyperglycemia Management), illness prevention (e.g. Fall Prevention), and health promotion (e.g. Exercise Promotion). Interventions are for individuals or for families (e.g. Family Integrity Promotion). Indirect care interventions (e.g. Emergency Cart Checking) and some interventions for communities (e.g. Environmental Management: Community) are also included.

Each NIC intervention has a unique number which can facilitate computerization. NIC interventions have been linked with NANDA nursing diagnoses and the Omaha System problems and are in the process of being linked with Nursing Outcomes Classification (NOC) patient outcomes. There is a form and a review system for submitting suggestions for new or modified interventions.

Developing Organization

The classification work is part of the Center for Nursing Classification at the University of Iowa College of Nursing. Research methods used to develop the Classification include content analysis, expert survey, focus group review, similarity analysis, hierarchical cluster analysis, multidimensional scaling, and field testing. More than 40 national nursing organizations have reviewed NIC and assisted with intervention development and validation and taxonomy construction and validation. The research, conducted by a large team of investigators, has been partially supported for the past seven years by the National Institute of Nursing Research, National Institutes of Health.

ANSI Accreditation:

NIC is not a standard. It is a standardized language organized in a 3 level taxonomic structure for ease of use. It is published by Mosby Year Book who owns the copyright. Neither the University of Iowa which produces NIC nor Mosby is involved in the development of standards.

Name

Nursing Interventions Classification (NIC)

F

Contact For More Information:

William Donahue, Program Associate
Center for Nursing Classification
College of Nursing
The University of Iowa
Iowa City, IA 52240
Phone: 319-335-7054/7051
Fax: 319-335-7051
E-mail: william-donahue@uiowa.edu
OR classification-center@uiowa.edu

Description

NIC contains 433 interventions each with a definition and a detailed set of activities that describe what it is a nurse does to implement the intervention. Each intervention is coded with a unique number. The interventions are organized in 26 classes and 7 domains. NIC facilitates the implementation of a Nursing Minimum Data Set. The use of NIC to plan and document care will facilitate the collection of large data bases which will allow us to study the effectiveness and cost of nursing treatments. The use of standardized language provides for the continuity of care and enhances communication among nurses and among nurses and other providers. NIC provides nursing with the treatment language that is essential for the computerized health care record. The domains and classes provide a description of the essence of nursing. NIC is helpful in representing nursing to the public and in socializing students to the profession. The coded interventions can be used in documentation and in reimbursement. The language is comprehensive and can be used by nurses in all settings and in all specialties.

Readiness

NIC is available in the following print publication: Iowa Intervention Project (1996). Nursing Interventions Classification (NIC), 2nd ed. St. Louis: Mosby Year Book.
The following vendors are licensed to distribute NIC:
- ERGO, Mission, Kansas, 319: 384-3377.
- JRS Clinical Technology, Stamford, CT, 203:322-1823.
In addition, there are numerous journal publications about NIC that detail aspects of development or use. An anthology of NIC publications and an implementation manual containing helpful guides and forms related to implementation from selected user agencies are available from the Center for Nursing Classification.

Indicator of Market Acceptance

NIC is recognized by the American Nurses' Association and is included in the National Library of Medicine's Metathesaurus for a Unified Medical Language. Both the Cumulative Index to Nursing Literature(CINAHL) and Silver Platter have added NIC to their nursing indexes. NIC is included in the Joint Commission on Accreditation for Health Care Organization's (JCAHO) as one nursing classification system that can be used to meet the standard on uniform data. The National League for Nursing has made a 40 minute video about NIC to facilitate teaching of NIC to nursing students and practicing nurses. Many health care agencies are adopting NIC for use in standards, care plans, and nursing information systems; nursing education programs are beginning to use NIC; authors of major texts are beginning to use NIC to discuss nursing treatments; and researchers are using NIC to study the effectiveness of nursing care. Interest in NIC has been demonstrated in several other countries, notably, Canada, Denmark, Iceland, Japan, Korea, Switzerland, and The Netherlands.

Level of Specificity

NIC groups approximately 13,000 nurse activities into 433 standardized intervention terms each with a unique code. NIC has numerous uses including in care planning, documentation, standards construction, critical paths, competency evaluation, job descriptions, curriculum and course syllabus construction. The use of NIC in nursing information systems allows for the collection of standardized data to be used in effectiveness research and in determining the costs of nursing.

Identifiable Costs

NIC is available in book form to individuals for a single fee, which in January 1997 was $35.95. In addition, licenses are granted to distribute NIC for commercial or institutional use by contacting Robin Carter at Mosby Year Book, 800:325-4177, ext. 4412 (robin.carter@mosby.com) Licensing fees are determined by the number of users per site and are renewed with each new edition of the book (approximately every 4 years). Permission to use NIC in printed material can be obtained by contacting Liz Fathman at Mosby Year Book, 800:325-4177, ext. 4866 (liz.fathman@mosby.com).

International Conference on Harmonization

Representation includes:
Food and Drug Administration
European Union
Japan's Ministry of Health and Welfare
PhRMA (Pharmaceutical Research and Manufacturers of America)
JPMA (Japanese Pharmaceutical Manufacturers Association)
EFPIA (European Federation of Pharmaceutical Industries Association)

ANSI Accreditation

Not ANSI Accredited

International Medical Terminology (IMT)

Contact For More Information:

Kathryn A. Huntley
Standardized Nomenclature Program Manager
Food and Drug Administration
HF-21 Rm 16B-45
5600 Fishers Lane
Rockville, MD 20857
Voice mail: (301) 594-6491
Fax: (301) 594-0829
E-mail: khuntley@bangate.fda.gov

F

Description of Standard

The International Medical Terminology (IMT) is a medical terminology designed to support the classification, retrieval, presentation, and communication of medical information throughout the medical product regulatory cycle. The foundation of the IMT is the Medical Dictionary for Drug Regulatory Affairs (MEDDRA) developed by the UK Medicines Control Agency (MCA) in its Adverse Drug Reactions On-line Information Tracking System (ADROIT).

The IMT is superior to other medical terminologies in its scope, size, and specificity. Included in the IMT are terms describing diseases, diagnoses, signs, symptoms, therapeutic indication names, and qualitative results of investigations (e.g. laboratory tests, radiological studies), medical and surgical procedures, and terms describing medical, social, and family history. The IMT consists of a five level hierarchy, starting with 26 System Organ Classes (SOCs), that represent the highest level groupings of the terminology. Including all levels it contains approximately 40,000 terms. The Preferred term (PT) is the internationally agreed upon level at which regulatory information is to be exchanged. The IMT contains approximately 8,800 PTs, vastly improving the specificity of exchanged regulatory information over previous thesauri.

The current version of the IMT is available in multiple formats:
- ASCII text files
- Access Database
- On the FDA's Standardized Nomenclatures Database (SND)
- The thesaurus is also available in paper format.

Readiness of Standard

A) This is not a guideline
B) The implementable version will be a combination of products, the terminology and a maintenance organization. The terminology will be completed March 1997 the maintenance organization will be operational December 1997.
C) The 1.5 version of the terminology is obtainable through the FDA at no cost. The final version will be available through the maintenance organization.
D) There will be a user manual, help desk support etc. through the maintenance organization.
E) There will be a single version, multiple translations i.e. Japanese, Spanish, French and German to begin.
F) No
G) No.
H) None
I) The 1.5 version of the terminology is available for review. The FDA has rewritten 8 of the 26 System Organ Classes. The structure of terminology will not change just the terms populating the various levels below the System Organ Class level.
J) The final review of the US proposals, and the review and repopulation of the mid-levels to aid in data aggregation and display as well as the assignment of codes.
AA) ICH Expert Working Group meeting the first week of January 1997, the presentation to the ICH Steering Committee the first week of March 1997.
BB) ICH Steering Committee meeting March 1997, Selection of the Maintenance Organization July 1997, Terminology available December 1997
CC) None

Indicator of Market Acceptance

A) 308 copies of Version 1.0 and 386 copies of Version 1.5 have been distributed in North America to date. There are also distribution points in Japan and Europe.
B) none currently
C) A closely related product is currently being used in the ADROIT system of the UK's Medicines Control Agency.
D) The development of this standard under the ICH umbrella is very important in that once agreed upon by the regulators they are committed to implementing it. That means the regulatory authorities of Europe, United states and Japan will implement therefore the industries in those regions will also implement it. It is being reviewed by the World Health Organization for use by WHO countries and also by the WHO Drug Monitoring Program in Upsala Sweden.

Within the US, the National Cancer Institute's Cancer Therapy Evaluation Program *is planning to* adopt this terminology for use in collecting cancer clinical trial data.

Level of Specificity

A) The IMT is not a guideline.
B) The IMT's hierarchy consists of five levels and was designed to facilitate both coding and retrieval of medical information. These levels include System Organ Class (SOC), the broadest term; High Level Group Term (HLGT); High Level Term (HLT); Preferred Term (PT); and Lowest Level Term (LLT). Concepts in the vocabulary are grouped based upon inclusive relationships. The hierarchy can be used to locate concepts at a desired degree of specificity.

The following is a description of the IMT hierarchical levels from the most specific, or granular, to the broadest.

LLT - The Lowest Level Terms provide the most specific terms in the vocabulary. The LLTs are not used for reporting, but help define the scope of the preferred term to which they are linked, and provide a collection of terms used in verbatim reports to describe adverse experiences or medical history. In the IMT, the LLTs contain both synonyms and quasi-synonyms. In a strictly controlled thesaurus, the finest division of vocabulary consists only of synonyms and lexical variants (spelling and word order variations). In practical medical coding vocabularies, however, this rule is not rigorously enforceable. Terms that have similar meanings, or which describe similar concepts, are often grouped under the same preferred term.

PT - The preferred term is the internationally agreed upon level at which regulatory information is to be exchanged. The PT represents a single, unambiguous, clinical concept. Terms at this level should be at a level of specificity to code regulated indications and to capture signals of specific significant adverse events. The LLTs under each PT indicate the intended scope of the term. A PT may be linked to one or more SOCs, but is assigned to only one Primary SOC under which it is grouped for cumulative data outputs to prevent duplicate counting.

HLT - A High Level Term groups together PTs which are related by anatomy, pathology, physiology, etiology or function for data retrieval and presentation purposes only. An HLT may be linked to one or more HLGT(s) or SOC(s).

HLGT - High Level Group Terms, like the HLTs, are broad concepts used for grouping clinically related terms for data retrieval and presentation. They may be linked to one or more SOC(s).

F

SOC - The System Organ Class represents the broadest collection of concepts for retrieval in the vocabulary. SOCs group concepts according to anatomical or physiological system, e.g. Gastrointestinal disorders; body organ, e.g. Disorders of the eye; mechanism, e.g. Infections and infestations; and purposes, e.g. Surgical and medical procedures.

It does not reference other standards.

FDA recommendation for the IMT coding scheme (this is only a recommendation and has not been finalized):
- IMT use a sequential numbering (non-expressive, numeric code) method with a length of at least 8 for the terminology coding scheme.
- Unique codes be applied to all terms across all categories.
- After term changes to MEDDRA Version 1.5 are complete, a numeric code be applied to terms sequentially by alphabetical order as the last step in the development process for the IMT.
- Use 10000001 as the first code applied to the first term sorted alphabetically in order to enforce a length of 8.

User Guide to be developed.
Schedule for IMT Implementation:
- ICH approval - 3/97
- Wide Availability - 12/97

Relationships with Other Standards

Terms from other commonly used medical thesauri have also been added to the IMT to make the transition from these other vocabularies to the IMT easier. These include the Food and Drug Administration Coding Symbols for a Thesaurus of Adverse Reaction Terms (COSTART), the World Health Organizations Adverse Reaction Terminology (WHO-ART), the International Classification of Diseases, version 9, Clinical Modifications (ICD-9-CM), the Japanese Adverse Reaction Thesaurus (JART), and the Hoechst Adverse Reaction Terminology (HARTS).

There are some medical concepts that are not included in the IMT. The following areas are considered outside the scope of this regulatory terminology:
- Drug product terminology (i.e., complete listing of drug names);
- Equipment, device or diagnostic product terminology (i.e., complete listing of medical devices, diagnostic equipment or in vitro diagnostic products);
- Device failure terminology;
- Clinical trial study design terminology;
- Patient demographic terminology;
- Qualifiers that refer to populations rather than individual patient results (e.g., rare, frequent);
- Numerical values associated with investigations or observations (e.g., numeric laboratory test results)
- Descriptors of severity (e.g., severity, mild).

Identifiable Costs

Cost of licensure is yet undetermined but the goal is to make the internationally maintained terminology as inexpensive and readily available as possible. In all regions consideration must be given to the developing nations under WHO as well as the start up and specialty industries throughout the world.

Health Care Claim Adjustment Reason Code/Health Care Claim Status Code Committee

ANSI Accreditation:

Health Care Claim Adjustment Reason Codes and Health Care Claim Status Codes are considered external codes by ANSI ASC X12, and the Committee is not an SDO. The committee was formed in 1994 by industry representatives to X12, to create a mechanism for management of the codes used for the enumerated transactions.

Health Care Claim Adjustment Reason Codes

A series of standard alphanumeric codes, and messages, that detail the reason why the payer made and adjustment to the health care claim payment. These codes are used in the ANSI ASC X12 Claim (837) and Payment/Advice (835) transaction sets, and in the UB92 and NSF flat file claim and associated payment transactions.

Developing Organization

These codes are developed and maintained by the Health Care Claim Adjustment Reason Code/Claim Status Code Committee. This committee is comprised of one voting member from the following groups:
- American Dental Association
- American Hospital Association
- American Medical Association
- Blue Shield Plans
- Blue Cross Plans
- Commercial Health Insurance Carriers
- Health Care Financing Administration - Medicaid
- Health Care Financing Administration - Medicare
- Health Insurance Association of America
- National Council for Prescription Drug Programs
- Property and Casualty Insurance Industry
- American Association of Health Plans
- Association For Electronic Healthcare Transactions (AFHECT)
- One X12N workgroup co-chair from each affected workgroup (835, 837, 276/277)

The committee is responsible for maintaining the quality and business applicability of the code lists for an electronic data interchange environment. It's objective is to meet the business needs of the user community while eliminating redundancy in the codes. The Blue Cross and Blue Shield Association serves as Secretariat for the committee.

F

Contact for more information:

Frank Pokorny
Manager, Electronic Commerce and National Standards
Blue Cross and Blue Shield Association
676 North St. Clair
Chicago, IL 60611
Phone: 312-330-6223
Fax: 312-440-5674
E-mail: us993fjp@ibmmail.com

Description

A series of approximately 175 standard numeric and alphanumeric codes, and messages, that detail the reason why the payer made and adjustment to the health care claim payment. An individual code may be up to three characters long. A set of that apply equally to services, products, drugs and equipment. Codes for Medicare A have the letter "A" in the first position; Medicare B show the letter "B".

Readiness

Codes are currently in use and revisions are made thrice annually, effective on February 28, June 30 and October 31 of each year. The most recent version of the code list will be able to be applied to all versions of the ASC X12 Draft Standards, except as limited within the code lists.
Health Care Claim Adjustment Reason Codes and the Health Care Claim Status Codes are available in electronic and print formats:

Electronic file -
Washington Publishing Company World Wide Web Site
http://www.wpc-edi.com
Paper Copy -
Blue Cross and Blue Shield Association
Inter-Plan Teleprocessing Service
676 North St. Clair
Chicago, IL 60611

Indicator of Market Acceptance

Health Care Claim Adjustment Reason Code is currently in wide use within the health care community for both EDI and flat file transactions, and for both private/commercial and government programs. Codes are developed and agreed upon by committee action

Level of Specificity

A set of approximately 175 numeric and alphanumeric codes that apply equally to services, products, drugs and equipment. Codes for Medicare A have the letter "A" in the first position; Medicare B show the letter "B". Codes are available on lists in simple ascending order, and by functional groups: treatment; insurance procedural; insurance contractual; other.

Identifiable Costs

Code lists are available at no charge from either the Washington Publishing Web Site or the Blue Cross and Blue Shield Association.

Health Care Claim Status Codes

A series of standard alphanumeric codes, and messages, that detail the status of a claim that has been submitted for payment. These codes are used in the ANSI ASC X12 Claim Status Response (277) and Payment/Advice (835) transaction sets, and in the flat file transactions associated with the UB92 and NSF formats.

Description

A composite data element comprised of the following alphanumeric and numeric data elements:
- Health Care Claim Status Category Code -- Mandatory
- Health Care Claim Status Code -- Mandatory
- Entity Identifier Code -- Optional - Used when an entity is associated with the Health Care Claim Status Code

An individual code may be up to seven (7) characters long.

Readiness

Health Care Claim Adjustment Reason Code and Health Care Claim Status Codes are available in electronic and print formats:
Electronic file -
Washington Publishing Company World Wide Web Site
http://www.wpc-edi.com
Paper Copy -
Blue Cross and Blue Shield Association
Inter-Plan Teleprocessing Service
676 North St. Clair
Chicago, IL 60611

Indicator of Market Acceptance

Health Care Claim Status Code is currently in wide use within the health care community for both EDI and flat file transactions, and for both private/commercial and government programs. Codes are developed and agreed upon by committee action.

Level of Specificity

Health Care Claim Status Category Code is a 2 position alphanumeric field that is mandatory. These codes are divided into six broad categories:
1. supplemental messages

2. acknowledgments
3. pending
4. finalized
5. requests for additional information
6. general questions

Health Care Claim Status Code is a three position numeric code that is mandatory. There are approximately 450 codes currently available. Each code's description is understood to automatically refer to service, procedure, treatment, supply, test, visit and medication.

Entity Identifier Code is a two position alphanumeric field that is optional - Used when an entity is associated with the Health Care Claim Status Code

An individual code may be up to seven (7) characters long.

Identifiable Costs

Code lists are available at no charge from either the Washington Publishing Web Site or the Blue Cross and Blue Shield Association.

Logical Observation Identifier Names and Codes (LOINC) Consortium

Logical Observation Identifier Names and Codes (LOINC)

Developing Organization

LOINC is a consortium of laboratories, system vendors, hospitals, and academic institutions organized by the Regenstrief Institute and supported by grants from the John A. Hartford Foundation of New York, the Agency for Health Care Policy and Research, and the National Library of Medicine.

ANSI Accreditation:

LOINC is a consortium, not a formal SDO. However, it is designed to work in conjunction with the HL7/ASTM and CEN observation (result) messages.

Name

Logical Observation Identifiers Names and Codes (LOINC).

Contact For More Information:

Stan Huff <coshuff@ihc.com>
36 South State St, Suite 800
Salt Lake City, UT 84111
Phone: 801 442 4885
Fax: 801 263 3657

Clem McDonald <clem@regen.rg.iupui.edu>
Regenstrief Institute

Indiana University School of Medicine
1001 W. 10th St. 5th fl RHC
Indianapolis, IN 46202
Phone: 317 630 7070
Fax: 317 630 6962

To obtain the Users' Guide, and full LOINC database in report, ASCII text, or dBase formats:
http://www.mcis.duke.edu/standards/termcode/loinc.htm

DESCRIPTION

(1) Laboratory LOINC
LOINC concentrates on the identification and naming of test and clinical observations, things like diastolic blood pressure, serum glucose, blood culture, or "heart physical exam." LOINC does not deal formally with the values reported for these observations/measurements, some of which are valued as numbers, and some of which are valued as codes or text. Most of these coded answers are expected to be provided from other sources, such as SnoMed, CPT4, ICD9CM, and other code systems.
The laboratory component of the data base is fairly complete with respect to the tests listed in Table 1.

Table 1 Subject matter covered by Lab LOINC

Chemistry
Coagulation
Hematology
Microbiology including cultures, microscopic examinations, RNA and DNA probes,
Antibody and antigen measures
Antimicrobial susceptibility testing
Toxicology and drug testing
Surgical pathology
Blood banking
Blood counts and Urinalysis
Fertility

Each record in the LOINC data base identifies one distinct observation. Each record contains the LOINC identifier, which is a meaningless number with a self check digit, and a multi-part formal name which includes component (e.g., glucose, intra-arterial diastolic), type of property (e.g., mass concentration, pressure), timing (e.g., point measure 24 hour), system (e.g., serum, brachial artery), scale (e.g., quantitative, qualitative), and method (e.g., dip stick, ausculatory).

In addition, the data base contains related names (near synonyms), molecular weights, indicators of terms that have been retired, a pointer to the terms that replace them, and related codes from other systems, e.g., the chemical abstract code for chemical substances.

With the data base comes a manual that provides formal rules for naming the parts of an observation, and a full definition of the data base.

LOINC does not yet include names for order sets, e.g., CHEM12.

F

Figure 1 Example Laboratory LOINC codes

1919-0 ASPARTATE AMINOTRANSFERASE:CCNC:PT:FLU:QN
3255-7 FIBRINOGEN:MCNC:PT:PPP:QN:COAG
4531-0 COMPLEMENT TOTAL HEMOLYTIC:PT:BLD:QN
9782-4 ADENOVIRUS SP IDENTIFIED:PRID:PT:XXX:QL:ORGANISM SPECIFIC CULTURE
4991-6 BORRELIA BURGDORFERI DNA:ACNC:PT:XXX:SQ:AMP/PROBE
6324-8 BRUCELLA ABORTUS AB:TITR:PT:SER:QN:AGGL
6337-0 CANDIDA ALBICANS AG:ACNC:PT:SER:SQ:ID
9822-8 MICROORGANISM IDENTIFIED PRID:PT:DIAF:QL:STERILE BODY FLUID CULTURE
6981-5 AZITHROMYCIN:SUSC:PT:ISLT:SQN:GRADIENT STRIP
5573-1 ALUMINUM:MFR:PT:HAR:QN
6473-3 MICROSCOPIC OBSERVATION:PRID:PT:TISS:QL:TRICHROME STAIN

The same general approach has been applied to common clinical measures as to laboratory observations. The same six major parts of the name, some with subparts, are used.

Table 2 Subjects covered in clinical LOINC

Blood pressure (systolic, diastolic, and mean)
Heart rate (and character of the pulse wave)
Respiratory rate
Critical care measures
(Cardiac output, resistance, stroke work, ejection fraction, etc.)
Body Weight (and measures used to estimate ideal body weight)
Body Height
Body temperature
Circumference of chest, thighs, legs, etc.
Intake and output
Major headings of history and physical
Major headings of discharge summary
Major headings of an operative note
Electrocardiographic measures

Clinical LOINC code numbers are taken from the same sequence of numbers as the Lab LOINC codes.

For many clinical measures, measurements are distinguished for estimated, reported, and measured values. (E.g., a patient's report of his or her body weight is a different variable from a measured result or the physician's estimate.) Also varying degrees of pre-coordination are provided for the observation, the body site at which it was obtained, and the method. E.g., a cardiac output based on the Fick method is distinguished from a cardiac output based on a 2D cardiac echo.

Physiologic measures are often monitored continuously over time, and the instrument reports summary "statistics" over that reporting period. The summary statistics can include minimum, maximum, and mean over a time period for vital signs measurements and fluid intake and output. When we address measures taken over time, we usually include 1 hour, 8 hour, 10 hour, 12 hour, and 24 hour summaries. The middle three durations are included to cover the varying durations of work shifts within and across institutions.

The parts of clinical measurement names are the same as for laboratory measures. The fourth part, the system, usually identifies an organ system or a particular part of the anatomy. For a measure of systolic left ventricular pressure, the system would be "Cardiac ventricle.left." In contrast to laboratory tests, where the component is usually some chemical entity, the clinical measurement component usually identifies the specific aspect of a property that is measured. For example, the property type might be pressure. Then the component would identify the pressure measured as intravascular diastolic. In general the component is used to distinguish the various points or ranges, or inflections of a physiologic tracing, and to define precisely which of a number of possible dimensions of length or area are being measured in imaging.

Laboratory measures tend to be more regular than clinical measures. The system is usually a specimen and the component a chemical or molecular moiety. For most clinical measurements, the component is also an attribute of a patient or an organ system within a patient. However, attributes of non-patient entities are often of interest in the case of clinical measurements. For example, we might want to know the class of instrument used to obtain the measurement.

Figure 2 Example Clinical LOINC terms

8285-5 CIRCUMFERENCE.OCCIPITAL-FRONTAL:LEN:PT:HEAD:QN:TAPE MEASURE
8496-2 INTRAVASCULAR DIASTOLIC:PRES:PT:BRACHIAL ARTERY:QN
9940-8 Q WAVE DURATION:TIME:PT:LEAD V1:QN:EKG
8660-3 HISTORY OF SYMPTOMS & DISEASES:FIND:PT:CARDIOVASCULAR
SYSTEM:QL:REPORTED
8651-2 HOSPITAL DISCHARGE DX:IMP:PT:^PATIENT:QL
9129-8 FLUID OUTPUT.CHEST TUBE:VOL:PT:PLEURAL SPACE:QN

Readiness

The LOINC database of over 10,000 observations/measurement/test result codes is available for free use on the Internet.
There is only one official version of the LOINC standard. Codes are never re-used when the meaning of a term changes. Updates and additions are made at two to three month intervals.

Indicators of Market Acceptance

The laboratory component of LOINC was installed on the Internet in April of 1995, and has been greeted enthusiastically since. It has been endorsed by the American Clinical Laboratory Association (ACLA) and recommended for adoption by its members. The ACLA is the association of large referral laboratories, and its members are responsible for more than 60% of US outpatient laboratory volume. Corning MetPath and LabCorp, two of the largest commercial laboratories, have adopted LOINC as their code system for reportable test results, as has LifeChem and Associated Regional and University Pathologists (ARUP). In addition, Indiana University labs, University of Colorado, Intermountain Health Care, University of Missouri, and Barnes/Jewish Hospital are in the process of converting their reporting to LOINC codes. The province of Ontario, Canada has made a tentative commitment to the LOINC codes for a province-wide coding standard.

The LOINC codes have been used as the basis for HCFA's ICD10-PCS laboratory codes. They have been incorporated in HCFA's quality assurance testing pilot software, and they have been adopted by the Centers for Disease Control and Prevention/State and Territorial Epidemiologist project for transmitting communicable diseases reports electronically.

F

Level of Specificity

The identifiers are specific in up to eight dimensions. The goal is to match the level of specificity provided by the master files of the systems that report these kinds of results. Laboratory test results are distinguished (and specific) to the analyte (e.g., glucose), the type of property (e.g., mass concentration), the timing aspects (e.g., 24 hour specimen), the specimen, (e.g., urine), and the method - as needed. In the case of serology tests, which tend to include method information in their name, LOINC includes the methods. In the case of chemistry tests, that tend not to include method information in their name, the LOINC codes tend not to be specific about method. The data base now includes over 10,000 laboratory and clinical observations.

Identifiable Costs

The LOINC data base and Users' Guide is available for free use for any purpose by users and vendors from the Internet Web site listed above. It is copywritten in order to prevent the development of multiple variants.

Georgetown University Home Care Project

Home Health Care Classification (HHCC) System

Home Health Care Classification (HHCC) System is a system designed to assess and document home health and ambulatory care using its standardized HHCC nomenclature. Its documentation method tracks home health and ambulatory care. It is based on a conceptual framework using the nursing process to access a patient holistically. HHCC nomenclature consists of six data dictionaries:
- 20 home health care components to assess and classify care;
- 145 nursing diagnoses (50 major categories & 95 subcategories);
- 3 expected outcome goals that modify nursing nursing diagnoses;
- 160 nursing interventions (60 major & 100 subcategories);
- 4 nursing action types that modify nursing interventions and converts the dictionary to 640 unique nursing interventions;
- 3 actual outcomes that evaluate the care process.

A patient/client is also assessed using 20 medical diagnoses and/or surgical procedure categories, and 10 socio-demographic data elements.

HHCC System can be used to identify: (a) care needs in terms of care components and their respective nursing diagnoses and interventions; and (b) resource use in terms of nursing and other health providers (physical, occupational, and speech therapy, medical social worker, and home health aide). The medical assessment categories and socio-demographic data elements are descriptive variables that can be correlated with clinical care data.

HHCC is also designed to record the clinical care pathways for an entire episode of care. The care events can be used to determine care costs, and can provide a payment method for managed care services. HHCC System runs on microcomputer using a portable notebook to facilitate ease of use for data collection and then downloaded to a computer-based workstation for processing.
References are available upon request.

Purpose: The Home Health Care Classification (HHCC) - Nursing Diagnoses and Nursing Interventions was developed by Saba as part of the Georgetown University Home Car Project. It was developed to classify, code for computer processing and analyze study data. The HHCC is being used to document and describe home health nursing care, as well as determine cost and measure outcomes.

Structure: The Home Health Care Classification (HHCC) - Nursing Diagnoses and Nursing Interventions are classified according to 20 Home Health Care Components:

1. Activity 11. Physical Regulation
2. Bowel Elimination 12. Respiratory
3. Cardiac 13. Role Relationship
4. Cognitive 14. Safety
5. Coping 15. Self-Care
6. Fluid Volume 16. Self-Concept
7. Health Behavior 17. Sensory
8. Medication 18. Skin Integrity
9. Metabolic 19. Tissue Perfusion
10. Nutritional 20. Urinary Elimination

HHCC of Nursing Diagnoses: The scheme consist of 145 nursing diagnoses (50 two digit major categories and 95 three-digit subcategories). Each nursing diagnosis has a modifier to code three possible expected outcomes: **1=improved, 2=stabilized, or 3=deteriorated.**

HHCC of Nursing Interventions: It consists of 160 unique nursing interventions (60 two digit major categories and 95 three-digit subcategories). Each nursing intervention has a modifier to code four types of nursing action: **1=access, 2-direct care, 3=teach, and/or 4=manage**. The type of action modifier adds the implementation facet to the HHCC of Nursing Intervention Taxonomy expanding it to **640 possible nursing intervention codes.**

The HHCC is structured according to the Tenth Revision of the International Classification of Diseases (ICD-10). Each classification label consists of a five character alphanumeric code. The HHCC Care Component is alphabetic and the first character, the Nursing Diagnosis or Nursing Intervention is represented by a second and third digit for major categories, and in some instances a fourth numeric digit for minor subcategories, and the fifth digit is used to represent a modifier for each scheme.

Availability:
Virginia K. Saba, EdD, RN, FAAN
Georgetown University
School of Nursing
3700 Reservoir Road, NW
Washington, DC 20007
Tel: (202) 687-46479

F

Perspective on Code Sets within Transaction Standards

This perspective was presented to the ANSI HISB on December 13, 1996 by Christopher Chute, M.D., co-chairman of the Codes and Vocabulary Sub-committee of the ANSI HISB TCC.

Analysis of Code Sets within Transaction Standards

Data Standards Roster
Code Sets within Transaction Standards

The Codes and Vocabulary Sub-committee reports the obvious finding that existing Transactions Standards have embedded within their specification scores of implicit and explicit value tables for data elements. Common examples include values for demographic variables such as race, gender, or marital status. More clinically pertinent codes include Admission Type and Condition Codes. Some standards contain large numbers of specified codes, for example the ANSI X12 837 Health Care Claim template includes or references 441 discreet code tables within that single standard.

Two problems present themselves: 1) Cross mapping named fields or elements among transaction standards; and 2) for each cross mapped element, resolving the code set values among embedded codes sets across transaction standards. The Table below simplistically illustrates a result of this process for one of the 441 code tables in X12N 837 - Admission Type.

Admission Type

UB-92	X12N	HL/7	Values
		A	Accident
1	=UB92	E	Emergency
		L	Labor and Delivery
		R	Routine
2	=UB92		Urgent
3	=UB92		Elective

Table: Code values for fields "Admission Type"

This subcommittee recommends that HHS assume or commission a detailed evaluation of the complex problem of embedded code sets among transactions standards. For the major transaction standards and their clinical systems sources (e.g. X12N, UB-92, NSF, HL/7, and ASTM E-1384) we suggest:

1. Embedded Code Sets be identified and characterized.
2. Code sets should be clustered across standards for similarity on the basis of element name, table content, or semantic function.
3. For each cluster of similar code sets, the values should be tabulated in a way to clearly represent overlap, discord, and union. The Table layout above might provide a practical format.
4. An analysis of content conflict on the basis of these similarity tables should be presented.
5. Recommended resolutions of code table conflicts should be proposed.

The resultant report would be an enormously valuable resource for Standards Developer Organizations and the overall ANSI HISB to review and collaboratively revise. DHHS might then act upon the revised recommendations from the Standards community to adopt common code table standards across transaction records and their clinical source systems.

F

Unique Identifiers (including allowed uses)

Purpose & Scope

The purpose of the Unique Health Identifiers is to uniquely identify Individuals, Employers, Health Plans and Health Care Providers within the health care system.

1. Individuals

Current practice consists of Medical Record Numbers issued and maintained by individual provider organizations which is also known as Master Patient Index (MPI). HIS vendors have begun to develop software to facilitate cross reference to MPIs across an enterprise often known as Corporate MPI.

1.1. Unique Identifier Standards for Individuals:

1.1.1. UHID by ASTM

ASTM is the only Standards Development Organization that has developed and published standards in this area. Other options listed below are candidate identifiers frequently discussed by industry experts.

1.2. Other Unique Identifier Options for Individuals:

1.2.1. Social Security Number (SSN)

1.2.2. Biometrics IDs

1.2.3. Directory Service

1.2.4. Personal Immutable Properties

1.2.5. Patient Identification System based on existing Medical Record Number and Practitioner Prefix

1.2.6. Public Key - Private Key Cryptography Method

2. Employers, Health Plans and Health Care Providers

None of the Standards Developing Organizations have developed standards in the area of identifying employers, health plans and health care providers. However, HCFA and several other organizations have developed identifiers in this area with input from Federal and state agencies that administer health programs and other stake holders of the industry including standards developing organizations (SDOs).

Employers:

2.1 Unique Identifier Standards for Employers:
    None Exists
2.2 Unique Identifier Options for Employers:
2.1.1. PAYERID

Health Plans:

3.1 Unique Identifier Standards for Health Plans:
    None Exists
3.2 Unique Identifier Options for Health Plans:
3.2.1. PAYERID

Health Care Providers:

4.1. Unique Identifier Standards for Health Care Providers:
    None Exists

4.2. Unique Identifier Options for Health Care Providers:

4.2.1. National Provider Identifier

4.2.2. Unique Physician Identifiers (UPIN)

4.2.3. NABP Pharmacy Number (NABP#)

4.2.4. Health Industry Number (HIN)

1. Individuals

1.1. Unique Identifier Standards for Individuals:

1.1.1. UHID by ASTM

- Category/Classification of Standard:

  Unique Identifiers (including allowed uses) for Individuals

- Standard Development Organization (SDO):

  ASTM

- ANSI Accreditation, ANSI Accreditation applied for or not:
  ANSI Accredited

- Name of the Standard:

  Standard Guide for Properties of a Universal Health Identifier (UHID) "E1734"

- Contact for more information:

  Name: Terry Luthy
  Address: ASTM 100 Barr Harbor Drive
  West Conshohocken, PA 19428
  E-mail: tluthy@local.astm.org
  Phone: 610-832-9737
  Fax: 610-832-9666

- Description of Standard:

  The UHID Scheme consists of a sequential identifier, a delimiter, check digits and an encryption scheme to support data security. This Standards Guide covers a set of requirements outlining the properties of a national system of Universal Health Identifier (limited to the population of United States). It includes positive identification of patients, automated linkage of various computer-based records, mechanism to support data security of privileged clinical information and the use of technology to keep health care operating cost at a minimum.

- Readiness of Standard:

  The Guide provides a detailed implementation sample for the UHID and evaluates the implementation against the criteria outlined by the standards. The method is being implemented by two (2) VA hospitals in Florida.

F

- Indicators of Market Acceptance:

  ASTM E1714 is an approved American National Standard. Regarded as an ideal standards guide for the Unique Patient Identifier. The VA hospital network (VISN) is planning to expand the implementation of ASTM Standards based identifier. More than 350 copies of the standards have been distributed.

- Level of Specificity:

  The UHID Scheme consists of a sequential identifier, a delimiter, check digits and an encryption scheme to support data security. It supports multiple encrypted IDs for an individual.

- Relationship with Other Standards:

  N/A

- Identifiable Costs:

  ASTM Standards volume 14.01 for Health care informatics that include this Standards Guide can be purchased for a nominal fee.

1.2. Other Unique Identifier Options for Individuals:

1.2.1. Social Security Number (SSN)

- Description of Standard:

  The original scope of SSN was to function as a Social Security Account Number (SSAN). Its scope since the 1935 legislation has been expanded. It is now in use as a personal identifier in a wide area of applications including use by local, state and federal authorities, financial institutions, and numerous consumer organizations.

- Readiness of Standard:

  Strength: The existing SSA structures, trained personnel, detailed standard procedural guidelines, cost economies, rapid implementation etc. are all in favor of the use of SSN as a valid patient identifier.
  Weakness: Many organizations including those who support the use of SSN as a Health Identifier have identified several serious defects that must be fixed before it can be used as a valid Unique Health Identifier. Examples are:
    1. Not unique
    2. No exit control
    3. Lack of check-digits
    4. Significant error level
    5. Privacy & confidentiality risks
    6. Lack of legal protection
    7. Lack of capacity for future growth
    8. Lack of mechanism for emergency use and timely issue.
    9. Provision for non citizens, etc.

The Computer-based Record Institute (CPRI) supports a modified SSN with important changes to the process of issue of SSN including check-digits, encryption scheme, a trusted authority, and legislative measures, etc.

- Contact for more information:
Social Security Administration
6401 Security Blvd, Baltimore, MD 21235

- Indicators of Market Acceptance:
Used by VA hospitals and Medicare Administration as a patient identifier. Used by many health care organizations as part of the patient demographic information.

- Identifiable costs:
Expenditure borne by the Government.

1.2.2. Biometrics IDs

- Description of Standard:

    Several sophisticated methods of biometrics identification methods have been proposed, including finger print, retinal pattern analysis, voice pattern identification and DNA analysis.

- Readiness of Standard:
Law enforcement and Immigration departments use some of the biometrics identification methods. However, the necessary standards, procedures, and guidelines are non-existent for use in health care. Some of the concerns relating to this option are organ transplant, amputation and diseases affecting organs e.g. retinopathy.

- Contact for more information:
N/A

- Indicators of Market Acceptance:
N/A

- Identifiable costs:
Considered very expensive. Specific details not available.

1.2.3. Directory Service

- Description of Standard:
This method is proposed by Dr. William L. McMullen of Mitre Corporation. It will use existing patient identifiers to provide linkages to records of individuals across systems. The system includes social characteristics (name, SSN, address, driver license etc.) human characteristics (finger print, retina scan etc.) and other groupings such as sex, race, DOB, etc. The directory service would reconcile interactively and heuristically the proper association of the patient identification data at the current point of care with any one of the other prior points of care. This step would be supported by automated capabilities that would facilitate locating the other patient records for which a record linkage is valid. The current point of care location would then be linked with any of the other selected point of care locations by electronically exchanging their network addresses.

- Readiness of Standard:
N/A

F

- Contact for more information:
  The Mitre Corporation
  7525 Colshire Drive
  McLean, VA 22102-3481

- Indicators of Market Acceptance:
  N/A

- Identifiable costs:
  Considered expensive. Specific details not available.

1.2.4. Personal Immutable Properties

- Description of Standard:
  Dr. Paul Carpenter and Dr. Chris Chute of Mayo Clinic have proposed a model Unique Patient Identifier (UPI) which consists of a series of three universal immutable values plus a check digit. The three values are a seven-digit date of birth field, a six-digit place of birth code, a five-digit sequence code (to identify the individual born on the same date in the same geographic area) and 4) a single-check digit. For emergency situations the use of temporary UPI with the prefix "T" is recommended.

- Readiness of Standard:
  N/A

- Contact for more information:
  Dr. Paul Carpenter or Dr. Chris Chute
  Mayo Clinic
  Rochester, MN 55905

- Indicators of Market Acceptance
  N/A

- Identifiable costs:
  N/A

1.2.5. Patient Identification System Based on Existing Medical Record Number and Practitioner Prefix:

- Description of Standard:
  Medical Records Institute proposes the use of existing provider institution generate medical record number with a provider number prefix. The solution requires consensus on a practitioner identification system but eliminates the cost of creating, implementing and maintaining nationwide (patient) numbering system. The unique practitioner ID would identify the location of the patient database, and the medical record number would identify the patient's record within that database. The solution also includes the patient designation of a practitioner of choice to be the curator who functions as the gateway for the linking and updating of information.

- Readiness of Standard:
  N/A

- Contact for more information:
  Medical Records Institute
  567 Walnut Street, P.O. Box 600770
  Newton, MA 02160

- Indicators of Market Acceptance:
  N/A

- Identifiable costs:
  N/A

1.2.6. Public Key - Private Key Cryptography Method

- Cryptography-based health care identifiers:
  Dr. Peter Szolovits, Massachusetts Institute of Technology proposes a Health care Identifier System based on public-key cryptography method. Anyone who wants to use this method needs to acquire two keys that allow arbitrary messages to be encoded and decoded. These two keys contain mathematical functions that are inverses of each other. The method consists of a patient private-key and a organizational (provider) public-key together generating and maintaining IDs that are both organization specific as well as unique to individual patients within that organization. The ID can be revealed to other institutions or practitioners only with the private-key of the patient. Both centralized and decentralized controls are possible. Under the decentralized scheme the patient has the ultimate control over the degree to which the lifetime collection of medical information is made available to others. Under the centralized scheme an umbrella organization (trusted authority) handles all patient private-keys via an ID Server, and the patient will have the public-key.

  At the request of authorized institutions the ID Server will generate Patient ID with the use of both the patient's private-key and public-key. Under both schemes, the use of smart card and computer are required.

- Readiness of Standard:
  N/A

- Contact for more information:
  Dr. Peter Szolovits
  Massachusetts Institute of Technology
  Laboratory for Computer Science
  545 Technology Square
  Cambridge MA 02139

- Indicators of Market Acceptance:
  N/A

- Identifiable costs:
  N/A

F

2. Employers

2.1 Unique Identifier Standards for Employers:
  None Exists

2.2 Unique Identifier Options for Employers:

2.1.1. PAYERID

- Description of Standard:
  The PAYERID has a nine numeric digit identifier which includes a 6-digit base number, a 2-digit suffix and a check digit. For those plans and employers requiring many different numbers the ID is issued as a 6-digit base number, a 2-digit suffix and a check digit. For those not requiring different numbers, it is issued in the form of one or more 8-digit numbers with a check-digit. The PAYERID was planned a national identification system to facilitate health care claims. In view of the HIPAA 1996 Legislation, HCFA will be proposing PAYERID as the standard health identifier for both health plans and employers.

- Readiness of Standard:
  HCFA's Schedule for implementing PAYERID is listed below.
  - Notice of Proposed Rule Making (NPRM) February '97
  - Voluntary use of PAYERID for Medicare Claims April '97
  - Publish Final Regulation July '97
  - Require for Medicare January '98
  - Require for Industry July '99
  -

- Contact for more information:
  Robert Moore
  HCFA
  7500 Security Blvd.
  Baltimore, MD 21244

- Indicators of Market Acceptance:
  N/A

- Identifiable costs:
  N/A

3. Health Plans

3.1 Unique Identifier Standards for Health Plans:
  None Exists

3.2 Unique Identifier Options for Health Plans:

3.2.1. PAYERID
Same as 2.2.1 above.

4. Health Care Providers

4.1. Unique Identifier Standards for Health Care Providers:
   None Exists

4.2. Unique Identifier Options for Health Care Providers:

4.2.1. National Provider Identifier (NPI)

- Description of Standard:
  The NPI is an eight-position alphanumeric identifier. The eighth position is an International Standards Organization-approved check digit, which will allow a calculation to detect keying or transmission errors. The National Provider System will assign the NPI and will also assign two-position alphanumeric location identifiers to indicate practice locations of the provider. Neither the NPI nor the location identifiers will have embedded intelligence. That is, information about the provider, such as the type of provider or state where the provider is located, will not be conveyed by the NPI. This information will be recorded in the system, but will not be part of the identifier. Individual and group providers will receive location identifiers for their office practice locations. Individuals and groups will not receive location identifiers for the hospitals or other organization providers where they practice, since these organization providers will receive their own NPIs. The NPIs of individual providers who are members of a group will be linked to the NPI of the group. The relationships defined among organization providers differ, depending upon the specific business rules of different health programs. The National Provider System will enumerate organization providers at the elemental level, so that different health programs can link these providers according to their program-specific business rules. Each organization provider in a separate location will receive a separate NPI. Each member of an organization chain and each part of an organization provider that needs to be identified will receive a separate NPI. The National Provider System will have a query facility that will link organization providers that have a common Employer Identification Number. Organization providers will have only one active location identifier.

- Readiness of Standard:
  HCFA's schedule for implementation of NPI is listed below.
  - Notice of Proposed Rule Making Published in
  - Federal Register 02/21/97
  - Final Regulation Published in Federal Register 07/02/97
  - NPIs Issued to Medicare Providers No Later Than 08/01/97
  - Required Use of NPI for Medicare claims 12/01/97

- Contact for more information:
  Robert Moore
  HCFA
  7500, Security Blvd.
  Baltimore, MD 21244

- Indicators of Market Acceptance:
  N/A

- Identifiable costs:
  None

F

4.2.2. Unique Physician Identifier Number (UPIN)

- **Description of Standard**
  HCFA created UPIN as required by COBRA to identify physicians who provide services for which payment is made under Medicare. UPIN is a six-place alphanumeric identifier. The UPIN Registry is the carrier that maintains the UPIN. A total of 704,926 UPINs have been assigned to 2,088,309 physicians.

- **Readiness of Standard**
  UPIN addresses only a small segment of the provider community i.e. physicians with dedicare practice. HCFA's current proposal of National Provider File/NPI replaces UPIN with NPI.

- **Contact For More Information**
  Robert Moore
  HCFA
  7500, Security Blvd.
  Baltimore, MD 21244

- **Indicators of Market Acceptance**
  N/A

- **Identifiable costs**
  None

4.2.3. National Association of Boards of Pharmacy Number (NABP Number)

- **Description of Standard**
  Each licensed pharmacy in the United States is assigned a unique seven-digit number by the National Council for Prescription Drug Programs (NCPDP), in cooperation with the National Association of Boards of Pharmacy. The purpose of this system is to enable a pharmacy to identify itself to all third-party processors by one standard number. The first two digits of the NABP Number denotes state designation. The second group four digits identify the pharmacy and assigned sequentially from 0001 up. The last digit is a check-digit.

- **Readiness of Standard**
  NABP Number is currently in use by pharmacies in United States.

- **Contact for more information**
  Noe Gomez
  NCPDP/NABP
  4201 North 24th Street, Suite 365
  Phoenix, AZ 85016

- **Indicators of Market Acceptance**
  NABP Number is currently in use by pharmacies in United States.

- **Identifiable Costs**
  None

4.2.4. Health Industry Number (HIN)

- Description of Standard
  HIN is used as an identifier for contract administration in the health industry supply chain, as a prescriber identifier for claims processing and for market analysis applications. It enumerates prescriber by location, provider establishments and other entities in the health industry supply chain. The Identifier includes a "base HIN" consisting of seven (7) character identifier and a two (2) character suffix to identify the location of the prescriber.

- Readiness of Standard
  HIN has been in use since 1987 in the health industry supply chain and in state-administered claims processing.

- Contact for more information
  Robert A. Hankin, Phd, President,
  HIBCC
  5110 North 40th Street, Suite 250
  Phoenix, AZ 85018

- Indicators of Market Acceptance
  According to HIBCC, HIN is endorsed or being implemented by the following:
  - American Hospital Association (AHA)
  - American Medical Association (AMA)
  - American Nurses Association (ANA
  - American Society for Automation in Pharmacy (ASAP)
  - American Veterinary Distributors Association (AVDA)
  - Animal Health Institute (AHI)
  - Centers for Disease Control & Prevention (CDC)
  - Health Industry Distributors Association (HIDA)
  - Health Industry Group Purchasing Association (HIGPA)
  - Health Industry Manufacturers Association (HIMA)
  - Healthcare Information and Management Systems Society (HIMSS)
  - National Wholesale Druggists' Association (NWDA)
  - Pharmaceutical Research and Manufacturers Association (PhRMA)
  - State of Tennessee, TennCare Program
  - US Department of Defense (DoD), Defense Personnel Support Center (DPSC)
  -

- Identifiable Costs
  There is no cost to entities enumerated on the database.

Security, Safeguards and Electronic Signatures

Overview of Health Care Security and Confidentiality Standards Development Efforts and Status - January 1997

Standards Development Organizations (SDOs) and governmental entities in the United States, Europe, Japan, Singapore, Australia, and New Zealand are currently developing standards to insure the security, confidentiality, and privacy of health care data as it resides in systems or as it is being passed in message transactions between systems. The focus of these groups is to develop security policies and procedures related to threats to system security and also to define security services. Threats to system security include disclosure, deception, disruption, and usurpation. Security services

F

include authentication, confidentiality, integrity, availability, authenticity, authorization, non-repudiation, security administration, audit and digital signatures.

Health care specific security efforts have primarily focused on the utilization of security technologies from the general computer industry, adopting existing technologies, and providing further definition and clarification only in regard to specific domains and attributes that are unique to health care. In analyzing threat, security services, and confidentiality in the health care environment, there are only five key areas where health care security differs somewhat in analysis, definition, or requirements outside of existing non-health care specific security technologies:

1. Health care documents can have multiple signatures and have specific signature rules defined by user role;
2. Health care is a domain where a common framework for interoperability requires a greater degree of uniformity over access control (confidentiality) than most other domains;
3. Auditing in health care serves a legal as well as a security function.
4. Threats to privacy and confidentiality in health care are primarily from inside the domain ("insider threat" is greater than 75 to 80% of risk in health care), rather than from outside the domain.
5. Security, privacy and confidentiality of existing records (essentially paper records) is provided by a generally uniform, across state, and informal set of ethics of professional practice among the associated health care professions.

In addressing these health care specific "exceptions" the following steps are underway, or require action:

a) In setting standards for digital signatures in the health care domain additional signature attributes to support multiple signatures and signature rules are being defined;

b) Comprehensive adoption of security standards in health care, not piecemeal implementation, is advocated to provide security to data that is excahnged between health care entities;

c) Audit and audit trail data (so called, "derivative data" from direct data access, and system use) needs to be considered in the legal establishment of privacy and access rights under privacy legislation;

d) Again, in addressing threat, as under (b) above, a comprehensive implementation of security standards across a domain or system is important, as a piecemeal approach, such as the implementation of point-to-point security alone (message-based security), will not provide privacy and confidentiality protection from insider threat within a domain;

e) Confidentiality policy, as well as access control and authorization policies are an essential part of secure systems. Their establishment is being addressed within the framework of security standards efforts through the direct participation of health care specialty representatives composed of clinical health care professional organizations and societies, medical records professionals, health care transcription professionals, regulatory organizations, government agencies, the JCAHO and NCQA, insurance providers and health plans, and health care information system vendors and consultants.

Even taking into account the above issues, health care security standards efforts are perhaps best analyzed and reviewed in relation to a general system security framework, not essentially oriented to health care, as follows:

a) Identification and Authentication
b) Authorization and Access Control (Confidentiality)
c) Accountability (Non-Repudiation and Auditing)
d) Integrity and Availability
e) Security of Communication
f) Security Administration

By definition, if a system, or communications between two systems (such as health care transactions), where implemented with technology(s) meeting standards in each of the categories of this framework, that system would be essentially secure. This is an important distinction in that no single SDO is addressing all aspects of health care information security and confidentiality, and specifically, no single SDO is developing standards that cover every category of this framework. Cooperation between SDOs developing health care security standards, coordinated in the US through ANSI HISB, and between ANSI HISB and CEN TC251 regarding European standards efforts, is very active at this time, in an attempt to end up with a comprehensive standards framework to match the security framework outlined above. Please note that there is security standards work underway in each category of the framework above that should be completed by the middle to end of 1997, providing, when taken together, a complete set of standards for security in the health care domain.

The most comprehensive health care security standards development is currently being carried out by CEN TC251 in Europe and by the ASTM E31 in the United States. The American Standards Committee (ASC X12), Health Level 7 (HL7), and ACR NEMA / DICOM are currently involved in the development of standards for secure transmission of data and transactions. Health care organizations that are not accredited SDOs, such as the Computer-based Patient Record Institute (CPRI) and CORBAmed are active in assisting and promoting the standards development process through their participation in ANSI HISB and through the development of policy within documents (CPRI) and standards certification by (CORBAmed).

What follows is an overview of work being done by SDOs and other entities in the United States and Europe (in alphabetic order, by organization):

ACR NEMA / DICOM

The DICOM Committee (formerly known as the ACR/NEMA committee) has created a Working Group on Security that is considering additions to the DICOM standard to support the secure exchange of medical images and related information between two entities communicating over a public network (e.g. the Internet). The Working Group was asked to provide short term solutions using existing technology while developing long term strategies for utilizing DICOM within a secure environment based on anticipated clinical and regulatory needs. The Working Group has been coordinating its work with work being done by a similar Ad Hoc committee set up by CEN TC 251 WG 4 in Europe, as well as with work being done by groups affiliated with JIRA and MEDIS-DC in Japan who are developing demonstrations of secure image data transmissions to meet the needs of the Japanese health care institutions. The DICOM, European, and Japanese groups held a series of meetings and teleconferences in the later half of 1996 where a joint work plan was formulated and common goals set.

The CEN TC 251 WG 4 Ad Hoc on Security, in cooperation with the DICOM Working Group on Security and the Japanese groups, is developing usage scenarios which will direct long term planning towards comprehensive security within the health care field, and in particular within medical imaging. Realizing that a comprehensive secure environment may be many years away, the DICOM Working Group decided to pursue a short term goal of providing limited security using existing technology. It is hoped to incorporate such solutions in technology demonstrations being planned by the Japanese through MEDIS-DC and JIRA. The short term goal of the DICOM Working Group on Security is to draft extensions to DICOM which embed digital signatures in DICOM data objects for data source authentication and as data integrity checks. In addition, the extensions would provide an option to layer DICOM message exchange services on top of a secure transport protocol such as SSL 3.0 in order to provide confidentiality during data transfers, to authenticate the parties involved in the information exchange, and to further insure integrity during transmission. When practical, these

F

extensions to DICOM would use existing technology in order to expedite implementation. The Ad Hoc Committee hopes to finalize a draft of these extensions in 1997.

ACR NEMA / DICOM contact:
Lawrence Tarbox, Ph.D.
Imaging Department
Siemens Corporate Research
755 College Rd. East
Princeton, NJ 08540
ltarbox@scr.siemens.com
(609) 734-3396 [voice]
(609) 734-6565 [fax]

Accredited Standards Committee (ASC) X12

The American Standards Committee X12, Electronic Data Interchange (EDI)/EDIFACT, has a number of security standards under development that are primarily targeted at messaging. X12's work in message security takes a non-health care-specific approach and is managed by X12 Subcommittee C (X12C) the data security task group of X12 that is co-chaired by Don Petry, and which coordinates efforts with the UN/EDIFACT Security Joint Working Group, chaired by Terry Dosdale of the United Kingdom.

Current X12C efforts include:

X12.42, Cryptographic Service Message (815) (usually referred to as the 815). The 815, which has been published and has a Reference Model in development, is used to provide the data format required for cryptographic key management in support of authentication and encryption. 815 includes the automated distribution and exchange of keys.

X12.376 Secure Authentication & Acknowledgment (993) (usually referred to as the 993). Currently in development, 993 is used by the recipient of a transaction set to authenticate and acknowledge the origin, content, or sequence of data received with the originator of the transactions.

X12.58 Security Structures, which has been published and has a Reference Model in development, is used to define the data formats required for authentication and encryption to provide integrity, confidentiality and verification of the originator at the functional group and transaction set levels.

ISO/IEC 9735, under the general title *Electronic data interchange for administration, commerce and transport (EDIFACT) - Application level syntax rules*, which is currently in draft form, to be reviewed at the X12 meetings in San Francisco in early February of this year, has five parts specifically targeting message security. These parts are: *Part 5 - Security rules for batch EDI (authenticity, integrity and non-repudiation of origin); Part 6 - Secure authentication and acknowledgment message; Part 7 - Security rules for batch EDI (confidentiality); Part 9 - Security key and certificate management message;* and *Par 10 - Security rules for interactive EDI.* The security aspects of ISO 9735 are targeted for finalization by march of 1997, and will be forwarded to ISO for final approval through the ISO Fast Track process.

American Standards Committee (ASC) contact:
Regina Girouard
Manager, Secretariat Services
Data Interchange Standards Association, Inc. (DISA)
1800 Diagonal Road, Suite 200

Alexandria, VA 22314
rgirouard@disa.org
703-548-7005 (x165) [voice]
703-548-5738 [fax]

ASTM

The American Society for Testing and Materials (ASTM) Committee E31 on Computerized Systems established a Division on Security and Confidentiality in early 1996 to facilitate the acceleration of health care security and confidentiality standards development within the ASTM and to coordinate security standards development efforts with other SDOs. The Division on Security and Confidentiality primarily coordinates the efforts of three sub-committees:

E31:17 - Privacy, Confidentiality, and Access
E31:20 - Data and System Security for Health Information
E31.22 - Medical Transcription and Documentation.
These three sub-committees within ASTM currently have seventeen (17) standards either under ballot or in draft or outline form that are targeted for completion by spring and summer 1997.

The objective of ASTM sub-committee E31.17 - *Privacy, Confidentiality, and Access*, is to establish a set of guidelines and standards for the procedural, technical, and administrative management of health information. In addition, the sub-committee is charged with identifying the rights and privileges of individual users, and the subjects of, health information. This latter focus is oriented towards taking a comprehensive view of "confidentiality" as incorporating the protection, not only of the "subject" of patient-specific health information (the patient), but also of health care providers and health care organizations. It is important to note that E31.17 is not concentrating on a definition of the rights of "privacy". Privacy is the domain of legislation, and ethical and moral professional practice of health care providers. Confidentiality, involves the framework in which to protect data privacy to meet legislative and professional practice guidelines.

One of the critical issues that has come up in the work of E31.17 over the last few years is a recognition of a lack of uniform standards, not only for the management of computer based health records (electronic, automated, et. al.), but explicitly for the management of paper-based, and derivative paper-based (photocopy, FAX, computer printed) health records. E31.17 efforts, therefore, are targeted at defining uniform standards for the management of health information, regardless of the "media" used for access, display, exchange, or administration of health records. In addition, the E31.17 sub-committee is treating all health information, including financial and administrative health information, under the same standards and guidelines, so that all health information is covered by a comprehensive set of confidentiality, security, disclosure, and access guidelines, appropriate to the type of data (clinical, administrative, financial).

E31.17 security standards completed or under development are as follows:
Balloted

Standard Guide for Confidentiality, Privacy, Access and Data Security Principles for Health Information Including Computer Based Patient Records

Draft

Documentation of Access for Individually-Identifiable Health Information

- *Standard Guide for Confidentiality and Security Training of Persons Who Have Access to Health Information*
- *Standard Guide for Amendments/Additions to Health Information by Health Care Providers, Administrative Personnel, and by the Subjects of Health Information*
- *Standard Guide to the Transfer/Disclosure of Health Information in an Emergency Treatment Event*
- *Standard Guide for the Use and Disclosure of Health Information*
- *Policy Guide for the Transfer/Re-disclosure of Health Information Between Health Plans*

Rights of the Individual in Health Information

Standard Guide to the Use of Audit Trails, and for Access and Disclosure Logging/Tracking in the Management of Health Information

The objective of ASTM sub-committee E31.20 - *Data and System Security for Health Information*, is to establish a technical framework and infrastructure, outlined in a set of guidelines and standards, to specify security and confidentiality implementations that will protect the privacy of health care information. The sub-committee, through its strong representation of industry experts, is focused on using existing techniques and technologies, such as digital signatures, to build a health care security infrastructure. In addition, the sub-committees efforts are directed at providing standards for health care security and confidentiality that are based upon existing and emerging standards in other industries.

E31.20 security standards completed or under development are as follows:

Published (ANSI Approved)
- *E 1762 - Standard Guide for Authentication of Healthcare Information*
  Ballot Pending
- *Standard Specification for Authentication of Healthcare Information Using Digital Signatures*
  Draft
- *Authentication and Authorization to Access Healthcare Information*

Internet and Intranet Security for Healthcare Information and Secure Timestamps for Healthcare Information

- *Data Security, Reliability, Integrity, and Availability for Healthcare Information*
- *Distributed Authentication and Authorization to Access Healthcare Information*

The objective of ASTM sub-committee E31.22 - *Medical Transcription and Documentation*, is to establish a set of guidelines and standards for the procedural, technical, and administrative management of dictated and transcribed health information. In addition, the sub-committee is charged with identifying the rights and privileges of individual users (transcriptionists, health records personnel, and health care providers), and the subjects of, health information. This latter focus is oriented towards taking a comprehensive view of "confidentiality" as incorporating the protection, not only of the "subject" of patient-specific health information (the patient), but also of health care providers, transcriptionists, health records personnel, and health care organizations.

E31.22 security standards completed or under development are as follows:

Draft
- *Security and Confidentiality of Dictated and Transcribed Health Information*

American Society for Testing and Materials (ASTM) contact:
Teresa Cendrowska
ASTM
100 Bar Harbor Drive
West Conshohocken, PA 19428-2959
tcendrow@astm.org
610-832-9500 [main office number]
610-832-9718 [voice - direct]
610-832-9666 [fax]

Computer-based Patient Record Institute (CPRI)

The Computer-based patient Record Institute (CPRI) through its Work Group on Confidentiality, Privacy and Security, under co-chairs Kathleen Frawley, JD and Dale Miller, has, under ongoing development, a set of security-related efforts oriented towards the establishment of guidelines, confidentiality agreements, security requirements, and frameworks. The CPRI, while not currently an ANSI accredited SDO, works very closely with accredited SDOs in the establishment of security and medical record standards, and enjoys significant cross-representation on SDO security committees.

CPRI security and framework development is completed, or underway, in the following areas:

Published

- *Guidelines for Establishing Information Security Policies at Organizations Using Computer-based Patient Record Systems*
- *Guidelines for Information Security Education Programs at Organizations Using Computer-based Patient Record Systems*
- *Guidelines for Managing Information Security Programs at Organizations Using Computer-based Patient Record Systems*
- *Glossary of Terms Related to Information Security for Computer-based Patient Record Systems*
- *Security Features for Computer-based Patient Record Systems*
- *Sample Confidentiality Statements and Agreements for Organizations Using Computer-based Patient Record Systems*

Computer-based Patient Record Description of Content
- *Computer-based Patient Record System Description of Functionality*

F

Computer-based Patient Record Project Evaluation Criteria and Computer-based Patient Record Project Scenarios

Under Development

- *Guidelines for Access Control in Computer-based Patient Record Systems*
- *Guidelines for Implementation of Electronic Authentication in Computer-based Patient Record Systems*

Under Consideration (tentatively targeted for development in the second half of 1997)

- *Guidelines for the use of the Internet for Computer-based Patient Record Systems*
- *Ethics Related to Health Information Security and Confidentiality in Computer-based Patient Record Systems*
- *Guidelines for Conducting Audit Control in Computer-based Patient Record System Security*
- *Guidelines for Business Resumption Planning in Computer-based Patient Record Systems*

Computer-based Patient Record Institute (CPRI) contact:
Margret Amatayakul
Executive Director
Computer-based Patient Record Institute
1000 E. Woodfield Rd., Suite 102
Schaumburg, IL 60173
cprinet@aol.com
847-706-6746 [voice]
847-706-6747 [fax]

CEN TC251 Working Group 6 on Security, Privacy, Quality and Safety

CEN TC251 Working Group 6 (WG6), under the Chairmanship of Dr. Gunnar Klein of Sweden (recently appointed to chairman for CEN TC251) is charged with managing the development of security and confidentiality standards for the European Commission. CEN TC 251 WG6 represents a consolidated effort to develop comprehensive standards in security and confidentiality for health information. CEN TC251 WG6 has completed a pre-standard *Security Categorization and Protection of Healthcare Information Systems* (COMPUSEC) and a digital signature standard. The digital signature standard mandates the use of RSA's digital signature and authentication algorithm. Additional standards work is currently underway in CEN TC251 WG6 in trusted systems in conjunction with TRUSTHEALTH a project within the Telematics Applications Program, supported by the European Commission. TRUSTHEALTH is a project to build and test technical security services to support data confidentiality, document origin authentication, time stamps, access authentication, and professional authorization access controls.

Additional CEN TC 251, and/or European Commission health care security-related projects include: ISHTAR (Implementation of Secure Healthcare Telematics Applications in Europe); HAWSA; DAICARD3; MEDSEC; EUROMED-ETS (distributed trusted third party services); and, SEMRIC (Secure Medical Record Information Communication).

European Committee for Standardization Technical Committee CEN TC251 contact:
Gunnar Klein
Chairman CEN TC251
GKAB
Renstiernas Gata 14
S-116 28 Stockholm
Sweden
gunnar@klein.se or 73754.2411@compuserve.com
46-8-702 93 60 [voice]
46-8-702 93 61 [fax]

Health Level Seven (HL-7)

Health Level Seven (HL-7) formed the Secure Transactions Special Interest Group (SIGSecure) to address the development of secure HL7 transactions at its August 1996 meeting. This SIG will focus on the use of HL7 in communications environments where there is a need for authentication, encryption, non-repudiation, and digital signature. This group will direct its efforts on insuring the mechanisms are available for implementing a secure HL7 transactions and not on standardizing security policies. The HL7 organization is also interested in participating with the efforts of the Internet Engineering Task Force. A CommerceNet trial using email protocols (MIME) to encapsulate HL7 messages is being explored for feasibility.

SIGSecure will identify user requirements and a threat model, the services needed to meet those requirements, the mechanisms for providing those services, and the specific implementations for those mechanisms. The scope will be limited to providing network and Internet security mechanisms for HL7 transactions at the application level, independent of underlying transport. SIGSecure has a stated goal of leveraging existing standards to the maximum extent possible with a priority given to International, National (ANSI), and Publicly Available Specifications. It addition it will coordinate with other SDOs to avoid duplication and to promote harmonization.

Health Level Seven HL7 SIGsecure contacts (Co-Chairs):
Jack Harrington
Hewlett Packard Company
3000 Minuteman Road
Andover, MA 01910-1085
jackh@an.hp.com
508-687-1501 [main office]
508-659-3517 [voice - direct]
508-686-1319 [fax]

Mary E. Kratz
University of Michigan Medical Center
B1240 Taubman Center
1500 E. Medical Center Drive
Ann Arbor, MI 48109-0308
mkratz@umich.edu
313-763-6871 [voice]
313-763-0629 [fax]

F

IEEE

The Institute of Electrical and Electronic Engineers (IEEE) Medical Data Interchange (MEDIX) does not currently have an active group addressing security and confidentiality issues. This, according to Bob Kennelly of MEDIX, is due to the focused domain of IEEE/MEDIX that is essentially the sub-nets between bedside monitoring devices and monitors in intensive care, operating room, and inpatient settings. IEEE/MEDIX is interested in participating in cooperative efforts in the development of secure messaging standards.

National Council for Prescription Drug Programs (NCPDP)

The National Council for Prescription Drug Programs (NCPDP), as with IEEE/MEDIX, does not currently have an active group addressing security and confidentiality. This is also due to the focused domain under which they are currently working. The NCPDP is also interested in participating in cooperative efforts in the development of secure messaging standards.

Low Cost Distribution Mechanism

No input was received for this section.

REFERENCE 4

Consumer Requirements in Relation to Information and Communications Technology Standardization

ANEC97/ICT/012
April 1997 - GL

ANEC - European Association for the Co-ordination of Consumer Representation in Standardization

36 Avenue de Tervueren, box 4 -- B-1040 Brussels
Ph. +32 2 743 2470 - Fax +32 2 736 9552
http://www.citizen.be/standard/anec.htm
anec@anec.org

Executive Summary
Consumer Requirements and Priorities in ICT

Generic Consumer Requirements

In the first section of this document ANEC identifies a number of generic consumer requirements applicable to all standardization projects in Information and Communications Technology. This includes issues such as ease of use, functionality of solution, design for all amongst others. Further details can be found in chapter 8. It is proposed that these recommendations could be promoted as a joint CEN/CENELEC/ETSI memorandum to ensure their application across all the standardization work in the ICT sector. This would contribute to the production of a coherent and consistent catalogue of standards even where consumer representatives are not actually present.

F

Specific Consumer Priorities

The following consumer priorities are identified and further explained later in this report:

Specific ICT Priority Project	Consumer Priority	Key Aspects for Standardization
Electronic Purchasing	Encryption systems Electronic signatures Security	Security of transaction Error tolerance Transparency of costs Privacy
Interlinking technology	Horizontal standards	Interoperability Compatibility
Information kiosks	Categorized list of information Consistent user information	Ease of use Reliability of information
Digital broadcasting	Electronic programming guide Encryption systems	Access control Cost transparency Grading systems Backward compatibility
Set-top units	Single distributable and adaptable standard	Interoperability Expandability Upgradability
Mobile communications	Minimum service level Transparency of geographical coverage area	Cost transparency Interoperability Suppression of call-line identification
Generic Internet issues	Standard for the categorization of sites Access control system Minimum service level	Privacy Rating system

Smart cards	Access to smart card systems Electronic purses	Privacy Clear legal responsibilities
Smart houses	Interoperability Single standardized home bus	Ease of use Guaranteed minimum service in case of system failure
Self-service systems	Standard for uniform design of system Coding of user profiles	Access for all Ease of use Privacy
Public transport informatics	Access to information Billing/ ticketing	Transparency of costs
Research/ test methods	Benchmark standard for testing Tools for life-cycle analysis	Standardized test methods to provide consumer information before purchase
Power consumption	Standard method for testing power consumption	Access to comparative information on energy usage
Information to consumers	Standard on what information is given (time/ type/ means) Standard product profile	Standardized information provision before sale, at point of sale and while using ICT

Background

The vast opportunities offered by the advent of the Information Society are revolutionizing the daily lives of citizens across the world. It has been acknowledged however at the highest political levels in Europe that not only industry but in particular the consumer should benefit from the information society. The desire to put the citizen first is driving the current political agenda. This has emphasized the urgent need to incorporate consumers, with their requirements and expectations of user friendly ICT products into a rapidly changing ICT standardization process.

In response to this, ANEC, the European Association for the Co-ordination of Consumer Representation in Standardization has decided to become more active in the area of Information and Communications Technology. This document is one part of a project undertaken by a specifically set up ANEC group of European consumer experts on ICT. The aim of the project is to identify generic consumer requirements, ICT areas of interest to the

F

consumer and to define ways how consumer input can be most efficiently achieved in the European ICT standardization process. Considering the speed of developments in ICT this document will be updated regularly.

This document states consumer requirements and priority projects in ICT standardization.

Scope

The purpose of this document is to provide the ICT standardization process with consumer requirements that should be incorporated when producing ICT standards and to provide an overview of areas ANEC recommends for standardization.

About this document

These consumer requirements have been identified and consolidated from several sources including:

- the ISO/ IEC User/ Consumer Manifesto and ANEC/ Consumers International contributions to this JTC1 initiated document

- Several rounds of contributions from the ANEC Ad Hoc Group of European Consumer Experts on Information and Communications Technology.

- Several rounds of contributions from the ANEC General Assembly and Co-ordination Group (comprising all European consumer organizations and where existing consumer Councils of the national standards bodies)

- the GII meeting on ICT standards in Geneva, January 1996;the Workshop on ICT and Services at the ANEC General Assembly in 1995;

- ANEC PARTICIPATION IN THE WORK OF THE information SOCIETY FORUM

- MONITORING OF THE WORK OF THE EPN STANDARDS BODIES AND THE European INSTITUTIONS BY THE ANEC SECRETARIAT

- ANEC contributions to the ETSI User Group on Mobile Communications;

- the literature;

Definitions

For the purposes of this document, the following definitions apply:

Consumer: The consumer is a natural person or group of persons using products and/or systems for purposes which are outside his or her trade, business or profession. The consumer is the end user of the products/ systems and is usually the one paying for them.

Dialogue: Interaction between a consumer and a system to achieve a particular goal.

System: A configuration of hardware and software, which is designed to perform tasks in a particular environment. The system typically interacts with consumers via some form of dialogue.

Interoperability: The ability of equipment from different manufacturers (or different systems) to communicate together on the same infrastructure (same system).

Consumer Requirements in Standardization

ANEC

ANEC, the European Association for the Co-ordination of Consumer Representation in Standardization was set up following an agreement in 1993 between the Consumer Consultative Committee of the European Commission and its EFTA counterpart for the setting up of a single voice for EU and EFTA consumers in European standardization. The Association has on top become an associate member of CEN, fully accepted into the CENELEC family, a full member of ETSI, European member of EOTC and is in liaison with the ICT Standards Board. The objective of ANEC shall be to ensure that consumer interests are represented in the work of the European standardization bodies and any similar bodies who are concerned with standards directly or indirectly affecting consumers.

ANEC's policy framework is laid out in its strategic program.

The general aims, which ANEC pursues at the political level, are the following:

- ensure consumer interests are given their full weight at the political level in the work of the European standards bodies and European institutions

- improve participation at the national level

- Enhance professionalism and effectiveness of consumer observers through training and access to expertise e.g. comparative testing results, product safety research, accident data and consultants.

The aims, which ANEC pursues at the technical level, are the following

- improving consumer safety by

F

- preventing accidents

- mitigating the effects of accidents

- promoting and maintaining health and hygiene

- enhancing product/service performance

- improving product/service information for consumers

- facilitating consumer choice

- contributing to environmental protection

-

General Consumer Principles

The following "Consumer Principles" elaborate on those fundamental consumer rights previously identified by President J.F. Kennedy, the United Nations and the European Commission. These key consumer tests, which guide ANEC's work and this submission to the ICT Standards Board, are:

Access: Can people actually get the goods or services they need or want?

In the generality of consumer work this is a function of consumers' ability to afford to buy the things they need or want and of their availability to all consumers regardless of location, social and economic considerations. For ANEC, this may lead to considerations of whether the use of national, rather than international or European, standards inhibits access to national markets throughout the community.

Choice: Is there any? And can consumers affect the way goods or services are provided through their own decisions?

Promoting consumer choice is fundamental to consumer policy. In standardization, this supports the principle that a standard should not favor any one particular manufacturer or supplier or be unnecessarily restrictive as to the design of or materials used in a product's manufacture.

Safety: Are the goods or services a danger to health or welfare?

The safety of products used by consumers has always been the first priority of consumer representatives active in standardization. A detailed discussion on the implications of this and the ways it can be pursued is given later in this document.

Information: Is it available, and in the right way to help consumers make the best choices for themselves?

The provision of adequate information, both to assist in consumer choice and to support the safe and effective use of the product/service, is a key consumer concern. Allied to this is a concern regarding the dangers of providing more information than consumers can readily absorb and, hence, reducing the impact of vital messages.

Equity: Are some or all consumers subject to arbitrary or unfair discrimination?

ANEC has adopted the specific aim of looking after the interests of various groups of consumers who are felt to be at particular risk.

Redress: If something goes wrong, is there an effective system for putting it right?

Ensuring that consumers can be confident in claims of compliance with standards is an important concern. This means that, in their technical committee work, consumer representatives should aim to ensure that tests are repeatable and reproducible. At a policy level it requires influence on systems for product certification.

Representation: If consumers cannot affect the supply of goods or services through their own decisions, are there ways for their views to be represented?

By definition, individual consumers cannot materially influence the content of product standards. ANEC and consumer representatives on national delegations are the main conduits for representing their interests and, whatever resource constraints there may be, must participate effectively in key areas of consumer concern.

Generic consumer requirements for ICT Standardization

When designing, selecting, commissioning, modifying and standardizing ICT systems, certain generic consumer requirements need to be taken into account.

Proposal

It is recommended that these generic consumer requirements should be addressed in a joint CEN'CENELEC'ETSI memorandum to ensure their application across all the standardization work in the ICT sector. Industry and consumers alike demand consistency in the standardization process and this initiative could contribute enormously to the production of a coherent and consistent catalogue of standards even where consumer representatives are not actually present.

The specific requirements identified by ANEC are the following

- Ease of use

- Design for all

- Functionality of solution

- Multi-cultural and multi-linguistic aspects

- Terminology

- Comprehensible standards

F

- Interoperability and compatibility

- Consistent user interface

- Adaptability

- Provision of system status information

- Error tolerance and system stability

- Ease the consumer's need to remember system operation

- Explorability

- Privacy and security of information

- Cost transparency

- Quality of service, system reliability and durability

- Reliability of information

- Health and safety issues

- Environmental issues

- Rating and grading systems

Note 1. It should be noted that it is important to see all the requirements in relation to each other as they are interlinked. Resolving just one or two of the issues will not ensure that consumer interests are satisfactorily taken account of.

Note 2. Requirements are not presented in any hierarchical order of importance. This is because the relevance and thereby importance of each and every requirement is situation dependant. In some situations some of the requirements may not be applicable.

Ease of use

ICT must be easy to use for all intended user groups stated in the scope of the standard (see above). Following ergonomics software principles for user interface design should help achieve ease of use.

ICT standards should address ergonomical aspects of ICT hardware, software, services and support. Existing standards should be applied.

Note: Ease of use can be measured in terms of performance (e.g. the time taken by users to complete a predetermined task, and/or number of errors, and/or satisfaction with a service: see EN 29241 -11 Guidance of usability). Goals for ease of use (known as usability statements) should be developed.

Design for all

ICT standards should support the principle of "Design for all. This is a process of creating products, systems, services which are accessible and usable by people with the widest possible range of abilities operating within the widest possible range of situations.

There may however be occasions where a system is not intended for all users. In these instances, the standard should state which users and tasks the system is not designed for and why these groups' requirements are not taken into account.

Functionality of solution

With regard to functionality of solution, one has to ensure that the standard addresses the problems actually faced by consumers and will actually help solve those problems. There should be advice on which user groups and tasks the system should be used for, and in which operating environments. This advice should be in the scope of the standard. The advice should be open for review.

Multicultural and multi-linguistic aspects

Multicultural and multi-linguistic aspects need to be considered when developing global ICT standards.

Terminology

As part of a consumer centered design, the terminology used in user interfaces, (this includes brochures, user instructions and information presented by the system) should meet the basic generic consumer requirements.

Comprehensible standards

Standards must be unambiguous and easy to understand, i.e. written in plain language so that non-technical people can comprehend them and contribute to the standardization process.

Inter-operability and compatibility

Different services must be interoperable so that, in practice, any service can be accessed on any appropriate network on any relevant device, thus avoiding the acquisition of access to several different networks and terminals for similar services (i.e. portability is achieved). Compatibility within a system should be ensured for example new versions of systems should be compatible with previous versions of the same system and components for systems originating from different manufacturers should also be compatible. Different systems should be compatible, so as to allow their joint operation.

F

Consistent user interface

The systems must have a consistent user interface. It is especially important that the method of processing storing and accessing the systems is consistent for the user.

Note. A consistent user interface can be achieved by different means e.g.:

- All components of the user interface are uniform.

- The user interface adapts to the user, so that the user always meets a personalized uniform interface. This principle is the subject of the TIDE project 1040 "SATURN", where the feasibility of using a smart card to trigger a personalized user interface is being evaluated and promoted for standardization.

Adaptability

The system should be adaptable to meet a user's specific requirements and abilities. For example, provide output in a format and at a pace that meets the individuals' needs.

Note 1: This is a way of achieving consistency for the user: see above

Note 2: This principle could be applied to prevent unintended users gaining access to a system.

Note 3: This principle could be applied in the case of custom upgrading of systems.

Provision of system status information

The status of the system (e.g. waiting for input, checking, fetching, etc.) should be always available for the consumer. Different mechanisms should be employed to give complete feedback to the consumer e.g. audio/visual for error messages data input required. All messages should be positive and not place blame on the consumer.

Error tolerance and system stability

The system should anticipate errors of operation and be forgiving. Informative error messages should lead the consumer forward. The system should be robust and should remain stable if consumers try services, which cannot be delivered or make choices that are redundant.

Minimize consumer's need to remember system operation

Systems should display dialogue elements to the consumer and allow them to choose from items generated by the system or to edit them. Menus are a typical technology to achieve this goal.

Explorability

The system should allow consumer to discover its functions.

Privacy and security of information

The system should ensure privacy of the individual. It should not be possible for unauthorized people to follow a user's activities on an electronic network. Electronic footprints are to be avoided. Standards should help provide methods for checking this, especially in open and decentralized networks (Internet). Inevitable footprint data must be deleted after an appropriate time. The system should not allow disclosure of information about the consumer to unauthorized people and should indicate clearly to whom information is given.

Security of information, sent, stored or received or deleted, must be ensured. The level of security should be clearly stated to the consumer.

Cost transparency

The system must be transparent regarding all costs involved. Cost information should be presented in a standardized way. This includes both initial costs involved for the user and costs in terms of subscribing to and operating the system, especially when interworking on networks, or when using on-line help or other fundamental services (e.g. directory enquiries, short message service on a mobile phone). Disconnecting from a service must be free of charge or the charge must be stated in a standardized way at point of purchase.

Quality of service, system reliability and durability

There should be a standardized way to determine and present quality of service, and systems reliability and durability. This should include the development of standardized performance indicators. This information should be displayed at the point of sale. Batteries are an example of products that consumers need such information at point of sale (durability and reliability).

Reliability of information

The system should indicate reliability of information (possibly by quoting sources) provided on the system. (e.g. Balance of account is xxx ECU at 1000 hours on ddmmyy. Note: bank clearing system has been out of action last two days).

Health and safety issues

When developing ICT standards any health & safety issues should be assessed. Existing standards should be applied.

F

Environmental issues

ICT standards should indicate that environmental issues, such as power consumption have been addressed. A clean life-cycle from manufacturing to disposal should be the goal of all ICT systems/products. Possible environmental risks that may arise in the product/system life cycle should be identified and indicated to the consumer.

A standardized way of assessing and indicating environmentally friendly ICT products, services and systems should be developed.

Rating and grading systems

ICT standards should allow the application of rating and grading systems.

Further work

In order to fulfil the above consumer requirements, standards for calculating and presenting ICT systems in terms of ease of use, cost, durability, system reliability and information reliability (source and content) will need to be developed.

Active consumer participation MUST be ensured throughout all phases of the standardization process in order to ensure "consumer friendly" systems. This includes the programming of standardization work, priority setting and participating in the technical work.

Consumer priorities in relation to ICT standardization

Definitions

For the purposes of this section, the following definitions applies:

Consumer: The consumer is a natural person or group of persons using products and/or systems and/or services for purposes which are outside his or her trade, business or profession. The consumer is the end user of the products/ systems/services paying or not paying for them. Consumers are not homogeneous and have a wide variety of needs and abilities.

Explorability: systems should enable the consumers to "discover" the content of a system intuitively.

Robustness: systems should remain stable if consumers try services which cannot be delivered or make choices that are redundant.

Redundancy: the same (important) information should (if possible) be offered/presented by different media (text, Audio, video).

General ANEC Priorities for ICT standardization

The design of user-friendly information systems is important for consumers. This includes aspects of how the different technologies are set up and what specific area is being dealt with - because a software solution can not be more user or consumer friendly than the applications it is supposed to support (this applies to both consumer and professional applications).

Ergonomic software design became necessary because of the ever-increasing development in the ICT area. Computers have become an every-day working tool and a new industry has been created in hard- and software development. The increasing use of information technology and the huge range of different products available (from word-processing to multimedia software) has made the design and regulation of this area a prime objective. Therefore it is important to find general requirements.

Key aspects for standardization

Ecological aspects: Developments must be sustainable in an ecological sense. Scientific and objective methods help to assess environmentally friendly products under regard of the whole lifetime -circle. This information should be indicated in a standardized way.

Ethical aspects: Scientific and objective methods should help to assess ethical sound products (e.g. no child labor, no support of ideologies based on discrimination or violence). This information should be indicated in a standardized way.

Design for all: Any publicly accessed terminal/ ticket machine should have a default selection, i.e. if a consumer does not understand what options are offered a "safe" result can be reached by using the default options.

ANEC Priorities for ICT standardization work

ANEC priorities for ICT standardization are as follows:

- Electronic Purchasing

- Interlinking Technology

- Information Kiosks

- Digital Broadcasting

- Set-top units

- Mobile Communications

- Generic Internet Issues

F

- Smart Cards

- Smart Houses

- Self Service Systems

- Public Transport Telematics

- Research/test methods for ICT

- Power consumption

- Information to consumers

Note:

The numbered list above does not indicate any order of preference.

Many of the project areas overlap

The ANEC group of consumer experts on information and communications technology is currently (summer 1997) working on this section.

SPECIFIC ICT PROJECTS

ELECTRONIC PURCHASING

Ordering and payment of commodities by means of mass market ICT products and services (such as PC and WWW).

Why it is important for consumers

Electronic purchasing may be the only way certain products or services will be offered for sale in the future. It may be the best access for people living in remote areas or for disabled consumers. The market forces for the introduction of electronic trade and purchasing systems is very strong and a number of incompatible payment systems on Internet have already emerged. Electronic purchasing will have legal, ethical and technical implications for the consumer.

Consumer Priorities

Encryption systems

Electronic Signatures

Security

Key aspects for standardization

Main consumer issues for standardization are security of transaction, error tolerance, transparency of costs incurred and privacy.

Interlinking technology

The Interlinking of telephones, TVs, set top units and home computers.

Why it is important for consumers

The consumer must be able to access services by use (in principle) of component parts from any manufacturer. A consumer should not have to buy for example different TV sets or set top units to access different services/ broadcasts. Standard services should be available without the need for upgrading or changing existing systems for example: it should be possible to listen to stereo broadcasting with a simple mono radio with no loss of information.

Consumer Priorities

Horizontal standards

Key aspects for standardization

In particular with view to the merging areas of information technology, communications and broadcasting it needs to be ensured that interlinking technology is in place and different systems are compatible so that the consumer does not have to by different devices. Interlinking technology also has to be interoperable.

Information kiosks

The provision of public information via information kiosks (currently PC's) currently in a public environment.

Why it is important for consumers

As the name implies, public information (which can be of considerable importance - e.g. information about voting, taxes, legislation) must be available to all members of the public and on equal terms. There must be no barriers (technical or economic) that hinder members of the public gaining access to the information; otherwise a two-tier society will be created.

Consumer Priorities

Categorized list of information must be provided

Consistent user information

Key aspects for standardization

A key aspect for the standardization of information kiosks is ease of use. The information provided needs to be reliable.

F

DIGITAL BROADCASTING

Digital broadcast is the broadcast of digital audio, video (including TV) and data signals transmitted either by air (terrestrial broadcast), satellite or cable (from a single source to multiple receivers).

Why it is important for consumers

The consumer must be able to access services by use (in principle) of component parts from any manufacturer. A consumer should not have to buy for example different TV sets to access different services/ broadcasts (MPEG/ASTRA). It must be possible to connect video systems (recorders/ cameras) to different television sets/set top units especially in the digital domain. Standard services should be available without the need for upgrading or changing existing systems. Privacy should be ensured.

Consumer Priorities

Electronic programming guide

Encryption systems

Key aspects for standardization

Access control against unintended users (minors, children; with regards to both costs, time of day and themes e.g. sex, crime, advertisements). Cost transparency, grading systems, backward compatibility (the consumer should not be obliged to buy new technology).

Set-Top Units

Set-top units (STUs) are required in order to de-scramble signals in digital cable and satellite television. Set-top units can store information and may in future be connected to in-house digital networks (smart houses).

Why it is important for consumers

The consumer is faced with different, mainly proprietary decoding systems to access cable and satellite television and broadcasting as well as multimedia services using conventional television sets. Different systems exist both on national and on the European level. The consumer must be able to access services by use of set-top units/ decoders from any manufacturer. A consumer should not have to buy different set-top units to access different services/ broadcasts

Consumer Priorities

A single distributable and adaptable STU standard should be drafted

Key aspects for standardization

Interoperability of different systems, expandability and upgradability (the consumer should not be forced to buy a new STU with progressing technology or new services), distribution of signals.

Mobile Communications

Mobile communications provide access to telecommunications services at any terminal in different locations and whilst in motion. It also provides the capability of identifying and locating a particular terminal and or associated user. It builds upon interworking between public and private networks.

Why it is important for consumers

Mobile communications offer personal mobility, defined as: "Being able to access telecommunication services at any terminal on the basis of a personal telecommunications identifier, and the capability of the network to provide those services according to the users service profile".

Mobile communications also allows communications in emergencies (could be lifesaving). Mobile systems have distinct advantages (costs and technical) in countries with difficult geographical topology (e.g. Norway, Italy) allowing the connection of people in otherwise remote regions. Mobile communications are much cheaper to maintain than the traditional landlines. These cost savings should be passed on to the consumer.

Adverse aspects with mobile communications include use of mobile phones whilst driving, the nuisance of mobile phones ringing in public places, the effects of the electromagnetic fields when held next to the brain, obtaining mobile phone numbers from different operators, effect on technical equipment including: hearing aids, ATMs, medical equipment and allegedly train signaling equipment.

Consumer Priorities

Minimum service level

Transparency of geographical coverage area

Key aspects for standardization

The actual cost should be transparent to the consumer, different systems should be interoperable, for reasons of privacy it should be possible to suppress call-line identification, key aspects for minimum service should be developed.

Generic Internet Issues

Internet is an undefined, unregulated and uncontrolled network that allows worldwide communication between different people.

Why it is important for consumers

Since it is anticipated that Internet can be one of the main media for home and public information purposes, it is essential that all consumers can have easy access to the system and the information required. Research (see "3 I" project below) indicates that today's Internet and e-mail systems are too

F

complicated for consumers, especially elderly consumers (a growing user group). Home shopping, one of the many services offered by Internet usually includes transfer of money and data. This raises legal issues, including warranty. The use of Internet is taking off - it is therefore important for consumer representation in this area before it becomes firmly established.

Consumer Priorities

Standard for the categorization of Internet sites

Access control system

Minimum service level

Key aspects for standardization

A key issue for the consumer is privacy (electronic footprints should be not possible = trackability). Standardized rating system for information provided via Internet should be developed.

Smart Cards

Why it is important for consumers

Card based systems have started to permeate key facets of the information society: they are the key to bank services (at ATMs or via telephone), are the key to telephoning (phone cards, GSM), transport (tickets) and identity cards electronic passports/machine readable visas), health (patient cards/ health care professional cards) TV cards, Road tolls, electronic purses, IEP, access control, social security cards, etc. In order to avoid a two-tier society of those that are card literate and those that are not, it is important that any barriers to use (economic or technical) exist.

Consumer Priorities

Access to smart card systems

Electronic purses

Key aspects for standardization

A major consumer issue is privacy (personal information should not be disclosed to third parties, electronic footprints). The legal responsibilities (service provider/ intermediary/ consumer) must be clear.

Smart Houses

Why it is important for consumers

Could be an integral part of all houses in future. Those "owning" the infrastructure will dictate the preconditions. Consumers are a major stakeholder in smart houses, and yet they are underrepresented (with a few exceptions). A key consideration is the possibility of depending upon a single provider for all facilities (what happens if it goes bankrupt/ abuses monopolistic position?). If the technology is difficult for consumers to operate, some consumers will be disadvantaged, i.e. will not be able to enjoy the potential benefits (alarms, etc) offered by the system. Ironically the groups (elderly) that might gain the most benefit from such systems might be the very ones that cannot operate them.

Consumer Priorities

Interoperability

One standardized home bus

Key aspects for standardization

Given that there is ONE standardized home bus the main consumer issue is ease of use (system must be easily upgradable, maintenance friendly).

In case of failure of the electronic system a minimum of services must be available (heating, water, light)

Self Service Systems

A public or private service where the consumer operates an ICT based device, which delivers a product or service without involvement of other people. Self-service systems are usually to be found in a public environment. Self-service systems can be free, coin, note, token or card - operated.

See also: Smart cards, Information kiosks, Electronic purchasing.

Why it is important for consumers

Key societal functions, such as telecommunications, public transport, public administration, banks, post offices are increasingly introducing self service systems in an effort to reduce personnel costs. The consumers are expected to operate a technical system themselves, i.e. without the assistance of another human. Failure to operate the system correctly can result in no service or product being delivered. This could have considerable consequences. It is therefore vital that all persons in all environments can operate self-service systems.

Consumer Priorities

Standard for uniform design of system

Coding of user profiles on cards

Key aspects for standardization

Self-service systems should be easily accessible and accessible for all. Privacy should be ensured if user profiles are given on cards.

F

Public transport informatics

The coupling of information technology and communications in road transport is already helping to make travel easier, more comfortable, more efficient and safer. This wide area includes real-time traffic and travel information, in-vehicle guidance systems, traffic/transit/parking information collection and distribution, traffic management systems and co-ordination, human interfaces and ergonomics and vehicle/highway automation.

Why it is important for consumers

Standardized traffic information systems could allow the consumer to travel anywhere in Europe and receive transmissions containing information on congestion and incidents.

Consumer Priorities

Access to information

Billing/ ticketing

Transparency of costs

Key aspects for standardization

Public transport informatics systems must provide for transparent costs.

Research/ test methods

Why it is important for consumers

From the consumer's point of view, quality specifications for the design of software are necessary in order to compare and evaluate products. Both the great diversity of nearly similar products (e.g. software) and the great number of application software make it very difficult for the consumer to find the individually suitable program. In addition, commercially available products have a confusing number of functions requiring detailed studying of the technical specifications and user manuals and sometimes even detailed instruction courses.

For these reasons it would be useful to test the usability of products with different types of users during the design stage of a system and upon its completion.

Consumer Priorities

A benchmark standard for testing

Suitable tools for life-cycle analysis

Key aspects for standardization

Test methods should be standardized to provide data to consumers for easy comparison before purchase. E.g. energy consumption cost in standard mode, necessary equipment/knowledge, restrictions, safety, instructions.

Power Consumption

All devices using power supplies or batteries, specially that ones that run all the time in operation or stand-by mode: television sets, VCRs, receivers, amplifiers, computers, monitors, telephone and fax machines, terminals etc.

Why it is important for consumers

Power consumption is an important environmental issue both due to production and disposal of used energy and energy sources. Power consumption is also affecting the consumer in terms of costs.

Consumer Priorities

Standard method for testing power consumption

Key aspects for standardization

ICT devices should aim to use as little energy as possible. The level of power consumption should be indicated. Access to comparative information on energy usage must be ensured.

Information to consumers

This topic covers the provision of relevant information to the consumer about all types of ICT products, services and systems before the sale (e.g. contracts), at the point of sale (costs) and whilst using products, systems and services (user support).

Why it is important for consumers

A prerequisite for consumers to make appropriate decisions regarding the purchase and use of ICT products, systems and services is having the right information at the right time and right place.

For example, at point of sale the consumer needs to compare and contrast different alternatives and fully understand the implications of purchasing "packages" (e.g. free modem with 2 years Internet subscription - the price of which can alter...). The consumer also needs to understand and analyze his/her needs in relation to technological solutions. Purchasing inappropriate ICT solutions may have considerable consequences both long and short term.

Consumer Priorities

Standard on what information should be given (at what time, type of information, means of information), one standard product profile

Key aspects for standardization

Standardization of information presentation before sale, at point of sale and whilst using ICT. All types of information presentations must be easy to comprehend and relevant to the users tasks.

F

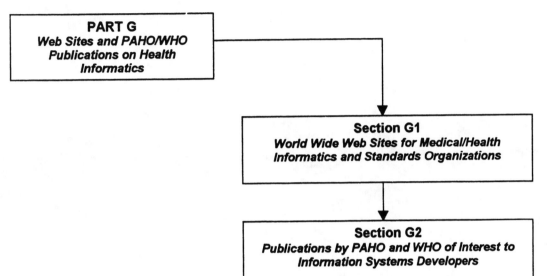

PART G
Web Sites and PAHO/WHO
Publications on Health
Informatics

Section G1
World Wide Web Sites for Medical/Health
Informatics and Standards Organizations

Section G2
Publications by PAHO and WHO of Interest to
Information Systems Developers

G

Part G. Web Sites and PAHO/WHO Publications on Health Informatics

G

World Wide Web Sites for Medical/Health Informatics Organizations and Standards

WEB SITE	WEB ADDRESS
American Health Information Management Association	http://www.ahima.org
American Medical Association	http://www.ama.assn.org
American Medical Informatics Association/General Health & Medical Web Resources	http://amia2.amia.org/lkres.html
ANSI - American National Standards Institute	http://www.ansi.org
Asociación Argentina de Informática Médica (AAIM)	http://www.pccp.com.ar/aaim
ASTM - American Society for Testing and MaterialS	http://www.astm.org
AVICENNA - The Medical Information Supersite of the WWW	http://www.avicenna.com
BioMedNet-For Biological and Medical Researchers	http://www.biomednet.com/home
BIREME – Regional Library of Medicine PAHO/WHO	http://www.bireme.br/
Brazilian Society for Health Informatics (SBIS)	http://www.sbis.epm.br/sbis/index.html
British Medical Informatics Society (BMIS)	http://www.cs.man.ac.uk/mig/people/medicine/bmis
British Medical Journal	http://www.bmj.com
CEN/TC 251 -- European Standardization Activities in Medical Informatics	http://www.centc251.org
Health Informatics Center, School of Medicine, Federal University of São Paulo, Brazil	http://www.epm.br/cis/CIS1.HTM
CIHI - Canadian Institute for Health Information	http://www.cihi.ca
CMA CPGInfobase/Canadian Medical Association	http://www.cma.ca/cpgs/index.htm
Cyberspace Hospital – access to health information resources on the Internet via a virtual hospital setting	http://ch.nus.sg/CH/ch.html
Cyberspace Telemedical Office – gateway to healthcare information, products, and services	http://www.telemedical.com

G

Data Interchange Standards Association	http://www.disa.org/
DICOM - Digital Imaging and Communications in Medicine Standard	http://www.xray.hmc.psu.edu/dicom/dicom_intro/DICOMIntro.html
Duke University Medical Center Division of Medical Informatics	http://dmi-www.mc.duke.edu/dukemi/misc/links.html
EDI – Electronic Data Interchange	http://www.premenos.com
European Federation for Medical Informatics (EFMI)	http://www.cxwms.ac.uk:80/Academic/AGPU/staffpag/robinson/interest/efmi_wg7/efmiaims.html#Index
European Health Telematics Observatory	http://www.ehto.be
European Telecommunications Standards Institute (ETSI)	www.etsi.fr
Grateful Med - search the National Library of Medicine	http://igm.nlm.nih.gov
GT Saude, Brazil	http://gts1.incor.usp.br/news_eng.html
Health Care Information Systems Directory of U.S. Services and Product Vendors	http://www.health-infosys-dir.com/
Health Care IT Services-Wales	http://www.gwent.nhs.gov/PubMed/medline.html
Health Gate-medical research	http://www.healthgate.com
Health Industry Bar Code Supplier Labeling Standard	http://www.hibcc.org
Health Informatics Center - Federal University of São Paulo (in Portuguese)	http://www.epm.br/cis
Health Informatics Worldwide - links to medical informatics activities at universities and other institutions around the world	http://www.imbi.uni-freiburg.de/medinf/mi_list.htm
Health Market International Implementing ICD-10	http://www.healthmkt.com/hmi/icd10.htm
Health on the Net Foundation	http://www.hon.ch
Health Web/Health Information	http://healthweb.org
Healthcare Informatics Standards Guide	http://www.mcis.duke.edu/standards/guide.htm
HIMSS Health Care Information and Management Systems Society	http://www.himss.org
HL7 - Health Level Seven	http://www.hl7.org
International Electrotechnical Commission	www.iec.ch
International Medical Informatics Association (IMIA)	www.imia.org
International Medical Informatics Association (IMIA) Federation for Latin American and the Caribbean	http://www.imia-lac.org/what_e.htm
International Telecommunication Union	www.itu.ch
Internet Medical Terminology Resources	http://www.gsf.de/MEDWIS/activity/med_term.html
Internet Mental Health	http://www.mentalhealthhelp.com
Internet Resources In Medical Informatics - Health Sciences Information Service, University of California, Berkeley	http://www.lib.berkeley.edu/HSIS/medin.html
Inventory of Standards	http://www.ehto.be/scripts/imiawg16/see_standards.cfm
ISO - International Standards Organization	http://www.iso.ch

Joint Commission on Accreditation of Health Care Organizations	http://www.jcaho.org/
Journal of Medical Internet Research (JMIR)	http://www.symposion.com/jmir/
LOINC - Duke University-Logical Observation Identifiers	http://www.mcis.duke.edu/standards/tercode/loinc.htm
MedExplorer-Health Medical Internet Search	http://www.medexplorer.com
Medical Informatics Institutions - World Wide. This is a comprehensive Home Page with links to all countries in the world, maintained by the Department of Medical Informatics, University of Freiburg, Germany.	http://www.imbi.uni-freiburg.de/medinf/mi_list.htm
Medical Records Institute	http://www.medrecinst.com/
Medical World Search-Medical Intelligence	http://www.mwsearch.com
Medline PubMed	http://www4.ncbi.nlm.nih.gov/pubmed/
National Center for Emergency Medicine Informatics	http://ncemi.org
U.S. National Library of Medicine	http://www.nlm.nih.gov
New England Journal of Medicine	http://www.nejm.org
NSW Health Enterprise Information Model – Australia	http://www.health.nsw.gov.au
Object Management Group (OMG)	www.omg.org
Organizing Medical Networked Information (OMNI Biomedical Internet Resources)	http://omni.ac.uk
Pan American Health Organization	http://www.paho.org
PaperChase-Access to Medline and more	http://www.paperchase.com
Primary Health Care Informatics Home Page	http://s1.cxwms.ac.uk/Academic/AGPU/staffpag/robinson/interest/medcomp/homepage.html
References About the Quality of Medical Information /Mnegri	http://www.irfmn.mnegri.it/oncocare/it/quality.htm
SLACK Incorporated-Medical Information	http://www.slackinc.com/chilidchome.html
SNOMED International	http://www.snomed.org
Society for Internet in Medicine (SIM)	http://www.mednet.org.uk/mednet/contents.html
Technology in Medical Education – Centre of Medical Informatics, Monash University	http://www.monash.edu.au/informatics/techme/index.htm
Telemedicine Glossary and Links	http://www.hscsyr.edu/~telemed/glossary.html
The Combined Health Information Database-NIH	http://www.chid.nih.gov
The Community Health Management Information Systems (CHMIS) Resource Center - an information clearinghouse with downloadable documents on a variety of subjects	http://www.chmis.org
The Lancet	http://www.thelancet.com

The Medical Information System Development Center – Japan	http://www.medis.or.jp/e_index.html
United States Department of Health and Human Services – Agency for Health Care Policy and Research	http://www.ahcpr.gov
Univ. of Sheffield School of Health Related Research	http://www.shef.ac.uk/~scharr/ir/netting.html
University of Hull Medical Informatics Group(MIG)	http://www.enc.hull.ac.uk/CS/Medicine
Uruguayan Health Informatics Society	http://www.chasque.apc.org/suis/
VA Veteran's Health Administration-Decentralized Hospital Computer Program	http://www.va.gov/dhcp.htm
World Health Organization	http://www.who.ch
World Journal Association-open peer review	http://www.journalclub.org

PUBLICATIONS BY
THE PAN AMERICAN HEALTH ORGANIZATION
AND THE WORLD HEALTH ORGANIZATION
OF INTEREST TO INFORMATION SYSTEMS DEVELOPERS

Acuña, H. R. (1982). *La informatica medica y los paises en desarrollo.* Bol Oficina Sanit Panam 93(4): 283-287.

Alleyne, G.A.O. (1995). *Prospects and Challenges for Health in the Americas,* Bull Pan Amer Health Org 29(3): 264-271.

Bobadilla, J.L.; Cowley, P; Musgrove, P. and Saxenian, H. (1994*). Design, content and financing of an essential national package of health services.* Bull WHO, 72 (4): 653-662.

Casas, J.A. (1992). *La Informática como Paradigma de Organización. Documento de Trabajo, Reunión Regional de Informática de Salud* (mimeo). PAHO/WHO Guatemala, Agosto 1992.

Pan American Health Organization (1982). *Health for All By the Year 2000: Plan of Action for the Implementation of Regional Strategies.* Washington, DC, PAHO.

Pan American Health Organization (1988a). *El Sistema de Información en los Sistemas Locales de Salud: Propuesta para su Desarrollo.* Programa de Desarrollo de Servicios de Salud/Grupo Interprogramatico, Washinton, DC.

Pan American Health Organization (1988b*) Los Servicios de Salud en las Americas - Analisis de Indicadores Basicos.* Cuaderno Tecnico No. 14, Washington, DC.

Pan American Health Organization (1989a). *Development and Strengthening of Local Health Systems in the Transformation of National Health Systems.* Washington DC, ISBN 92 75 12018 8.

Pan American Health Organization (1989b). *Primary Health Care and Local Health Systems in the Caribbean. Proceedings of the Workshop on Primary Health Care and Local Health Systems.* Tobago,7-11 November 1988, ISBN 92 75 120 22 6.

Pan American Health Organization (1989c). *BITNIS, una vja de acceso al mundo de la información biomédica.* Bol Oficina Sanit Panam 107(5): 449-450.

Pan American Health Organization (1990a). *La informática y la telemática en el campo de la salud: Usos actuales y potenciales.* OPS. Publicación Científica # 523. Washington DC.

Pan American Health Organization (1990b). *Health in Development. Document prepared by the Executive Committee of the Directing Council, Subcommittee on Planning and Programming,* SPP15/4, November 9, 1990, Washington, DC.

Pan American Health Organization (1992a). *Desarrollo y Fortalecimiento de los Sistems Locales de Salud en la Transformación de los Sistemas Nacionales de Salud - La Administración Estrategica.* HSD SILOS-2, Washington, DC, ISBN 92 75 32073 X.

G

Pan American Health Organization (1992b). *Proyecto convergencia encuentro regional: informe final. Cooperación técnica entre países para el desarrollo tecnológico en salud (CTPD) / Proyect convergence regional encounter: final report. Technical cooperation between countries for the technological development in health.* Santiago, OPS, SELA, PNUD. Presented in: Encuentro Regional Convergencia, Santiago de Chile, 6-10 julio.

Pan American Health Organization (1995a). *Health Situation in the Americas: Basic Indicators 1995.* Health Situation Analysis Program. Washington, DC.

Pan American Health Organization (1995b). *Health Conditions in the Americas, 1994 Edition*, Volumes I and II. Scientific Publication # 549. Washington, DC.

Pan American Health Organization (1995c). *Implications of the Summit of the Americas for the Pan American Health Organization; Framework for Health Sector Reform.* Provisional Agenda Item 5.7, XXXVIII Meeting of PAHO Directing Council. September 25-30, Washington, DC.

Pan American Health Organization (1995d). *Grupo de Trabajo para la Conformación de una Red de Información y Cooperación para el Desarrollo de la Informática de los SILOS y Proyectos de Colaboración de la OPS. Chapala, 23-24 enero 1995. Reporte preliminar.* Washingtonn, DC.

Pan American Health Organization (1996a). *Leadership of the Ministries of Health in Sector Reform.* Executive Committee of the Directing Council, Provisional Agenda Item 10 for the 27th Meeting of the Subcommittee on Planning and Programming, December 4-6, Washington, DC.

Pan American Health Organization (1996b). *Health Sector Reform: Proceedings of a Special Meeting.* ECLAC/IBRD/IDB/OAS/PAHO/WHO/UNFPA/UNICEF/USAID. Washington, DC, September 29-30.

Pan American Health Organization (1996c). *Rethinking International Technical Cooperation in Health.* Final Report of Technical Discussions Held March, 1996. Ritch Series Technical Report PAHO/DAP/96.11.29.

Pan American Health Organization (1996d). *PAHO and the Sectoral Reform Processes: Reference Document for Technical Cooperation* (draft). Washington, DC.

Pan American Health Organization and Caribbean Latin American Action(1996e). *Survey of telemedicine projects in Latin America and the Caribbean: Americas Healthnet.* Washington, DC.

Pan American Health Organization (1997a). *La Cooperación de la Organización Panamericana de la Salud Ante los Procesos de Reforma del Sector Salud.* Marzo, ISBN 92 75 07374 0.

Pan American Health Organization (1997b). *Strengthening the process of NGO-Government Collaboration for Health and Human Development 1996-2000. Summary Report and Recommendations.* PAHO Technical Discussions, September 1996. Office of External Relations, Washington, DC.

Pan American Health Organization (1997c). *Salud, Equidad y Transformación Productiva en América Latina y el Caribe.* Published in collaboration with the Comisión Económica para América Latina y el Caribe. Cuaderno Técnico no. 46. Washington, DC.

Pan American Health Organization (1997d). *Directory of Hospitals of Latin America and the Caribbean.* Division of Health Systems and Services Development, HSO. Washington, DC.

Pan American Health Organization (1997e). *Tecnologías de Salud Uniendo a las Américas - Impulsando una visión: la implantación y el uso de la tecnología y los sistemas de información en el mejoramiento de la salud y la atención de salud.* Documento de discusión para la Segunda Cumbre de las Américas. Programa de Información sobre Servicios de Salud, HSP/HSI, Agosto 1997.

Pan American Health Organization (1997f). *Nuevo paradigma para el desarrollo y la evaluación de la telemedicina: un enfoque prospectivo basado en un modelo.* Washington, DC. Series 2/ Health Services Information Systems Program, Division of Health Systems and Services Development, Pan American Health Organization.

Pan American Health Organization (1997g). *Registros médicos electrónicos para tres países de Centroamérica.* Washington, DC. Series 3/ Health Services Information Systems Program, Division of Health Systems and Services Development, Pan American Health Organization.

Pan American Health Organization (1997h). *La descentralización, los sistemas de salud y los procesos de reforma del sector. Informe final de la Reunión de Valdivia, Chile 17-20 de marzo de 1997 .* Washington, DC. Series 1/ Health Systems and Services Management Program, Division of Health Systems and Services Development, Pan American Health Organization.

Pan American Health Organization (1997i). *Informe del taller regional sobre gestión descentralizadora de Recursos Humanos en las reformas Sectoriales en Salud .* Washington, DC. Series 7/ Human Resource Development Program, Division of Health Systems and Services Development, Pan American Health Organization.

Pan American Health Organization (1997j). *Línea basal para el seguimiento y evaluación de la reforma sectorial .* Washington, DC. Series 1/ Reforma del Sector Salud, División de Desarrollo de Sistemas y Servicios de Salud, Pan American Health Organization.

Pan American Health Organization (1998a). *Recursos humanos: un factor crítico de la reforma sectorial en salud.* Informe de la Reunión Regional, San José, Costa Rica, 3-5 diciembre, 1997. Serie 8/ Desarrollo de Recursos Humanos, Pan American Health Organization.

Pan American Health Organization (1998b). *Sistemas de Información y Tecnología de Información en Salud: Desafíos y Soluciones para América Latina y el Caribe.* Programa de Sistemas de Información sobre Servicios de Salud / División de Desarrollo de Sistemas y Servicios de Salud. Washington, DC., Junio 1998, ISBN 92 75 12246 5

Pan American Health Organization (1998c). *Information Systems and Information technology: Challenges and Solutions for Latin America and the Caribbean.* Health Services Information Systems Program / Division of Health Systems and Services Development. Washington, DC., July 1998, ISBN 92 75 12246 6

Rodrigues, R.J. and Goihman, S. (1990). *Sistemas de informação para a gestão dos Sistemas Locais de Saúde.* Bol Of Sanit Panam 109 (5-6): 488-501.

Rodrigues, R.J. and Israel, K. (1995). *Conceptual Framework and Guidelines for the Establishment of District-based Information Systems.* PAHO/WHO Office of Caribbean Program Coordination, Barbados. PAHO/CPC/3.1/95.1, ISBN 976 8083 75 1.

G

Rodrigues, R.J.; Novaes, H.M.; Oxman, G.; Israel, K. and Priale, R.F. (1996a). *Manual de pautas para el establecimiento de sistemas locales de información - v.2* .Organización Panamericana de la Salud, Serie HSP-UNI / Manuales Operativos PALTEX 2/8). Washington, DC.

Rodrigues, R.J; Crawford, C.M.; Koss, S. and McDonald, M. (Eds.) (1996b). *Telecommunications in Health and Health Care for Latin America and the Caribbean. Preliminary Report of an Expert Consultation Meeting.* Washington, DC. Series 1/ Health Services Information Systems Program, Division of Health Systems and Services Development, Pan American Health Organization.

Saltman, R. (1995). *Applying planned market logic to developing countries' health systems: an Initial exploration. Forum on Health Sector Reform*, Discussion Paper 4, WHO, Geneva, (Draft, mimeo).

Sapirie, S.A. (1994). *Strengthening Country Health Information: A New Strategy for Strengthening National Health Information Systems, Procedures and Networks* (draft). Geneva, WHO/SCI.

Sosa-ludicissa, M.; Levett, J.; Mandil, S. And Beales, P.F. (Eds) (1995). *Health, Information Society and Developing Countries*. Studies in Health Technology and Informatics Volume 23. European Commission DG XIII and WHO. IOS Press/Ohmsha, Amsterdam, ISBN 90 5199 226 2.

Sosa-ludicissa, M.; Oliveri, N.; Gamboa, C.A. and Roberts, J. (Eds) (1997). *Internet, Telematics and Health*. Studies in Health Technology and Informatics Volume 36. PAHO/WHO and IMIA. IOS Press, ISBN 90 5199 289 0.

Tarimo, E. (1991). *Towards a Healthy District*. WHO, Geneva, ISBN 92 4 154412 0.

World Health Organization (1981*). Development of Indicators for Monitoring Progress Towards Health for All by the Year 2000*. Health for All Series No.4, Geneva.

World Health Organization (1982). *The Place of Epidemiology in Local Health Work*. WHO Offset Publication No.70, Geneva.

World Health Organization (1987*). Report on Working Group on Application of Informatics in Health*, Manila, Philippines. Regional Office for Western Pacific.

World Health Organization (1988). *Informatics and Telematics in Health: Present and Potential Uses*. Geneva, ISBN 92 4 156117 3.

World Health Organization (1989*). Strengthening Information Support for Management of District Health Systems. Report of an Interregional Meeting*. Surabaya, Indonesia, 30 October-3 November 1989. Geneva.

World Health Organization (1992a). *The Hospital in Rural and Urban Districts: Report of a WHO Study Group on the Functions of Hospitals at the First Level of Referral*. WHO Technical Report Series, 819. Geneva.

World Health Organization (1992b). *Health Dimensions of Economic Reform*. Geneva.

World Health Organization (1993a). *Research for Health: Principles, Perspectives and Strategies. Report of the Advisory Committee on Health Research*. WHO/RPD/ACHR (HRS)/93, Geneva.

World Health Organization (1993b). *Evaluation of Recent Changes in the Financing of Health Services: Report of a WHO Study.* Technical Report Series 829. Geneva.

World Health Organization (1995). *The World Health Report, 1995: Bridging the Gaps.* Geneva.

World Health Organization (1997a). *The World Heath Report 1997: Conquering Suffering, Enriching Humanity.* Geneva.

World Health Organization (1997b). *WHO Cooperation in Strengthening National Health Information Systems. A Briefing Note for WHO Country Representatives and Ministries of Health.* Publication WHO/HST/97.2, Geneva.

World Health Organization (1997c). *Cooperación de la OMS para el fortalecimiento de los sistemas nacionales de información en salud: nota de instrucciones para representantes de la OMS en los países y Ministerios de Salud.* Publication WHO/HST/97.2, Geneva.

World Health Organization (1998). *A Health Telematics Policy in support of WHO's Health-for-All Strategy for Global Health Development.* Report of the WHO Group Consultation on Health Telematics, December 11-16, 1977. Publication WHO/DGO/98.1.

G